Visceral Pain

Ming Xia • Bifa Fan • Hong Jiang
Editors

Visceral Pain

From Bench to Bedside

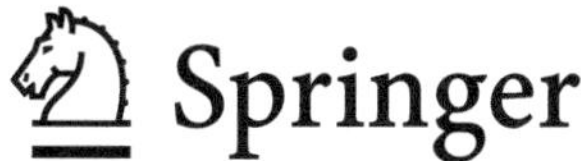

Editors
Ming Xia
Anesthesiology
Shanghai Ninth People's Hospital
Shanghai, China

Bifa Fan
Pain Medicine
China-Japan Friendship Hospital
Beijing, China

Hong Jiang
Anesthesiology
Shanghai Ninth People's Hospital
Shanghai, China

ISBN 978-981-99-9169-3   ISBN 978-981-99-9167-9 (eBook)
https://doi.org/10.1007/978-981-99-9167-9

This Springer imprint is published by the registered company Springer Nature Singapore Pte Ltd.
The registered company address is: 152 Beach Road, #21-01/04 Gateway East, Singapore 189721, Singapore

Paper in this product is recyclable.

Contents

Contributors

Editors

Ming Xia Department of Anesthesiology, Shanghai Ninth People's Hospital, Shanghai Jiao Tong University School of Medicine, Shanghai, China

Bifa Fan Department of Pain Medicine, China-Japan Friendship Hospital, Beijing, China

Hong Jiang Department of Anesthesiology, Shanghai Ninth People's Hospital, Shanghai Jiao Tong University School of Medicine, Shanghai, China

Associate Editors

Daying Zhang Department of Pain Clinic, The First Affiliated Hospital, Nanchang University, Nanchang, Jiangxi, China

Haipeng Liu Department of Pain Management, Gansu Provincial Hospital, Lanzhou, Gansu, China

Ningning Ji Department of Anesthesiology, Shanghai Ninth People's Hospital, Shanghai Jiao Tong University School of Medicine, Shanghai, China

1 Introduction

Hong Jiang

1.1 An Overview of Visceral Pain

1.1.1 Concept of Pain

Pain varies in intensity, quality, and duration, as well as in its pathophysiologic mechanisms and implications. It is therefore a challenge to define the concept of pain succinctly and accurately. The International Association for the Study of Pain (IASP) defines pain as an unpleasant sensory and emotional experience associated with tissue damage or injury [1], which has been widely and long accepted by the health care professionals. This definition suggests that pain has two important characteristics. One is that pain is an awareness that occurs in the brain and an experience that induced by the activity of multiple cortical sites. Nociception, on the other hand, refers to peripheral or central nervous system activities triggered by noxious stimuli. However, not all nociception brings the sensation of pain. Thus, pain requires the individual's autonomous consciousness, the participation of intact nervous system as well as the activity of the cortical nociceptive circuitry of the nervous system affecting specific cortical currents. The other is that pain has both sensory and emotional components which are supported by brain imaging studies of patients with specific brain injuries. Imaging results demonstrated that nociception can also lead to activation of corresponding cortical areas that process emotions, such as the amygdala and anterior cingulate cortex which can be controlled by the perceived experiment and further produces different sensations. In addition, patients who suffer from the above-mentioned cortical damage alone may also go through a loss of corresponding sensation, but not lead to the disappearance of pain. They may still feel a vague unpleasant experience when the corresponding brain is injured and the contralateral body part receives noxious stimuli.

Criticisms of the IASP definition have been prompted from different perspectives. For examples, some pointed out that the definition emphasizes the sensation of conscious human only, separating the connection between mind and body and being highly subjective. For other populations and species, such as neonates, animals and so on, they may be deprived of the right to develop pain since they are unable to report it verbally. Moreover, it neglects the cognitive and social factors that contribute to the pain experience, meaning that pain has certain intentionality which influences the patient's sensational and emotional experience [2]. Additionally, the term "unpleasant" has been debated as potentially trivializing the intense pain and suffering associated with many acute and chronic clinical pain states and failing to capture "all the words that can be used to describe the experience" and its associated pain [2,

H. Jiang (✉)
Department of Anesthesiology, Shanghai Ninth People's Hospital, Shanghai Jiao Tong University School of Medicine, Shanghai, China

M. Xia et al. (eds.), *Visceral Pain*, https://doi.org/10.1007/978-981-99-9167-9_1

3]. In addition, it was disputed that pain is more than a symptom and that chronic pain may be a disease with its own clinical course, and therefore the definition should convey this view [4, 5].

A revised IASP definition of pain has been published based on the criticisms and discussions collected and researched and with tremendous deliberation. The definition is that pain is "An aversive sensory and emotional experience typically caused by, or resembling that caused by, actual or potential tissue injury" [6]. It reserves the emphasis on pain as an experience from the previous definition, while giving prominence to tissue injury-like experience which may be any sign of pain that requires no verbal description. The revised definition of pain highlights the pain as a critical health condition and is going to transform pain study and care [6].

1.1.2 Classification of Pain

Clinically, degrees, causes, and manifestations of pain vary from person to person. The classifications of pain involve different criteria or methods.

1. Classification of pain according to locations

   Pain belonging to this category includes somatic pain, visceral pain, and central pain.

   Somatic pain, also called superficial pain, refers to the pain that appears on the surface of the body, is localized, intense, mostly pins and needles, knife-like, sharp pain, and can clearly indicate the site of pain, such as frozen shoulder, arthritis, etc.

   Visceral pain, also known as deep pain, is usually hard to identify the site of the pain. The biliary colic, renal colic, stomach pain, etc. are examples of this type of pain, showing the nature of pain can be colic, pulling pain, vague pain, distension, etc.

   Central pain refers to pain caused by diseases in the nerve center, such as pain caused by brain hemorrhage and brain tumors.

2. Classification of pain according to characteristics

   Based on pain characteristics, pain can be divided into injury pain, inflammatory pain, neuropathic pain, cancer pain, neurological pain, and psychological pain. Injurious pain is pain caused by noxious stimuli. Inflammatory pain refers to pain mediated by inflammatory factors in the inflammatory response. Neuropathic pain is a lesion occurring anywhere in the nervous system that is burning-like, intense diffuse and persistent, and may be associated with nociceptive hypersensitivity and unusual pain. Cancer pain, also known as advanced cancer pain, generally refers to the pain that occurs with advanced tumors or tumor metastatic pain. Psychogenic and psychological pain is pain generally without organic lesions or other physical diseases, mainly caused by psychological or spiritual factors.

3. Classification of pain according to courses

   According to the course of the disease, pain can be divided into acute pain, chronic pain, intractable pain, and special pain categories. Acute pain refers to acute injury pain in soft tissues and joints, post-surgical pain, obstetric pain, acute herpes zoster pain, gout, etc. Chronic pain is generally soft tissue and joint strain pain or degenerative pain, discogenic pain, neurogenic pain, etc. Intractable pain mainly includes trigeminal neuralgia, post-herpetic neuralgia, disc herniation, intractable headache, etc. Special pain mainly refers to thrombotic vasculitis, intractable angina pectoris, idiopathic chest and abdominal pain, etc.

Though the above classification standard can be referred to, clinical pain is not necessarily bound to these criteria when it comes to specific situations, as pain may fall into one of several categories together at the time of occurrence, or be superimposed by several different types of pain.

1.2 Concept and Classification of Visceral Pain

Visceral pain has a significant systemic impact, accounting for a large proportion of all forms of chronic pain [7]. Surveys have shown that the prevalence of chest pain among adults was 20%, intermittent abdominal pain was 25%, and pelvic pain in women was 16–24% [8]. Visceral pain, despite its ubiquity, is poorly understood due to the complexity of the interactions between the visceral organs, the autonomic nervous system, and the central nervous system. For instance, not all visceral organs respond to stimuli as some organs are more sensitive than others, and not all stimuli cause pain. Besides, emotions and stress can affect visceral pain via the hypothalamic-pituitary-adrenal axis. Thus, multiple factors play a role in the development of visceral pain. Visceral pain signals can be transmitted to multiple locations within the central nervous system and can converge with somatic afferent nerves, which may lead to modulation of referred pain and signals within the central nervous system. Dysregulation may also happen, resulting in hyperalgesia. Physical responses to visceral pain such as spasticity may also be produced. Recent studies have manifested that the gut microbiome can modulate pain and that probiotics can lead to improvements in pain in irritable bowel syndrome (IBS) patients. While in contrast, pathogenic bacteria may contain or secrete substances that cause inflammation and pain [9].

There are various classifications of visceral pain [8, 10]. The classification criteria include nerve conduction mechanisms, etiology, anatomy, and manifestation modalities. According to nerve conduction mechanisms, visceral pain can be divided into nociceptive conduction through visceral afferent nerves, conduction through spinal nerve afferent fibers such as mural pleura, peritoneum, mediastinum and mesentery, and visceral pain produced through distal sites with certain types of somatic pain or nociceptive hypersensitivity, i.e., true visceral pain, pseudo-visceral pain, and visceral referred pain. According to the etiologies, visceral pain can be classified as functional, inflammatory, and cancerous visceral pain. And according to the anatomical features, visceral pain includes thoracic pain, abdominal pain, and pelvic pain. Last but not least, pain originating from internal organs may manifest in several different ways. The main phenomena associated with visceral nociception can be schematically summarized as: (a) true visceral pain; (b) referred pain without hyperalgesia; (c) referred pain with hyperalgesia; (d) visceral hyperalgesia; and (e) viscero-visceral hyperalgesia. Careful assessment of the characteristics of the symptoms and accompanying signs is essential for a correct diagnosis.

1.3 Clinical Features of Visceral Pain

1.3.1 Clinical Visceral Pain

Visceral pain is characterized by the lower density innervation of visceral structures comparing with the sensory innervation of other tissues and the differentiation of sensory input in the peripheral and central nervous systems, resulting in less diffuse and localized pain. In clinical practice, the mechanisms behind visceral pain vary widely, including distension or muscle contraction of hollow organs, ischemia, traction of the mesentery, chemical irritants, and nerve compression due to malignant tumor [11].

The abdominal viscera are innervated by two systems: the vagus nerves and the spinal visceral sensory nerves. Most viscera receive dual afferent innervation via sympathetic and parasympathetic nerves, which ultimately project to the central nervous system. In noxious events, the spinal tract and dorsal column are two main ascending fiber tracts in the spinal cord that transmit sensory input from the viscera to the brain. Subsequent projections to the medial thalamus are closely associated with pain-triggered emotional and autonomic responses, whereas projections to the lateral ventral thalamus are associated with pain perception, both in terms of location and intensity. Visceral pain also preferentially increases activity in the anterior cingulate cortex, which may explain the strong emotional response to visceral pain. In addition, in response to ongoing injury or inflammation, visceral afferents lead to peripheral and central sensitization due to increased neuronal excitability, finally bringing increased sensitivity, such as hyperalgesia, and an enlargement of the metastatic pain areas seen in some visceral pain syndromes, such as IBS, dyspepsia, and interstitial cystitis [11].

Visceral pain usually has a temporal evolution and varies in clinical features at different stages of pathology. "True visceral pain" is a diffuse, ill-defined sensation, usually perceived in the midline, lower sternum or upper abdomen of the body. Pain in visceral organs may present in different areas, such as the bladder pain may present in the perineal region, the heart pain may present in the left arm and neck, and the left ureter pain may present in the left lower abdomen and low back. This diffusivity and difficulty in localizing visceral pain is due to the low density of visceral sensory innervation and the extensive differentiation of visceral input within the central nervous system. Thus, visceral pain is more diffuse than noxious cutaneous stimuli in terms of location and timing [12].

Subsequent symptom development may require the transfer of pain to parietal somatic structures within the same metadomain as the affected organs. Thus, spatial discrimination of visceral pain usually involves superficial structures, producing secondary hyperalgesia in superficial or deep body wall tissues due to the fusion of visceral sensations (discussed later). Referred pain with or without hyperalgesia is more acute, more precisely localized, and less likely to be accompanied by autonomic signs, making it difficult to distinguish from pain of somatic origin. Unlike somatic or superficial pain, the main characteristic of visceral pain is that it is more sensitive to stimuli such as mechanical pulling, organ ischemia or spasm, and inflammation, while it is insensitive to stimuli such as cutting and burning [13].

Visceral pain is often associated with marked autonomic phenomena, including pallor, profuse sweating, nausea, digestive disturbances, and changes in body temperature, blood pressure, and heart rate [13]. Pain occurs slowly but persists for a long time, is difficult to localize and often accompanied by referred pain, emotional or defensive reactions.

When the internal organ system is in a healthy state, it may cause a minimal level of sensation. During daily activities, fullness, belching, and venting derive from digestion or excretion process will not cause discomfort. In general, they often lead to minor discomfort, but when lesions or inflammation of internal organs occur, stimuli that normally induce no harmful reaction may be amplified and cause serious effects on the patient, further leading to more severe discomforts or pain. In visceral pain, there is a high incidence of nausea, in addition to possible autonomic reactions such as night sweats, profuse sweating, and shortness of breath. The strong emotional response that accompanies visceral pain is also one of the challenges, and the occurrence rate often depends on the patient's perception of pain. Strong emotional changes induced by visceral sensations may be accompanied by further changes in visceral sensations, generating anxiety due to pain and in turn, anxiety causes more severe pain, thus potentially creating a positive feedback pathway that further exacerbates the pain level. Therefore, the correlation between the degree of pathological changes in visceral pain and the intensity of the pain they cause is poor [14].

1.3.2 Specific Types of Visceral Pain or Abdominal Pain Syndrome

Many surveys indicated that most of chronic and recurrent pain occurred in the chest, abdomen, and pelvic regions. For example, intermittent abdominal pain was present in about 25% of adults and chest pain in about 20%, while more than 24% of women were often bothered by pelvic pain [15]. For more than 23% of patients, pain was considered part of daily life and symptoms were often managed by patients themselves; while a smaller percentage sought medical help. Visceral pain conditions are strongly associated with declined quality of life, and both the cost of medical care and the impaired ability to work due to the disease place a significant burden on the patient's life.

Abdominal pain is the most common clinical form of visceral pain and may be a manifestation of a specific disease, but in many patients, all diagnostic tests may turn out to be normal or negative. This pain of visceral origin usually presents as vague sensation, spasmodic pain, and indefinite localization. Surgeons call it non-specific abdominal pain, older textbooks just called it non-organic pain, and abdominal pain in children is mostly recurrent abdominal pain (RAP). Currently, the majority of patients have simple abdominal pain, but some patients who visit health care institutions with severe pain may be diagnosed as chronic functional abdominal pain syndrome.

The general incidence of abdominal pain is as high as 22–28%, with more women than men, and only about 20% of all abdominal pain patients select to seek medical attention [10]. A significant proportion of those surveyed, however, suffer from pain that influences their daily life, and there is no significant gender difference in the degree of impact. This also means that in many undiagnosed populations, abdominal pain is also an important factor that interferes daily life. The natural course of abdominal pain in adults is largely unknown. In a follow-up study on the recurrence and remission of abdominal manifestations in populations, it was found that the overall incidence of recurrence remained constant, being approximately 10%, but the symptoms of the vast majority of patients got improved. The remission rate was 35%, and the ratio of overall incidence versus remission rate were unchanged [10].

Functional abdominal pain is the main clinical presentation of patients admitted to hospital with abdominal pain. Back decades ago, abdominal pain without a clear cause ranked tenth among the most common causes of hospitalization in men and sixth in women. This situation has not been improved to date, with up to 67% of consecutive admissions to surgical wards in hospitals being "non-specific" abdominal pain [10].

1. Irritable bowel syndrome (IBS)

   IBS represents a group of symptoms including abdominal pain and altered bowel movement patterns, but lacks any evidence of an underlying organic injury. These symptoms can persist for a long time, often up to several years. Depending on whether constipation or diarrhea occurs, IBS can be divided into four main types, namely diarrheal IBS, constipated IBS, mixed IBS (diarrheal and constipated), or uncertain IBS. Disorders such as anxiety, major depression, and chronic fatigue syndrome are also common in patients with IBS.

   Currently, the etiology of IBS is not fully understood. Related theoretical studies include altered brain-gut axis, intestinal dysmotility, changes in pain sensitivity, infections (including small intestinal bacterial overgrowth, neurotransmitters, genetic factors, and food sensitivities), etc.

   The diagnosis of IBS is based on signs and symptoms, and high-risk factors include age over 50 years, weight loss, fecal blood loss, or a family history of inflammatory bowel disease. However, similar symptoms may be seen in other conditions, including celiac dis ease, colitis, inflammatory bowel disease, bile acid malabsorption, and colon cancer.

   Currently, IBS is incurable, and its treatments target at relieving symptoms. Lifestyle modification, changes in diet, medications, pain management, probiotics, and psychological counseling are adopted to treat IBS patients. Among them, dietary treatment methods include increasing the intake of soluble fiber and limiting the intake of fermentable oligosaccharides, disaccharides, monosaccharides, and polyols. Pharmacological treatment includes antidiarrheal, laxatives, and antidepressants.

2. Chest pain

   In the clinical setting, chest pain is a common symptom and one of the most common reasons for seeking medical care in emergency department. Chest pain caused by cardiovascular disease should be considered first. Acute chest pain is often considered a warning sign of myocardial ischemia. However, chest pain that mimics angina may be non-cardiac in nature. The most common causes of chest pain in adults include gastrointestinal disease (42%), coronary artery disease (31%), musculoskeletal disease (28%), pericarditis (4%), and pulmonary embolism (2%). Other less common causes include pneumonia, lung cancer, and aortic aneurysm. In addition, panic attack is one of psychological causes of chest pain. It can be seen that non-cardiogenic factors may trigger more chest pain situations than cardiogenic factors. Functional chest pain is also called non-cardiac chest pain (NCCP), and it has been reported that the incidence of NCCP in China was as high as 13.9%, but the research and investment on it was relatively small and much lower than that of cardiac chest pain [16].

In children, the most common causes of chest pain are musculoskeletal disorders (76–89%), exercise-induced asthma (4–12%), gastrointestinal disorders (8%), and psychological causes (4%). In addition, chest pain in children may also be caused by congenital factors [10].

It is currently believed that non-cardiogenic chest pain should also be treated with different strategies in clinical practice according to its etiologies. Therefore, a correct understanding of the source of the disease that contributes to a correct diagnosis, is a key prerequisite for effective treatment of NCCP.

3. Functional abdominal pain syndrome (FAPS)

FAPS differs from other functional bowel disorders in that it is less common. Its symptoms are mostly irrelevant to food intake and bowel movements, and there is a high rate of comorbidity with psychiatric disorders. Its etiology and pathophysiology are not fully understood. Because FAPS may represent a heterogeneous group of disorders, peripheral neuropathic pain mechanisms, alterations in the endogenous pain modulation system, or a combination of these may show together in one patient. The diagnosis of FAPS is based on positive symptom criteria and a long history of symptoms; in the absence of alarm symptoms, an extensive diagnostic evaluation is not required. Treatment is determined by a therapeutic relationship between physician and patient and an empirical treatment algorithm using various types of centrally acting medications, including antidepressants and anticonvulsants. The choice, dosage, and combination of medications are influenced by psychiatric comorbidities. Psychotherapy options include psychotherapy, relaxation techniques, and hypnosis. Patients with refractory FAPS can benefit from a multidisciplinary outpatient approach to pain [17].

4. Recurrent abdominal pain in children (RAP)

Abdominal pain is one of the most common symptoms in children. The pain is often acute and the possible causes are classified as gastrointestinal or extraintestinal factors, specifically including gastrointestinal infections, dietary mydriasis, urinary tract infections and other more dangerous surgical conditions, such as acute appendicitis. If properly managed, this acute abdominal pain usually does not lead to long-term sequelae. However, there are often some difficulties in the treatment of pediatric abdominal pain. First, in young children, the history of pain is usually "second-hand", i.e., children are unable to describe the location and nature of the pain precisely and it is often relayed by the parents or caregivers. Fortunately, most parents can be helpful in providing information about the cause of their child's abdominal pain. In addition, the physical examination of pediatric abdominal pain is often difficult due to factors such as the child's poor cooperation.

RAP is very common in children and can affect up to 10–20% of school-age children. In the mid-twentieth century, RAP in children was first reported by Apley and Naish, who noted that in the vast majority of cases RAP has no definite etiology and was therefore thought to be the result of psychological influence in children [18]. In young children, abdominal pain is often vaguely localized, with the child usually indicating that the pain comes from the central region of the abdomen. Moreover, the severity and frequency of pain are not associated with the cause. The term "recurrent" refers to the duration and frequency of the pain, which is usually considered to be at least 3 months, during which at least three episodes of pain are severe enough to interfere with the child's daily activities. Over the years, with advances in medical technology and a better understanding of the pathophysiology of abdominal pain, an increasing number of organic causes have been identified. However, it is currently believed that the most common etiology of RAP in children remains functional.

5. Chronic pelvic pain (CPP)

   Pelvic pain is broadly defined as pain in and around the pelvic area and is usually more common in acute pain than in chronic pain. When the pain persists for more than 6 months, it is considered to be CPP. Relatively speaking, CPP is associated with comorbidities such as IBS, major depressive disorder, or pelvic inflammatory syndrome. CPP is not only common in female patients, but also common in male patients. Reviewing the literature, Sibert et al. published in 2010 a prevalence of chronic pelvic pain syndrome (CPPS)/chronic prostatitis in men of approximately 10%; bladder pain syndrome/interstitial cystitis (in both sexes) 0.24–0.31%; post-vasectomy, testicular and epididymal pain 15–20%; and ejaculation or orgasm-related pain in men 1–9% [19].

   CPP is a form of concentrated pain in which the body produces a low threshold for pain, which is often the result of chronic pain. For example, if a woman has endometriosis, over a period of 3–6 months, the acute pain associated with this condition may become concentrated pain, as the pain becomes chronic. In concentrated pain, previously mild to moderate pain is experienced as severe pain (hyperalgesia), or tenderness can be interpreted as pain (ectopic sensation). In addition, CPP is strongly associated with previous physical or emotional trauma. Therefore, the etiology of CPP may also be related to functional somatic pain syndromes.

   The diagnosis of CPP is made after 3–6 months of pelvic pain and is usually based on history or physical examination; there are many associated symptoms or precipitating factors that help establish the diagnosis. Although imaging and laboratory findings are often inconclusive in the diagnosis of CPP, they are often helpful in diagnosing comorbidities that contribute to the development of CPP.

   Treatment of CPP is often complex, with limited evidence-based options. Treatment usually focuses on suspected causes of CPP, such as treatment of comorbid mood disorders, neuropathy, or uterine dysfunction. The prevalence of CPP is estimated to be 5.7–26.6% [20]. Given its prevalence, patients experiencing CPP must be treated with a high degree of suspicion. The management of CPP requires an interprofessional team approach; collaboration between multiple specialties is needed to provide adequate pain relief. Some patients with CPP may benefit from cognitive behavioral therapy and hormone replacement. Conversely, others may require more invasive therapeutic interventions such as spinal cord stimulation or total hysterectomy. Pelvic pain is broadly defined as pain in and around the pelvic area and is usually more common in acute pain than in chronic pain. When the pain persists for more than 6 months, it is considered CPP. Relatively speaking, CPP is associated with comorbidities such as IBS, major depressive disorder, or pelvic inflammatory syndrome.

6. Cancer visceral pain

   Cancer visceral pain is a special type of visceral pain caused by tumor, which is more complicated than general visceral pain, and is easily affected by patients' emotion, cognition and other spiritual factors, and spiritual factors are influenced by culture and religion, so it is still very difficult to diagnose or treat. According to incomplete statistics, about 50% of cancer patients have inadequate pain treatment, and in a few types of tumor patients, the proportion of inadequate pain treatment is even higher, which greatly affects the survival quality of cancer patients and is one of the important reasons why many patients are afraid to talk about cancer. Contrary to the public perception, untreated pain is not insignificant, but long-term chronic pain can change the immune system and even organ function, increase patients' anxiety and depression, which can seriously affect health and quality of life, and may even accelerate patients' death.

Globally, the degree of treatment for cancerous visceral pain is highly inconsistent; even in China, patients with the same degree of pain may receive widely varying pain-related treatments due to economic factors, patients' education level, psychological factors influence, and physicians' cognitive factors. A few patients and elderly people may be more reluctant to talk about their pain with their doctors, believing that pain is a sign of cancer deterioration, convinced that pain cannot be relieved, unresolved concerns about addiction and side effects of medication, and possibly because they cannot afford to pay for the treatment of analgesic drugs. In fact, the prevalence of cancerous visceral pain varies depending on the location of the primary tumor. The incidence and extent of pain also vary at different stages of tumor development. Usually, the more advanced the cancerous visceral pain is, the higher the incidence of pain and the greater the intensity of pain, and it is often the most difficult to control pain at the advanced stage of the disease. In addition, pain caused by tumor metastasis is also very common, and is more common and severe in progressive and end-stage cancer. However, regardless of the degree and nature of cancer pain caused by any of these causes, patients have the right to safe, effective pain treatment with few side effects, and this requires that all physicians should properly understand and treat cancer visceral pain in order to treat every patient with cancer visceral pain with the most optimal method available.

1.4 Summary

This chapter focuses on a review of several commonly seen visceral pain disorders in clinical practice and their epidemiology. As opposed to the detailed and specific coverage in subsequent chapters, the main purpose of this chapter is to provide a preliminary understanding of visceral pain-related disorders and research, to lay the initial foundation for future in-depth understanding and research, and to help the reader quickly understand the general scope of the coverage in the subsequent sections of this book. Although the diagnosis of visceral organic pathology has not been ruled out in many patients, current studies in the literature mostly suggest that most patients do have functional problems. Because of the difficulty in classifying and treating these diseases, it is important to further understand the etiology and pathogenesis of visceral pain, and then to investigate and explore the corresponding treatment countermeasures and their clinical efficacy, in order to reduce patients' suffering and introduce unnecessary medical costs. Meanwhile, in addition to the specific types of visceral pain or abdominal pain mentioned above, many different types or mixed occurrence of visceral-related pain in clinical practice will be illustrated in detail in subsequent relevant chapters from multiple perspectives based on the etiology and mechanism, epidemiology, diagnosis and treatment, and research progress of various types of visceral pain and visceral pain-related disorders, respectively.

References

1. Merskey H, Bogduk N. Classification of chronic pain. 2nd ed. Seattle: IASP Task Force on Taxonomy, IASP Press; 1994. http://www.iasp-pain.org/Education/content.aspx?ItemNumber=1698
2. Williams AC, Craig KD. Updating the definition of pain. Pain. 2016;157:2420–3.
3. Cohen M, Quintner J, van Rysewyk S. Reconsidering the International Association for the Study of Pain definition of pain. Pain Rep. 2018;3:e634.

4. Loeser JD, Treede RD. The Kyoto protocol of IASP Basic Pain Terminology. Pain. 2008;137:473–7.
5. Treede RD, Rief W, Barke A, Aziz Q, Bennett MI, Benoliel R, Cohen M, Evers S, Finnerup NB, First MB, et al. Chronic pain as a symptom or a disease: the IASP Classification of Chronic Pain for the International Classification of Diseases (ICD-11). Pain. 2019;160:19–27.
6. Raja SN, Carr DB, Cohen M, Finnerup NB, Flor H, Gibson S, Keefe FJ, Mogil JS, Ringkamp M, Sluka KA, Song XJ, Stevens B, Sullivan MD, Tutelman PR, Ushida T, Vader K. The revised International Association for the Study of Pain definition of pain: concepts, challenges, and compromises. Pain. 2020;161(9):1976–82. https://doi.org/10.1097/j.pain.0000000000001939. PMID: 32694387; PMCID: PMC7680716.
7. Halder SLS, Locke GR. Epidemiology and social impact of visceral pain. In: Visceral pain. Oxford University Press; 2009. p. 1–8.
8. Giamberardino MA. Visceral pain. Oxford University Press; 2009.
9. Katz BL, Van Houten T, Sassan Sabouri A. Chapter 2—Neuroanatomy and mechanisms of visceral pain. In: Pak DJ, Yong RJ, Shah KB, editors. Interventional management of chronic visceral pain syndromes. Amsterdam: Elsevier; 2021. p. 5–15.
10. Zhijie L. Visceral pain—basic and clinical. Beijing: Science Publishing House; 2018.
11. Ahmed HS, Shah KB, Pak DJ. Chapter 1—Epidemiology of chronic visceral pain syndromes. In: Pak DJ, Jason Yong R, Shah KB, editors. . Interventional management of chronic visceral pain syndromes: Elsevier; 2021. p. 1–3.
12. Procacci P, Zoppi M, Maresca M. Visceral sensation. In: Cervero F, Morrison JFB, editors. Progress in pain research. Amsterdam: Elsevier; 1986. p. 21–8, 39.
13. Sikandar S, Dickenson AH. Visceral pain: the ins and outs, the ups and downs. Curr Opin Support Palliat Care. 2012;6:17–26.
14. Millham FH. Acute abdominal pain. In: Sleisenger and Fordtran's gastrointestinal and liver disease, vol. 11. Amsterdam: Elsevier. p. 144–57.
15. Kapural L, et al. Chronic abdominal pain: an evidence-based, comprehensive guide to clinical management, vol. 13. New York: Springer Science+Business Media; 2015. https://doi.org/10.1007/978-1-4939-1992-5_2.
16. Wong WM, Lam KF, Cheng C, et al. Population based study of non-cardiac chest pain in southern Chinese: prevalence, psychosocial factors and health care utilization. World J Gastroenterol. 2004;10(5):707–12.
17. Clouse RE, Mayer EA, Aziz Q, Drossman DA, Dumitrascu DL, Mönnikes H, Naliboff BD. Functional abdominal pain syndrome. Gastroenterology. 2006;130(5):1492–7. https://doi.org/10.1053/j.gastro.2005.11.062. PMID: 16678562.
18. Feuerstein M, Dobkin PL. Recurrent abdominal pain in children. In: Gross AM, Drabman RS, editors. Handbook of clinical behavioral pediatrics. Applied clinical psychology. Boston, MA: Springer; 1990. https://doi.org/10.1007/978-1-4613-0505-7_18.
19. Sibert L, Rigaud J, Delavierre D, Labat JJ. Chronic pelvic pain: epidemiology and economic impact. Prog Urol. 2010;20:872–85.
20. Ahangari A. Prevalence of chronic pelvic pain among women: an updated review. Pain Physician. 2014;17(2):E141–7. PMID: 24658485.

2 Anatomy of the Visceral Nerves

Bifa Fan

To give a clear and concise description of visceral pain, it is necessary to start by introducing the anatomy of the visceral nerves which are complicated and closely related to the activation of sensations. The visceral nerves are divided into visceral motor nerves and visceral sensory nerves. A comparison of visceral motor nerves and somatic motor nerves will be made to reveal the unique features of visceral motor nerves. Then, sympathetic nerve, parasympathetic nerve, visceral plexuses, and enteric nervous system will be introduced, as they all play an indispensable and crucial role in consisting of the visceral motor nerves. The visceral sensory nerves section covers the concepts of interoceptor and neural pathways. Besides, referred pain is also illustrated as it is an important physiological characteristic of visceral sensation. It is a sensory hypersensitivity or nociception phenomenon in a certain area of the body surface. The detailed classification and explanation of visceral nerves will lay a solid foundation for further discussion of visceral pain and diseases.

The visceral nervous system is a component of the entire nervous system and can be divided into central and peripheral parts according to their distribution.

The central part of the visceral nervous system is located in the spinal cord, brainstem, mesencephalon, and cerebral cortex. Visceral stimulus signals are transmitted to the central nerve, triggering two different physiological responses in the organism, one that does not cause subjective sensations but is accessible by scientific means, such as blood pressure fluctuations, lung expansion, intestinal peristalsis, etc., i.e., autonomic activity in the traditional sense. These reflex activities can be achieved, in part, by short-circuit reflex arcs within the visceral wall. Another visceral signaling impulse transmitted to the central nervous system causes sensory awareness in the brain, the most typical of which is visceral pain.

The peripheral part is mainly located in the visceral, cardiovascular, and glandular areas, hence named as visceral nerves. Visceral nerves, like somatic nerves, can be divided into sensory and motor fiber components according to the nature of the fibers. The visceral motor nerves regulate visceral and cardiovascular movements and glandular secretion, which are usually not controlled by human will and are not random, so they are also called the autonomic nervous system; because they mainly control and regulate the metabolic activities of substances common to plants and animals, they do not govern the movements of skeletal muscles unique to animals. Therefore, they are also called the vegetative nervous system. According to the morphological, functional, and pharmacological characteristics, the visceral motor nerves can be divided into two parts: sympathetic and parasympathetic nerves. The enteric nervous system is structurally and

B. Fan (✉)
Department of Pain Medicine, China-Japan Friendship Hospital, Beijing, China

M. Xia et al. (eds.), *Visceral Pain*, https://doi.org/10.1007/978-981-99-9167-9_2

functionally distinct from the sympathetic and parasympathetic nervous systems, but it is also part of the autonomic nervous system as it participates in and mediates the voluntary movements of the intestine. The primary sensory neurons of the visceral sensory nerves are also located in the cerebral nerves and spinal ganglia, while the peripheral branches are distributed in the visceral and cardiovascular internal sensory apparatus, transmitting the perceived information to the centers at all levels and also reaching the cerebral cortex. This plays an important role in maintaining the dynamic balance of the internal and external environment of the organism and maintaining normal life activities.

2.1 Visceral Motor Nerves

2.1.1 Differences Between Visceral Motor Nerves and Somatic Motor Nerves

Generally speaking, somatic motor nerves are under volitional control, while visceral motor nerves are not. There are also major structural and functional differences between them, which are summarized in Table 2.1.

Table 2.1 Differences between visceral motor nerves and somatic motor nerves

Differences	Visceral motor nerves	Somatic motor nerves
Innervated organs	Smooth muscle, cardiac muscle, and glands	Skeletal muscle
Fiber composition	Sympathetic nerves and parasympathetic nerves	Only one type
Number of neurons from low-level centers to effectors	Two neurons: the preganglionic neuron and the postganglionic neuron	Only one
Fiber thickness	Thin medullary (pre-nodal fibers) and non-medullary (post-nodal fibers) thin fibers	Thick medullary fiber
Postganglionic fiber distribution form	Climbing of organs or blood vessels to form plexuses, which in turn branch to effectors	Distribute in the form of nerve trunks
Controlled by will or not	No	Yes

2.1.2 Sympathetic Nerve Anatomy

The sympathetic nerve is part of the visceral motor nerve, and together with the parasympathetic nerve and the enteric nervous system, it forms the autonomic nervous system.

1. Physiological functions of sympathetic nerve

   The main function of sympathetic nerves is to stimulate the "fight or flight" response of the body. Sympathetic excitation will cause pupil dilatation, increased heart rate, skin and visceral vasoconstriction, coronary artery dilation, increased blood pressure, small bronchial diastole, gastrointestinal peristalsis, bladder wall muscle relaxation, reduced saliva secretion, sweat gland secretion, and contraction of the erector spinae. When the body is in a state of nervous activity, sympathetic nerve activity plays a major role.

2. Composition of sympathetic nerves

   The low-level center of sympathetic nerves is located in the lateral nucleus of the middle band (preganglionic neuron) in the T_1–$L_{2/3}$ segment of the spinal cord. The preganglionic neurons send preganglionic fibers out of the intervertebral foramen via the anterior roots, which terminate in the corresponding postganglionic neurons (sympathetic ganglia), which then send postganglionic fibers to the effectors. The peripheral part of the sympathetic nerve includes the sympathetic trunk, the sympathetic ganglion, and branches from the ganglion and the sympathetic plexus. Depending on their location, sympathetic ganglia can be divided into paravertebral ganglia and prevertebral ganglia.

   (a) Paravertebral ganglia: The ganglia of the sympathetic trunk is located on both sides of the spine and is connected to the left and right sympathetic trunks by the interganglionic branch. The sympathetic trunk is distributed from the base of the skull to the coccyx, and the two trunks merge in front of the coccyx. The sympathetic trunk is divided into five parts: cervical, thoracic, lumbar, sacral, and caudal. The number of sympathetic ganglia in each part is similar to the number of vertebrae in each part, except for 3–4 ganglia in the cervical part and 1 ganglion in the caudal part, and the total number of sympathetic ganglia on each side is 19–24. The sympathetic trunk ganglion consists of multipolar neurons of different sizes, and some of the postganglionic fibers of the sympathetic nerve originate from these cells.

(b) Prevertebral ganglia: Irregular nodular masses located anterior to the spine, at the root of the visceral branch of the abdominal aorta. The prevertebral ganglia include celiac ganglia, superior mesenteric ganglion, inferior mesenteric ganglion, and aorticorenal ganglia.

3. Communicating branch between sympathetic nerve and spinal nerve

Each sympathetic ganglion is connected to the corresponding spinal nerve by a communicating branch. The communicating branch is divided into the white communicating branch and the gray communicating branch. The white communicating branch is mainly composed of preganglionic fibers with myelin sheath and is white in color, so it is called the white communicating branch. The cytosol of preganglionic neurons exists only in the lateral horn of the spinal cord in T_{1-12} and L_{1-3} segments, and the white communicating branch also exists only between the anterior branches of each spinal nerve from T_1 to L_3 and the corresponding sympathetic trunk ganglion. The gray communicating branch is connected between the sympathetic trunk and 31 pairs of anterior spinal nerve branches, and consists of postganglionic fibers emanating from the sympathetic trunk ganglion cells, which are mostly unmyelinated and grayish in color, hence the name gray communicating branch.

4. The general itinerary of sympathetic nerves

(a) The preganglionic fibers of the sympathetic nerve: The preganglionic fibers emanate from the lateral nucleus of the intermediate zone of the spinal cord and enter the sympathetic trunk via the anterior spinal nerve roots, the spinal nerve trunk, and the white communicating branch, and then have three kinds of destinations:

- Terminating in the corresponding paravertebral ganglion and changing neurons.
- Ascending or descending within the sympathetic trunk to terminate in the paravertebral ganglion above or below.

  It is generally believed that preganglionic fibers from the middle band of the lateral nucleus in the upper thoracic segment of the spinal cord (T_{1-6}) ascend within the sympathetic trunk to the cervical region and exchange elements in the cervical paravertebral ganglion; those in the middle thoracic segment (T_{6-10}) ascend or descend within the sympathetic trunk to exchange elements in the sympathetic ganglion of the other thoracic segments: those in the lower thoracic and lumbar segments (T_1–L_3) descend within the sympathetic trunk and exchange elements in the lumbosacral sympathetic ganglion.
- After crossing the paravertebral ganglion, it goes to the prevertebral sympathetic ganglion for neurons.

(b) The destination of postganglionic fibers of sympathetic nerves:

- Postganglionic fibers originating from the sympathetic trunk ganglia return to the spinal nerves via the gray communicating branch and are distributed with the spinal nerves to the blood vessels, sweat glands, and erector spinae of the head and neck, trunk, and extremities. Thirty-one pairs of spinal nerves are connected to the sympathetic trunk by the gray communicating branch, and their branches generally contain postganglionic fibers of sympathetic nerves.

- Climbing arteries travel, forming corresponding plexuses in the arterial epicardium, such as the internal and external carotid plexus, the ventral plexus, and the superior mesenteric plexus, and distributing with the arteries to the organs they innervate.
- Directly distributed by sympathetic ganglia to the innervated organs.

5. Local distribution of sympathetic nerves
   (a) Neck: The cervical sympathetic trunk is located posterior to the carotid sheath and anterior to the transverse processes of the cervical vertebrae. Generally, there are 3–4 sympathetic ganglia on each side, and as many as 6, which are called superior, middle, and inferior cervical ganglia. The superior cervical ganglion is the largest, shuttle-shaped, and is located anterior to the $C_{2,3}$ transverse process and posterior to the internal carotid artery. The middle cervical ganglion is the smallest, sometimes absent, and is located at the C_6 transverse process. The inferior cervical ganglion is located anterior to the C_7 transverse process and posterior to the beginning of the vertebral artery, and often merges with the T_1 ganglion to form the cervicothoracic ganglion (also known as the stellate ganglion).

   The distribution of postganglionic nerve fibers emanating from the cervical sympathetic ganglion is as follows:

   The cervical nerve joins eight pairs of cervical nerves via the gray traffic branch, and distributes with the cervical nerve branches to the blood vessels, sweat glands, and lissencephalic muscles of the head, neck, and upper limbs.

   Branches from the ganglion to the internal and external carotid arteries, subclavian artery and vertebral artery, etc., climbing on the surface of the arteries and forming the corresponding arterial plexus, accompanying the branches of the arteries to the glands of the head and neck (lacrimal glands, salivary glands, mucosal glands in the oral and nasal cavities, thyroid gland, etc.), the erector spinae, blood vessels, pupil opening muscle, smooth muscle of the eye and face, etc.

   The pharyngeal branches from the ganglion, which enter the pharyngeal wall directly, together with the pharyngeal branches (containing parasympathetic fibers) from the vagus and swallowing nerves, form the pharyngeal plexus, which is distributed in the pharyngeal wall and has branches to the glottis of the larynx and carotid artery.

   Three pairs of cervical sympathetic ganglia give off separate branches of the supracardiac, cardiac, and subcardiac nerves, respectively, which enter the thoracic cavity and participate in forming the cardiac plexus.

   (b) Thorax: There are 10–12 (11 are most common) thoracic ganglia on each side. They are connected upward to the cervical sympathetic trunk and continue downward through the diaphragm to the lumbar sympathetic trunk. The upper thoracic sympathetic ganglia are located on both sides of the spine, anterior or slightly lateral to the head of the ribs, crossing in front of the intercostal vessels and nerves, and gradually moving downward to the front of the vertebral body. The paravertebral ganglia of the thoracic sympathetic trunk are small in size. The thoracic sympathetic trunk emits the following branches:

   - Via the gray traffic branch, it is connected to 12 pairs of thoracic nerves and distributed with them to the blood vessels, sweat glands, and lissencephalic muscles of the thoracic and abdominal walls.
   - From the upper five pairs of thoracic sympathetic trunk ganglia, many branches are sent out to participate in

the thoracic aortic plexus, esophageal plexus, pulmonary plexus and cardiac plexus, etc.

- The visceral greater splanchnic nerve starts from the T_5 or $T_{6–9}$ sympathetic trunk ganglia and consists of preganglionic fibers that pass through these ganglia, synthesizes a trunk in the anterior and inferior course, and descends along the anterior inclination of the vertebral body, penetrates the foot of the diaphragm into the abdominal cavity, and terminates in the ventral ganglia. The lesser splanchnic nerve originates from the preganglionic fibers of the sympathetic trunk ganglia from T_{10} to T_{12}, descends through the pedicle of the diaphragm into the abdominal cavity, and terminates in the aorto-renal ganglion. The postganglionic fibers after the neuron exchange in the celiac ganglion and the aorticorenal ganglion are distributed to the substantive organs such as the liver, spleen, kidney, and the digestive tube above the left flexure of the colon.

  It is noteworthy that the visceral major and minor nerves, although passing through the paravertebral ganglion, do not change neurons in that ganglion, but go to the abdominal cavernous ganglion and the aortic renal ganglion to change neurons, respectively, and then innervate the corresponding visceral organs. Therefore, they belong to the preganglionic fibers of the sympathetic nerves.

(c) Lumbar: The lumbar sympathetic travels downward between the anterolateral aspect of the lumbar vertebral body and the medial border of the psoas major muscle, and the lower end enters the pelvis via the posterior aspect of the common iliac vessels. The right side is located lateral to or partially covered by the inferior vena cava: the left side is located lateral to the abdominal aorta. The lumbar paravertebral ganglia are usually four per side, but can be as few as two, irregular in shape and all small. The branches are as follows:

- The gray communicating branch connects five pairs of lumbar nerves and is distributed among the lumbar nerves.
- The lumbar splanchnic nerve consists of preganglionic fibers that pass through the lumbar ganglion and terminate in the prevertebral ganglion in the abdominal aortic plexus and the inferior mesenteric plexus, and replace the neurons. The postganglionic fibers are distributed to the alimentary canal and pelvic organs below the left curvature of the colon, and some fibers are distributed to the lower extremities along with the blood vessels. When lower extremity vasospasm is present, the lumbar sympathetic trunk can be surgically removed to obtain relief.

(d) Pelvis: The pelvic sympathetic trunk descends medially along the anterior sacral foramen to the front of the coccyx, with two to three pairs of sacral ganglia and one ganglion impar. Its branches are as follows:

- The gray communicating branch, joining each neighboring sacral nerve, distributes to the blood vessels, sweat glands and lissencephalic muscles of the lower limbs and perineum.
- Some small branches join the pelvic plexus and distribute to the pelvic organs.

  It can be seen that the sympathetic preganglionic and postganglionic fibers are distributed with some regularity. The preganglionic fibers from the middle lateral nucleus of $T_{1–5}$ segments of the spinal cord, after neuron replacement, innervate the head, neck, thoracic organs and blood vessels of the upper limbs, sweat glands, and the erector spinae. The preganglionic fibers from the lateral nucleus of the middle band of the upper lumbar segment of the spinal cord, after replacing neurons, innervate the digestive ducts below the left curvature of the colon, the pelvic organs and the blood vessels of the lower limbs, sweat glands, and the erector spinae.

2.1.3 Anatomy of Parasympathetic Nerves

1. Physiological functions of the parasympathetic nerve

   The role of the parasympathetic nervous system is opposite to that of the sympathetic nerve, and the two are in mutual balance. The parasympathetic nervous system can maintain the physiological balance of the body in a quiet state, and its role is threefold: first, to enhance gastrointestinal activity, secretion of digestive glands, promote the discharge of urine and feces, and maintain the body's energy; second, to narrow the pupils to reduce stimulation and promote the production of liver glycogen to save energy; third, to slow down heart rate, lower blood pressure and narrow bronchial tubes to save unnecessary consumption, and to assist reproductive activities, such as causing dilation of reproductive blood vessels and increased secretion of fluids from sexual organs.
2. Composition of parasympathetic nerves

   The parasympathetic nerves include preganglionic neurons, preganglionic fibers and postganglionic neurons, postganglionic fibers, and their low-level centers are located in the parasympathetic nucleus of the brainstem and the sacral parasympathetic nucleus (preganglionic neurons) in the gray matter of segment S_{2-4} of the spinal cord. The peripheral parasympathetic ganglia, called parasympathetic and intra-organ ganglia, are located in the cranial region and are larger and visible to the naked eye, including the ciliary ganglion, submandibular ganglion, pterygopalatine ganglion, and auricular ganglion. The preganglionic fibers of the cranial parasympathetic nerves exchange neurons in these ganglia, and then send out postganglionic fibers to the innervated organs with the corresponding brain nerves. Sympathetic and sensory nerve fibers pass through the ganglia (without exchanging neurons) and are called sympathetic and sensory roots, respectively. The parasympathetic ganglia located in other parts of the body are so small that they can only be seen with the aid of a microscope. For example, ganglia are located in the cardiac plexus, pulmonary plexus, bladder plexus, and uterovaginal plexus, as well as ganglia located in the walls of the bronchi and digestive tubes.
3. Distribution of parasympathetic nerves
   (a) Cranial parasympathetic nerves: Their preganglionic fibers travel within the III, IX, and X pairs of cerebral nerves, as outlined below.
   - The parasympathetic preganglionic fibers from the parasympathetic nucleus of the oculomotor nerve exit the cranium with the oculomotor nerve, enter the orbital cavity and reach the ciliary ganglion to exchange neurons, and their postganglionic fibers enter the wall of the eye and distribute to the pupillary sphincter and ciliary muscle.
   - The parasympathetic preganglionic fibers from the superior salivary nucleus exit the cranium with the facial nerve, and part of the preganglionic fibers exchange neurons via the great rocky nerve to the pterygopalatine ganglion in the pterygopalatine fossa. Another part of the preganglionic fibers passes through the bulbar cord, joins the lingual nerve, and then goes to the submandibular nerve ganglion, and the postganglionic fibers are distributed in the submandibular and sublingual glands.
   - The parasympathetic preganglionic fibers from the inferior salivary nucleus exit the skull with the glosso-

pharyngeal nerve, transfer to the auricular nerve ganglion below the foramen ovale via the bulbar nerve, and the postganglionic fibers are distributed to the parotid gland via the auriculotemporal nerve.

- The parasympathetic preganglionic fibers from the dorsal nucleus of the vagus nerve in the medulla oblongata follow the vagus nerve out of the cranium and branch to parasympathetic ganglion neurons near or in the walls of the thoracic and abdominal organs, and the postganglionic fibers are distributed in the cardiac muscle, smooth muscle, and glands. Among them, the preganglionic fibers to the heart are in the cardiac plexus or intramural nerve ganglia: the preganglionic fibers to the digestive canal are in the wall of the digestive canal and participate in forming the submucosal plexus (Meissner's plexus) and the intermuscular plexus (Auerbach's plexus), and send postganglionic fibers to innervate the corresponding organs in the intramural ganglia or interplexus nerve ganglia.

(b) Sacral parasympathetic nerve: The preganglionic fibers originate from the sacral parasympathetic nucleus in the S_{2-4} segment of the spinal cord, and then branch out from the sacral nerve to form the pelvic splanchnic nerve, which joins the inferior abdominal plexus, i.e., the pelvic plexus. The pelvic plexus branches to the digestive ducts and pelvic organs below the left curvature of the colon, and in the paramedian or intramural ganglia of these organs, postganglionic fibers are distributed to the smooth muscles and glands of these organs. Some of the parasympathetic fibers are distributed to the penis or clitoris, causing vasodilation of the cavernous body to make it erect, so the pelvic visceral nerve is also called the erectile nerve.

2.1.4 Main Differences Between Sympathetic and Parasympathetic Nerves

Both sympathetic and parasympathetic nerves are visceral motor nerves and often innervate an organ together, forming a dual innervation of the visceral organs. However, the sympathetic and parasympathetic nerves have their own characteristics in terms of origin, morphological structure, distribution range and function, as summarized in Table 2.2.

Table 2.2 Main differences between sympathetic and parasympathetic nerves

Differences	Sympathetic nerve	Parasympathetic nerve
Low-level nociceptors	Lateral nucleus of the intermediate band of gray matter in the thoracolumbar region of the spinal cord	Parasympathetic nucleus of the brainstem cerebral nerve and parasympathetic nucleus of the sacral part of the spinal cord
Location of peripheral ganglia	Both sides of the spine (paravertebral ganglia), anterior spine (anterior vertebral ganglia)	Near organs (paranodes), within the walls of organs (intra-organ nodes)
Ratio of preganglionic to postganglionic neurons	Axons of one preganglionic neuron can form synapses with many postganglionic neurons	Axons of one preganglionic neuron form synapses with fewer postganglionic nerves
Distribution	In addition to the head and neck, thoracic and abdominal organs, it also covers the blood vessels, glands, and trichomes of the body	The distribution is relatively limited, and most of the blood vessels, sweat glands, erector spinae, and adrenal medulla are not parasympathetically innervated
Effects on organs	The two act differently, antagonizing and unifying each other	

2.1.5 Visceral Plexus

Sympathetic, parasympathetic, and visceral sensory nerves are intertwined in the process of distribution in the viscera to form the visceral plexus (autonomic or vegetative plexus). These plexuses mainly climb around the head, neck and internal thoracic and abdominal arteries, or are distributed near organs and within organs. All visceral plexuses are composed of sympathetic and parasympathetic nerves, except for the internal carotid plexus, external carotid plexus, subclavian plexus, and vertebral artery plexus, in which no parasympathetic nerves participate. In addition, there are visceral sensory fibers passing through these plexuses. The important plexuses in the thoracic, abdominal, and pelvic-sacral regions are described below.

1. Cardiac plexus

   The cardiac plexus is composed of the superior, middle, and inferior cervical segments of the sympathetic trunk and the cardiac branches emanating from $T_{1-4/5}$ segments and the cardiac branches of the vagus nerve. The superficial plexus is located below the aortic arch and the deep plexus is located between the aortic arch and the tracheal fork. The plexus contains the cardiac ganglion (parasympathetic ganglion), where the parasympathetic preganglionic fibers from the vagus nerve exchange neurons. The branches of the plexus in turn form the atrial plexus and the left and right coronary plexus, which are distributed to the myocardium along with the arterial branches.
2. Pulmonary plexus

   The pulmonary plexus is located anteriorly and posteriorly to the pulmonary roots, and there are also small ganglia within the plexus. The pulmonary plexus is composed of the bronchial branches of the vagus nerve and branches of the T_{2-5} nodes of the sympathetic trunk, whose branches follow the branches of the bronchi and pulmonary vessels to the lungs.
3. Celiac plexus

   The celiac plexus is the largest visceral plexus and is located around the roots of the celiac artery and superior mesenteric artery. It is mainly composed of the celiac ganglion, superior mesenteric ganglion, aortic renal ganglion, etc., as well as branches of the major and minor visceral nerves from the thoracic sympathetic trunk and the ventral branches of the posterior vagus trunk and the upper lumbar sympathetic ganglion. The ventral plexus, along with the branches of the arteries, can be divided into many subplexuses, such as the hepatic plexus, gastric plexus, splenic plexus, renal plexus, and superior mesenteric plexus, and each subplexus reaches each organ along the eponymous vascular branches.
4. Abdominal aortic plexus

   The abdominal aortic plexus is located on both sides of the abdominal aorta and is a continuation of the abdominal plexus down the surface of the abdominal aorta, which also receives branches from the L_{1-2} sympathetic ganglia. This plexus divides into the inferior mesenteric plexus, which distributes along the branches of the eponymous artery below the left curvature of the colon to the superior rectum. A portion of the fibers descends into the pelvis and participates in the composition of the infra-abdominal plexus, and another portion is distributed along the common iliac artery and external iliac artery to the vessels of the lower extremities, sweat glands, and the erector spinae.
5. Hypogastric plexus

   The hypogastric plexus is divided into the superior and inferior hypogastric plexus. The inferior hypogastric plexus is located in front of the Ls vertebrae, between the end of the abdominal aorta and the two common iliac arteries, and is the downward continuation of the abdominal aortic plexus. The pelvic plexus continues from the inferior hypogastric plexus to the sides of the rectum and also receives postganglionic fibers from the sacral sympathetic trunk and parasympathetic preganglionic fibers from the S_{2-4} nerves. The hypogastric plexus is accompanied by branches of the internal iliac artery to form the rectal plexus, spermatic plexus, ureteral plexus, bladder plexus, prostatic plexus, and vaginal plexus of the uterus, and is distributed with the arteries to the pelvic organs.

2.1.6 The Enteric Nervous System

The enteric nervous system is a reticular system composed of neurons, neurotransmitters, and proteins located in the wall of the gastrointestinal tract (including the pancreas and gallbladder) and its supporting cells, which has the function of regulating and controlling the function of the gastrointestinal tract. The enteric nervous system is structurally and functionally different from the sympathetic and parasympathetic nervous systems in that its neurons are interconnected to form an independent system with the ability to integrate and process information similar to the brain and spinal cord, but it is still a component of the autonomic nervous system, also known as the "second brain".

The enteric nervous system consists of two major internally interconnected plexuses that begin in the lower esophagus and extend to the level of the dentate line of the anal canal. The larger is the myenteric nerve plexus or Auerbach's plexus, which surrounds the entire alimentary canal and mainly innervates smooth muscle, transmits stimulus information such as pulling and distension of the intestinal wall, and regulates the relaxation and contraction of the longitudinal and circular muscles and peristalsis of the intestinal canal; the smaller is the submucous plexus or Meissner's plexus, which mainly innervates the intestinal mucosa, transmits impulses from various stimuli in the gastrointestinal lumen and regulates secretion of the intestinal epithelium, relaxation and contraction of the intestinal vasculature, and water-electrolyte metabolism. These two plexuses are interconnected and jointly regulate gastrointestinal function.

The enteric nervous system is structurally and functionally encapsulated by glia similar to astrocytes of the central nervous system [1]. In addition to the neurons and glia of the enteric nervous system, the intestinal wall also contains Cajal interstitial cells (interstitial cell of Cajal, ICC), which form synaptic-like contacts with the axon terminals of interstitial plexus neurons. The ICC is the pacemaker and conductor of gastrointestinal slow-wave activity and serves as a "bridge" and "link" between the enteric nervous system and the smooth muscle of the intestine. The ICC serves as a "bridge" and "link" between the enteric nervous system and intestinal smooth muscle. So far, it is believed that ICC has three functions: (1) pacemaker of the basic gastrointestinal electrical rhythm; (2) mediator of enteric neurotransmission; and (3) mechanoreceptor [2].

The total number of human enteric neurons has been found to reach about 10, which is equivalent to the total number of neurons contained in the entire spinal cord. There are three types of neurons: sensory neurons, interneurons, and motor neurons, which constitute the complete reflex pathway. The enteric nervous system contains intrinsic primary afferent neuron (IPAN). The projection targets of the IPAN in the interosseous and mucosal plexuses are the interneurons. Intermediate neurons modulate intestinal motility and secretory reflexes. It can be seen that IPAN, interneurons and effector neurons constitute the reflex microcircuit of the enteric nervous system, which allows the gastrointestinal tract to receive stimulus signals and generate reflexes in the absence of external innervation. However, the modulatory action of the enteric nervous system on the gastrointestinal tract requires its perception of pressure and chemical stimuli in the intestinal lumen without intrinsic or extrinsic nerve fibers reaching the mucosal epithelium. This process is mediated by intestinal chromophores, which release large amounts of 5-hydroxytryptamine after sensing intestinal luminal stimuli, which activates submucosal primary afferent nerve fibers [3]. 5-Hydroxytryptamine stimulates intrinsic primary afferent neurons, which form synapses with upstream and downstream interneurons in the intermuscular plexus, thereby regulating local excitation and inhibition. In addition, a large number of enteric glial cells are distributed in the enteric nervous system. Previously, it was thought that enteric glial cells were only support cells for enteric neurons, but recent studies have revealed that enteric glial cells in the gastrointestinal tract are a unique class of peripheral glial cells distributed throughout the intestinal tract, with different subpopulations representing their unique functions in digestive and non-digestive diseases, especially in the epithelial barrier, neuroprotection, and mediation of intestinal inflammatory immunity important role [4, 5].

2.2 Visceral Sensory Nerves

The visceral organs of the human body are innervated by visceral motor nerves as well as sensory nerves. The visceral sensory nerve receives stimuli from the viscera and converts them into nerve impulses for transmission to the center. The center can regulate visceral activity by completing visceral-visceral or visceral-somatic reflexes directly through visceral motor nerves or somatic motor nerves. Visceral sensory nerves can also undergo complex conduction pathways to transmit impulses to the cerebral cortex, eliciting conscious responses and producing visceral sensations.

2.2.1 Characteristics of Visceral Sensory Nerves

Although visceral sensory nerves are morphologically and structurally similar to somatic sensory nerves, they still have some unique features.

1. The number of visceral sensory fibers is small, and the majority of fine fibers, and the pain threshold is high. For normal visceral activities, they generally do not cause subjective sensation, but stronger visceral activities can cause certain sensations, such as hunger sensation when the stomach undergoes strong hunger contraction, and rectal and bladder filling to a certain extent can cause bowel movement and urination.
2. The viscera are not sensitive to stimuli such as cutting, but they are sensitive to stimuli such as chemical inflammation, pulling, distension, and ischemia.
3. The afferent pathways of visceral sensation are diffuse, with sensory fibers from one organ entering the center through multiple segments of the spinal nerve, and one spinal nerve containing sensory fibers from several organs, e.g., segment T_{1-5} can receive sensory afferents from several organs such as the heart, lung, trachea, bronchus, and esophagus. Therefore, the visceral sensation is often diffuse and difficult to locate accurately.

2.2.2 Endoreceptors

Endoreceptors (interoceptors) are distributed in various layers within the organ wall and in the walls of blood vessels, etc. They receive physical and chemical stimuli such as osmotic pressure, pressure, temperature, ion, and compound concentrations. The thick medullary visceral afferent fibers terminate in the annulus: the small medullary or non-medullary visceral afferent fibers terminate in the diffuse endoreceptors. There are three main types of endoreceptor morphological structures: (1) Free sensory nerve endings are formed by repeated branching of sensory fiber endings, usually found in the epithelial and plasma membrane layers of mucous membranes, the endomysium of organ muscle layers, and organ connective tissue. These end receptors sense nociceptive and other stimuli, while the free endings distributed in the mucosa are chemoreceptors and those located in the muscular layer are mechanoreceptors, and the mechanoreceptors in the gastrointestinal tract are similar to "tensor receptors". (2) Nerve fiber endings form a complex network that is visible on the surface of the plasma membrane and within the muscular layer of the organ. (3) Circumferential vesicles, mostly round or oval in shape, are composed of flattened connective tissue cells and fibers forming concentric lamellae, and the interlamellae are filled with gel-like material, which are found in the mesentery, visceral layer of mesentery, supporting tissues of organs, extravascular membrane and pancreas.

Depending on their functions, the receptors can be classified as follows:

1. Chemoreceptors

   The main ones are aortic sinus and carotid sinus, which are oxygen and carbon dioxide concentration receptors; gastric mucosa has pH-sensitive receptors; chemoreceptors in the small intestine are sensitive to different solutions and osmotic pressure and are involved in food absorption: taste buds have the function of sensing acid, sweet, bitter, and salty; olfactory receptors are sensitive to gases, volatile oils, and acids.
2. Mechanoreceptors

   Circumferential vesicles belong to pressure receptors, mesenteric circumferential vesicles are sensitive to mechanical stimuli; aortic arch and carotid sinus have traction receptors, which sense blood pressure changes.
3. Injury receptors

   They sense injurious stimuli and produce nociception.
4. Temperature receptors

   Animal studies have confirmed that raising the temperature of abdominal organs, respiratory rate is accelerated, this is not related to the temperature regulation of the skin, spinal cord, and hypothalamus, but this response disappears after removal of visceral nerves, which may be located in the venous canal wall of the small intestine and mesentery, connected to the afferent fibers of visceral nerves.

2.2.3 Visceral Sensory Nerve Conduction Pathway

Visceral sensory conduction pathways are divided into general visceral sensory conduction pathways and special visceral sensory conduction pathways. The former refers to all cardiac, vascular, glandular, and visceral sensory conduction pathways other than olfaction and gustation; the latter refers to olfaction and gustation conduction pathways.

1. General visceral sensory conduction
   (a) Conduction pathway via cerebral nerves: Visceral sensation is transmitted via facial nerve, glossopharyngeal nerve, vagus nerve to primary neurons such as geniculate ganglion, glossopharynx, and inferior vagus nerve. Its secondary neurons are located in the solitary bundle nucleus of the brainstem, from which crossed solitary spinal tracts emanate, follow the reticulospinal tract or intrinsic tract, and terminate in the gray matter of the spinal cord. In addition to constituting the visceral-visceral and visceral-somatic reflexes, the nucleus of the solitary fasciculus emits superior fibers that, after possibly exchanging neurons in the reticular formation, travel up through the midbrain perineurium and terminate in the ventral posterior medial nucleus of the thalamus, the midline nucleus, the inner platysmal nucleus, and the hypothalamus. Fibers emanate from the thalamus to the frontal and parietal cortices, and from the hypothalamus project to the cortical structures of the limbic system.
   (b) Trans-spinal conduction pathways: Visceral sensation is transmitted to the center via sympathetic nerves and pelvic-sacral parasympathetic nerves. The cytomes of primary neurons are located in T_1–L_3 and S_{2-4} spinal ganglia, respectively, and are pseudo-unipolar neurons, as are the somatosensory ganglion elements. Their peripheral protrusions are distributed to visceral organs and cardiovascular via spinal nerves, anterior spinal nerve branches, traffic branches, sympathetic trunks and their branches, and secondary neurons in the middle frame protrusions into the posterior horn of the spinal cord or the posterior commissure nucleus. It is believed that there are three routes of transmission: (1) The neurons are replaced in the posterior commissure nucleus in the dorsolateral part of the central canal of the spinal cord, then in the

parabrachial nucleus, then up to the thalamus, and then to the cerebral cortex. (2) Neurons are replaced in the gray matter of the spinal cord, ascending in the ipsilateral or contralateral anterolateral spinal cord, accompanying the spinal thalamic tract up to the ventral posterior lateral nucleus of the thalamus, and then projecting to the postcentral gyrus and upper lateral sulcus of the cerebral cortex. (3) Ascending along the intrinsic tract of the spinal cord, it changes neurons multiple times within the spinal cord and brainstem reticular formation, ascending to the dorsal medial nucleus of the thalamus and then projecting to the limbic lobe of the brain.

It is now believed that nociception in the general organs is mainly transmitted to the center with sympathetic nerves. Nerve impulses via parasympathetic afferents are mainly associated with visceral reflexes, such as respiration, vomiting, and pressure reflexes. There are also some nociceptive sensations of some organs that are transmitted to the center with parasympathetic nerves, such as the nociceptive sensations of trachea and esophagus that are partially transmitted to the center via the vagus nerve, and the nociceptive sensations of bladder, prostate, urethra, cervix, and lower rectum that are mainly transmitted to the center via pelvic visceral nerves.

2. Special visceral sensory transmission
   (a) Taste receptors and taste conduction pathways: Taste receptors, namely taste buds, are distributed in the contour papillae, fungiform papillae, lobe papillae and epithelium of the soft palate and epiglottis of the tongue mucosa, and have the function of feeling sour, sweet, bitter, and salty taste. The taste buds are oval in shape and reach the substrate at the bottom, which can convert taste sensations into nerve impulses and then transmit them to the center through specific conduction pathways [6, 7].

   The taste conduction pathway is composed of three levels of neurons. The first level neurons are located in the geniculate ganglion of the facial nerve, the inferior ganglion of the glossopharyngeal nerve, and the inferior ganglion of the vagus nerve. The central synapses of these ganglion cells enter the human medulla with their respective cerebral nerves to join the solitary tract and form synapses with secondary neurons in the nucleus of the solitary tract, where taste impulses are relayed superiorly. The nucleus of the solitary tract sends out secondary taste fibers, most of which cross left and right, and then travel upward with the medial thalamic tract, terminating in the medial apical part (parabasal nucleus) of the ventral posterior medial nucleus of the thalamus (arcuate nucleus) of tertiary neurons, which send out taste fibers that finally project to the central posterior gyrus 43 area of the cerebral cortex and insula cortex.
   (b) Olfactory receptors and olfactory conduction pathways: Olfactory receptors (olfactory organ) are located in the upper part of the nasal cavity, i.e., the superior turbinate and the relative septum, and are composed of olfactory cells, supporting cells, and basal cells. The olfactory cells are nerve cells that receive stimuli and generate nerve impulses to the olfactory brain. The mammalian olfactory organ is very sensitive and is an important tool for foraging, courtship, and escape from the attack [8–10].

   The olfactory conduction pathway consists of two levels of neurons: primary neurons are located in the olfactory cells and the central synapses form olfactory filaments (about 20) that cross the sieve plate of the sieve bone into the olfactory bulb: secondary neurons are cells within the olfactory bulb and form the olfactory bundle, which conducts to the telencephalon via the olfactory bundle. The olfactory bundle divides into three bundles of fibers in the dorsolateral part of the anterior perineurium: the lateral olfactory stripe, the medial olfactory stripe, and the middle olfactory stripe. Most of the olfactory impulses are transmitted to the hook gyrus, insula, part of the amygdala, and the internal olfactory area via the lateral olfactory stripe, mainly transmitting conscious olfactory perception; some of the olfactory impulses are transmitted to the septal area via the medial olfactory stripe, which then sends nerve fibers to communicate with the limbic system and hypothalamus, mainly transmitting instinctive emotional olfactory experience; some of the olfactory impulses are transmitted to the olfactory node via the middle olfactory stripe, which then sends nerve fibers back to the olfactory bundle. The olfactory nerve is regulated internally by the olfactory bulb.

It should be noted that, so far, the understanding of the afferent pathways of the visceral nerves is still in the "dark", and it will take time to fully understand their conduction pathways.

2.2.4 Referred Pain

1. Overview of referred pain

   When lesions occur in certain internal organs, they often produce sensory allergy or nociception in certain areas of the body surface, which is called referred pain. Sometimes referred pain occurs in the skin adjacent to the diseased viscus, and sometimes it occurs in the skin distant from the diseased viscus. For example, in the early stage of appendicitis, pain often occurs in the upper abdomen or around the umbilicus; in angina pectoris, pain is often felt in the anterior chest area, the left shoulder, and the inner body surface of the left arm; in hepatobiliary disease, pain often occurs in the body surface of the right shoulder, etc.

2. Anatomical bases of referred pain

   Referred pain is an important physiological characteristic of visceral sensation, and the structural bases that cause involvement pain may be the following [11].

   (a) The primary sensory fibers of the diseased organ enter the spinal cord and terminate in the unique secondary neurons on the one hand, and in the neurons related to the sensory transmission of the somatic structures by lateral branches on the other hand.
   (b) The primary sensory fibers of the diseased organ and the corresponding somatic structure terminate in the same secondary neuron.
   (c) The peripheral synapses of primary sensory neurons have different lateral branches distributed in visceral and corresponding somatic structures.

3. Mechanistic hypothesis of referred pain

   There are several hypotheses about the mechanism of referred pain, but it has not been possible to confirm which hypothesis is correct.

   (a) Convergent projection theory: One of the earliest hypotheses about the mechanism of involved pain was proposed based on the research results of W. A. Sturge and J. Ross in 1888, and T. C. Ruch in 1961. This theory suggests that nociceptive afferent fibers from the visceral and somatic surfaces converge at the same neuron at the same level of the spinal cord before being uploaded to the cerebral cortex, and since most painful stimuli normally originate from the somatic surface, the brain continues to habitually mistake visceral pain for somatic pain, and implicated pain occurs. There is research evidence that when local pain increases, so does the referred pain. However, the doctrine has encountered some challenges in that it does not explain the presence of a delay between involvement pain and local pain stimulation [12].
   (b) Convergent facilitation theory: This theory suggests that the lateral branches of visceral afferent fibers form synaptic connections in the spinal cord with the same dorsal horn neurons that receive somatic nociceptive afferents. The impulses from the visceral lesion can increase the excitability of this neuron and thus produce a

facilitatory effect on the surface afferent impulses, making a weak surface stimulus a nociceptive stimulus and thus producing involvement pain. In recent years, the term "central sensitization" can be used to summarize this theory. The repeated nerve afferents from peripheral neurons increase the excitability of neurons in the dorsal horn of the spinal cord or brainstem, resulting in central sensitization, when even a weak stimulus can cause pain sensation.

(c) Visceral hypersensitivity theory: This theory suggests that there is no central mechanism involved in the formation of referred pain, but it has central characteristics. Due to the opening of potential convergent afferent fibers in the dorsal horn of the spinal cord, a new receptive field appears in the distal part of the primary stimulus, and the signal afferent from the new receptive field is then considered as referred pain.

(d) Axonal reflex theory: The afferent fibers contain two parts before entering the dorsal horn of the spinal cord, one part is distributed in visceral organs and the other part is distributed in muscles, skin and intervertebral discs, and other tissues. This theory also cannot explain the delayed appearance of referred pain, the difference in threshold between local pain and referred pain, and the change in somatosensory sensitivity at the site of referred pain.

(e) Thalamic convergence theory: This theory suggests that nerve impulses from the affected visceral and involved pain sites overlap in the brain rather than the dorsal horn of the spinal cord. There is a lack of evidence from relevant studies to support this theory. However, in pain studies in monkeys, some neural pathway convergence was found in cortical and subcortical neurons.

References

1. Farrell KE, Keely S, Graham BA, Callister R, Callister RJ. A systematic review of the evidence for central nervous system plasticity in animal models of inflammatory-mediated gastrointestinal pain. Inflamm Bowel Dis. 2014;20(1):176–95.
2. Martinucci I, Blandizzi C, de Bortoli N, Bellini M, Antonioli L, Tuccori M, et al. Genetics and pharmacogenetics of aminergic transmitter pathways in functional gastrointestinal disorders. Pharmacogenomics. 2015;16(5):523–39.
3. Spencer NJ, Zagorodnyuk V, Brookes SJ, Hibberd T. Spinal afferent nerve endings in visceral organs: recent advances. Am J Physiol Gastrointest Liver Physiol. 2016;311(6):G1056.
4. Yoo BB, Mazmanian SK. The enteric network: interactions between the immune and nervous systems of the gut. Immunity. 2017;46(6):910–26.
5. Smith TK, Koh SD. A model of the enteric neural circuitry underlying the generation of rhythmic motor patterns in the colon: the role of serotonin. Am J Physiol Gastrointest Liver Physiol. 2017;312(1):G1.
6. Matsumoto I. Gustatory neural pathways revealed by genetic tracing from taste receptor cells. Biosci Biotechnol Biochem. 2013;77(7):1359–62.
7. Li C-S, Lu D-P, Cho YK. Descending projections from the nucleus accumbens shell excite activity of taste-responsive neurons in the nucleus of the solitary tract in the hamster. J Neurophysiol. 2015;113(10):3778–86.
8. Courtiol E, Wilson DA. Neural representation of odor-guided behavior in the rat olfactory thalamus. J Neurosci. 2016;36(22):5946–60.
9. Courtiol E, Wilson DA. The olfactory thalamus: unanswered questions about the role of the mediodorsal thalamic nucleus in olfaction. Front Neural Circuits. 2015;9:49.
10. Sanda P, Kee T, Gupta N, Stopfer M, Bazhenov M. Classification of odorants across layers in locust olfactory pathway. J Neurophysiol. 2016;115(5):2303–16.
11. Arendt-Nielsen L, Svensson P. Referred muscle pain: basic and clinical findings. Clin J Pain. 2001;17(1):11–9.
12. Roman CW, Sloat SR, Palmiter RD. A tale of two circuits: CCK NTS neuron stimulation controls appetite and induces opposing motivational states by projections to distinct brain regions. Neuroscience. 2017;358:316–24.

3 Physiological Mechanisms of Visceral Pain

Ming Xia

3.1 Introduction

Pain is a complex sensory experience significantly modulated by the central nervous system (CNS). Despite the high prevalence of chronic visceral pain and its profound negative impact on patients' quality of life, the understanding of the mechanisms underlying the physiology of visceral pain has prominently lagged behind the understanding of non-visceral pain (e.g., neuropathic and inflammatory). This was partly due to the complexity of the interactions between the visceral organs, the autonomic nervous system, and the CNS, and partly because early clinicians disagreed about whether the viscera received any sensory innervation and later, whether this innervation included nociceptors. The mechanisms of visceral pain share many features with pain occurred in other parts of the body. However, the anatomical basis with dual innervation and a central projection to areas controlling emotion, as well as the associated clinical data showing significant effects on mood, distinguish visceral pain from skin or other somatic pain. The fact that the viscera are more inaccessible than the skin and other tissues also hinders the understanding of visceral pain mechanisms. Therefore, in this review, an introduction to the basis for discussing the anatomical complexity of visceral sensory innervation was provided first. Then, considering recent and emerging knowledge about the location and functional characteristics of sensory receptive terminals in visceral organs, the impact of nociception/pain and nociceptor sensitization on chronic visceral pain conditions was explored. This chapter concludes with a brief description of central processing of visceral pain.

M. Xia (✉)
Department of Anesthesiology, Shanghai Ninth People's Hospital, Shanghai Jiao Tong University School of Medicine, Shanghai, China
e-mail: xiaming1980@xzhmu.edu.cn

3.2 Visceral Sensory Nerves

The visceral nerves are the peripheral nerves that control and regulate the functional activities of the visceral organs. They are composed of the nerve fibers of the spinal nerves and the brain nerves that innervate the smooth muscle, cardiac muscle and glandular activities, and their function is to regulate the visceral organs to adapt to changes in the internal and external environment, maintain the normal physiological functions of the human body and promote body growth and development.

The visceral nervous system is an integral part of the nervous system and can be divided into central and peripheral parts according to their distribution sites. According to the nature of the fibers, visceral nerves can be divided into visceral sensory nerves and visceral motor nerves. Like somatosensory nerves, the cell bodies of visceral sensory neurons are located in brain ganglia and spinal ganglia, and are also pseudo-unipolar

M. Xia et al. (eds.), *Visceral Pain*, https://doi.org/10.1007/978-981-99-9167-9_3

neurons. The spinal nerve enters the spinal cord from the dorsal root or enters the brainstem along the cerebral nerve, and transmits visceral sensory nerve impulses to the center. In the centers, visceral sensory fibers are linked with visceral motor neurons to complete visceral-visceral reflexes or with somatic motor neurons to form visceral-somatic reflexes; on the other hand, the impulses are transmitted to the cerebral cortex through more complex conduction pathways to form visceral sensations. The ganglia involved in the composition of visceral sensory nerves include the geniculate ganglion, the hypoglossal nerve and the vagus nerve. The peripheral synapses of the ganglion cells are distributed to the visceral organs along with the facial nerve, the hypoglossal nerve and the vagus nerve, and the central synapses enter the brainstem and terminate in the nucleus of solitary tract (NST).

In many studies, the visceral motor nerves are considered to be composed by sympathetic and parasympathetic nerves, which regulate visceral and cardiovascular movements and glandular secretion. Usually not controlled by human will and are not random, they belong to the autonomic nervous system. From the visceral nerve anatomy, it can be seen that the visceral sensory nerve travels mainly with sympathetic and parasympathetic nerves, and sympathetic, parasympathetic and visceral sensory nerves often intertwine to form the visceral plexus in the process of distribution in the viscera.

However, Gebhart and Bielefeldt clarified in their work that referring to the visceral spinal innervation as the sympathetic nerve is a mistake [1]. They explained that Langley described the visceral spinal innervation as "afferent sympathetic fibers" [2]. Whereas, others modified it to "sympathetic afferents". In contrast, vagus and pelvic nerve afferents were referred to as parasympathetic because they are anatomically related to the parasympathetic division of the autonomic nervous system. In light of the anatomical evidence, it can be inferred that the presumed function of "parasympathetic" afferent innervation focused on autonomic control rather than sensation and perception, while visceral pain and other sensations were thought to be conveyed to the CNS by afferent "sympathetic" fibers. The experimental data did not support this functional distinction between these anatomically defined afferent pathways. Therefore, the authors concluded that visceral afferent fibers are best described by their nerve names to avoid the presumed function implied by confusing terminology (e.g., "sympathetic afferents", an unfortunate oxymoron) [2].

Visceral afferent pathways are usually distinguished as cranial (i.e., vagus nerve) and spinal components according to the termination of their central processes. The vagus nerve is the most far-reaching sensory nerve in the body, innervating essentially all visceral organs in the chest and abdomen and even extending to some pelvic structures [3]. Notably, at least 80% of the axons in the vagus nerve are afferent, with cell bodies contained in the nodal and more distal cervical ganglia. The neurons of the cervical ganglia are derived from the neural crest and, based on their origin and properties, are more similar to those of the dorsal root ganglia [4]. The central terminals of vagal afferents project mainly to the nucleus of the solitary fasciculus of the dorsal medulla. Approximately 5% of the vagal afferent terminals are in the upper cervical spinal cord (C_{1-2}) and may contribute to the ontogenetic mechanisms of referral sensation as well as nociceptive odor [5]. Consistent with this role, vagal afferent stimulation modulates nociceptive transmission in the thoracic and lumbar spine of the spine and has an analgesic effect on the body. Although vagal afferents are considered not participating in visceral nociception, there is growing evidence that vagal afferents play a role in chemical nociception and, importantly, contribute to aversive sensations such as bloating, nausea, and apnea, as well as the emotional dimensions and unpleasantness associated with visceral pain.

3.3 Physiological Features of Visceral Pain

Visceral pain is a common clinical condition. The physiological characteristics of visceral pain are listed as follow.

1. The pain is widespread and difficult to locate accurately, being the most important physiological feature of visceral pain. When patients with abdominal pain seek medical attention, they are often unable to specify the location of pain production because the distribution of nociceptors is sparser in the viscera than in the somatic level. Also, the afferent pathways of visceral sensation are more diffuse and lack specific conduction pathways.
2. Not all organs can produce visceral pain.
3. Visceral pain is often manifested as chronic pain, but sometimes it can rapidly turn into severe pain.
4. The pain threshold is high. Stimulation of general intensity does not cause subjective sensation; when sensation is induced, the response is insensitive.
5. Visceral pain is very sensitive to stimuli such as pulling, dilatation, ischemia and spasm, while it is insensitive to common stimuli that cause somatic or skin pain such as burning, cutting, and needling.
6. Visceral pain is often accompanied by motor and autonomic reflexes, such as renal colic when accompanied by nausea and vomiting.

3.4 Visceral Nociception

The characteristics of visceral pain are often complex. The origin of visceral pain in the abdomen can begin in the visceral or parietal peritoneum, or both. The parietal peritoneum is usually innervated by somatic nerves that contain the cell bodies of the dorsal root ganglia. This allows pain to be localized to a specific area. The visceral peritoneum and the visceral organs themselves are heavily innervated by autonomic nerves, which leads to occult or involved pain [6]. Adequate, noxious stimulation leading to visceral pain is different from adequate noxious stimulation of the skin [7]. Activation of visceral nerves rarely leads to conscious sensations, but the sensations produced are usually those of discomfort or pain. Clinical findings highlight the incongruity between perceived pain and the lack of actual or potential tissue damage, as there is a group of chronic, painful "functional" visceral disorders that exist in the absence of an obvious pathological explanation. It is now widely recognized that adequate toxic stimulation of the skin, muscles, bones/joints, and viscera are different [1].

Pain from visceral organs is produced by stimuli that are exceptionally complex, including stretching of hollow organs, traction on the mesentery, organ hypoxia/ischemia, and chemical stimuli. However, not every stimulus is perceived as painful and nociceptors can become sensitive to persistent stimuli. This occurs because various nociceptors are modulated by various inflammatory and anti-inflammatory mediators, if the signal is strong enough to overcome the intrinsic threshold and eventually lead to the generation of action potentials [8]. In addition, various hormones may influence abdominal pain and sensation.

Visceral nociception is provoked by multiple stimuli and elicits several downstream effects depending on the intensity of the stimulus. Abdominal visceral nociceptors include chemoreceptors, thermoreceptors, and mechanoreceptors. Visceral afferent nerves utilize neuropeptides such as calcitonin gene-related peptide (CGRP), somatostatin, vasoactive intestinal peptide, and substance P. Organ distension, ischemia, and inflammation can all bring about different responses depending on the intensity of the stimuli. There are two types of afferent fibers, sympathetic and parasympathetic afferents. Based on research, parasympathetic afferent nerves appear to modulate pain signals rather than transmitting pain signals directly. Sympathetic afferent nerves appear to be responsible for transmitting pain signals back to the spinal cord. However, the vagus nerve may also respond to some of the same neurotransmitters that affect sympathetic afferent nerves, such as 5-hydroxytryptamine, adenosine triphosphate, prostaglandins, and capsaicin. Activation of vagal afferents by visceral stimuli associated with the above substances may lead to symptoms such as nausea and vomiting. This is because some of these nerves project to the brainstem. This may help explain the link between pain and some of these autonomic responses [6].

3.4.1 Noxious Visceral Stimuli

Lewis reviewed the general ineffectiveness of cutting, cauterizing, or squeezing visceral tissue to produce pain in humans in a study on pain, noting that the most reliably effective pain-producing stimuli are mechanical, including traction on the mesentery, hollow organ distension, and compression of some solid organs such as testes [9]. Dilated stimuli within the intestine were reported to be most painful when the longer, continuous intestine is dilated, implying that spatial summation is important for sensory production, consistent with the relatively sparse innervation of the distal intestine. Because the digestive tract is easily accessible through natural orifices, human clinical studies have long documented that distension of hollow organs is toxic which were supported by experimental evidence [10, 11]. These investigators also linked sensation to distended volume and pressure, establishing the importance of luminal pressure rather than volume as the appropriate distending stimulus for pain. Because all hollow organs are somewhat compliant and may even actively adapt to changes in volume (e.g., stomach, distal intestine, and bladder), stimulus intensity is unstable when distended volume remains constant. Initially toxic volumetric stimuli of constant intensity will cause the organ to swell to accommodate a larger volume, thereby altering transmembrane pressure and resulting in a net decrease in stimulus intensity. Later investigators confirmed that controlled constant pressure stimuli are "sufficient" toxic stimuli for swelling hollow organs. Thus, the correlation between pressure (rather than volume) thresholds and "pain" thresholds is more reliable and reproducible when studying hollow organ pain. Pain induced by constant pressure organ expansion in human subjects has been reported to replicate the location (referred sensation), quality, and intensity of pathological pain associated with the same organs [1].

Nonhuman animal studies of visceral nociception have swollen the gallbladder, esophagus, stomach, small intestine, colorectum, vagina, uterus, and bladder. The most characteristic model is colonic distention, which has been employed in rodents, cats, dogs, and nonhuman primates, with studies in mice and rats being the most common. Distention of the stomach and bladder has also been characterized [12, 13]. An important advantage of colon distension is that it can be performed in animals without anesthesia and/or after inflammation or organ injury. Animal models of other organ distension usually require sedation or anesthesia, thus complicating the assessment of whether the stimulus is toxic. For a distended stimulus (or any stimulus) to be considered toxic in intensity, its application must evoke a nociceptive reflex or nociceptive behavior, which may be a nociceptive withdrawal or pseudo-response, passive or active avoidance of the stimulus, or other learned behavior. If there is no evidence of a nociceptive behavioral response to a stimulus, it is inconclusive to conclude that the stimulus is toxic [1].

Schwartz et al. summarized the visceral stimulus in formulating visceral pain model used in nonhuman animals in their study [14]. The stimulus (1) must be an adequate (in the Sherringtonian sense) noxious stimulus that would produce pain when applied to humans and be related to human pathological pain; (2) must be reliable, reproducible, and ethical in that it is under experimenter control with respect to duration and intensity and can be readily terminated either by the experimental subject or experimenter; (3) should affect behavior consistent with it being aversive to the experimental subject; (4) should evoke pseudaffective reflexes consistent with those evoked in humans (e.g., increase in heart rate, blood pressure, and/or respiration); (5) should produce responses that are modulated by known antinociceptive/analgesic drugs [14]. They added that this classification applies to controlled, provocative stimuli that produce responses that can be reliably measured and quantified.

3.5 Visceral Afferent Fibers

The relatively low density of innervation in visceral organs has limited our understanding of the structural specialization and possible transduction mechanisms of visceral afferent terminals. Most visceral afferent fibers are thinly myelinated Aδ or unmyelinated C fibers, which are thought to form unencapsulated "free" nerve endings in their target organs. This view is mainly based on the presumed similarity between visceral and non-visceral somatic Aδ and C fibers. Early observations showed a small number of pachytene cells in the mesentery, which are associated with Aβ fibers [7]. More recent investigations have revealed a more specialized structure and function of vagal and spinal afferents in the proximal GI tract and rectum. The focus of these studies has been on mechanosensation, as distension of hollow organs is a commonly used experimental, physiologically meaningful, adequate, and potentially toxic visceral stimulus [15, 16]. Depending on the nature of the triggering stimulus, the sensory components that respond to stretch or tension are thought to be located in the smooth muscle layer of the intestine. Based on earlier and ongoing work [17–20], a recent review of exogenous primary afferent signals to the gut suggested that there are five structurally distinct sensory endings in the intestinal wall that account for sensation from the gut: inner ganglion laminae endings (IGLEs), mucosal endings, muscle-mucosal endings, intramuscular endings, and vascular endings [21].

3.5.1 Vagal Afferents

Detailed tracing studies of rodent vagal afferents revealed two distinct structures in the esophagus, stomach, and small bowel, namely, IGLEs and intramuscular arrays (IMAs). The IGLEs run parallel to the myenteric layer and interleave with structures within the myenteric ganglion [22]. As previously mentioned, the density of IGLEs decreases in more distant regions, but they can be found throughout the length of the GI tract [23]. The finding that vagal fibers branch into shorter terminals within their target organ, each forming a cluster of IGLEs or even IGLEs, is consistent with physiological studies suggesting that visceral afferents may have multiple and sometimes distant receptive fields [24]. The preferential distribution of IGLEs in the proximal and very distal GI tract suggests a potential regulatory role in food intake and defecation, which is associated with conscious perception but not with pain. Gautron and his colleagues used fluorescent labels genetically labeled to the voltage-gated sodium channel $Na_v1.8$ to describe other vagal afferents that branch within the enteric ganglion but do not form such specialized structures as IGLEs. The specific function of these intrinsic and extrinsic contacts between the nervous system is not fully understood.

IMAs are also thought to have mechanosensory specificity, but differ from IGLEs in morphology, distribution, and possibly physiological properties. As their name implies, IMAs form long and partially interconnected arrays within the muscular layer of the GI tract and run parallel to the circular or longitudinal muscles. In contrast to IGLEs, vagal IMAs are found primarily in the sphincter structures of the proximal stomach and upper GI tract and are uncommon in the intestine [22, 23]. Although not supported by direct experimental evidence, differences in structure and distribution suggest that IGLEs respond to muscle tone and may detect rhythmic motor activity, whereas IMAs may function as stretch receptors. Since these specific structures are associated with vagal afferents in the CNS and the contribution of vagal afferents to visceral nociception remains to be discussed, IGLEs and IMAs may contribute to visceral sensations such as satiety, but not likely to pain during gastric or intestinal distention [1].

Vagal afferents are the most distant receptor nerves in the body, innervating almost all the trachea in the chest, abdomen and even the pelvis, and mainly responding to chemical stimuli. At least 80% of the axons of vagus nerves are afferent nerves, and their cell bodies are located mainly in the vagal ganglion, but also partially in the anastomotic jugular ganglion. Since the jugular vein ganglia originate from the neural crest, they are more similar to the dorsal root ganglion neurons based on their origin and properties. Also, approximately 3% of the vagal afferents terminate in C_1, C_2, which may be related to intrinsic spinal mechanisms involving sensory and sharp sensory regulation. The central end of vagal afferents terminates mainly in the dorsal medulla of the NST, and there is evidence supporting that the vagal afferents is associated with chemically injurious sensations, which leads to adverse somatic responses such as bloating, nausea, and apnea and visceral pain associated with emotional properties and unpleasant emotions.

3.5.2 Spinal Afferents

As with all spinal sensory pathways, the cell body of visceral afferent neurons is located in the dorsal root ganglion (DRG) of the spinal cord; however, unlike somatic nerves, many visceral afferent fibers have prevertebral and paravertebral ganglia before entering the spinal cord, and the paravertebral ganglia may send branches to make synaptic connections with prevertebral ganglion neurons, thereby modulating visceral function. Visceral afferent fibers also extend ventral and/or dorsal to the sympathetic trunk, and thus often send nerve endings in many spinal cord segments, with different segments or levels of the spinal cord acting differently.

The gray matter of the spinal cord can be divided into ten laminae, which are numbered from posterior to anterior as I–X respectively. Lamina I–IV corresponds to the posterior horn and continues upward with the caudal end of the nucleus of the spinal tract of the trigeminal nerve, which is the main receptive area for the terminal and lateral branches of the primary afferent fibers of cutaneous extrasensory (pain, temperature, touch, pressure sensation) and belongs to the extrasensory area. The specific afferents of visceral afferent nerve locate in the superficial layers of the dorsal horn of the spinal cord (e.g., lamina I and II), which are also the primary sites of somatic injury sensory afferent nerves to the spinal cord. Lamina II occupies a large part of the posterior horn of the gray matter and consists of a large number of dense small neurons. This layer contains almost no myelinated fibers and plays an important role in the analysis and processing of sensory information from the spinal cord, especially nociceptive information. Lamina V–VI receive posterior fundamental somatosensory primary afferent fibers, as well as a large number of downstream fibers from cortical motor areas, sensory areas, and subcortical structures; therefore, these two layers are closely related to the regulation of movement. Lamina VII accounts for the bulk of the middle band and extends to the anterior horn at the cervical and lumbar expansions. This layer contains easily distinguishable nuclei: the nucleus thoracicus, also known as the dorsal nucleus or Clarke's column, is only found in the C_8–L_1 segment and is located medial to the base of the posterior horn, sending fibers up to the cerebellum.

The intermediomedial nucleus is the most medial nucleus in lamina VII and lateral to lamina X. It occupies the entire length of the spinal cord and receives visceral sensory fibers from the posterior roots. The intermediolateral nucleus is located in the lateral horn of segments T_1–L_2 (or L_3) and is the site of the sympathetic preganglionic neuronal cell, sending fibers through the anterior spinal nerve roots into the spinal nerve and C through the white communicating branch to the sympathetic trunk. In the lateral part of lamina VII of segments S_2–S_4, there is sacral parasympathetic nucleus, which is the site of parasympathetic preganglionic neuronal cell body. The lamina VII consists of cells of different sizes, and the cells in this lamina are interrogative neurons. The lamina IX is a complex arrangement of columns of nuclei composed of anterior horn motor neurons and interneurons, located in the ventral most part of the anterior horn. The anterior horn motor neurons are the lower motor neurons of the pyramidal conduction pathway and the terminus of some of the other descending conduction tracts and some fibers of the posterior roots. Laminar X is located around the central canal and includes the anterior and posterior gray matter connections where certain fibers of the posterior roots terminate.

3.6 Mechanisms of Visceral Pain

3.6.1 Peripheral Mechanisms of Visceral Pain Production

1. Role of ion channels in production and regulation of visceral pain

   Ion channels can be classified into mechanical, thermal, and chemical ion channels according to their gating properties. Based on the type of ions passing through, they can be classified as sodium channels, potassium channels, and calcium channels, etc. During the occurrence of visceral pain, ion channels may undergo covalent or non-covalent regulation, with up- or down-regulation of expression. The roles of different ion channels are different, and the voltage-gated sodium channels and ligand-gated channel are introduced here as examples.

   (a) Voltage-gated sodium channels

   The activation of voltage-sensitive sodium channels constitutes the fast-rising branch of action potential, and different subunits of voltage-sensitive sodium channels have been studied, usually referred to as $Na_v1.1$–$Na_v1.9$.

   In an experimental model of intestinal colitis in rats, DRG neurons innervating the bladder were isolated and cell culture revealed an increase in capsaicin-excited $Na_v1.8$ inward currents, and encapsulated amplification of tetrodotoxin-resistant sodium currents further led to increased excitability of bladder DRG neurons, suggesting that $Na_v1.8$ is involved in the process of visceral pain development [25, 26].

   Studies have shown that $Na_v1.9$ plays multiple roles in visceral afferents to noxious inflammatory stimuli, mechanical stimuli, and disease-specific stimuli in humans [26]. Overexpression of $Na_v1.9$ in DRG sensory neurons is required in normal mechanoreception, direct excitation, and sensitization of mouse colonic afferents, a role that works through mediators of inflammatory intestinal tissues and the presence of noxious inflammatory mediators themselves. The excitatory response to ATP or PGE2 was reduced in $Na_v1.9$ knockout mice, and mechanical hypersensitivity of their plasma membrane and mesenteric visceral nociceptors was alleviated by the application of bradykinin, ATP, histamine, PGE2, and 5-HT. Responses to mechanical stimulation of mesenteric afferent nerves were also reduced by $Na_v1.9$ knockout, yet there was no effect on the response to rapid high-intensity phase expansion of the intestinal junction. These results suggest that $Na_v1.9$ is required in the maintenance of intense mechanical stimulation responses and inflammatory mediator activation and could serve as an efficient target in the development of visceral analgesia.

   (b) Ligand-gated channel

   The expression and properties of ligand-gated channels are also altered in animal models of visceral nociception. Ischemia is the most common cause of cardiac pain. Tissue acidosis due to lactate accumulation activates inferior cardiac nerve afferents and may trigger ischemic pain. A study of cardiac sensory neurons and randomly selected noncardiac sensory neurons from the same DRG reported that a higher proportion of cardiac sensory neurons express acid-sensing ion channels (ASICs) than noncardiac sensory neurons, which is consistent with ischemia-induced acidosis as a trigger for cardiac pain [27]. Depending on the properties of the proton-evoked currents, most visceral sensory neurons express different members of ASICs as well as the H^+-sensitive vanilloid receptor TRPV1. A high percentage (60–80%) of mouse and rat colonic sensory neurons express TRPV1, which has been reported to be the main detector of extracellular acidosis in the mouse colon [28–31]. Serotonin, which is present in colonic mesenteric cells and released at high concentrations in response to mucosal stimulation, acutely alters TRPV1 function in mouse colonic sensory neurons, converging the temperature activation profile of TRPV1 to normal body temperature [31]. This may be relevant because several studies in patients with functional intestinal disorders, such as irritable bowel syndrome (IBS), suggest changes in 5-hydroxytryptamine release and/or reuptake within the intestinal mucosa, raising the question of whether modulation of TRPV1 function may contribute to enhanced responses to normal subconscious physiological stimuli in these patients. In addition, animal models of visceral inflammation and a variety of human diseases ranging from gastroesophageal reflux disease and painful bladder syndrome (PBS) to rectal emergencies have been associated with increased TRPV1 expression [32–34].

2. Role of neuronal plasticity in production and regulation of visceral pain

   Sensory nerve endings convert information from mechanical, thermal, or chemical stimuli into electrical signals by expressing specific receptor molecules, which may trigger one or more action potentials that propagate along the axon, causing the neuron to release neurotransmitters to synaptically connected secondary neurons and continue to deliver this information upward, and eventually sensory information is processed by the CNS leading to the generation of conscious perception. In vivo and in vitro experiments have demonstrated that primary sensory neurons have significant plasticity and can lead to the development of nociceptive hypersensitivity (peripheral sensitization). Primary sensory neurons have significant plasticity, including up- or down-regulation of receptor molecule expression and activation or inhibition of signaling pathways.

   (a) Activation of Visceral Nociceptors

   After visceral injury, the release of pain-causing chemicals such as ATP, H^+, K, 5-HT, and bradykinin formed by enzymatic degradation of plasma proteins acts directly or indirectly to activate the nociceptors P2X3, TRPV1, TRPV2, DRASIC, etc. in the peripheral nerve terminals, resulting in membrane depolarization. The impulse transmits up to the cerebral cortex to cause pain sensation and down to the motor neurons in the anterior horn of the spinal cord to cause the flexor reflex, which is a physiological pain process and acts as a defense alarm. If the tissue injury is treated promptly, pain can be eliminated. At the same time, the increased activity and continuous release of nociceptors results in the release of SP, which leads to vasodilation and tissue edema, thus facilitating the recovery from inflammation.

   (b) Inflammatory mediators enhance the sensitized state of peripheral nociceptors

   On the basis of the above-mentioned mechanisms, if the tissue injury is severe and the anti-infection is not promptly conducted, the inflammation will be triggered. As a result, increased blood flow to the injury site; exudation of plasma polymorphic granulocytes, lymphocytes, platelets, etc. release large amounts of proinflammatory mediators such as TNF-α, IL-1β, IL-6, IL-8; skin glioblast cells release large amounts of neurotrophic factors such as NGF and BDNF, etc. These substances further promote the release of inflammatory mediators from tissue mast cells such as prostaglandins, leukotrienes, BK, 15-di-HETE, 5-HT, histamine, NO, etc. participate in the inflammatory process and enhance the sensitization state of peripheral nociceptors, so that peripheral injury sites continue to produce injurious impulses transmitted to the spinal cord, and at the same time, IL-1β and other substances stimulate the synthesis of NGF, further reinforcing sensitization and forming a positive feedback regulatory loop. In addition, the overexpression of TTX-insensitive $Na_v1.8$ and $Na_v1.9$ channels specific to the injured C-fibers further discharges continuously and spontaneously to allow excitatory impulses to be continuously transmitted to the dorsal horn of the spinal cord.

(c) Dorsal root and axonal reflexes of spinal nerves

In recent years, it has been found that the enhanced continuous and spontaneous progressive discharge originated from the visceral injury can keep the spinal cord-injured neurons continuously excited or spinal cord neurons hyper excited, and this process will generate primary afferent depolarization mediated by the intermediate GABA neurons in the dorsal horn of the spinal cord, causing the spinal nerve dorsal root reflex. As a result, primary afferent depolarizing impulses are transmitted retrogradely along the dorsal root of the spinal nerve to the nerve end innervating the peripheral tissue injury site or its adjacent sites, causing the release of neuropeptides such as SP, CGRP, and excitatory amino acids such as glutamate and aspartate. The released neuropeptides enhance the neurogenic inflammation caused by canal dilation and exudation. While on the other hand, with excitatory amino acids, it further sensitizes the nociceptors by acting on NMDA/non-NMDA and NK receptors distributed on the peripheral nerve fiber terminals.

(d) Sympathetic nerve activation

Visceral tissue injury may cause the activation of sympathetic nerves at the site of injury as well as sympathetic nerves to grow basket-like outgrowth fibers wrapping around primary afferent nerve cell cytosol in the DRG. The subcutaneous injection of sympathetic neurotransmitters epinephrine and norepinephrine do not cause pain when the injection site is normal, but under the circumstances of tissue injury and inflammation, there will be pain, suggesting that sympathetic nerves also play a regulatory role in peripheral receptor sensitization, and this process has been proved to be mediated by α_2 receptors. In addition, neuropeptide Y and arachidonic acid metabolites may also participate in this process.

Hyperalgesia is one of the manifestations of neuron plasticity, and there are three forms of plastic changes in neurons associated with peripheral sensitization of nociceptors: activation, modulation, and modification.

(a) Activation of nociceptors: Activation-dependent sensitization is a rapid and reversible pathological change in nociceptors that occurs after an injury stimulus when specific receptors and ion channels are activated and their own properties are altered and the opening threshold is lowered, making the nociceptors more sensitive to subsequent stimuli.
(b) Modulation of nociceptors: Modulation refers to the process by which mediators released from local tissues before hyperalgesia play a role in visceral hyper-responsiveness to stimuli during inflammation. Various chemicals and inflammatory mediators such as K^+, BK, histamine, ATP, NGF, etc. released from damaged tissue cells and inflammatory cells infiltrating into the damaged tissue phosphorylate the receptors/ion channels of the nociceptors through a cascade mechanism of intracellular signaling, further reducing the threshold of sensation of the nociceptors and increasing the excitability of the cell membrane. These substances directly activate the afferent fiber endings to release some neuroactive substances such as SP and glutamate, and cause the release of pain-sensitive mediators, which induce peripheral sensitization.
(c) Modification of nociceptors: Modification refers to prolonged changes in the number or structure of transmitters, receptors, and ion channels of primary sensory neurons and are associated with the survival of neurons. For example, peripheral nerve injury at the spinal cord level is usually terminated at the dorsal horn in the form of synaptic connections, and

deep Aβ fibers sprouting establishes synaptic connections with superficial neurons at this time, resulting in altered connections between neurons. And such connections hinder the cure of intractable pain.

3.6.2 Central Processing of Visceral Pain

Recent developments in functional brain mapping have enabled more systematic studies of brain activation during visceral stimulation, leading to a more detailed understanding of the central processing of visceral sensation and pain. Viscerally evoked cortical potentials were first recorded in healthy subjects using electrical stimulation of the rectal mucosa [35]. Localization of activated regions in the brain was made possible by dipole mapping, which led to the demonstration of somatosensory and insula cortical activation during esophageal stimulation [36]. In combination with functional magnetic resonance imaging and positron emission tomography, rather stereotypical brain activation patterns emerged during stimulation of the esophagus, stomach, colorectum, and bladder distension [37–41]. The brain regions involved largely represent different components of the subjective experience during visceral pain. The thalamus, insula, and more dorsal portions of the anterior cingulate cortex may discriminately assess visceral sensory information; the amygdala, secondary source portions of the cingulate cortex, and thalamic locations regulate emotional arousal, whereas the frontal and parietal cortices are associated with cognitive assessment [42]. These regions overlap with those activated in other bodily regions when stimulated by pain, hence the term "neural matrix of pain", and the relatively subtle differences between visceral and somatic pain are associated with activation of regions within insular cortex, cingulate, and prefrontal cortex [43]. Interestingly, the activity of this functional network has increased in response to subconscious stimulation, suggesting its specific role in nociception [36]. Indeed, these regions are also activated in other subjective experiences, such as hunger or itching, and may reflect the processing of interoceptive, equilibrium or allosomal signals that are related to survival and therefore closely associated with arousal and emotion [44].

As emotion and stress were modulators of visceral pain, experimental studies have shown enhanced activation of brain regions involved in visceral sensory and emotional arousal when visceral stimuli are applied under conditions of aversion or stress [45, 46]. The plasticity of pain processing goes beyond the moderating influence of such contextual factors, as the classical conditioning paradigm may produce similar activation patterns in response to real and anticipated visceral stimuli [47, 48]. In contrast, placebo or no-placebo effects may reduce or increase pain scores and associated changes in brain activation during experimental stimulation [49]. In addition to such acute experimental studies, epidemiological data suggest that the effects of stressors may be more persistent, especially during periods of high plasticity like early in life or in the presence of traumatic events. Patient interviews and population-based studies suggest an association between a history of sexual and/or physical abuse and functional GI disorders associated with pain [50]. Such adverse or traumatic events may play a more important role if they occur early in life, a period of high neurological plasticity [51]. These observations prompted mechanistic studies in animal models, confirming that perinatal maternal deprivation, mild gastritis, or bladder/colonic stimulation (mechanical and chemical) all lead to enhanced responses to visceral stimuli in adulthood [52–54]. Although earlier studies showed relatively specific effects on visceral sensory pathways [55, 56], more recent data suggest more general changes in pain tolerance and lead to activation of the hypothalamic-pituitary-adrenal axis [57, 58].

Quantitative studies of gray and white matter density have revealed more prevalent changes that overlap with regions activated during acute pain stimulation and correlate with pain grade, duration, or associated anxiety components [59–62]. These results not only testify the function of these regions in the subjective experience of pain, but also underline the plasticity of the central nervous system, with functional and structural changes associated with the chronic pain experience [1].

Many studies have investigated differences in brain area activation in patients with chronic visceral pain syndrome. Although variations in experimental paradigms, underlying disease, brain imaging techniques, and analytical methods limit comparisons, currently available evidence suggests that differences between patients and healthy controls are more quantitative than qualitative [63, 64]. Altered activation patterns in the brainstem have been associated with hyperresponsiveness [63] and anxiety [65]. Consistent with the role of central control mechanisms of emotional arousal in functional bowel disease, scores of anxiety and depression were associated with increased pain scores and enhanced activation of the cingulate cortex [66 68]. Interestingly, this increase in pain scores and brain activation appears to be independent of stimulus modality and location, suggesting that experimental stress and stress tolerance have a broader effect on central processing and pain perception in these patients [69]. This interpretation is supported by repeated assessment experiments spaced several months apart that showed a decrease in acute pain intensity scores during visceral distension, which was mediated by a decrease in state anxiety [70]. Consistent with these findings, a recent meta-analysis concluded that patients with IBS exhibit enhanced activation of brain regions associated with emotional arousal and endogenous pain regulation, whereas regions responsible for discriminating visceral processing are involved to a similar extent as controls, suggesting that dysregulation of emotional rather than sensory mechanisms contributes to disease manifestations in these individuals [71].

Changes in neuroendocrine responses to stress in patients with visceral pain syndrome have been extensively studied based on enhanced activation of brain regions associated with emotional arousal and the known effects of stress hormones on primary afferent neurons. Results have been mixed, but suggest that increased levels of corticotropin-releasing hormone (CRH) or cortisol are more closely related to anxiety than to pain ratings [72, 73]. CRH injections lower pain thresholds only when repeated "detonation" of swelling is followed by visceral swelling, supporting some modulation of visceral sensation by the hypothalamic-pituitary-adrenal axis. In contrast, administration of nonspecific CRH antagonists reduces anxiety and visceral pain scores in response to stimuli. Although peripheral expression of CRH receptors may contribute to these effects, recently published brain imaging studies have highlighted the effect of CRH receptors on emotional arousal, as administration of CHR receptor subtype 1 antagonists attenuated the high activation of relevant brain regions in IBS patients [74, 75].

Preclinical data show similar modulation of anxiety and stress responses via neurokinin 1 (NK-1) receptors [76]. In a small proof-of-concept trial, a selective NK-1 receptor antagonist reduced anxiety and pain scores during rectal distension and decreased activation in the insula and anterior cingulate cortex in patients with IBS [69]. Interestingly, recent ligand binding studies have shown reduced NK-1 binding potential throughout the brain in patients with visceral pain, thus further supporting a role for this signaling pathway in the central regulation of visceral sensation and pain [77].

3.7 Summary

Chronic visceral pain conditions are often difficult to be managed effectively, the primary reason of which is the poor understanding of visceral sensory mechanisms and factors contributing to the development of visceral pain. Understanding of mechanisms is particularly problematic in functional visceral disorders, where there are no obvious pathological changes and pain is usually the main complaint. We review here the anatomical organization of visceral sensory innervation, which distinguishes the viscera from the innervation of all other tissues of the body. The viscera are innervated by two nerves that overlap in function, but also have distinctly different functions. In addition, visceral innervation is sparse compared to the sensory innervation of other tissues [78]. As a result, visceral sensation is often diffuse and usually refers to non-visceral somatic structures and is therefore difficult to localize. Early debates on whether viscera are innervated ("sensory"), and later on whether they are innervated by nociceptors, can be answered by progress in understanding the anatomical and functional properties of the receptor endings in the viscera that contribute to visceral pain (i.e., visceral nociceptors). In the case of persistent and chronic visceral pain, the contribution of plasticity (sensitization) of peripheral and central visceral nociceptive mechanisms is considered.

References

1. Gebhart GF, Bielefeldt K. Physiology of visceral pain. Compr Physiol. 2016;6(4):1609–33. https://doi.org/10.1002/cphy.c150049. PMID: 27783853.
2. Langley J. The autonomic nervous system. Cambridge: Heffer; 1921.
3. Cervero F. Sensory innervation of the viscera: peripheral basis of visceral pain. Physiol Rev. 1994;74(3):95–138.
4. Undem BJ, Chuaychoo B, Lee M-G, Weinreich D, Myers AC, Kollarik M. Subtypes of vagal afferent C-fibres in Guinea-pig lungs. J Physiol Lond. 2004;556(3):905–17.
5. Foreman RD. Mechanisms of cardiac pain. Annu Rev Physiol. 1998;61:143–67.
6. Katz BL, Van Houten T, Sassan Sabouri A. Chapter 2—Neuroanatomy and mechanisms of visceral pain. In: Pak DJ, Jason Yong R, Shah KB, editors. Interventional management of chronic visceral pain syndromes. Elsevier; 2021. p. 5–15. https://doi.org/10.1016/B978-0-323-75775-1.00020-9. ISBN 9780323757751.
7. Sherrington C. The integrative activity of the nervous system. New York: Charles Scribner's Sons; 1906.
8. Sagami Y, Shimada Y, Tayama I, Nomura T, Satake M, Endo Y. Effect of a corticotropin releasing hormone receptor antagonist on colonic sensory and motor function in patients with irritable bowel syndrome. Gut. 2004;53:958–64.
9. Lewis T. Pain. New York: The Macmillan Press; 1942.
10. Hertz A. The sensibility of the alimentary tract in health and disease. Lancet. 1911;1:1051–6.
11. Payne W, Poulton E. Visceral pain in the upper alimentary tract. Q J Med. 1923;17:53–80.
12. Ozaki N, Bielefeldt K, Sengupta JN, Gebhart GF. Models of gastric hyperalgesia in the rat. Am J Physiol. 2002;283(3):G666–76.
13. Ness TJ, Elhefni H. Reliable visceromotor responses are evoked by noxious bladder distention in mice. J Urol. 2004;171:1704–8.
14. Schwartz ES, Gebhart GF. Visceral pain. Curr Top Behav Neurosci. 2014;20:171–97. https://doi.org/10.1007/7854_2014_315. PMID: 24850079.
15. Ness TJ, Metcalf AM, Gebhart GF. A psychophysiological study in humans using phasic colonic distension as a noxious visceral stimulus. Pain. 1990;43:377–86.
16. Ness TJ, Randich A, Gebhart GF. Further behavioral evidence that colorectal distension is a 'noxious' visceral stimulus in rats. Neurosci Lett. 1991;131(3):113–6.
17. Berthoud H-R, Blackshaw LA, Brookes SJ, Grundy D. Neuroanatomy of extrinsic afferents supplying the gastrointestinal tract. Neurogastroenterol Motil. 2004;16(Suppl 1):28–33.
18. Kyloh M, Spencer NJ. A novel anterograde neuronal tracing technique to selectively label spinal afferent nerve endings that encode noxious and innocuous stimuli in visceral organs. Neurogastroenterol Motil. 2014;26(3):440–4.
19. Song X, Chen BN, Zagorodnyuk VP, Lynn PA, Blackshaw LA, Grundy D. Identification of medium/high-threshold extrinsic mechanosensitive afferent nerves to the gastrointestinal tract. Gastroenterology. 2009;137(1):274–284.e1.
20. Zagorodnyuk VP, Brookes SJH, Spencer NJ. Structure-function relationship of sensory endings in the gut and bladder. Auton Neurosci. 2010;153(1–2):3–11.
21. Brookes SJH, Spencer NJ, Costa M, Zagorodnyuk VP. Extrinsic primary afferent signalling in the gut. Nat Rev Gastroenterol Hepatol. 2013;10(3):286–96.
22. Fox EA, Phillips RJ, Martinson FA, Baronowsky EA, Powley TL. Vagal afferent innervation of smooth muscle in the stomach and duodenum of the mouse: morphology and topography. J Comp Neurol. 2000;428:558–76.
23. Wang FB, Powley TL. Topographic inventories of vagal afferents in gastrointestinal muscle. J Comp Neurol. 2000;421:302–24.
24. Berthoud H-R, Lynn PA, Blackshaw LA. Vagal and spinal mechanosensors in the rat stomach and colon have multiple receptive fields. Am J Physiol Regul Integr Comp Physiol. 2001;280(3):R1371–81.
25. Goodwin G, McMahon SB. The physiological function of different voltage-gated sodium channels in pain. Nat Rev Neurosci. 2021;22(5):263–74. https://doi.org/10.1038/s41583-021-00444-w. Epub 2021 Mar 29. PMID: 33782571.
26. Benn SC, Costigan M, Tate S, Fitzgerald M, Woolf CJ. Developmental expression of the TTX-resistant voltage-gated sodium channels $Na_v1.8$ (SNS) and $Na_v1.9$ (SNS2) in primary sensory neurons. J Neurosci. 2001;21(16):6077–85. https://doi.org/10.1523/JNEUROSCI.21-16-06077.2001. PMID: 11487631; PMCID: PMC6763192.

27. Benson CJ, Sutherland SP. Toward an understanding of the molecules that sense myocardial ischemia. Ann N Y Acad Sci. 2001;940(3):96–109.
28. Malin SA, Christianson JA, Bielefeldt K, Davis BM. TRPV1 expression defines functionally distinct pelvic colon afferents. J Neurosci. 2009;29(3):743–52.
29. Robinson DR, McNaughton PA, Evans ML, Hicks GA. Characterization of the primary spinal afferent innervation of the mouse colon using retrograde labelling. Neurogastroenterol Motil. 2004;16(3):113–24.
30. Christianson JA, Traub RJ, Davis BM. Differences in spinal distribution and neurochemical phenotype of colonic afferents in mouse and rat. J Comp Neurol. 2006;494:246–59.
31. Sugiura T, Bielefeldt K, Gebhart GF. Mouse colon sensory neurons detect extracellular acidosis via TRPV1. Am J Physiol. 2007;292:C1768–74.
32. Akbar A, Yiangou Y, Facer P, Brydon WG, Walters JRF, Anand P. Expression of the TRPV1 receptor differs in quiescent inflammatory bowel disease with or without abdominal pain. Gut. 2010;59(3):767–74.
33. Akbar A, Yiangou Y, Facer P, Walters JRF, Anand P, Ghosh S. Increased capsaicin receptor TRPV1 expressing sensory fibres in irritable bowel syndrome and their correlation with abdominal pain. Gut. 2008;57:923–9.
34. Matthews PJ, Aziz Q, Facer P, Davis JB, Thompson DG, Anand P. Increased capsaicin receptor TRPV1 nerve fibres in the inflamed human oesophagus. Eur J Gastroenterol Hepatol. 2004;16:897–902.
35. Collet L, Meunier P, Duclaux R, Chery-Croze S, Falipou P. Cerebral evoked potentials after endorectal mechanical stimulation in humans. Am J Physiol Endocrinol Metab. 1988;254:G477–82.
36. Aziz Q, Furlong P, Barlow J, Hobson A, Alani S, Bancewicz J. Topographic mapping of cortical potentials evoked by distension of the human proximal and distal oesophagus. Electroencephalogr Clin Neurophysiol. 1995;96:219–28.
37. Kern M, Hofmann C, Hyde J, Shaker R. Characterization of the cerebral cortical representation of heartburn in GERD patients. Am J Physiol Gastrointest Liver Physiol. 2004;286(3):G174–81.
38. Lu CL, Wu YT, Chen LF, Chang FY, Lee SD, Ho LT. Neuronal correlates of gastric pain induced by fundus distension: a 3T-fMRI study. Neurogastroenterol Motil. 2004;16:575–87.
39. Van Oudenhove L, Dupont P, Vandenberghe J, Geeraerts B, Van Laere K, Bormans G. The role of somatosensory cortical regions in the processing of painful gastric fundic distension: an update of brain imaging findings. Neurogastroenterol Motil. 2008;20(3):479–87.
40. Silverman DH, Munakata JA, Ennes H, Mandelkern MA, Hoh CK, Mayer EA. Regional cerebral activity in normal and pathological perception of visceral pain. Gastroenterology. 1997;112(3):64–72.
41. Matsuura S, Kakizaki H, Mitsui T, Shiga T, Tamaki N, Koyanagi T. Human brain region response to distention or cold stimulation of the bladder: a positron emission tomography study. J Urol. 2002;168(3):2035–9.
42. Labus JS, Naliboff BN, Fallon J, Berman SM, Suyenobu B, Bueller JA. Sex differences in brain activity during aversive visceral stimulation and its expectation in patients with chronic abdominal pain: a network analysis. NeuroImage. 2008;41(3):1032–43.
43. Strigo IA, Duncan GH, Boivin M, Bushnell MC. Differentiation of visceral and cutaneous pain in the human brain. J Neurophysiol. 2003;89(3):3294–303.
44. Craig AD. A new view of pain as a homeostatic emotion. Trends Neurosci. 2003;26(3):303–7.
45. Coen SJ, Yágüez L, Aziz Q, Mitterschiffthaler MT, Brammer M, Williams SCR. Negative mood affects brain processing of visceral sensation. Gastroenterology. 2009;137(1):253–61.e2.
46. Rosenberger C, Elsenbruch S, Scholle A, De Greiff A, Schedlowski M, Forsting M. Effects of psychological stress on the cerebral processing of visceral stimuli in healthy women. Neurogastroenterol Motil. 2009;21:740–5.
47. Song GH, Venkatraman V, Ho KY, Chee MWL, Yeoh KG, Wilder-Smith CH. Cortical effects of anticipation and endogenous modulation of visceral pain assessed by functional brain MRI in irritable bowel syndrome patients and healthy controls. Pain. 2006;126(1–3):79–90.
48. Yágüez L, Coen S, Gregory LJ, Amaro E, Altman C, Brammer MJ. Brain response to visceral aversive conditioning: a functional magnetic resonance imaging study. Gastroenterology. 2005;128(3):1819–29.
49. Schmid J, Theysohn N, Gaß F, Benson S, Gramsch C, Forsting M. Neural mechanisms mediating positive and negative treatment expectations in visceral pain: a functional magnetic resonance imaging study on placebo and nocebo effects in healthy volunteers. Pain. 2013;154:2372–80.
50. Talley NJ, Fett SL, Zinsmeister AR, Melton LJ III. Gastrointestinal tract symptoms and self-reported abuse: a population-based study. Gastroenterology. 1994;107:1040–9.
51. Bradford K, Shih W, Videlock EJ, Presson AP, Naliboff BD, Mayer EA. Association between early adverse life events and irritable bowel syndrome. Clin Gastroenterol Hepatol. 2012;10(4):385–90.e3.
52. DeBerry J, Randich A, Shaffer AD, Robbins MT, Ness TJ. Neonatal bladder inflammation produces functional changes and alters neuropeptide content in bladders of adult female rats. J Pain. 2010;11(3):247–55.
53. Liu L-S, Winston JH, Shenoy MM, Song G-Q, Chen JDZ, Pasricha PJ. A rat model of chronic gastric sensorimotor dysfunction resulting from transient neonatal gastric irritation. Gastroenterology. 2008;134(3):2070–9.
54. Ren T-H, Wu J, Yew D, Ziea E, Lao L, Leung W-K. Effects of neonatal maternal separation on neurochemical and sensory response to colonic distension in a rat model of irritable bowel

syndrome. Am J Physiol Gastrointest Liver Physiol. 2007;292(3):G849–56.

55. Coutinho SV, Plotsky PM, Sablad M, Miller JC, Zhou H, Bayati AI. Neonatal maternal separation alters stress-induced responses to viscerosomatic nociceptive stimuli in rat. Am J Physiol Gastrointest Liver Physiol. 2002;282(3):G307–16.
56. Lin C, Al-Chaer ED. Long-term sensitization of primary afferents in adult rats exposed to neonatal colon pain. Brain Res. 2003;971(3):73–82.
57. Videlock EJ, Adeyemo M, Licudine A, Hirano M, Ohning G, Mayer M. Childhood trauma is associated with hypothalamic-pituitary-adrenal axis responsiveness in irritable bowel syndrome. Gastroenterology. 2009;137(3):1954–62.
58. Wang J, Gu C, Al-Chaer E. Altered behavior and digestive outcomes in adult male rats primed with minimal colon pain as neonates. Behav Brain Funct. 2008;4:28.
59. Blankstein U, Chen J, Diamant NE, Davis KD. Altered brain structure in irritable bowel syndrome: potential contributions of pre-existing and disease-driven factors. Gastroenterology. 2010;138(3):1783–9.
60. Frøkjær JB, Bouwense SAW, Olesen SS, Lundager FH, Eskildsen SF, van Goor H. Reduced cortical thickness of brain areas involved in pain processing in patients with chronic pancreatitis. Clin Gastroenterol Hepatol. 2012;10(4):434–8.e1.
61. Frøkjær JB, Olesen SS, Gram M, Yavarian Y, Bouwense SAW, Wilder-Smith OHG. Altered brain microstructure assessed by diffusion tensor imaging in patients with chronic pancreatitis. Gut. 2011;60(3):1554–62.
62. Seminowicz DA, Labus JS, Bueller JA, Tillisch K, Naliboff BD, Bushnell MC. Regional gray matter density changes in brains of patients with irritable bowel syndrome. Gastroenterology. 2010;139:48–57.
63. Berman SM, Naliboff BD, Suyenobu B, Labus JS, Stains J, Ohning G. Reduced brainstem inhibition during anticipated pelvic visceral pain correlates with enhanced brain response to the visceral stimulus in women with irritable bowel syndrome. J Neurosci. 2008;28(3):349–59.
64. Mertz H, Morgan V, Tanner G, Pickens D, Price R, Shyr Y. Regional cerebral activation in irritable bowel syndrome and control subjects with painful and nonpainful rectal distension. Gastroenterology. 2000;118:842–8.
65. Dunckley P, Wise RG, Fairhurst M, Hobden P, Aziz Q, Chang L. A comparison of visceral and somatic pain processing in the human brainstem using functional magnetic resonance imaging. J Neurosci. 2005;25(3):7333–41.
66. Elsenbruch S, Rosenberger C, Bingel U, Forsting M, Schedlowski M, Gizewski ER. Patients with irritable bowel syndrome have altered emotional modulation of neural responses to visceral stimuli. Gastroenterology. 2010;139(4):1310–9.e4.
67. Elsenbruch S, Rosenberger C, Enck P, Forsting M, Schedlowski M, Gizewski ER. Affective disturbances modulate the neural processing of visceral pain stimuli in irritable bowel syndrome: an fMRI study. Gut. 2010;59(3):489–95.
68. Ringel Y, Drossman DA, Leserman JL, Suyenobu BY, Wilber K, Lin W. Effect of abuse history on pain reports and brain responses to aversive visceral stimulation: an fMRI study. Gastroenterology. 2008;134(3):396–404.
69. Tillisch K, Labus J, Nam B, Bueller J, Smith S, Suyenobu B. Neurokinin-1-receptor antagonism decreases anxiety and emotional arousal circuit response to noxious visceral distension in women with irritable bowel syndrome: a pilot study. Aliment Pharmacol Ther. 2012;35(3):360–7.
70. Naliboff BD, Berman S, Suyenobu B, Labus JS, Chang L, Stains J. Longitudinal change in perceptual and brain activation response to visceral stimuli in irritable bowel syndrome patients. Gastroenterology. 2006;131(3):352–65.
71. Tillisch K, Mayer EA, Labus JS. Quantitative meta-analysis identifies brain regions activated during rectal distension in irritable bowel syndrome. Gastroenterology. 2011;140(3):91–100.
72. Chang L, Sundaresh S, Elliott J, Anton PA, Baldi P, Licudine A. Dysregulation of the hypothalamic-pituitary-adrenal (HPA) axis in irritable bowel syndrome. Neurogastroenterol Motil. 2009;21:149–59.
73. Stasi C, Bellini M, Costa F, Mumolo M, Ricchiuti A, Grosso M. Neuroendocrine markers and psychological features in patients with irritable bowel syndrome. Int J Color Dis. 2013;28(3):1203–8.
74. Larauche M, Gourcerol G, Wang L, Pambukchian K, Brunnhuber S, Adelson DW. Cortagine, a CRF1 agonist, induces stress-like alterations of colonic function and visceral hypersensitivity in rodents primarily through peripheral pathways. Am J Physiol Gastrointest Liver Physiol. 2009;297(3):G215–27.
75. Hubbard CS, Labus JS, Bueller J, Stains J, Suyenobu B, Dukes GE. Corticotropin-releasing factor receptor 1 antagonist alters regional activation and effective connectivity in an emotional–arousal circuit during expectation of abdominal pain. J Neurosci. 2011;31(3):12491–500.
76. Ebner K, Muigg P, Singewald G, Singewald N. Substance P in stress and anxiety. Ann N Y Acad Sci. 2008;1144(3):61–73.
77. Jarcho JM, Feier NA, Bert A, Labus JA, Lee M, Stains J. Diminished neurokinin-1 receptor availability in patients with two forms of chronic visceral pain. Pain. 2013;154(3):987–96.
78. Sharma GS, Tillisch K. Chapter 4—Visceral pain: mechanisms, syndromes, and treatment. In: Pangarkar S, Pham QG, Eapen BC, editors. Pain care essentials and innovations. Elsevier; 2021. p. 45–58. https://doi.org/10.1016/B978-0-323-72216-2.00004-1. ISBN 9780323722162.

4 Pathophysiological Mechanisms of Visceral Pain

Hong Jiang

For this chapter, based on the previous introduction of visceral pain from the anatomy and physiology perspectives, further exploration of the etiology and the receptor and regulation of visceral pain will be done to enable the perception of visceral pain from a pathophysiological perspective.

The etiology of visceral pain is various and complicated, and normally an organ- and system-based way of discussion will be taken. To be specific, there are internal chest pain (involving the respiratory system, circulatory organ, esophageal diseases, etc.), abdominal visceral pain (related to gastrointestinal diseases, pancreatic diseases, hepatobiliary diseases, urinary system diseases, vascular disease, etc.), obstetrical and gynecological visceral pain (pain at parturition, dysmenorrhea, endometriosis, leiomyoma, etc.), and cancerous pain (due to cancer development, pain after cancer treatment, and cancer pain syndrome).

In the receptor and regulation of the visceral pain part, features of visceral sensory receptors and regulatory mechanisms will be demonstrated. It refers to the receptors of different viscera, central receptors, regulatory mechanisms (feedback regulation of sensory receptors, inhibition between synapses, multisynaptic transmission), regulation of nociception by the central nervous system at all levels (cerebral cortex, diencephalon, brain stem, spinal cord), and the concept of hyperalgesia.

A final pathophysiological mechanism of visceral pain section concludes the chapter with neurophysiology mechanism, endogenous biochemical mechanism, and psychological mechanism.

4.1 Etiology of Visceral Pain

Visceral pain can be divided into true visceral, pseudo (mural) visceral, and referred pain according to the nerve pathways that conduct pain [1]. Generally speaking, pain in which the lesion is located in the visceral organs of the thoracic, abdominal, and pelvic cavities is called true visceral pain. Spinal sensory nerve endings are distributed on the wall pleura, on the peritoneum, and on the mediastinum and diaphragm, as well as on the mesentery and the lesser omentum, and the pain that occurs when the lesion involves the above-mentioned parts is called pseudo (mural) visceral pain. The pain or nociceptive hypersensitivity in some somatic parts of the distal compartment caused by visceral pain is called referred pain.

Visceral organs are innervated by parasympathetic nerves consisting of the vagus and pelvic nerves and sympathetic nerves emanating from the thoracolumbar segment, which are very sensitive to stimuli such as dilation, ischemia,

H. Jiang (✉)
Department of Anesthesiology, Shanghai Ninth People's Hospital, Shanghai Jiao Tong University School of Medicine, Shanghai, China

M. Xia et al. (eds.), *Visceral Pain*, https://doi.org/10.1007/978-981-99-9167-9_4

inflammation, pulling, and distension and can cause significant pain. Visceral pain varies slightly depending on the organ, and the following describes the etiology of visceral pain and the characteristics of pain perception of different organs in the thoracic, abdominal, and pelvic viscera respectively [1].

4.1.1 Chest Visceral Pain

Chest pain is a group of common non-specific symptoms in clinical practice, and its concept has been extended with the deepening of clinical practice, and now the concept of chest pain in a broad sense is gradually accepted by clinicians, that is, chest pain includes any discomfort in the anatomical range due to any cause, and also includes pain in other parts of the body that may be caused by chest diseases. The extension of the concept of chest pain expands the diagnostic thinking of clinicians, reduces the occurrence of missed diagnoses and misdiagnoses, and has important clinical practice significance.

The nerves, muscles, bones of the chest wall and organs and tissues in the chest cavity, and some organs of the diaphragm and subphrenic nerve can cause chest pain under the action of inflammation, ischemia, trauma, tumor, mechanical compression, physical and chemical stimulation, and other factors. The common clinical chest visceral pain is mainly caused by diseases of the respiratory organs, circulatory organs, esophagus, and mediastinum, which are described in the following sections.

4.1.1.1 Respiratory Organ Diseases

1. Lung tissue lesions
   (a) Pulmonary inflammatory chest pain

   Inflammation of the lung caused by pathogenic microorganisms, physicochemical factors, immune injury, allergy, and drugs, of which bacterial pneumonia is the most common pneumonia. Pneumonia-induced pulmonary pain is often accompanied by cough, sputum, fever, and dyspnea. Half of the patients may have chills and may have rust-colored sputum.

   (b) Lung cancer chest pain

   A total of 34–62% of lung cancer patients are accompanied by different degrees of pain [2]. Generally, as the tumor progresses, irritating cough, chest tightness, croup, fever, and mild chest pain will appear. In the late stage, due to the compression of adjacent organs and tissues or distant metastasis, symptoms such as diaphragm paralysis, hoarseness, superior vena cava obstruction, and pleural effusion may appear. When the tumor invades the chest wall, it may cause severe chest pain. Pulmonary atelectasis and irritant gas inhalation may also cause chest pain.
2. Tracheobronchial lesions

   Trachea and bronchitis can cause mild and moderate retrosternal pain, which is often burning, accompanied by cough, sputum, dyspnea, fever, and other symptoms.
3. Pulmonary vascular lesions

   Acute pulmonary hypertension can cause chest pain, often centrally located, crushing, and colicky, and is easily confused with myocardial infarction. In contrast to the latter, acute pulmonary hypertension does not radiate to the jaw and arm and is rarely located in the back. Pulmonary embolism is an acute clinical syndrome with various emboli blocking the pulmonary arteries as the cause, including pulmonary vascular embolism, amniotic fluid embolism, air embolism, and fat embolism syndrome [3]. Common causative factors include blood stasis, venous vessel wall injury, and hypercoagulable state. Patients often present with pleuritic-like chest pain, which is more intense in severity and duration than pneumonia. Patients with large infarcts usually have severe visceral or retrosternal crushing pain, similar to the local ischemia of myocardial infarction except that it does not radiate. The classic triad of pulmonary embolism—hemoptysis, pleuritic-like chest pain, and pleural friction sounds—is uncommon.

4. Pleural disease

   Pleurisy is usually an inflammation of the pleura caused by irritation of the pleura following a viral or bacterial infection. There may be fluid accumulation in the pleural cavity (exudative pleurisy) or no fluid accumulation (dry pleurisy), and the etiology includes infection, tumor, connective tissue disease, pulmonary embolism, etc. The chest pain is characterized by a sudden onset and varies greatly in degree. The typical chest pain is stabbing pain, which is aggravated by coughing and deep breathing, and may be combined with coughing, chest tightness, shortness of breath, and even dyspnea [4]. In case of infectious pleurisy or pleural effusion secondary infection, there may be chills and fever. The visceral pleura is painless, and the pain is caused by the inflammation of the wall pleura. When the diaphragmatic pleura is diseased, the pain may radiate to the shoulder and abdomen; adhesion pleurisy may have long-term dull pain, and the chest pain caused by tuberculous pleurisy is mostly located below the anterior or posterior axillary line where the respiratory motion is large, and the chest pain increases when breathing deeply or coughing. In dry pleurisy, chest pain is heavier, with shallow and fast breathing and decreased tidal volume: in exudative pleurisy, pain is reduced instead. If a large amount of fluid accumulation occurs, leading to the separation of the two layers of pleura from each other, chest pain may disappear.

5. Pneumothorax

   Pneumothorax is a phenomenon in which the lung tissue and its dirty layer pleura are ruptured, or the chest wall and wall layer pleura are penetrated, resulting in the air entering the pleural cavity to make air accumulate in the pleural cavity. It can cause sudden onset of inflammatory pain in the pleura, which may occur to the affected shoulder or wall, with difficulty in breathing. If accompanied by mediastinal displacement, it is likely to cause deep central pain and a feeling of heaviness behind the sternum.

4.1.1.2 Circulatory Organ Diseases

1. Acute coronary syndrome

   The most common acute chest pain is acute coronary syndrome caused by ischemic heart disease, including unstable angina pectoris and acute myocardial infarction, which account for most of the acute chest pain. Diseases such as arteriosclerosis, occlusive vasculitis, rheumatic arteritis, and syphilitic aortitis can lead to the formation of thrombosis, embolism, and intimal hemorrhage in the coronary arteries, all of which can cause myocardial infarction [5].

   Cardiac pain is afferent via sympathetic nerves from T_{1-5} and enters the spinal cord through the posterior roots [6]. Stimuli such as ischemia and hypoxia can cause the release of pain-causing substances such as K^+, H^+, histamine, 5-HT, adenosine, lactate, kinin, etc. from the tissues, which in turn, by acting on sensory nerve endings, transmit information about injurious stimuli to the corresponding spinal cord posterior roots' conversion neurons, leading to nociception. The typical site of ischemic chest pain is usually behind the sternum, but sometimes there is pain in the left shoulder and arm, left upper extremity, or even in the jaw, neck, and upper abdomen, because the sensory afferent fibers in these areas terminate at the same time as the sensory fibers innervating the heart on the same transition neurons, and the cortical center sometimes "misjudges" them.

2. Pericarditis

   Acute non-specific pericarditis is a plasma fibrinous pericarditis that may be associated with viral infection or allergic or autoimmune reactions. The pain is mostly located in the posterior sternum of the precordial region and is stabbing or dull. The radiating sites are similar to angina pectoris for the neck, left shoulder, left scapula, epigastrium, etc. The pain may increase with deep breathing, coughing, or chest movement.

3. Aortic disease

   Chest pain of aortic origin is commonly associated with aortic coarctation aneurysm and saccular aneurysm. Aortic coarctation is a critical cardiovascular emergency in which blood enters the middle layer of the aorta to form a coarctation hematoma and peels off along the aortic wall. The chest pain is similar to myocardial infarction, and the pain is sudden, intense, tear-like, and relatively widespread. Chest pain caused by aortic aneurysm compressing surrounding tissues is mostly in the upper part of the chest or neck, and its characteristics vary according to the compressed organ, among which the pain is most significant when the aneurysm compresses bones and nerves.

4. Cardiac neurosis

   Cardiovascular, respiratory, and neurological symptoms are the main manifestations, and there is no organic lesion in clinical and pathological aspects. The chest pain is mostly located in the left chest or apical region, and can also be radiated to the left shoulder, manifesting as stabbing or tearing pain of short duration; it can also manifest as persistent dull pain lasting for several hours or even days, which is not related to activities or is not clearly related.

5. Other

   Heart valve disease, hypertrophic cardiomyopathy, myocarditis, etc. may also cause chest pain.

4.1.1.3 Esophageal Disease

Gastroesophageal reflux is the most common cause of esophageal-derived chest pain, and the others are, in order, infectious diseases, systemic diseases, physical factors, and esophageal mucosal lesions caused by trauma.

1. Gastroesophageal reflux

   Reflux esophagitis is an inflammatory change caused by the continuous reflux of gastric and duodenal contents into the esophagus under the action of certain pathogenic factors, which irritates the esophageal mucosa for a long time, especially the mucosa of the lower esophagus. Once the esophageal mucosa is damaged, its permeability increases and the contents of the esophagus can penetrate into the intrinsic layer of the mucosa, stimulating the nerve endings and causing pain, with symptoms such as heartburn, burning pain behind the sternum or pain under the xiphoid process. The pain often occurs 30–60 min after meals, and in severe cases it is severe and can radiate to the back and chest, resembling the chest pain of angina pectoris or pleurisy. Lower esophageal sphincter tone is reduced or relaxed, the ability of the esophagus to remove refluxed material is reduced, and gastric emptying is impaired, making it easy for gastric contents to flow back into the esophagus. Bending, coughing, smoking, drinking alcohol, eating chocolate, drinking coffee, obesity, and pregnancy can cause or worsen esophageal reflux: standing, drinking water, or taking antacid preparations can reduce or temporarily relieve symptoms. Gastroesophageal reflux pain is characterized by increased pain when swallowing, accompanied by varying degrees of dysphagia or even vomiting, easily produced by solid food passing through the lesion area, and relieved by eating a liquid or soft diet.

   Other diseases that can cause inflammation of esophageal mucosa can also lead to chest pain, such as infectious diseases (*Candida albicans*, herpes simplex virus, cytomegalovirus, etc.), systemic diseases (herpetic epidermolysis bullosa, smallpox-like sores, scleroderma, etc.), and chemical burns of the esophagus.

2. Esophageal dysmotility diseases

   In addition to painful swallowing, pancreatic dysmotility disorder can also lead to gastroesophageal reflux and cause chest pain. The pain can be boring, burning, stabbing, cutting, or cone pain, mostly in the posterior sternum and upper middle abdomen, but also in the back of the chest, the right side of the chest, the right edge of the sternum, and the left quarter rib area. It may be accompanied by dysphagia, vomiting, reflux, and weight loss. In addition, there are esophageal peristaltic disorders, hypertonic esophageal chest pain, and irritable esophageal chest pain.

3. Esophageal cancer

When esophageal cancer develops, it causes progressive dysphagia and chest pain due to tumor obstruction, and the pain may be confined to the back of the sternum or may radiate to the back.

4. Esophageal rupture

   Esophageal rupture can be spontaneous or traumatic rupture, and the symptom is immediate chest pain, and in severe cases, the pain is unbearable, similar to angina. If the rupture is in the upper or middle part, the pain is located behind the sternum in the upper chest; if the rupture is in the lower part, the pain is located behind the sternum and in the upper abdomen. Patients with esophageal rupture are often associated with dyspnea, cyanosis, sweating, and shock.

5. Esophageal hiatal hernia

   Pain due to esophageal hiatal hernia is often located in the sternotomy plane, to the right or left side of the sternum, or behind the glabella. The pain may radiate to the back, shoulder, neck, upper arm, forearm, palm, jaw, and ear. The nature of the pain is mostly burning, occasionally colicky, or pins and needles. The pain often occurs 1 h after a full meal and may be accompanied by shortness of breath, palpitations, belching, eructation, heartburn, regurgitation, and dysphagia. Pregnancy, obesity, ascites, large abdominal tumors, violent coughing and vomiting, and eructation are common triggers of this disease. Flat lying, bending, squatting, and coughing can aggravate the pain: standing, semi-recumbent position, and walking can reduce the pain.

4.1.1.4 Referred Chest Pain Caused by Abdominal Visceral Pain

1. Gastrocardiac syndrome

   Gastrocardiac syndrome is a reflexive disorder of the cardiovascular system caused by gastric diseases, resulting in discomfort or vague pain in the precordial region, a few similar to angina pectoris, pinprick-like or crush-like pain, lasting from a few minutes to several hours. The treatment of coronary artery dilation is ineffective, and antispasmodic and acid-suppressing drugs can relieve the symptoms. The pathogenesis may be related to autonomic dysfunction, and the most common causes are peptic ulcer, chronic gastritis, gastric mucosal prolapse, gastric cancer, and smoking.

2. Chloe-heart syndrome

   Chloe-heart syndrome refers to the acute attack of biliary tract diseases such as cholecystitis and cholelithiasis, which, through visceral involvement reflex, causes ischemic changes in the heart and results in angina pectoris, arrhythmia, and other symptoms similar to coronary heart disease. The cause may be related to the innervation of the heart and biliary system. The heart is innervated by $T_{2–8}$ spinal nerves, and the gallbladder and common bile duct are innervated by $T_{4–9}$ spinal nerves, which are crossed [7]. Therefore, when inflammation occurs in the biliary tract and the internal pressure increases, it can reflexively cause coronary artery constriction and blood flow reduction through $T_{4,5}$ nerves, which induces cardiac dysfunction.

3. Colon-related pain

   Colonic hepatic flexure syndrome may produce right upper abdominal and right anterior chest radiating pain; in the case of colonic hepatic flexure syndrome, left upper abdominal pain and left anterior chest radiating pain.

4. Others

   Pancreatitis can irritate the diaphragm and produce pleuritic chest pain; hepatosplenomegaly and subdiaphragmatic infection can both produce chest pain: subdiaphragmatic abscess can inflame the diaphragm and cause pain in the chest or scapular area on the sick side.

4.1.1.5 Others

Chronic mediastinitis can cause persistent burning pain or pressure behind the sternum: mediastinal tumors can compress the surrounding tissues, causing persistent drilling pain in the back, both sides of the chest, or the anterior chest.

Spinal origin chest pain: misalignment of spinal joints can cause arrhythmia and coronary heart disease. The incidence of cervicogenic heart disease in China accounts for 13% of cervical spondylosis, and there is a trend of gradual increase [8].

In addition, anxiety, depression, hysteria, and other mental factors can also produce symptoms of chest pain, but the location of the pain is often not fixed, and its nature and duration are also elusive, independent of sleep and activity.

4.1.2 Abdominal Visceral Pain

Abdominal pain is an extremely common clinical symptom, and in 4–10% of our emergency patients, the reason for emergency visits is abdominal pain [9]. Its etiology is very complex, including inflammation, tumor, bleeding, obstruction, trauma, perforation, and functional disorders. According to the lesion causing abdominal pain, it can be divided into organic, functional, and psychological.

4.1.2.1 Pain of Gastrointestinal Diseases

Gastrointestinal tract can produce abdominal pain with signs and symptoms such as abdominal muscle tension, nausea, vomiting, lack of appetite, sweating and palpitations under the effect of distension, pulling, and chemical stimulation, as well as ischemic inflammatory factors.

1. Peptic ulcer

   Peptic ulcer is one of the common causes of abdominal pain. Its pain site is usually in the middle of the upper abdomen, located between the xiphoid process and umbilicus, but the pain site of duodenal ulcer is low and to the right, and the pain of ulcer near the cardia is located at the lower posterior end of the sternum, and the pain can radiate to the back and shoulder when there is chronic perforation or adhesion [10]. There is a clear regularity between ulcer pain and diet, with gastric ulcers showing postprandial pain and duodenal ulcers showing hunger pain, with midnight pain being another characteristic manifestation. If this rhythmic pain becomes persistent, it suggests that the ulcer may have penetrated the plasma membrane or is a precursor to malignancy. The common triggers of ulcer pain are work strain, mental stress, overeating, and heavy alcohol consumption. The nature of the pain is dull pain, burning pain, cone pain, pressure, and distension, which may be accompanied by hunger, vomiting, and bleeding.

2. Inflammatory factors

   Inflammatory factors such as chronic gastritis often manifest as vague pain in the upper abdomen, pain without obvious regularity, often accompanied by lack of appetite, postprandial fullness, and acid reflux. Biliary reflux gastritis often has obvious and persistent pain in the upper abdominal region, especially after meals, and may be accompanied by nausea and vomiting. Typical abdominal pain in appendicitis starts in the upper abdomen or around the umbilicus, with paroxysmal abdominal pain that gradually worsens and shifts to the right lower abdomen after a few hours. It is often accompanied by gastrointestinal symptoms such as nausea and vomiting.

   Inflammatory bowel disease and ulcerative colitis are mostly paroxysmal spasmodic pain along the course of the colon, with a pattern of "pain and defecation and relief", and persistent pain when the plasma membrane is involved. It may be accompanied by diarrhea, nausea, vomiting, and abdominal distension. The common symptoms of intestinal tuberculosis are vague abdominal pain and spasmodic pain, which is obvious in the right lower abdomen and around the umbilicus. The pain worsens after meals and may be relieved after defecation. It is often accompanied by symptoms such as bloating, vomiting, constipation, and diarrhea alternately.

3. Mechanical factors

   The typical abdominal pain of mechanical intestinal obstruction is paroxysmal colic, and the pain is mostly located around the umbilicus: strangulated intestinal obstruction mainly manifests as persistent severe pain even after the onset of colic, which cannot be relieved by general analgesics, and paralytic intestinal obstruction lacks colic symptoms and manifests as persistent abdominal distension. It is often accompanied by vomiting, abdominal distension, and stopping defecation.

4. Cancerous factors

   Depending on the location of the tumor and the degree of infiltration, it can be manifested as pain of different degrees. In an advanced stage of gastrointestinal cancer, with extensive metastasis or infiltration of the abdominal wall and retroperitoneum, the pain includes visceral pain as well as somatic pain.

5. Ischemic enteropathy

   Due to atherosclerosis narrowing or obstruction at the opening of the gastrointestinal branches of the abdominal aorta, the involved arteries mostly occur in the superior mesenteric artery. Postprandial pain in the upper or middle abdomen caused by ischemia in the intestine.

6. Other

   Free appendicitis is mainly manifested by recurrent episodes of dull pain in the right lower abdomen, and the pain is mostly caused by irritation of the mesentery due to swinging or twisting of the appendix. The pain often comes on in the morning, after strenuous activities or long walks, and the pain can be relieved by rest or local massage. In combination with appendicitis, there may be fever, nausea, vomiting, and other concomitant symptoms. When the appendix is strangulated and necrotic, there may be continuous severe pain, accompanied by intestinal obstruction, peritonitis, and other signs.

4.1.2.2 Pain in Pancreatic Diseases

1. Acute pancreatitis

   Acute pancreatitis is a common clinical emergency abdomen, and common attack triggers are overeating, alcohol abuse, biliary obstruction, etc. The main manifestation is persistent dull pain or colic in the middle of the epigastrium, which increases in paroxysms and radiates to the low back, ipsilateral shoulder, and both quarters of the rib cage. Patients are often unable to lie on their backs, and sitting and forward leaning positions can reduce the pain. It is often accompanied by fever, abdominal distension, nausea, vomiting, and even shock.

2. Pain of pancreatic cancer

   Pain is the most common and serious clinical symptom of advanced pancreatic cancer. Most patients' pain is due to tumor invasion of the abdominal plexus including autonomic nerves, which often occurs as severe pain in the abdomen and back, seriously affecting patients' diet and sleep, accelerating physical exertion, and causing a series of poor prognosis.

4.1.2.3 Pain of Hepatobiliary Diseases

1. Primary hepatocellular carcinoma pain

   Pain is the most common clinical symptom of hepatocellular carcinoma patients, especially those with advanced hepatocellular carcinoma, with an incidence rate of almost 100% [11]. Its pain is mostly manifested as intermittent or specific hidden pain, dull pain, or stabbing pain in the right rib area or under the saber. The pain is mainly caused by the rapid enlargement of the tumor, which compresses the liver pericardium and produces involvement pain. The sudden rupture and bleeding of cancer nodules on the liver surface may cause sudden and severe pain. The tumor growth site may vary. Tumor in the left lobe of the liver often causes pain in the middle and upper abdomen; tumor in the right lobe of the liver causes pain in the right quarter rib area; when the tumor involves the diaphragm, the pain radiates to the right shoulder or right back; tumor in the posterior part of the right lobe can cause lumbago.

2. Biliary colic

   It is mainly caused by spasmodic contraction of the gallbladder, bile duct, or sphincter of Oddi caused by bile duct stones, cholecystitis, biliary ascariasis, etc. It mostly occurs after a full meal or eating greasy food, drinking alcohol, and emotional excitement. Chronic cholecystitis often manifests as pain in the right upper abdomen, often triggered by eating greasy foods. If there are gallstones embedded in the gallbladder neck, the pain will be sudden onset of severe colic with paroxysmal intensification, often accompanied by pain radiating from the back of the right shoulder, left upper abdomen, and around the umbilicus. The pain may be relieved in prone position or right lateral position. It may be accompanied by indigestion, bloating, nausea, vomiting, diarrhea, jaundice, and palpitations. Gallstone disease mostly attacks at night with paroxysmal colic, mostly accompanied by nausea, vomiting, and fever. Biliary ascariasis has paroxysmal severe epigastric pain with nausea and vomiting, but intermittent quiet as usual.

4.1.2.4 Pain of Urinary System Diseases

1. Kidney stones

   Back pain is a typical symptom of kidney stones. When the stone is larger and less mobile in the renal pelvis, it is mostly vague and dull pain; when the stone is smaller, it is easy to cause renal colic due to obstruction in the ureteral junction of the renal pelvis. The pain is paroxysmal and varies in duration. It may be accompanied by dizziness, nausea, vomiting, hematuria, sweating, dry mouth, and even shock.
2. Ureteral stones

   Ureteral stones stimulate the smooth muscle to contract strongly and cause sudden and severe colic in the affected lumbar region. It radiates to the ipsilateral groin, inner thigh, and perineum, often accompanied by dizziness, nausea, vomiting, hematuria, etc. The special symptoms of ureteral bladder wall segment stones are urinary frequency, urinary urgency, and urinary pain.
3. Bladder spasmodic pain

   Disease factors such as cystitis, urethritis, prostatitis, bladder stones, bladder tumor, bladder foreign body, prostatic hyperplasia, and lower urinary tract surgery can cause bladder spasmodic pain. The characteristic manifestation is paroxysmal burning-like or knife-like pain in the upper pubic bone and pelvic area, which can radiate to the vulva and medial femur, and can be accompanied by symptoms such as urinary frequency, urinary urgency, urinary pain, urge incontinence, and strong urge to urinate.
4. Interstitial cystitis

   The pain caused by interstitial cystitis is often located in the lower abdomen, pelvis, groin and perineum, and may be accompanied by urinary frequency, urgency, and nocturia. Anxiety and depression are also common complications of interstitial cystitis.
5. Prostatitis

   The painful areas of prostatitis are located in the perineum, perianal area, suprapubic (lower) abdomen, groin, lumbosacral area, scrotum, inner thighs, and urethra. It may be accompanied by signs of urinary tract irritation, sexual dysfunction, and secondary symptoms.
6. Other

   Polycystic kidney, renal vein thrombosis, renal embolism, urethral syndrome, low back pain-hematuria syndrome, orchitis, epididymitis, etc.

4.1.2.5 Pain of Retroperitoneal Disease

Retroperitoneal diseases that can cause low back pain mainly include retroperitoneal fibrosis and retroperitoneal tumor.

1. Retroperitoneal fibrosis

   Retroperitoneal fibrosis is due to non-specific, non-suppurative inflammation of retroperitoneal fibrofatty tissue causing extensive fibrosis, which causes obstruction by compression of extraperitoneal cavity organs. Its etiology is unclear and may be associated with autoimmune or allergic vasculitis. It usually presents with non-specific back pain, abdominal pain, and cribriform pain, which is persistent and dull or vague. The onset is usually insidious and the duration is long. It may be accompanied by other symptoms such as anorexia, wasting, and fatigue.
2. Retroperitoneal tumor

   Primary retroperitoneal tumors can be divided into neurogenic and embryogenic, of which 60–85% are malignant [12]. Among benign tumors, fibroma, neurofibroma, and cystic teratoma are common;

among malignant tumors, fibrosarcoma, malignant nerve sheath tumor, and malignant lymphoma are common. Clinical symptoms are often manifested as gradually increasing discomfort, soreness, and swelling of the low back, which gradually evolves into low back pain, and pain in the perineum or lower limbs may occur. Causes of pain: (1) tumor compressing nerve; (2) tumor compressing ureter causing urinary obstruction; (3) bleeding inside the tumor and increasing volume causing high tension of envelope, etc.

4.1.2.6 Pain of Vascular Disease

The most common cause of an abdominal aortic aneurysm is atherosclerosis. Other causes include trauma, syphilis, tuberculosis, white stuffing syndrome, congenital dysplasia, or other infections. The incidence of aneurysms is currently increasing year by year. Most patients may have a passive mass palpable in the left side of the abdomen next to the umbilicus, with discomfort or pain in the upper abdomen. When the aneurysm invades the vertebral body or compresses the spinal nerve root, low back pain appears. The sudden onset of severe abdominal pain or low back pain is a sign of aneurysm rupture with massive intra-abdominal or retroperitoneal bleeding, and patients often die of hemorrhagic shock within a short period of time.

4.1.2.7 Abdominal Pain of Spinal Origin

Abdominal pain that cannot be explained by abdominal organ lesions should be considered as possible spinal origin abdominal pain, caused by anomalies in the anterior, spinal, and posterior spinal anatomical structures. The abdominal nerves are distributed by spinal nerves and visceral sensory nerves. The spinal nerves are distributed in the wall of the abdominal wall and the mural layer of the peritoneum from the T_6 to L_1 spinal cord segments, and the visceral sensory nerves are distributed in the organs of the abdominal cavity and the visceral peritoneum, and there is an inductive connection between the visceral nerves and the spinal nerves. Therefore, soft tissue lesions in the lumbar region can involve the abdominal wall tissues to cause abdominal pain.

4.1.2.8 Functional Abdominal Pain Syndrome

Functional abdominal pain syndrome, also known as chronic functional abdominal pain, is a functional disorder with persistent or frequent episodes of abdominal pain that lasts more than 6 months but is not related to or has little relationship with the gastrointestinal tract. Patients often have other general discomfort and psychological disorders such as anxiety and depression. The cause and pathogenesis of the syndrome are not very clear and may be related to abnormalities in visceral sensitivity, central pain regulation due to brain-gut interaction, and abnormal psychological states. Current research suggests that functional abdominal pain syndrome may be a kind of central pain, due to a variety of factors that affect the physiological regulation of normal intestinal function by the central nervous system, causing normal internal regulatory signals to be amplified in the central nervous system, resulting in abnormal sensations and thus abdominal pain.

4.1.3 Gynecological and Obstetric Internal Pain

About 1/3 of women's lower back pain is related to the physiological characteristics of women or gynecological diseases [13, 14]. Among them, the pain caused by childbirth and menstruation is the most distressing pain for women, and it directly affects physical and mental health.

4.1.3.1 Labor Pains

When the uterus contracted, the pressure inside the official rose significantly, the ligaments and peritoneum of the uterus were stretched, the blood vessels of the uterine wall were compressed to different degrees, and the surrounding tissues appeared temporary ischemia and hypoxia. The pain is mainly felt in the lower abdomen, lumbar region, and sometimes in the hip and sacral region. Continuous contractions of the uterus and partial descent of the fetal previa cause dilatation of the perineal tissues, pain in the back, thighs and calves, and distension of the perineum, accompanied by a strong, involuntary "defecation feeling".

4.1.3.2 Dysmenorrhea

Periodic intense paroxysmal, spasmodic pain and distension in the lower abdomen and lumbar region, radiating to the lumbosacral region, upper abdomen, pubic bone, inner thighs, perineum, and anus, accompanied by pallor, lumbago, headache, nausea, vomiting, diarrhea and weakness, around the time of menstruation or during menstruation. Dysmenorrhea is related to endocrine factors, uterine anatomical factors, and psychological factors, and can also be secondary to pelvic inflammatory disease, endometriosis, and submucosal fibroids. Dysmenorrhea is very common and about half of young women have symptoms during their periods, mostly in young unmarried women. The nature of the pain is mostly paroxysmal colic. When the outflow of menstrual blood is clear, the pain disappears, usually after 12–24 h, but also lasts for 2–3 days. The accompanying symptoms include headache, dizziness, breast distension, frequent urination, constipation or diarrhea, insomnia, irritability, etc. In severe cases, there may be pallor, cold sweat, chills in the hands and feet, nausea, vomiting and even syncope.

4.1.3.3 Supernumerary Ovary

The presence of extra ovarian tissue in an abnormal location is called supernumerary ovaries. They can cause chronic pelvic pain if they develop cystic or neoplastic changes. Patients with additional ovaries may have pelvic and lower abdominal pain. Symptoms of paratesticular ovaries are somewhat atypical and include dysmenorrhea, irregular uterine bleeding, and pelvic pressure pain.

4.1.3.4 Adenomyosis of the Uterus

The invasion of endometrial glands and mesenchyme into the myometrium of the uterus for growth is called uterine adenomyosis. Its general manifestation is excessive menstruation and dysmenorrhea in menstruating women.

4.1.3.5 Adhesions

Pelvic inflammatory disease, endometriosis, appendiceal perforation, history of pelvic and abdominal surgery or inflammatory bowel disease can lead to pelvic adhesions. Adhesions can cause pelvic pain, which is generally constant in location and can increase after sudden activity, sexual intercourse, and other activities.

4.1.3.6 Adnexal Cysts

Ovarian cysts do not usually cause chronic pelvic pain, except for endometriotic cysts.

4.1.3.7 Endometriosis

Endometriosis is the appearance of tissue with the structure and function of endometrial tissue in an abnormal location. It is one of the most common causes of gynecologic pain. The pain associated with endometriosis is located in the lower abdomen and pelvis and presents as cramping pain that may radiate to the anus, perineum, or thighs. It often begins with dysmenorrhea, and painful intercourse is a common manifestation of its associated pelvic pain. Some patients may involve the intestinal tract, showing symptoms such as urgency, constipation, diarrhea, blood in the stool, and intestinal obstruction; occasionally the urinary tract may be involved, showing symptoms such as urinary frequency, urgency, painful urination, hematuria, and obstruction; rarely the lungs are involved, showing symptoms such as dyspnea, pleural effusion, and pulmonary atrophy; endometriosis of the ovary, when the chocolate cyst ruptures, may cause acute abdominal pain and signs of peritoneal irritation.

4.1.3.8 Smooth Muscle Tumor

Some patients have painful symptoms, usually manifested as dysmenorrhea. Chronic pelvic pain due to tumor compression and invasion is usually progressive. Uterine fibroids in the rectal uterine sink can cause rectal compression and pelvic discomfort; compression of the ureter by the fibroid leads to hydronephrosis and back pain; and twisting of the fibroid tip can cause severe pelvic pain. Occasionally, it may manifest as painful percussive intercourse.

4.1.3.9 Preserved Ovary Syndrome

Preserved ovary syndrome occurs mostly after a hysterectomy with one or both ovaries preserved. The adhesions interfere with ovarian function and ovulation, preventing the ovaries from expanding and ovulating periodically and leading to pelvic pain. It manifests as chronic lower abdominal or pelvic pain, which can be cyclic or persistent dull pain, or cyclic colic or spasmodic pain that can radiate to the lower back and legs, and some patients have deep intercourse pain and also lower segment urethral symptoms.

4.1.3.10 Pelvic Stasis Syndrome

Pelvic stasis syndrome is pelvic pain and painful intercourse associated with pelvic varicose veins and stasis. Stasis dysmenorrhea or premenstrual cramping pain is one of the most common symptoms, mostly presenting as dull and chronic pain, which can occur as transient, severe acute pelvic pain. The location of the pain is wandering, mostly on both sides of the lower abdomen, in the suprapubic region, and involves soreness at the roots of both thighs or hips, low back pain, and vulvar and vaginal cramps. Walking, standing, lifting heavy objects, bending, and mental tension often make the pain worse, and there may be deep intercourse pain or post-coital pain.

4.1.3.11 Peritoneal Cysts

The cause of peritoneal cysts can be related to surgical adhesive disease or can be mesothelial reactive hyperplasia. The clinical presentation is chronic, recurrent abdominopelvic pain, which often develops gradually from lower abdominal fullness and discomfort and may be associated with constipation and difficulty in urination.

4.1.3.12 Symptomatic Pelvic Relaxation Disorder

Defective laxity or support function due to destruction or loss of strength of pelvic floor muscles and fascia. It can lead to pelvic pain, lumbosacral pain, and back pain. It often manifests as a feeling of pulling, heaviness, fullness, and insecurity. The symptoms are mildest in the morning, and the pain gradually worsens with prolonged standing and activity, and there may be painful intercourse.

4.1.3.13 Other

Tubal endometriosis, ovarian cancer, cervical cancer, endometrial cancer, cervical polyps, endometrial polyps, pelvic muscle spasm, pelvic floor pain syndrome, chronic pelvic inflammatory diseases, etc. can lead to pelvic pain.

4.1.4 Cancer Pain

Malignant tumors can invade adjacent tissues and organs and destroy their structures and functions, and can also spread or metastasize to distant parts of the body in various ways. When the primary tumor and its metastases compress or invade the nerves, blood vessels, and intestines, it can produce pain. For example, cancer infiltrates into pleura and peritoneum, and tumor cells invade blood vessels, both can cause pain; liver cancer invades the liver peritoneum, which can cause pain in the liver area; intra-abdominal implantation of the tumor can cause abdominal pain; intestinal tumor obstructs digestive tract, which can cause intestinal colic. In addition, the tumor itself can affect the metabolism, endocrine, and internal environment of the body, which makes the pain mechanism more complicated. Initially, cancer pain is mostly chronic, insidious, and dull, and gradually becomes sharp and knife-like pain, which can radiate along the innervation area.

It is currently believed that there are three mechanisms of cancer pain: pain directly caused by cancer development, pain caused by cancer treatment, and concurrent painful diseases in cancer patients.

4.1.4.1 Pain Caused by Cancer Development

1. Tumor invasion of nerves

   When tumor progression leads to the invasion of nerves, its pain is acute in nature and often radiates to the distribution range of nerves on the body surface. When the tumor infiltrates into the abdominal plexus, mesenteric plexus, and sacral plexus, the pain site is not clear and it is persistent.

2. Tumor invades cavity organs

   If the tumor invades the bile duct, pancreatic duct, intestinal duct, ureter, bladder, uterus, and other organs, it often shows periodic and recurrent severe pain, accompanied by nausea, vomiting, cold sweat, and other symptoms.

3. Tumor invades the vascular system

   If the tumor invades arteries, veins, and lymphatic vessels and causes obstruction of return flow to the affected organs, it may cause the aggregation of pain-causing substances or interruption of blood flow, resulting in local ischemic necrosis and severe pain.

4. Tumor itself secretes pain-causing substances

   Tumor tissues themselves can release pain-causing substances such as prostaglandins and peptides, which can lower the pain threshold and cause pain.

4.1.4.2 Pain Caused by Cancer Treatment

1. Post-surgical pain

   Post-operative scar and neuroma formation can produce pain, such as post-thoracotomy pain syndrome, etc.

2. Pain after radiotherapy

   Pain can be caused by lumbosacral plexus fibrosis and other lesions caused by radiotherapy.

3. Others

   Pain after cancer treatment also includes pain caused by treatment operations, acute pain caused by hormone treatment, acute pain caused by immunotherapy, acute pain caused by infection, etc.

4.1.4.3 Cancer Pain Syndrome

Due to the general rules of malignant tumor development, invasion and destruction of nerves, secondary infection, stretching of parenchymal organs, obstruction of blood flow of tissues and organs, and obstruction of hollow organs also produce some common cancer pain syndromes.

1. Pelvic cancer pain syndrome

   Pelvic cancer is more common and mostly originates from pelvic soft tissues. The most common primary tumor is colorectal cancer, followed by gynecological malignant tumors, and a few originate from extra-abdominal tumors. The swelling growth of tumors and invasion of nerves or ligaments are the causes of pain. If there is secondary infection, obstruction, or bleeding, the pain can be aggravated.

2. Cancerous liver pain syndrome

   Only a few patients with hepatocellular carcinoma have symptoms of pain in the liver area. The pain is persistent dull pain under the right quarter rib, which is aggravated when bending forward and moving, and can be slightly relieved by lying down or gently stroking the liver area; it can also be manifested as a paroxysmal stabbing pain in the right upper abdomen, lasting for several minutes, starting from the right quarter rib and radiating to the sides or back, and the patient often feels suffocated. The liver parenchyma is not sensitive to pain, and the main cause of pain comes from liver peritoneal traction, while the sudden increase in pain is mostly due to tumor bleeding or death.

3. Cancerous intestinal colic syndrome

   It can occur when an abdominal or pelvic tumor compresses, adhere, or erodes smooth muscle, vein, lymphatic tract, or autonomic nerve or causes intestinal obstruction. The pain is usually intermittent and can be aggravated by eating. When there is local intestinal strangulation or necrosis, the abdominal pain will increase.

4. Cancerous chest pain syndrome

   The primary cancer is mostly bronchial cancer, which manifests as paroxysmal or persistent chest pain.

4.2 Conduction of Visceral Pain

4.2.1 Visceral Pain Receptors

4.2.1.1 General Concept and Characteristics of Receptors

Most peripheral afferent nerve endings can respond to a variety of different stimuli, however, the differences in their location, morphology, and sensory area determine that they can more effectively sense one of the many types of stimuli. Due to this difference in specific sensitivity, receptors can be divided into mechanoreceptors, chemoreceptors, photoreceptors, and temperature receptors. According to the morphological and structural characteristics of the receptors, they can be divided into exposed nerve endings (pain and touch receptors), Krause vesicles (cold receptors), Ruffini terminals (thermoreceptors), Meissner vesicles (tactile receptors), Merkel discs (fine touch), hair follicle nerve endings (hair follicle touch), and special receptors (sight, hearing, smell, and taste). They can be divided into superficial receptors, deep receptors, and visceral receptors according to their distribution. Both Aδ and C fibers have free nerve endings that convert injurious or high threshold thermal, mechanical, and chemical stimuli. Aδ and C fibers respond to stimuli in the receptive area in a specific manner of slow adaptation and sustained impulses after stimulus fading. Class C fibers mediate Class II pain, or idiopathic pain, which is vaguely localized or difficult to localize and is described as burning or dull pain.

The nerve endings that serve as pain receptors have many branches and often overlap with areas innervated by other nerve endings emanating from their superior or inferior spinal cord segments. Most injurious receptors are polymorphic and can transduce different forms of injurious stimuli into action potentials. However, the pain specificity of free nerve endings cannot be absolutized, as they have also been found to be equally sensitive to cold, temperature, and touch, and there is even more information that other forms of receptors are also capable of sensing variable pain stimuli. The distribution density of pain receptors varies according to tissues, organs and sites, being most dense in the cornea and dental pulp, followed by the skin, and most sparse in muscles and viscera [15].

4.2.1.2 Characteristics of Visceral Pain Receptors

Visceral pain receptors are free endings of visceral sensory nerves, which are distributed on the perineurium, luminal walls, intertissues of visceral organs and the walls of vasculature entering visceral organ tissues. Visceral organs such as the heart, coronary vessels, lungs, gastrointestinal tract, urinary and reproductive systems contain Aδ fibers and C fibers. Visceral mechanoreceptors include annular lamellar vesicles, which are located in the mesentery and in the connective tissue surrounding the viscera.

Visceral pain receptors also have the same characteristics as general receptors, such as their own appropriate stimulus and threshold, transduction, encoding, and rhythmic discharge. The characteristic features of visceral pain receptors are that they have high excitation thresholds and produce little adaptation.

The nature of injurious receptors in different visceral organs is different, and the appropriate injurious stimuli are also different.

1. Thoracic organs

   Injury receptors in the heart are sympathetic afferent fiber endings that sense histamine, 5-HT, bradykinin and H^+ in the blood, which excite or sensitize sympathetic afferent fibers and produce pain.

   There are two types of injurious receptors in the lungs, one located around the capillaries and other located within the lung and bronchial epithelium. Pulmonary bruits, pulmonary embolism, pulmonary atelectasis, pneumothorax, and chemical stimuli can excite these receptors.
2. Digestive system organs

   The gastrointestinal tract has slow- and fast-response mechanoreceptors and chemoreceptors. Mechanoreceptors are located in the smooth muscles of the stomach, small intestine, large intestine, gallbladder,

bladder, uterus, and other cavernous organs. Excessive dilatation or spasm of the digestive tract can produce pain. Some afferent fibers reach the intestinal wall along the superior mesenteric artery and its branches and can respond to pulling on the mesenteric and visceral plasma membranes, contraction of smooth muscle, and distension of the viscera. There are also fibers distributed in the blood vessels, which can be excited by ischemia. C-polysensory receptors located in the rectal mucosa and anus respond to mechanical, thermal, and chemical stimuli.

Sympathetic nerves innervate the peritoneum on the surface of the liver and the blood vessels distributed in the liver. The rapid enlargement of the liver stretches the peritoneum on the surface of the liver and stimulates the afferent nerve fibers, which can produce pain. The peritoneum covering the surface of the pancreas also has sympathetic afferent fibers, which are mechanical receptors. The enlargement of the pancreas can cause pain, and pain sensitivity can occur when the receptor threshold is lowered in pancreatitis.

3. Urinary system organs

   The sympathetic nerve fiber endings that dominate the kidney contain injurious receptors, and pulling on the renal fascia and stimulating the renal parenchyma can cause pain. Injury receptors in the ureter are mainly C-fibers, which are particularly sensitive to pulling and spasm.

4. Genital organs

   The receptors in the prostate, ureter, ovary, uterus, and broad ligament are slow-reacting receptors, some of which respond to strong pressure, heat, and pain substances. C-polysensory receptors are widely distributed in the testis and epididymis and are slow to respond to pressure. Strong mechanical stimuli, noxious thermal stimuli, bradykinin and other pain substances, and hypertonic saline can excite them.

4.2.1.3 Injurious Stimuli and the Transduction of Injurious Receptors

1. Injurious stimulation

   When a certain threshold of stimulus intensity is exceeded, any stimulus can produce pain for most receptors. This particular threshold, called the injurious stimulus, can produce tissue damage, and this receptor is called the injurious receptor. Injury receptors are polymorphic and therefore can transduce different forms of injurious stimuli into action potentials. The main injurious stimuli that can cause visceral pain are smooth muscle spasm, dilation, ischemia, inflammation, chemical stimulation of hollow organs, mesenteric traction, compression, torsion, and direct nerve invasion due to envelope tension of substantial organs and malignant tumors. The most basic cause of visceral pain is ischemia and inflammation, while the destruction of visceral tissue itself does not cause pain, and the stimuli that can cause visceral pain are called visceral injurious stimuli.

2. The transduction of receptors

   The receptors receive injurious stimulus excitation, produce depolarization process, cause local potential changes, when the potential changes accumulate to the level of the threshold potential is generated action potential, also known as the generator potential, its potential amplitude and stimulus intensity, no latency, not affected by local anesthetics. The greater the receptor potential, the higher the frequency of afferent impulses elicited. The transduction of receptors allows the transformation of injurious stimuli into electrical activity on afferent nerves.

   The membrane permeability of receptor cells to Na^+, K^+, and Cl^- differs in the resting state, resulting in a difference in ion concentration inside and outside the cell membrane. When a receptor cell is stimulated, the membrane permeability to Na^+ increases, and the inward flow of Na^+ depolarizes the membrane potential and generates a receptor potential. In addition, K^+ and Cl^- are also involved in the occurrence of receptor potential.

The receptor potential is only a local potential, not an action potential. It differs from an action potential in that the receptor potential cannot be transmitted along the nerve fibers to distant areas, but only spreads to neighboring areas in the form of electrical tension spread, with a typical electrical tension decay: it does not appear in the "all" or "none" form, and the response is hierarchical, varying with the strength of the stimulus. The response is graded and varies in amplitude depending on the strength of the stimulus, and there is no inactivity period, and the response is not affected by local anesthetics or sodium blockers.

4.2.2 Visceral Pain Afferent to Nerve Fibers

The conduction of nerve fibers refers to the conduction of action potentials along the course of nerve fibers, and its conduction function has the following characteristics: insulating conduction, bidirectional conduction, non-attenuating conduction, fast conduction speed, and relatively non-fatiguing nature.

4.2.2.1 Visceral Pain Afferent Fibers

The neural regulation of visceral activity is all done by the autonomic nervous system, which is divided into two major parts: sympathetic and parasympathetic nervous systems [16]. The peripheral fibers that transmit visceral pain travel along the sympathetic and parasympathetic nerves, in which the sensory fibers in the sympathetic nerve are transmitted from the receptors of the viscera, along the sympathetic nerve fibers that travel through the paravertebral sympathetic ganglion in the white traffic branch, and from the posterior root into the posterior horn of the spinal ganglion of T_{1-3}, and the parasympathetic nerve travels in the ganglion and transmits to another neuron near the visceral organs, along the vagus nerve to the intracranial vagal nucleus or the parasympathetic nucleus of S_{2-4}.

1. Sympathetic nerves

   Sympathetic nerves are widely distributed in all organs, and almost all organs have sympathetic innervation. Sympathetic nerves originate from the lateral horn of the gray matter in the T_{1-3} and L_{1-3} nodes. The preganglionic fibers emanate from the lateral horn of the spinal cord and reach the paravertebral ganglion via the white traffic branch, forming the sympathetic trunk, where the preganglionic fibers form synaptic connections with the postganglionic fibers, and the postganglionic fibers are distributed to all organs. There are also a few preganglionic fibers that pass through the sympathetic trunk without replacing neurons until the prevertebral ganglion. Preganglionic fibers are called white traffic branches and are generally myelinated; postganglionic fibers lose their myelin sheaths and are called gray traffic branches. A single sympathetic preganglionic fiber often makes synaptic connections with multiple postganglionic neurons, allowing for a wide range of sympathetic activity. In general, different organs receive sympathetic fibers emanating from specific spinal cord segments, but there are interlocking innervation of nerve fibers coming from different segments in the same visceral organ, which determines the complexity of visceral pain symptoms.

2. Parasympathetic nerves

   The parasympathetic nerves come from the nuclei of the third, VII, IX, and X pairs of brain nerves in the brainstem and S_{2-4} are equivalent to the lateral horn parts of the gray matter. After the parasympathetic nerves are emitted from the center, they are replaced in the organ wall or in the plexus near the organ, and then send out postganglionic fibers to innervate the effector organs, so their preganglionic fibers are longer and postganglionic fibers are shorter. The parasympathetic nerves that innervate the thoracic viscera and the abdominal viscera above the splenic flexure of the transverse colon have preganglionic fibers that begin in the dorsal nucleus of the vagus nerve on both sides of the medulla and pass through the plexus in front of the spine and under the diaphragm, with the terminal fibers distributed next to the organs, where they form synapses with the shorter postganglionic fibers and are distributed to all organs. The parasympathetic nerves that innervate the colon, rectum, perineum, and bladder emanate from the S_{2-4} spinal cord segments and are distributed to the above organs along with the intrapelvic nerves.

4.2.2.2 Differences Between Visceral Pain Afferent Fibers and Somatic Pain Afferent Fibers

Dorsal root ganglia are found in the dorsal or posterior roots of all spinal nerves, and their central synapses are capable of transmitting sharp pain originating from specific cutaneous areas to the central nervous system via the corresponding spinal ganglia, and this one-to-one relationship allows sharp pain in the cutaneous area to produce a clear localization. Unlike sharp pain in the dermatomes, visceral pain is less closely related to the nerve roots. The segmental division of visceral pain is known as the spinal ganglion, and pain fibers emanating from one spinal ganglion enter the spinal cord through several posterior roots, thus producing more widespread or unlocalized pain. Moreover, the presence of interlocking innervation of nerve fibers coming from different segments in the same organ determines the complexity of visceral pain. Visceral pain is mainly conducted by C-fibers, which are unmyelinated nerve fibers with a higher excitation threshold, the thinnest and slowest conduction velocity, a more diffuse pain range, poorly localized, and insensitive to sharp stimulation, cutting and burning and touch and pressure, while mechanical pulling, distension, ischemia, spasm, inflammation, and chemical stimulation can cause severe pain, and these injurious stimuli are the main causes of visceral pain [17]. The pain is usually persistent and slow and has a distinct emotional overtone. Because visceral injurious stimuli can provoke central nervous system reactivity, visceral pain can trigger strong autonomic reflexes and skeletal muscle spasms.

4.2.2.3 Visceral Sensory Nerves

Visceral sensory nerve cells are found in the posterior horn of the spinal cord, and their axons travel in the autonomic nerves, with endings located in the viscera, the tracts of cavernous organs, and the perineurium of parenchymal organs, and are connected to the receptors of these organs. They can sense information about blood flow, tension, traction, kinking, tissue structure, chemical properties of vascular contents, etc. of visceral organs, and transmit the information to the center through visceral sensory nerve afferent fibers to produce sensation, which becomes the afferent part of the autonomic reflex arc. The posterior roots of visceral sensory nerves enter the spinal cord and travel up the same pathway as cutaneous nociception.

Various visceral sensory pathways composed of visceral sensory nerve afferent fibers are involved in the reflex regulation of visceral function.

1. Visceral-visceral reflex

   Reflexes that rely on visceral information for the regulation of visceral function are called visceral-visceral reflexes. Most of these reflexes are mediated by parasympathetic nerves.

   (a) Vagus reflex: It regulates the activity of visceral function and transmits gastric dilation and gastric filling. When the dilation and filling of the stomach is overloaded, it causes nausea and vomiting reflexes.
   (b) Intestinal reflex: It consists of afferent and efferent fibers of visceral nerves. It transmits nociception of the viscera and is often a common cause of intestinal paralysis after surgery or after nerve block, etc.
   (c) Parasympathetic pelvic reflex: It transmits the sensation of filling of the bladder and rectum, and reflexively regulates urination, defecation, and erection.

2. Viscerosomatic reflex

   The viscerosomatic reflex is a reflex of the somatic motor system caused by afferent information from visceral pain. For example, when appendicitis occurs, there is often tension in the affected abdominal muscles.

3. Somatovisceral reflex

The somatovisceral reflex refers to somatic sensations that can cause autonomic reflexes, such as stimulation of the skin that can cause visceral and vascular reflexes. When gastrointestinal spasmodic pain is present, warming the skin in a specific area can relieve the pain.

4.2.2.4 Excitability of Visceral Afferent Neurons

Voltage-sensitive ion channels are the basis for action potential formation, so the expression, properties, and density of these channels determine the excitability of neurons. Voltage-sensitive sodium channels (Na_V) are associated with the rapid rising phase of action potentials [18, 19]. At least six known subunits of sodium channels exist in primary afferent neurons, including Na_Vl.8 and Na_V1.9, which are not readily blocked by the neurotoxin-tetrodotoxin. In the dorsal root ganglion, Na_Vl.8 is mainly distributed in small-diameter neurons with demyelinated axons, and the latter plays an important role in the development of pain. It was found that the visceral pain behavior was significantly reduced in animals after knocking out the Na_Vl.8 gene. Other sodium channels have also been associated with altered neural excitability and the development of peripheral and/or central sensitization formation.

Multiple voltage-sensitive calcium channels are also present in visceral sensory neurons. Calcium ion flow activates calcium-dependent potassium channels and also triggers neurotransmitter release, which creates interneuronal messaging. Calcium ions can modulate protein kinase and phospholipase activities to act on different ion channels, ultimately altering the excitability of the cell membrane.

There are also several different potassium currents in visceral sensory neurons, including a specific transient potassium current, which is significantly reduced in gastrointestinal inflammation with visceral hypersensitivity, suggesting an important role of potassium channel expression and regulation in influencing visceral action potential timing and firing patterns.

In addition, many ligand-gated ion channels are involved in the mechanism of visceral pain, such as 5-hydroxytryptamine receptors and purinoceptors. Acid-sensitive ion channels have also been implicated in the development of visceral pain.

4.2.3 Visceral Pain Conduction Pathway

Afferent impulses from visceral injurious receptors terminate in the posterior horn of the spinal cord via the first-level neurons that conduct pain, which are initially integrated by the posterior horn neurons; the second-level neurons cross in the spinal cord to the opposite side and travel upward in the thalamic tract of the spinal cord within the lateral cords to reach the thalamus, where they are processed by the third-level neurons that project injurious information from the thalamus to the cerebral cortex, where they produce nociception.

4.2.3.1 Synapse-Mediated Conduction Mechanism

In the conduction pathway of visceral pain, neuron-to-neuron information transmission is based on neurosynapses, which ensure that neurons are functionally connected to each other [20]. According to the synaptic contact site, synapses can be divided into axon-dendritic synapses, axon-cytosolic synapses, Axon-axon synapse, dendrite-dendritic synapse, cytosolic-cytosolic synapse, dendrite-cytosolic synapse, and cytosolic-dendritic synapse; according to their effects on the activity of the next neurons, synapses can be divided into excitatory and inhibitory synapses; according to the nature of synaptic transmission, synapses can be divided into chemical, electrical, and mixed transmission synapses [21]. The synaptic connections in the CNS have four main types of contacts: spokes, aggregates, chains, and loops, in addition to single-wire connections.

The general characteristics of synaptic transmission are: unidirectional conduction, synaptic delay, summation, fatigue susceptibility, susceptibility to changes in the internal environment and drugs, and postrelease effects.

Synapses are characterized by excitatory postsynaptic potentials (EPSP) or inhibitory postsynaptic potentials (IPSP) via calcium-mediated release of synaptic transmitters, which manifest as excitation or inhibition of postsynaptic neurons.

4.2.3.2 Conduction Pathways

Nociceptive impulses from thoracic and abdominal organs are transmitted to the center via sympathetic nerves, while nociceptive impulses from pelvic organs are transmitted to the center via parasympathetic nerves. Visceral pain signals enter the posterior horn of the spinal cord via nociceptive afferent fibers and are transmitted to higher centers along the same pathways as cutaneous nociception. The transmission mechanisms and pathways are particularly complex, and the following pathways are related to visceral pain transmission but are not specific to visceral pain transmission bundles [22, 23].

1. Spinal thalamus bundle

   The spinal thalamic tract is a major pathway for the transmission of pain perception. The first two levels of neurons permute in the gray matter of the posterior horn of the spinal cord in plates IV–VIII and then ascend to the contralateral side via the anterior joint crossing, terminating in the thalamus. The lateral tract can be divided into lateral and ventral tracts. The lateral tract projects to cortical sensory areas via the internal capsule after permutation in the ventral posterior lateral nucleus of the thalamus, while the ventral tract has some fibers that project to a wide area of the brain and liaise with the hypothalamus and limbic system after permutation in the medullary nucleus of the thalamus via the brainstem reticular formation.

2. Spinal reticular tract

   The spinal reticular tract starts from the gray matter of the posterior horn of the spinal cord in the IV, V, and VII laminae, and is composed of short, multisynaptic fibers that travel ventrally upward from each medullary ganglion, with most fibers entering the ipsilateral reticular formation of the brainstem and a few fibers traveling contralaterally, before reaching the thalamus. The spinal reticular fasciculus is diffuse, receives extensive peripheral afferent convergence, often intermingles with some fibers of the anterior spinal thalamic fasciculus, and travels bilaterally to the nonspecific nuclei of the thalamus through the reticular switch neurons of the medulla oblongata.

3. Spinal cervical tract

   The fibers of the spinal cervical tract originate from the gray matter V and VI lamina cells in the posterior horn of the spinal cord and travel ipsilaterally up the dorsolateral side to the level of the $C_{1,2}$ nodes and the lower medulla oblongata, then turn contralaterally and enter the ventral posterior lateral nucleus of the thalamus, where they project to the cortical sensory areas.

4. Dorsal medial tract

   The dorsomedial tract originates mainly from cells in layer VI of the posterior horn of the spinal cord, with a few originating in layers V and VI. It ascends in the ipsilateral dorsal cord to the posterior column nucleus of the medulla oblongata (the nucleus of the thin tract and the nucleus of the cuneus), then turns contralaterally and enters the ventral lateral nucleus of the thalamus along the medial thalamus, where it projects to the cortical somatosensory areas.

5. Intrinsic tract of the spinal cord

   The intrinsic tracts of the spinal cord are short fibers surrounding the gray matter of the spinal cord, mainly responsible for liaising with the conduction between the nodes, and are the liaison system for the reflex mechanism of pain, which also has diffuse upward middle fibers, reaching the brainstem reticular formation and the thalamus via multi-level neurons.

6. Spinal cord midbrain tract

   Spinal cord injurious neuronal afferents cross over the spinal cord to the contralateral side and pass through many nuclei of the midbrain reticular formation to the thalamic specific and non-specific nuclei after conversion neurons. The distribution of spinal midbrain tract neurons varies widely among animal species, projecting to the cuneate nucleus, parabrachial nucleus, periaqueductal gray matter, interthalamic nucleus, deep superior colliculus, and red nucleus of the midbrain. Its cells include three categories of non-injury neurons, non-specific injury neurons and specific injury neurons.

7. Spinal cord parabrachial amygdala

   Spinal cord injurious information afferents are mainly terminated by the contralateral dorsolateral tract in the parabrachial nucleus, which then projects to the amygdala after converting neurons.

8. Spinal parabrachial hypothalamic tract

   Spinal cord injurious information afferents are mainly terminated by the contralateral dorsolateral tract in the parabrachial nucleus, which converts neurons and then projects to the hypothalamus. After the synapse in the parabrachial nucleus, secondary neuronal axons terminate in the ventral medial nucleus of the hypothalamus.

9. Spinal hypothalamic tract

   Spinal cord injurious stimulus afferents project directly to the ipsilateral hypothalamus and cross over to the contralateral hypothalamus, which is closely linked to the limbic system and plays an important role in the processing of information about the emotional component of nociception.

4.2.4 Characteristics of the Visceral Pain Centers and Their Information Transmission

4.2.4.1 Subcortical Centers

The subcortical structures related to pain mainly include the spinal cord, thalamus, hypothalamus, and some nuclei and neurons of the brainstem.

1. Spinal cord

   The spinal cord is the primary center for nociceptive signal processing. The signal of an injurious stimulus is transmitted from afferent fibers to the posterior horn of the spinal cord, where it is processed and partly caused by spinal reflexes and partly continued to be transmitted. The spinal cord can perceive injurious stimuli, respond to injurious stimuli, and play a regulatory role for injurious stimuli.

2. Related nuclei of the thalamus

   The thalamus is composed of six major nuclei, some of which are involved in pain mechanisms. The nuclei that are closely related to pain transmission are the medial nucleus and the posterior lateral nucleus of the lateral nucleus, the posterior medial nucleus and the parabrachial nucleus and central nucleus of the medullary plate. The frequency and time course of neuronal firing in the thalamic nuclei are proportional to the change in stimulus intensity, so they can quantitatively reflect external stimuli. These neurons encode information about the site, extent, intensity, and timing of peripheral stimuli to the cortex and have a nociceptive discrimination function. The thalamus is the most important integration center before various sensory information enters the cerebral cortex to form the primary sensation, receiving projections from the spinal cord and brainstem, relaying and then projecting to the cerebral cortex. It can respond to injurious stimuli, regulate nociception, and is also involved in the emotional response to nociception.

3. Hypothalamus

   Some nuclei in the hypothalamus contain nociceptive nerves that are excitatory or inhibitory in response to injurious stimuli, and these neurons play a role, to a greater or lesser extent, in the regulation of pain. The hypothalamus consists of three major nuclei groups according to cell size: (1) the preoptic nucleus, funicular nucleus, dorsomedial nucleus, inferior anterior nucleus, and periventricular nucleus, which are composed of two small cells; (2) the ventral medial nucleus, lateral nodal nucleus, and papillary body nucleus, which are composed of three medium-sized cells; and (3) the supraoptic nucleus, paraventricular nucleus, dorsal nucleus, and posterior nucleus, which are composed of four large cells.

4. Brainstem reticular formation

   The reticular formation of the brainstem is located in the median brain, pons and midbrain, and is divided into the median, medial, and lateral parts. The nuclei in it are, from bottom to top, the extended reticular nucleus, pontine reticular nucleus, pontine covered reticular nucleus, cuneate nucleus, subcuneate nucleus, and pedunculopontine covered nucleus. The nuclei of the extended brain segment have cardiovascular and respiratory centers, as well as vomiting and swallowing centers. The brainstem reticular formation is where multiple sensory afferent impulses converge and is an important nociceptive regulator, and this structure has an important role in the regulation and integration of central nociception.

4.2.4.2 Higher Centers

The cerebral cortex is the higher center for sensory discrimination and response initiation integration of pain. Pain processes involve a wide range of areas, and pain impulses necessarily enter the domain of consciousness. The following cortical areas are generally considered to be involved in the whole process of pain.

1. First sensory area

   The first sensory area, i.e., areas 3, 1, and 2 of the postcentral gyrus, is distributed according to the inverted projection of the human body and mainly receives projection fibers from the ventral posterior nucleus of the thalamus, which is the sensory discrimination area of pain and is more explicit in the discrimination of pain on the surface of the body.

2. Second sensory area

   The second sensory area is the lowest part of the postcentral gyrus, the area between the precentral gyrus and the insula, and its body projection is distributed transversely, with the anterior end being the head and the caudal end in order, mainly receiving projections from the old spinal thalamic tracts relayed by the thalamus, with bilateral nature, and is related to visceral pain.

3. Third sensory area

   The third sensory area is the precentral gyrus. This area is a motor auxiliary area and also receives fiber projections from the thalamus and is involved in deep sensory discrimination and pain response activities.

4. Limbic system

   The limbic system includes the cingulate gyrus, hook gyrus, hippocampal gyrus, and related structures of the limbic system. The process of pain is closely related to this area and is associated with the strong emotional changes that accompany pain, especially the modulation of visceral pain and psychogenic pain. Stimulation of some areas of the limbic system increases the pain threshold and produces analgesic effects.

   The visceral projection area is the narrowest in the range of pain projections to the cerebral cortex. The response initiation system of pain and the integrated modulation of pain are activities in which a wide range of cortical areas are jointly involved in the interaction; therefore, the division of labor and localization of brain cortical areas are relative.

4.2.4.3 Characteristics of Visceral Information Central Transmission

1. Afferent nerve fibers from individual viscera can excite many spinal neurons, and most of these neurons receive projections from neighboring segments.
2. The stimulus-response curve induced by cavernous organ expansion is monotonically increasing with increasing pressure in both the non-injurious pressure range and the supraphysiological range.
3. Most spinal neurons, activated by visceral mechanical stimulation, also respond to chemical stimuli.
4. Visceral information is not transmitted through unique spinal channels, but through well-recognized somatosensory channels.
5. Somato-visceral convergence is common, somatic receptive fields often include injurious

components, and the segmental nature of somato-visceral convergence is the basis of referred pain.

6. Inflammation of visceral organs can lead to central sensitization of neurons in the posterior horn of the spinal cord when visceral and somatic input signals appear to be susceptible and may play an important role in the phenomenon of implicated nociceptive hyperalgesia.
7. The central transmission of visceral information is controlled by the downstream inhibitory system, and the activity of visceral afferent nerves can activate inhibition in different segments.

4.3 Perception and Regulation of Visceral Pain

4.3.1 Feeling Characteristics of Different Organs

1. Cavernous viscera

   Injury receptors exist in the smooth muscle walls of cavernous viscera such as the gastrointestinal tract, bile duct, uterus, ureter, and bladder. They show a moderate discharge response to active contraction of smooth muscle or dilatation of the organ. When the cavernous organ is obstructed, the smooth muscle undergoes isometric contraction and the discharge frequency of these receptors increases significantly and causes colic.
2. Heart

   Nociceptive information from the heart is transmitted via sympathetic nerves, not the vagus nerve. Myocardial ischemia due to coronary artery obstruction and the accumulation and hyperosmolarity of local chemicals such as adenosine, bradykinin, histamine, prostaglandins, 5-HT, potassium ions, lactate, etc. during myocardial contraction are suitable stimuli for cardiac nociceptive receptors.
3. Lung

   Both intracapillary and transcapillary receptors and pulmonary irritant receptors in the lungs are connected to nociceptive afferent fibers and are transmitted to the center via the vagus nerve. Pulmonary bruising, embolism, pulmonary atelectasis, pneumothorax, and irritant gas inhalation can activate these receptors and induce dyspnea and pain, and can reflexively cause bradycardia, shortness of breath, or apnea.
4. Other organs

   Pain receptors in the liver, kidney, spleen, and mesentery are mostly distributed on the peritoneum of the corresponding organ surface. They are not sensitive to sharp stimuli such as knife, needle, fire, etc., but react strongly to blunt stimuli such as pulling, rubbing, and swelling. They are often accompanied by nausea, vomiting, reflex bradycardia, or severe referred pain.

4.3.2 Central Sensory Characteristics

In the process of nociceptive sensation in the central nervous system, the centers at all levels have their own characteristics.

4.3.2.1 Performance of Pain Conduction Tracts

The nerve bundles that conduct pain also carry other sensory signals, and their travel and projection are not direct and have their specific limited forms.

1. Lateral conduction system

   The lateral conduction system includes the neospinothalamic tract, the spinal conduction tract, and the spinal cervical tract. They mainly project to the cortical sensory areas, and their common features are fewer permutations, more direct, faster conduction, and a localized projection conduction system. The neospinothalamic tract is larger, more sensitive to pain signals, and more discriminative; while the postsynaptic fibers of the spinal conduction tract can discharge continuously at high frequencies to injurious stimuli; the spinal cervical tract responds to injurious mechanical and temperature stimuli and has two points of discrimination.

2. Medial conduction system

   The medial conduction system includes the spinal reticular tract, the old spinal thalamic tract, and the intrinsic spinal tract, collectively referred to as the paracentral system. The common features are short fibers, multi-level neurons, diffuse pathways, slow conduction, ambiguous localization, and responses to injurious stimuli, with response frequency increasing with stimulus intensity and visceral and emotional-behavioral responses.

   There are many synaptic connections between these two conduction systems, so there are also mechanisms of interaction between their activities, as shown by the inhibitory effect of the lateral system on the medial system and the compensatory effect of the medial system on the lateral system, such that when the lateral system is blocked, pain impulses can still be transmitted to the center, which is a substitute for the medial system. The functions of the pain conduction tracts are not each individually manifested; their respective branches contact each other during transmission and converge and radiate at each synaptic level, and project in multiple directions, thus producing complex effects.

4.3.2.2 Performance of Subcortical Centers

1. Thalamus

   The thalamus is the main subcortical center for pain, in which both the central and parabasal nuclei receive slow pain projections from C-fibers of the brainstem reticular formation and can discriminate the temporal concept of pain, and is the most important nociceptive integration center in the brain.

2. Hypothalamus

   Some nuclei of the hypothalamus have pain-sensitive neurons, which present excitatory and inhibitory responses to injurious stimuli, along with emotional and visceral responses, and chronic pain also affects its regulation of the endocrine system.

3. The limbic system

   The limbic system has the function of receiving and modulating pain information. Pain impulses are projected from the limbic system to the cerebral cortex to produce the experience of pain and psychological responses. When the pain impulse is transmitted downward from the limbic system, it regulates the degree of instinctive emotional response.

4. Brainstem reticular formation

   The brainstem reticular formation is both a pathway for pain transmission and a low-level center for pain, with the medial part being the integration and effector areas and the lateral part being the sensory contact areas. Pain signals are regulated here (euphoria or inhibition) and are especially important for the visceral responses (changes in respiratory rhythm, heart rate, heart rhythm, blood pressure, and vomiting) triggered by the visceral centers (respiratory, cardiovascular, and vomiting) therein.

4.3.2.3 Performance of Higher Centers

The cerebral cortex has the function of sensory discrimination and response initiation to pain signals. The pain signal actually undergoes the whole process of perception, integration, modulation, and organismal response (including psychological response) in the cerebral cortex. These cortical activities are extensive, with the joint participation of many functional areas, including visual, auditory, olfactory, taste, and experiential memory, in addition to the cortices of sensory and motor areas. The localization of their functions is only relative and generally tends to be divided as follows.

1. Sensory discrimination system

   The sensory discrimination system mainly discriminates the form, nature, space, and intensity of pain. The postcentral gyrus has the discrimination of the form of painful stimuli, such as stabbing, cutting, burning, squeezing, and swelling. The precentral gyrus has the discrimination of pain space, which can identify the presence of stimulus, the site and the level of stimulus. The posterior lateral area of the postcentral gyrus can identify the intensity of pain, i.e., the degree of lightness, severity, intensity, etc. of pain.

2. Response initiation system

   The visceral pain response is driven by the limbic system, hypothalamus, brainstem reticular formation, and other central systems, and appears as a response and dysfunction of the autonomic, endocrine, humoral biochemical and even immune systems.

3. Cortical liaison system

   The functional areas of the cerebral cortex during pain are closely connected to each other through various lines, and the nerve fibers of these connections include the following three parts.

   (a) Connecting fibers: They are the lateral fibers that connect the two hemispheres with each other, including the anterior and posterior pincers of the corpus callosum and the blanket, which are connected to the frontal, parietal, parietal and occipital parts of the two hemispheres, followed by the anterior and posterior unions.
   (b) Contact fibers: They are the fibers connecting the cortices of this hemisphere, including the superior and inferior tracts, superior and inferior fronto-occipital tracts, cingulate tracts and hook tracts, which connect the functional areas of the lobes of this hemisphere, respectively.
   (c) Short fibers: There are also some "U"- or "V"-shaped proximal fibers, which are connected to the intercortical gyrus.

   The pain signals directed to the cerebral cortex can come from non-invasive forms in addition to directly intervening injurious stimuli, such as when an injurious stimulus is perceived by special senses such as sight, sound, smell or taste before contact or intervention, immediately awakening the conditioned reflexes of the cerebral cortex and producing nociception or increasing the intensity of pain in advance, as well as producing a visceral response to pain.

4.3.3 Regulatory Mechanisms of Visceral Pain

4.3.3.1 Feedback Regulation of Receptors

Nociceptive receptors can produce a series of nerve impulses and transmit them to the center along certain afferent nerve pathways after suitable stimulation, but the activities of the receptors themselves and their conduction parts are often regulated by the feedback of the central nervous system. Nociceptive impulses can be influenced by the activity of the peripheral part of the nervous system at their origin, which usually shows a positive inhibition process, and the nociceptive transmission pathway is often under the influence of this nervous inhibition. Negative feedback modulation of nociceptive receptors with cortical involvement prevents the production of excessive pain and allows a number of potential nociceptive components to be attenuated or eliminated in the early stages of central nociceptive modulation.

4.3.3.2 Inter-synaptic Inhibition

Inter-synaptic inhibition processes arise mainly at two different parts of the synapse: presynaptic inhibition and postsynaptic inhibition [24, 25]. The CNS exerts various inhibitory activities through these two forms of inhibition.

1. Presynaptic inhibition

   The release of inhibitory transmitters on the presynaptic membrane during excitation of the interneuron causes partial depolarization of the presynaptic membrane by opening Cl^- channels, resulting in a decrease in the membrane potential and a decrease in the peak action potential generated by the subsequent nerve impulses reaching the presynaptic membrane, and a decrease in the release of excitatory transmitters, which is not sufficient to excite the postsynaptic neuron and exhibits an inhibitory effect. In this case, the excitability of the postsynaptic membrane is not altered and no inhibitory postsynaptic potentials are generated, but only changes in presynaptic membrane properties are manifested.

2. Postsynaptic inhibition

   Changes in the properties of the postsynaptic membrane result in inhibitory postsynaptic potentials, causing the center to exhibit inhibitory effects. The process is that an excitatory neuron first excites an inhibitory neuron, which releases inhibitory neurotransmitters that act on other neurons to inhibit their activity. The significance of the presence of postsynaptic inhibition is that through its negative feedback control, neuronal activity can be terminated in time, promoting a consistent pace of activity among many neurons within the same central level.

4.3.3.3 Convergence

Despite the relative specificity of peripheral sensory neurons to perceive stimuli of different properties, afferent impulses evoked by stimuli of different properties or originating from different sites can converge in the same neuron at all levels of the central sensory transmission pathway, a phenomenon called convergence. The nerve cell in which convergence occurs requires a stronger level of stimulation or a greater number of afferent fibers to be stimulated at the same time in order to be excited. Incoming impulses via this neuron may lack precise localization information or even be mislocalized (entrapment pain).

4.3.3.4 Multisynaptic Transmission

The nociceptive non-specific conduction system in the spinal cord is a multisynaptic transmission pathway. Nociceptive afferent impulses travel up the spinal cord via many short fibers in succession, so that the excitation of one neuron causes the excitation or inhibition of many neurons at the same time through polysynaptic connections, expanding the range of influence. This multisynaptic transmission within the center allows for a large spatial expansion of excitation and a long duration. Multisynaptic transmission makes the localization of pain unclear, and the influence of different sources of impulses on each other makes the information from the same source uploaded by different pathways, causing different effects.

4.3.4 Modulation of Nociception by the Central Nervous System at All Levels

The whole process of pain is always under the regulation of the organism itself, which is in a sense a defense mechanism or a "compensatory" mechanism in a certain range of the organism against injurious stimuli. The pain modulation activities involve all levels of centers and synaptic transmission from the cerebral cortex to the spinal cord, but they differ in scope and mode.

4.3.4.1 Cortical Modulation

The cerebral cortex is the highest-level center for nociceptive integration and perception. Sensory areas of the cortex selectively inhibit the projective effects of injurious stimuli, which is particularly significant in chronic pain. It has been found that the cerebral cortex does inhibit the activity of pain neurons in subcortical centers, which can alter pain recognition processes through downstream modulation of the corticospinal tract and can also influence the activity of dorsal horn neurons through brainstem transit. The limbic system is not only involved in the formation of pain-emotion response processes but also has the function of modulating information afferents in the pain response mechanism and presents a downward inhibitory effect through its downward transmission.

4.3.4.2 Modulation of the Mesencephalon

Many nuclei located in the subcortex have a significant modulatory effect on pain. Some nuclei in the hypothalamus contain pain-sensitive neurons that are sensitive to injurious stimuli and are involved in the excitation or inhibition of pain. Stimulation of the anterior, middle, posterior, and supraoptic nuclei of the hypothalamus increases the pain threshold and produces significant pain suppression, with the supraoptic nucleus having a more pronounced effect. The central nucleus of the thalamus can inhibit the pain discharge of its adjacent parabrachial nucleus. This inhibition is actually the result of the central nucleus fibers inhibiting the cortical excitatory effect on the parabrachial nucleus, or the central nucleus producing the pain suppression effect through the modulation of the parabrachial nucleus by the caudal nucleus. The thalamus is the most important integrating center for pain modulation.

4.3.4.3 Modulation of the Brainstem

The brainstem is the center of the endogenous nociceptive modulation system, and the function of brainstem structures is more prominent in the downstream modulation mechanism of pain. The dorsal reticulospinal system, which originates from the medial part of the inferior brainstem reticular formation, has a downward inhibitory effect, a tonic inhibition that inhibits the response of posterior horn interneurons and superior tract transmission cells to injurious afferents.

The central gray matter of the midbrain and the median suture macronucleus of the delayed brain and its adjacent reticular formation and the reticular formation of the dorsolateral nucleus of the pons are thought to be specific nociceptive systems. This system receives both downward impulses from higher centers and upward impulses from the spinal cord; therefore, it selectively inhibits both the upward transmission of pain impulses and analgesic modulation by higher centers, whose downward pain-modulating fibers are mainly those of the central gray matter, the nucleus accumbens, and the reticular giant cell nucleus. Both can suppress pain and enhance it through antinociceptive inhibition.

While the brainstem reticular formation inhibits the electrical activity of dorsal horn pain transmission neurons, neurons that respond to non-injurious stimuli are not inhibited, and even if a strong analgesic effect occurs, it does not affect other sensory or motor processes. This analgesic effect is not only highly selective, but also characterized by a distinct somatic subdomain structure. The injurious brainstem downstream system selectively controls the upward transmission of injurious information into the brain, while being subject to downstream modulation by higher brain analgesic structures. Thus, the brainstem pain control system can be agonized by higher centers or exert pain suppression by negative feedback mechanisms agonized by peripheral inputs.

4.3.4.4 Modulation of the Spinal Cord

The spinal cord is both the first point of transmission of information from injurious stimuli to higher centers and the first point of integration and modulation of nociception before the information from injurious stimuli enters the higher centers. The spinal mechanisms of pain are important in neurotheology, neurophysiology, and neurological life.

The spinal cord has an extremely strong analgesic and nociceptive function, reducing or blocking the transmission of injurious information to the center through the gate effect, presynaptic inhibition, feedforward inhibition, and postsynaptic inhibition of upward projecting neurons, allowing pain relief. Pain signals are modulated in the spinal cord before they enter the higher centers, i.e., the amount, nature, and timing of pain information is regulated, transformed, or controlled. This function of the spinal cord is concentrated in the glial region of the posterior horn of the spinal cord, where the glial cells are central to the modulatory effect within each segment of the spinal cord, and is also subject to downstream modulation by higher centers.

4.3.5 Nociceptive Hypersensitivity

The phenomenon of reduced nociceptive threshold is called nociceptive sensitization. Sensitization refers to an increase in the intensity of the response. It is often manifested by increased activity in the resting state and decreased response thresholds in high-threshold visceral afferent fibers. Nociceptive sensitization is an important feature of tissue injury and inflammation and is also seen in the context of neuropathy. Most mechanosensitive visceral afferent fibers show sensitization in response to hollow organ guarding after preemptive non-injurious stimulation. This suggests that: sensitization of visceral afferent fibers can occur without tissue injury or inflammation; visceral sensory nerves are highly plastic and can undergo rapid and reversible excitability changes that may lead to changes in visceral sensation.

4.3.5.1 Peripheral and Central Mechanisms of Pain Sensitization

Both peripheral and central mechanisms are involved in the development of visceral sensitization. Injurious stimulation of peripheral injurious receptors releases chemical transmitters such as bradykinin, histamine, 5-HT, and prostaglandins, resulting in sensitization of injurious receptors, generating more nerve impulses to the central nervous system and increasing the excitability of central neurons at the level of the spinal cord, thus allowing previously injurious stimuli to be felt as more painful and forming visceral sensitization. The damaged nerve can produce high-frequency clustered discharges in the absence of any external stimulus, leading to nociceptive hypersensitivity and sensory abnormalities. During chronic pain, abnormal changes in nociceptive transmission ion channels and receptors occur, and abnormal expression and ectopic distribution of sodium channels, potassium channels, and calcium channels in nerve axons may occur, with a large number of ectopic and spontaneous non-coding afferent discharges contributing to nociceptive hypersensitivity and sensory abnormalities.

Activation of spinal excitatory amino acid receptors and their downstream effectors can cause central sensitization. Injury receptors are repeatedly and chronically stimulated prompting pathological changes in spinal dorsal horn cells, and glial cells and others are involved in the synthesis of new neurotransmitters and modulation of existing transmitters, leading to the integration of spinal dorsal horn and involvement in the formation of visceral nociceptive sensitization. The rostral ventromedial medulla (RVM) at the cephalic end of the medulla oblongata is an important site of the downstream conduction pathway regulating spinal nociception, which is involved in the formation and maintenance of central sensitization at the spinal cord level [26, 27]. It is involved in the formation of visceral nociceptive sensitization mainly through excitatory amino acid receptors, opioid receptors, and cholecystokinin receptors.

Unlike other forms of somatic sensation, nociception does not produce rapid adaptation to delayed stimuli, because sustained stimuli can produce stronger injurious sensations or can reduce the threshold or intensity of the stimulus.

4.3.5.2 Generation of Central Sensitization

Central sensitization is the increased excitability produced by the input impulses to peripheral injurious receptors, resulting in hypersensitivity to subsequent prick withdrawal. Activation of injurious receptors by electrical stimulation of fine afferent nerves, noxious stimuli, inflammation, or tissue damage, as well as increased ectopic peripheral dense impulses to nerves and posterior root ganglia, cause dorsal horn neurons to become hyperexcitable, resulting in an enlarged receptive area, increased amplitude and duration of response to suprathreshold stimuli and lowered thresholds. All these factors will cause enhanced activity of supraspinal neurons and produce central sensitization.

In low frequency, repetitive injurious receptor inputs, the Aδ fibers and C fibers of dorsal horn neurons produce slow synaptic potentials, and the sum of these slow potentials produces a progressive increase and sustained depolarization of posterior horn neurons. At the same time, axon terminals of spinal cord injury receptors release excitatory amino acid mediators and neuropeptides, which cause further depolarization by opening ion channels through complex second messenger action.

4.3.5.3 Primary and Secondary Nociceptive Hypersensitivity

Nociceptive hypersensitivity occurs not only at the site of injury but also in the surrounding uninjured area. Nociceptive allergy in the injured area is called primary nociceptive allergy, and nociceptive allergy in the uninjured area around the injury is called secondary nociceptive allergy.

Primary nociceptive hypersensitivity is the result of inflammation or stimulation of nerve endings in the damaged tissue by local mediators and chemical factors that increase the conduction sensitivity of primary sensory neurons of high threshold injury receptors as a direct result of altering the sensitivity of the peripheral endings of the damaged tissue. Injury receptor thresholds are reduced and sensitization to injurious stimuli occurs. The sensory field of the injure receptors extends to the adjacent area of the injury site, and due to this extension, more fibers can be activated by injurious stimuli after the injury, and this spatial summation produces more severe pain. Primary nociceptive hypersensitivity may be the result of injury to a low-threshold mechanoreceptor, leading to loss of central inhibition of injurious receptor input and thus enhanced pain.

Secondary nociceptive hypersensitivity has no reduction in nociceptive threshold and is characterized by significant nociception in the secondary nociceptive hypersensitive areas compared to normal sensory areas in response to an intense stimulus, resulting in enhanced pain that lasts no longer than 24 h. The extended sensitizing effect of injury receptors may be one of the mechanisms of secondary nociceptive sensitization. Activation of one injury receptor leads to the release of chemicals like substance P, which activates neighboring injury receptors, leading to the further release of chemicals and activation of additional injury receptors, producing secondary nociceptive sensitization. The generation of secondary nociceptive sensitization may be due to the diffusion of central excitation.

4.3.5.4 Hyperalgesia Due to Psychological Factors

Pain in visceral disease is influenced by psychological processes so that negative psychological effects are bound to increase the intensity of visceral pain, and this increased intensity is the psychologically induced hyperalgesic effect, often influenced by the patient's social role, family status, living conditions, personality tendencies, and temperament type.

Emotional behaviors such as stress, anxiety, preoccupation, and cognition can influence pain produced by peripheral events through neuromodulation in the cortex, amygdala, hypothalamus, and other brain parts, thus altering the pain experience.

The nature, extent, and duration of pain in this condition are difficult to explain by the pathological mechanism of the lesion and the use of analgesics alone does not produce the desired effect, accompanied by tension, anxiety, fear, or depression. It is classified into the following types according to its clinical characteristics.

1. Focal value-added type

   Patients over-exaggerate the degree of pathological pain of the actual lesion, and often have obvious "role disorder" and emotional coloring, with anxiety, tension, fear, and other emotional changes. This type is often seen in patients with sudden lesions, accidental injuries, and accidental trauma.
2. Lesion association type

   The lesion site and pathological mechanism are not likely to cause pain, but the patient's psychological association produces pain symptoms, such as gallbladder polyps, gastrointestinal polyps, benign tumors, etc. These diseases usually do not cause pain when they are not combined with other lesions or changes, so the pain in this case is the result of psychological association.
3. Memory replay type

   The original treated lesion or lesion has been removed, but the patient still has episodes of the original pain, or still feels the presence of the original organ.
4. Psychological rejection type

   All patients who receive allogeneic tissue or organ transplantation have immune rejection, which is physiological rejection, but at the same time, the patient also has a psychological rejection of the allogeneic tissue or organ, which is psychological rejection, manifested as chronic persistent pain or paroxysmal aggravation of the recipient site, and the pain cannot be explained by surgical trauma.

4.4 Pathophysiological Mechanisms of Visceral Pain

4.4.1 Neurophysiological Mechanisms of Visceral Pain

Some of the neurophysiological mechanisms of visceral pain have been discussed in the Sect. 4.2, and the mechanisms of signal transduction receptors and channels in the neurotransmission pathway of visceral pain are described below.

1. Acid-sensitive ion channel (ASIC)

   ASIC belongs to a member of the NaC/DEG family. Currently, six ASIC subunits (ASIC1a, ASIC1b, ASIC2a, ASIC2b, ASIC3, ASIC4) have been identified, which are highly expressed in receptor neurons in the peripheral and central nervous system [28, 29]. These channels have a function in mechanoreceptive signal transduction and play a crucial role in nociceptive sensation in particular. Inflammation induces transcription of this ion channel and generates post-transcriptional regulation, which affects neuronal excitability and participates in the sensitization process of nociceptive sensation.

   The six subunits of the ASIC family can form homomeric or heteromeric acid-sensitive ion channels, which exhibit different current phenotypes and channel properties. In contrast, the homodimers formed by ASIC2b or ASIC4 are nonfunctional, and they generally act as auxiliary or regulatory subunits to form heterodimers with other subunits.

   ASIC1a is widely expressed in the brain, spinal cord, and dorsal root ganglia, and its homodimeric channel is highly H^+-sensitive and the current exhibits only a rapid inactivation component. The channel is mainly permeable to Na^+, but is also permeable to Ca^{2+}. ASIC1b, a splice variant of ASIC1a, is expressed only in the dorsal root ganglion, and this channel has similar H^+ sensitivity and kinetic properties to ASIC1a, but it is permeable only to Na^+. ASIC2a is expressed in the brain, spinal cord, and dorsal root ganglion, and it is less sensitive to H^+ and has no steady-state current component. ASIC2b, a splice variant of ASIC2a, is widely distributed in vivo and is expressed in both brain and dorsal root ganglia; the homodimer of this subunit is nonfunctional and is usually co-expressed as an auxiliary subunit with other subunits into a heterodimer. ASIC4 is also widely distributed and does not form a functional homodimeric channel.

   Because tissue acidification is directly related to nociception, ASIC is thought to have an important role in nociceptive triggering or modulation.
2. Transient receptor potential channel (TRP channel)

   The TRP channel is an important class of cation channels located in the cell membrane. In mammals, 28 subtypes of TRP channels have been identified, belonging to six subfamilies, with different regulatory mechanisms and a wide range of functions.

   TRP channels have six transmembrane structural domains, as well as N and C termini located in the cytosol. TRP channels are nonselective cation channels, with Ca^{2+} and Na^+ as the main passing ions, but different TRP channels have different selectivity ratios for the two ions.

   The regulation of channels, including activation and inactivation, i.e., the opening or closing of channels. The activation mechanisms of various TRP channels can be classified as receptor activation, ligand activation, temperature change activation, osmolarity change activation, voltage-dependent activation, etc.
3. Temperature receptors

   Some TRP channels are also temperature-sensitive, which is the basis for sensory nerve cells to respond to injurious heat sensations. These channels have different temperature activation thresholds and are expressed in primary sensory neurons and in some tissues. Six temperature-related channels have been identified in mammals in recent years, four of which are members of the V subfamily of TRP channels. These channels have a very wide tissue distribution and are functionally calcium-permeable channels.

4. Sodium channels

   Neurological sodium channels can be divided into fast and slow channels in terms of current and action potential duration; they can be divided into riverine toxin-sensitive and riverine toxin-insensitive sodium channels according to their sensitivity to riverine toxin. The sodium channel is mainly a transmembrane glycoprotein consisting of a subunit constituting the pore and two accessory β subunits [30]. At least nine genes have been identified encoding voltage-gated sodium channel α subunits, named $Na_V1.1$ to $Na_V1.9$; and three β subunits, named β_1, β_2, and β_3. Voltage-gated sodium channels $Na_V1.8$ and $Na_V1.9$ are specifically expressed in the peripheral nervous system, mostly in injurious sensory neurons, and are targets for analgesic drug action. $Na_V1.7$, $Na_V1.3$, and a β subtype (β3) are upregulated in certain neuropathic pains, enhancing neuronal excitability and pain sensitivity. Sodium channel-blocking drugs such as lidocaine and snail toxin can attenuate or even eliminate acute pain, inflammatory pain, and neuropathic pain.

5. Potassium channels

   Mammalian potassium channels are composed of four transmembrane alpha subunits and four beta subunits within the membrane [31]. Potassium channels play an important role in maintaining the resting potential of neurons and regulating their excitability and response properties. Potassium channels mainly regulate membrane depolarization, resting potential, frequency of nerve impulse delivery, and release of neurotransmitters from sensory neurons. In neuropathic pain, potassium channels are differentially regulated at the transcriptional level, and K^+ currents play a role in determining pain threshold. Altered potassium channel expression after peripheral nerve injury is associated with excitation of the dorsal root ganglion and chronic pain.

6. Calcium channels

   At least six types of voltage-sensitive calcium channels (VSCC) exist in mammalian nerve tissue. Different subtypes of VSCCs are jointly involved in, and coordinate, the secretory activity of synapses. Activation of calcium channels results in Ca^{2+} inward flow and neuronal depolarization thereby altering synaptic receptors, cell membrane excitability, second and third messenger concentrations, and gene expression. These phenomena are present in normal injurious responses, primary or secondary nociceptive hypersensitivity, and painful responses to innocuous stimuli, and VSCC blockers, especially N-type VSCC blockers, inhibit the generation or development of these processes. N-type calcium channels play an important role in the generation and maintenance of secondary thermal nociceptive hypersensitivity. Voltage-gated calcium channels have an important role in the pathogenesis of neuropathic pain and have become targets for the analgesic effects of a wide variety of drugs.

4.4.2 Endogenous Biochemical Mechanisms of Visceral Pain

The neurotransmitters/modulators involved in the sensation and regulation of visceral pain include almost all neurotransmitters/modulators of the central and peripheral nervous system, such as acetylcholine, monoamines (5-HT, histamine, dopamine, epinephrine, norepinephrine), amino acids (γ-aminobutyric acid, glycine, glutamate, aspartate), peptides (endorphins, enkephalins, substance P, prostaglandins), and other neurotransmitters. Endogenous biochemical substances such as inorganic salts (K^+, H^+, Ca^{2+}) and adenosine (ATP, ADP, AMP). The properties of the main biochemical substances and their mechanisms of action are described below.

1. Substance P

   Substance P is a peptide composed of 11 amino acids, which can cause contraction of the isolated intestine and is not blocked by atropine, and is the most abundant among all hormones in the intestine.

Substance P has a dual effect on pain signaling: it is an excitatory mediator in afferent neurons and is an excitatory mediator for injurious afferent fibers of primary sensory neurons, with a high content in C fibers; it decreases pain sensitivity in higher central nerves and their downstream regulatory pathways. The release of substance P from peripheral terminals in response to reverse stimulation of sensory nerves causes vasodilatation, increased permeability of the canal wall, and plasma protein spillover in peripheral tissues, independent of sympathetic activity, and may even be inhibited by sympathetic activity. A small dose of substance P activates endorphin neurons, thus suggesting that substance P itself is not an endogenous morphine-like substance and can cross the blood-brain barrier, but its analgesic effect in the brain requires the involvement of the opioid receptor pathway.

In the spinal cord, substance P is involved in primary afferents to injurious stimuli, and afferent injury receptors lead to the release of substance P from the dorsal horn of the spinal cord, which is enhanced by the concomitant release of calcitonin gene-related peptide (CGRP). Substance P/NK1 receptors are an important pathway mediating spinal nociception, and high doses of morphine can counteract substance P-induced nociception through its analgesic mechanism. Substance P and NMDA are synergistic in increasing the excitability of spinal convergent neurons, and substance P enhances the excitatory amino acid pathway. Substance P and its metabolite P (5–11) act on NK1 receptors and are involved in the formation of nociceptive sensitization at the spinal cord level. They also act on sites other than NK1 receptors through themselves and their metabolite P (1–7), leading to a down-regulation of NK1 receptors, thus counteracting the pain-sensitive effect, and activating opioid receptors with an analgesic effect.

In conclusion, substance P is a very actively studied neuropeptide, which is very closely related to the processing of pain information, but also very complex. Substance P has an important role in the generation of injury information in peripheral tissues, in the primary afferent processes of injury signals, and in the processing of pain information in the spinal cord and brain. The functional variation of substance P varies widely in chronic pain disorders of different etiologies, which can exhibit analgesic properties as well as nociceptive and nociceptive properties, suggesting its involvement in different pain disorders through different mechanisms.

2. Endogenous morphine-like substances (MLF)

There are more than 18 neuropeptides with morphine activity in the brain, called MLF, which are widely distributed [32]. MLF can be synthesized in various parts of the body, but cannot cross the blood-brain barrier. MLF in the central nervous system is an important biochemical substance that controls pain transmission, and its content increases when the body is subjected to injurious stimuli, and it acts with neurons in the posterior horn of the spinal cord in a presynaptic inhibitory manner to inhibit the transmission of injurious stimuli.

(a) μ receptor: μ receptor in rat brain consists of 398 amino acids and has a high affinity for both β-endorphin and enkephalin. It is not only activated by exogenous morphine and plays an important role in morphine analgesia, but also the activation of μ receptors at the brain and spinal cord levels can antagonize the analgesic effect of κ receptors. It has also been shown that morphine enhances the evoked potentials in 31% of injury response-specific neurons in the dorsal horn of the spinal cord and inhibits the evoked potentials in another 31%, while 17% of neurons show a biphasic excitatory/inhibitory response, all of which can be blocked by naloxone, suggesting that μ receptors may have a bidirectional role in the regulation of pain [33]. In addition, some studies have also confirmed that the release of certain enkephalins in the brain may indeed be conducive to the production of pain sensitivity, and that small doses of naloxone block the pain-sensitive effects of these enkephalins, thereby producing analgesia.

(b) δ receptor: δ receptor consists of 371 amino acids and binds mainly to enkephalins, and also has some affinity with β-endorphins. The density is higher in the limbic system and brainstem, so its action may be related to pain behavior. Enkephalin/δ receptors also regulate pain perception in a bidirectional manner: naloxone induces the release of prednisolone from the spinal cord leading to analgesia, while δ receptors can ease pain perception in inflammatory states, and μ receptors are analgesic by inhibiting δ receptors, which further suggests that the δ receptor pathway can ease the transmission of pain perception.

(c) κ receptors: κ receptors are composed of 380 amino acids and are the receptors of prednisolone, which are more distributed in the brain, but the receptors in the spinal cord are more clearly related to analgesia. Its effect on pain perception process is bi-directional. κ receptors in the spinal cord are not only involved in mediating the downstream analgesic pathway of morphine but also play an anti-analgesic role. A variety of drugs can activate the antinociceptive effect of spinal cord prednisolone/κ receptors, which disappears after severing the spinal cord, suggesting that this antinociceptive effect can be expressed only when the connection with the brain is maintained. Subcutaneous or subarachnoid injection of prednisolone pretreatment also resulted in desensitization of this antinociceptive effect. In both normal and inflammatory pain models, prednisolone/κ receptors exhibited bidirectional modulation of the evoked firing of injurious electrical or mechanical stimulation of spinal cord dorsal horn neurons.

The bidirectional modulation of pain perception processes is a common feature of all types of opioid receptors. In the study of the effects of opioid agonists on the action potential time course of mouse dorsal root ganglion neurons, it was found that opioid peptides acting on the three types of opioid receptors, μ, δ, and κ, at doses below nanomolar levels all prolonged the action potential time course of spinal dorsal root ganglion neurons, showing excitatory effects, while when opioid peptide doses were at micromolar levels, they shortened the action potential time course of dorsal root ganglion neurons, showing inhibitory effect. This further suggests that all the above three types of opioid receptors have a bidirectional role in regulating pain sensory processes.

(d) Functional association of various opioid receptors: Endogenous enkephalins synergize with β-endorphin and prednisolone to produce analgesic effects at the brain and spinal cord levels, respectively. δ receptors may synergize with μ receptors to produce analgesic effects. The analgesic effect of stress-enhanced spinal μ receptor agonists is also mediated by activation of spinal δ receptors. δ receptors and κ receptors both have synergistic effects on the analgesic effect of μ receptors. Spinal μ and κ receptors can synergize with intracerebral μ receptors to produce stronger analgesic effects, whereas spinal δ receptors can only synergize with intracerebral δ receptors for analgesia. This suggests that synergistic analgesic effects may occur between the same or different types of opioid receptors in the center.

Another evidence for a functional link between various opioid receptors is the phenomenon of cross-tolerance. For example, cross-tolerance exists between κ and μ receptors, and morphine tolerance is followed by cross-tolerance in the spinal δ receptor pathway, but not in μ receptors. The presence of cross-tolerance suggests a functional link between the receptors.

The selectivity of the four types of opioid receptors mentioned above is relative and limited to low concentrations of opioid peptides, with no significant selectivity at higher concentrations. In the brain, 20–30% of opioid receptors are bound to endorphins and can be antagonized by naloxone [34]. The various opioid peptide messaging pathways do not simply act by transmitter, receptor, or central site, but their effects include not only involvement in analgesia and nociceptive transmission, but even in antianalgesia. The relationship between different sites or different transmitters/receptors is also both synergistic and antagonistic. Opioid transmitters/receptors do not work in a simple cellular population, but are interconnected to form networks and perform extremely complex functional connections.

Numerous experimental results have found that in different visceral pain disorders there is an increase or decrease in the amount of different types of opioid peptides in the body, suggesting that the function of the opioid peptide system is greatly altered in patients with chronic pain. Both analgesic and anti-analgesic activities of the prednisolone system are enhanced in inflammatory states. Enkephalins may act on μ receptors at afferent nerve endings to inhibit the transmission of injurious information, thus suggesting that enkephalin release is associated with the recovery from inflammation. The increase in spinal cord prednisins after nerve injury and the fact that prednisin/κ receptors no longer synergize with endogenous enkephalins to exert analgesic effects and produce nociceptive phenomena suggests that the increase in prednisins is related to nociceptive behavior.

3. 5-HT

   5-HT has different mechanisms of action in the central nervous system and in peripheral tissues, acting as a mediator of analgesia in the central nervous system. 5-HT neurons in the CNS inhibit cortical and spinal cord posterior horn neuronal firing and thus have an enhanced analgesic effect. 5-HT neurons' downstream conduction fibers make synaptic contact with endorphin neurons in the posterior horn of the spinal cord, causing endorphin neurons to release enkephalins, which act on opioid receptors on pain afferent nerves, thus creating presynaptic inhibition and reducing excitatory transmission of pain. This is an important downstream regulatory mechanism for pain. When peripheral tissues are damaged, 5-HT is released from dissociated platelets and causes pain, which is mainly involved in vascular pain and injury pain.

4. Bradykinin

   Bradykinin has a strong nociceptive effect in peripheral tissues, and it can cause pain in very small amounts, and it is involved in all inflammatory pain, and it increases capillary permeability and causes tissue edema, which leads to exudation of other nociceptive substances and aggravates the pain. Because of the rapid destruction of bradykinin in the body, the duration of potent pain-causing ability is short. Some studies have shown that acute peritonitis, pancreatitis, angina, and other severe pain are related to bradykinin.

5. Prostaglandins

   Prostaglandins are evenly distributed in the brain and play an important role in lowering the pain threshold. When nerves are stimulated by injury, prostaglandins are released from the nerve endings and the tissues in the region to which they belong, and their synthesis and release are increased during the inflammatory process, which can increase the sensitivity of nerve endings to other pain-causing substances such as bradykinin. Aspirin blocks the synthesis of prostaglandins in tissues throughout the body and relieves inflammatory pain. Prostaglandins are not directly involved in synaptic transmission, but only modulate it. It inhibits the release of epinephrine, which in turn inhibits the transmission of adrenergic synapses.

6. Ascending hormone

   Uplift is a hormone secreted by the preoptic and paraventricular nuclei of the hypothalamus, which enters the posterior pituitary gland via the pituitary bundle and is then released into the blood. It is secreted by the choroid and ventricular tract. Norepinephrine has a nociceptive effect and is involved in some parts of the pain response.

7. Norepinephrine

   Norepinephrine has a nociceptive effect in tissues other than nerve conduction, and has both excitatory and inhibitory effects in central neurons, with inhibition being the main one.

8. Acetylcholine

   Acetylcholine is widely distributed in the nervous system and plays an important role in transmission. The third level of afferent sensory nerve neurons is cholinergic neurons, and the downstream cholinergic neurons have an inhibitory effect on the spinal cord. Intracerebral injection of cholinomimetic drugs can produce analgesic effects, as they cannot cross the blood-brain barrier, and systemic administration has no analgesic effect. High concentrations of acetylcholine in peripheral tissues have analgesic effects.

9. Dopamine

   Dopamine is mainly concentrated in the striatum, pallidum, and substantia nigra of the extrapyramidal system, and is an important mediator of the extrapyramidal system. When the function of the dopaminergic system is enhanced, the nociceptive sensation is hyperalgesic and the effect of morphine is reduced: conversely, it is enhanced.

10. Potassium, hydrogen, and calcium

    These inorganic salts mainly play a nociceptive role in tissues; K^+ concentration up to 10 mmol/L can cause pain, H^+ also has a very strong nociceptive effect, and pain can be produced at pH <6.2 [35]. Tissue ischemia, cell destruction due to injury, and changes in pH in tissues lead to an increase in K^+ concentration and a decrease in pH, which can induce pain, and the above changes are more obvious during inflammation.

11. Cholecystokinin (CCK)

    CCK is the most abundant neuropeptide known in the brain, and it is widely distributed throughout the central nervous system except the cerebellum. There are two types of CCK receptors, named CCK_A receptors and CCK_B receptors. CCK may have an extremely close relationship with pain signal regulation. The analgesic effect of CCK is mainly achieved through CCK receptors. The analgesic effects of μ receptors and δ receptors may be associated may be closely related to the analgesic effects of CCK_A receptor pathway. In addition, CCK counteracts the analgesic effects mediated by endogenously released opioid peptides. CCK reduces the number of μ receptors and the affinity of κ receptors but does not affect the binding of δ receptors, so CCK counteracts the analgesic effects of μ- and κ-type opioid receptor agonists, but not those of δ receptor agonists. The central anti-opioid peptide analgesic effects of CCK are mainly achieved through CCK_B receptors. CCK is able to modulate endogenous opioid peptide activity through mechanisms including receptor and postreceptor levels, and opioid peptides can presynaptically modulate the release of various neuropeptides, including CCK, in the spinal cord. μ receptors in the spinal cord inhibit CCK release, δ receptors have a bidirectional excitatory/inhibitory effect, and κ receptors increase CCK release indirectly by blocking the inhibitory effect of μ receptors.

    Taken together, CCK and its receptors are important in central nociceptive information processing. CCK inhibits injury information afferents by acting on CCK_A receptors in concert with the endogenous opioid system, while by acting on CCK_B, receptors inhibit the analgesic effects of endogenous opioid receptors, thus regulating opioid activity and injury information afferents in a bidirectional manner. Opioid receptors can also achieve bidirectional modulation of CCK activity directly or indirectly, which together complete the central nociceptive information processing process.

12. Nitric oxide (NO)

    NO in peripheral tissues has a bidirectional effect on the regulation of nociception, and can be involved in both nociceptive and analgesic effects. NO is involved in nociceptive formation in the spinal cord, where it is a mediator of nociception induced by excitatory amino acid NMDA receptors. NO in the brain is also involved in the formation of pain sensitization.

13. Histamine

    Histamine is an active substance with strong biological effects and is highly abundant in the mast cells of connective tissue, and a histaminergic neuronal system exists in the brain. Injection of histamine into different brain regions has different effects on pain perception, which can produce both analgesia and nociceptive phenomena, suggesting that there is a bidirectional regulation of nociception by histamine in different brain regions. Histamine is released during peripheral nerve depolarization, which excites nociceptive neurons. Intracentral histamine enhances cortical perception of the nociceptive response.

14. Cytokines

    Cytokines play an important role in the production and persistence of peripheral inflammatory pain and injurious neuropathic pain. Cytokines associated with nociception are nerve growth factor, interleukin-1, interleukin-6, interleukin-8, and tumor necrosis factor. Most of the cytokines related to pain have dual regulatory effects, both nociceptive and analgesic effects.

15. Adenosine triphosphate (ATP)

    A variety of injurious stimuli cause the release of intracellular ATP outside the cell, which activates G protein-coupled receptors, ionotropic receptors, and purinergic receptors on sensory neurons and provides analgesic effects.

    In addition, it has been shown that human tissues contain degenerin, a mechanically activated molecule, which may play a role in the transmission of mechanical stimuli. A recent study found a mechanosensitive detrusor inactivation channel on small diameter sensory neurons that is inactivated by cellular wrinkling, so it may play a role in the exposure of the organism to hyperosmotic stimulus signals after injury.

    The endogenous biochemical mechanisms of pain are complex dynamic processes in the organism, including changes in multiple enzymes, the endocrine system and the immune system in addition to the described parts. It can be seen that various biochemical substances have a complex relationship with pain, with multiple substances exhibiting more or less multidirectional or even diametrically opposed effects. In addition, there are a wide range of synergistic or antagonistic effects between different substances and the same substance in different sites. This suggests that there is an intricate network among these substances involved in the integration of nociceptive information.

4.4.3 Psychological Mechanisms of Visceral Pain

Currently, the pathophysiological research of visceral pain and its related treatment are related to many medical fields, which also include psychology. Chronic visceral pain, like other chronic pain disorders, inevitably has a negative impact on patients' quality of life due to the prolonged presence of symptoms and can incur significant socioeconomic costs. In principle, although a wide variety of pharmacological, psychiatric, and other treatments exist, none of these treatments achieve the desired long-term outcome for many patients, and researchers attribute this to the fact that the mechanisms underlying chronic visceral pain have not been fully elucidated. In the last 30 years, researchers have found that psychological factors have an important influence on the pathophysiology of visceral pain and may provide appropriate psychological treatments. In the case of IBS, for example, a growing body of evidence (including functional brain imaging) suggests a correlation between stress and negative emotions on the frequency and severity of pain in patients.

Many previous studies have suggested that reduced pain thresholds in the corresponding visceral organs (i.e., nociceptive hyperalgesia) constitute the main pathophysiological mechanism of visceral pain; however, this opinion has been challenged by several recent studies. It was found that a significant proportion of BS patients had normal rectal sensations and did not exhibit hypersensitivity. In fact, it has been suggested that the increased sensitivity to visceral stimuli in BS is due to an increased tendency to report pain rather than enhanced neurosensory sensitivity. These interesting reports have also led to an unprecedented rise of psychological factors in the study of visceral pain mechanisms. Since then successive studies have reported findings supporting a change in the propensity to report pain in patients with BS, but with similar neurosensitivity compared to controls. This tendency to report pain, in turn, has been associated with psychological factors such as stress. In addition, anxiety and depressive symptoms in BS patients were also associated with pain scores but not with rectal sensory thresholds, suggesting that the assessment of visceral stimuli may be uniquely "sensitive" to emotional factors in BS patients. The psychological mechanisms of BS may include psychiatric co-morbidity, chronic emotional distress and altered stress responses, personality traits, and educational attainment. It is clear that all these factors may influence the organism's response to visceral stimuli, consistent with the biopsychosocial disease model. Considering that BS is often associated with affective disorders, including anxiety and depression, personality traits and/or emotional state factors become the "main suspect factors". Indeed, many studies have shown that negative emotions induced by psychological stress, mood-related medication, or hypnosis can affect rectal pain sensitivity in patients with BS.

Overall, pain as a subjective sensory process does not necessarily correlate strictly with external injurious stimuli, and as mentioned above, patients with visceral pain may not be hyperalgesic per se, but simply show an increased propensity to report pain, which determines the complexity of visceral pain and the high interindividual variability of pain complaints, and highlights the importance of psychological mechanisms in the mechanism of visceral pain. Thus, although the nature and causes of visceral pain may be similar, the response to the same injurious stimulus may vary between individuals, and the probability and severity of reporting the same injurious stimulus varies across psychological states. This also places a higher demand on the corresponding treatment approach, i.e., to focus on the psychological correlates of visceral pain and to develop highly individualized treatment plans.

4.4.4 Mechanism of Referred Pain

Pain in visceral organs often presents with pain or pain-sensitive areas at sites distant from the site of stimulation, usually reflected mostly in body surface areas innervated by the same or adjacent spinal cord segments, and this pain is called referred to as referred pain. Essentially, it means that pain originating in one part of the body is involved in other parts of the body that do not receive direct injurious stimulation. There is a certain regularity between the site of involvement and the internal organs, and the area of involvement of the organs is relatively fixed. However, there are a few involved pains that do not conform to the pattern of innervation of nerve segments, which are called habitually referred pains, that is, when a part of the body is stimulated, pain can appear in a somatic part that has had previous trauma or pathological process, and there is often nociceptive hypersensitivity and reduced pain threshold on the skin at the site where the involved pain occurs.

Regarding the mechanism of occurrence of referred pain, it can be summarized as follows.

4.4.4.1 Nerve Convergence

Pain afferent fibers from visceral organs and pain afferent fibers from somatic involvement areas both converge on secondary neurons in the same segment of the dorsal horn of the spinal cord. Since there are more nociceptive afferent fibers in the posterior roots than in the spinal thalamic tract fibers, this results in several nociceptive afferent fibers converging on the same spinal thalamic tract fibers. When pain actually comes from a visceral organ that is not easily localized, the cerebral cortex senses that the pain information comes from a somatic site in the same segment as the diseased visceral afferent nerve.

4.4.4.2 Convergence-Facilitation

When the pain impulses from the visceral organs are delivered at high frequencies, the excitation range of the posterior horn cell groups in the spinal cord is expanded and "stress foci" are established, which transmit the impulses to more neurons, i.e., the nerve impulses from the skin and into the same spinal cord segment are facilitated, the fibers of the spinal thalamic tracts are excited, and the corresponding sensations in the skin area appear.

4.4.4.3 Gate Mechanism

According to the hypnosis of the gate mechanism, the gate is open for a long time due to the impulses emitted from the site of injury or lesion of the body. The gate opens when the C fiber (visceral pain fiber) conducts, so that the conduction of Aδ fiber (somatic pain fiber) can easily pass through, thus the conduction of visceral pain creates the somatic pain-sensitive area in the corresponding region on the same spinal node.

4.4.4.4 Convergence-Projection

Sensory centers in the cerebral cortex cannot pinpoint visceral pain, but can clearly localize somatic pain, so the central projections of visceral pain impulses are often reflected in somatic areas at the same time. In addition, there is a convergence area of visceral and somatic afferent impulses in the cerebral cortex, and this area is thought to be the common station of pain pathways in deep organs and somatic tissues.

4.4.4.5 Axonal Reflex Theory

The presence of bifurcated axons in some primary sensory neurons, which are distributed both on the somatic and visceral organs, creates confusion about the source of afferent nerve impulses and may explain the segmental nature of involvement pain.

References

1. Sikandar S, Dickenson AH. Visceral pain. Curr Opin Support Palliat Care. 2012;6(1):17–26.
2. Zhang B, Li X, Ma Z, Zhang S, Song X, Gao H, et al. Prevalence and management of pain in lung cancer patients in northern China: a multicenter cross-sectional study. Thorac Cancer. 2022;13(11):1684–90.
3. Pulmonary embolism [Internet]. Pulmonary embolism. Johns Hopkins Medicine. 2021 [cited 2023 Apr 3]. https://www.hopkinsmedicine.org/health/conditions-and-diseases/pulmonary-embolism.
4. Thompson AD, Shea MJ. Chest pain—cardiovascular disorders [Internet]. MSD manual professional ed. MSD Manuals. 2023 [cited 2023 Apr 3]. https://www.msdmanuals.com/professional/cardiovascular-disorders/symptoms-of-cardiovascular-disorders/chest-pain
5. Dye JR, Kaul MS, St. Clair EW. Inflammatory diseases of the coronary arteries. In: Lanzer P, editor. PanVascular medicine. Berlin: Springer; 2014. https://doi.org/10.1007/978-3-642-37393-0_64-1.
6. White James C. Cardiac pain. Circulation. 1957;16(4):644–55.
7. Thoracic spinal nerves [Internet]. Physiopedia. [cited 2023 Apr 3]. https://www.physio-pedia.com/Thoracic_Spinal_Nerves.
8. Lv Y, Tian W, Chen D, Liu Y, Wang L, Duan F. The prevalence and associated factors of symptomatic cervical spondylosis in Chinese adults: a community-based cross-sectional study. BMC Musculoskelet Disord. 2018;19(1):325.

9. Cervellin G, Mora R, Ticinesi A, Meschi T, Comelli I, Catena F, et al. Epidemiology and outcomes of acute abdominal pain in a large urban emergency department: retrospective analysis of 5,340 cases. Ann Transl Med. 2016;4(19):362.
10. Peptic ulcer [Internet]. Mayo Clinic. Mayo Foundation for Medical Education and Research. 2022 [cited 2023 Apr 3]. https://www.mayoclinic.org/diseases-conditions/peptic-ulcer/symptoms-causes/syc-20354223.
11. Christian-Miller N, Frenette C. Hepatocellular cancer pain: impact and management challenges. J Hepatocell Carcinoma. 2018;5:75–80.
12. Al-Dasuqi K, Irshaid L, Mathur M. Radiologic-pathologic correlation of primary retroperitoneal neoplasms. Radiographics. 2020;40(6):1631–57.
13. Manyozo S. Low back pain during pregnancy: prevalence, risk factors and association with daily activities among pregnant women in Urban Blantyre, Malawi. Malawi Med J. 2019;31(1):71.
14. Backhausen MG, Bendix JM, Damm P, Tabor A, Hegaard HK. Low back pain intensity among childbearing women and associated predictors. A cohort study. Women Birth. 2019;32(4):e467.
15. Sacerdote P, Levrini L. Peripheral mechanisms of dental pain: the role of Substance P. Mediat Inflamm. 2012;2012:1–6.
16. Waxenbaum JA, Reddy V, Varacallo M. Anatomy, autonomic nervous system. Treasure Island, FL: StatPearls Publishing; 2023. https://www.ncbi.nlm.nih.gov/books/NBK539845/
17. Pain principles (section 2, Chapter 6) neuroscience online: an electronic textbook for the Neurosciences. Department of Neurobiology and Anatomy—the University of Texas Medical School at Houston [Internet]. [Cited 2023 Apr 3]. https://nba.uth.tmc.edu/neuroscience/m/s2/chapter06.html.
18. Wang J, Ou S-W, Wang Y-J. Distribution and function of voltage-gated sodium channels in the nervous system. Channels. 2017;11(6):534–54.
19. Renganathan M, Cummins TR, Waxman SG. Contribution of nav1.8 sodium channels to action potential electrogenesis in DRG neurons. J Neurophysiol. 2001;86(2):629–40.
20. Yam M, Loh Y, Tan C, Khadijah Adam S, Abdul Manan N, Basir R. General pathways of pain sensation and the major neurotransmitters involved in pain regulation. Int J Mol Sci. 2018;19(8):2164.
21. Südhof TC. The cell biology of synapse formation. J Cell Biol. 2021;220(7):e202103052.
22. Westlund KN. Visceral nociception. Curr Rev Pain. 2000;4(6):478–87.
23. Chen S, Wang S, Rong P, Wang J, Qiao L, Feng X, et al. Acupuncture for visceral pain: neural substrates and potential mechanisms. Evid Based Complement Alternat Med. 2014;2014:1–12.
24. Bardoni R, Takazawa T, Tong C-K, Choudhury P, Scherrer G, MacDermott AB. Pre- and postsynaptic inhibitory control in the spinal cord dorsal horn. Ann N Y Acad Sci. 2013;1279(1):90–6.
25. Zeilhofer HU, Wildner H, Yévenes GE. Fast synaptic inhibition in spinal sensory processing and Pain Control. Physiol Rev. 2012;92(1):193–235.
26. Vera-Portocarrero LP, Zhang E-T, Ossipov MH, Xie JY, King T, Lai J, et al. Descending facilitation from the rostral ventromedial medulla maintains nerve injury-induced central sensitization. Neuroscience. 2006;140(4):1311–20.
27. Latremoliere A, Woolf CJ. Central sensitization: a generator of pain hypersensitivity by central neural plasticity. J Pain. 2009;10(9):895–926.
28. Kweon H-J, Suh B-C. Acid-sensing ion channels (ASICs): therapeutic targets for neurological diseases and their regulation. BMB Rep. 2013;46(6):295–304.
29. Dulai JS, Smith ES, Rahman T. Acid-sensing ion channel 3: an analgesic target. Channels. 2021;15(1):94–127.
30. Isom LL, Ragsdale DS, De Jongh KS, Westenbroek RE, Reber BFX, Scheuer T, et al. Structure and function of the β2 subunit of brain sodium channels, a transmembrane glycoprotein with a Cam motif. Cell. 1995;83(3):433–42.
31. Kuang Q, Purhonen P, Hebert H. Structure of potassium channels. Cell Mol Life Sci. 2015;72(19):3677–93.
32. Pathan H, Williams J. Basic opioid pharmacology: an update. Br J Pain. 2012;6(1):11–6.
33. Mayer DJ, Mao J, Holt J, Price DD. Cellular mechanisms of neuropathic pain, morphine tolerance, and their interactions. Proc Natl Acad Sci U S A. 1999;96(14):7731–6.
34. Johansson J, Hirvonen J, Lovró Z, Ekblad L, Kaasinen V, Rajasilta O, et al. Intranasal naloxone rapidly occupies brain mu-opioid receptors in human subjects. Neuropsychopharmacology. 2019;44(9):1667–73.
35. Du X, Gamper N. Potassium channels in peripheral pain pathways: expression, function and therapeutic potential. Curr Neuropharmacol. 2013;11(6):621–40.

Evaluation and Examination of Visceral Pain

5

Ming Xia

5.1 Introduction

Pain is a subjective experience, and quantitative analysis of this subjective feeling is necessary for clinical work. Pain assessment refers to the determination and evaluation of the intensity and nature of pain in patients before and during pain treatment using certain methods. Generally, pain measurement refers to the measurement of pain intensity using measurement criteria (metric). Pain assessment, on the other hand, includes the measurement of the interaction of different factors in the whole process of pain occurrence. The purpose of pain assessment includes the following aspects: (1) to clarify the diagnosis, to determine the characteristics of pain more accurately, and to help determine the most effective treatment plan for pain control; (2) to provide a more objective basis for adjusting the treatment plan in a timely manner by combining changes in the patient's subjective feelings during the pain diagnosis and treatment process, and to reduce or avoid the bias caused by simply relying on the patient to make retrospective comparisons; (3) to use quantitative methods to estimate treatment effects, compare and summarize the efficacy of various methods for different treatments (including effective and non-effective treatments, pharmacological, physical, and psychological treatments), further select effective treatments, and determine future treatment guidelines according to the disappearance, reduction or relief of pain and its degree and ineffectiveness; and (4) in pain research, make judgmental analysis and comparisons of scientific findings.

The commonly used pain assessment methods are the indirect or the direct ones, with the former being more widely used. Because the indirect method is closely related to the patient's age, experience level, language expression and cognitive level, there are special methods and requirements for pain assessment of special patient's population, such as infants and the elderly. At the same time, because pain is not only related to physiology and pathology, but also influenced by emotional and psychological factors, so far, although there have been many pain assessment methods, none of them has reached the level of accuracy, objectivity, simplicity and convenience, and there is still a need for continuous improvement.

A thorough pain assessment is a prerequisite for managing pain in clinical practice and the basis for defining pain that requires treatment, whether with interventional or pharmacologic management methods. Understanding the characteristics of pain can also guide the selection and implementation of treating methods, while benefiting the comparison of the effectiveness of treatments. In a research setting, standardized pain evaluation is essen-

M. Xia (✉)
Department of Anesthesiology, Shanghai Ninth People's Hospital Affiliated to Shanghai Jiao Tong University School of Medicine, Shanghai, China
e-mail: xiaming1980@xzhmu.edu.cn

M. Xia et al. (eds.), *Visceral Pain*, https://doi.org/10.1007/978-981-99-9167-9_5

tial to improve comparability across studies and facilitate meta-analysis. Considering the importance of visceral pain evaluation as described above, this chapter will discuss methods of pain assessment, specifically assessment of visceral pain in animal models, assessment of visceral pain in humans, and specificities of visceral pain assessment.

Assessment of abdominal pain requires a method that relies on the likelihood of disease, patient history, physical examination, laboratory tests, and imaging studies. The location of the pain is a useful starting point that will guide further evaluation. Certain elements of the history and physical examination are helpful, such as constipation and bloating strongly suggest intestinal obstruction, while others are of little value. The American College of Radiology recommends different imaging studies to evaluate abdominal pain depending on the site of pain. Ultrasonography is recommended to assess right upper abdominal pain and computed tomography to assess right lower abdominal pain. It is also important to consider special populations, such as women, who are at risk for genitourinary disorders that may cause abdominal pain, and older adults, who may present with atypical symptoms of disease.

Most studies on pain evaluation have focused on somatic pain, and although chronic pain often has common features across etiologies, attention should be paid to the differences between visceral pain and somatic pain when assessing visceral pain. The differences are obvious as visceral pain is diffuse and difficult to localize, and in the clinical setting, the main models used are referred pain and autonomic dysfunction. These aspects should be taken into account when using pain evaluation tools. In addition, pain has both physiological and psychological characteristics, and psychophysiological perceptual testing methods are used to help understand visceral pain when evaluating pain. In the following discussion, different evaluation methods, including unidimensional measurement scales, multidimensional questionnaires, and quantitative sensory testing, and their strengths and challenges will be introduced.

5.2 Assessment of Visceral Pain in Animal Models

Pain is a subjective sensation in humans, which makes the study of pain in animal models difficult. The nociception and neural encoding and transmission of noxious stimuli are similar between animals and humans, but the cognitive expressions and perceptual features of humans are absent in animals. Therefore, except for verbal expressions, humans and animals share similar responses (e.g., muscle contractions, avoidance, and aversion).

As mentioned in previous chapters, viscera do not respond to all somatically noxious stimuli. In Sherrington's findings, visceral pain can be activated by stretching of the mesentery, ischemia, inflammation, and chemical stimulation-induced dilatation of the cavernous organs [1]. The use of animal models to assess pain and measure pain-related variables is quantifiable, and such variables are chosen from a wide range of methods, among which are methods of somatic pain assessment, such as the von Frey method or thermal radiation, as well as vascular and visceral contractions, respiratory reflexes and neurophysiological assessment among physiological reflex assessment, and expression of c-fos in the dorsal horn of the spinal cord or brainstem. However, considering the variety of animal models of visceral pain and correspondingly various assessment criteria, there is a lack of uniform measurement standards among all laboratories studying visceral pain. Several methods for measuring visceral pain in animal models will be briefly described below.

5.2.1 Recording of Abdominal Muscle Contraction

Abdominal muscle contraction is an objective and quantitative indicator of pain, and invasive recording methods such as force conduction equipment or electromyography, which takes into account the reflexes from the primary afferent neuron to the synapse and then to the dorsal roots of the spinal cord, may be chosen to allow for a more detailed assessment. However, some laboratories do not choose this method because it is an invasive indicator and may itself generate pain, which can interfere with the results.

5.2.2 Histological Analysis

The histological analysis method can be used for the study of tissue injury in pain pathology, but it is not an ideal method for pain description due to the pronounced variability among different animal species. For example, dextran sodium sulfate (DSS)-induced colitis is supposed to induce a significant inflammatory response, but colonic hyperreactivity was not seen in at least two different strains of mice.

5.2.3 Electrophysiology of Nerve Bundles or a Neuron

Electrophysiological recordings can reflect peripheral pain mechanisms, but it is not always possible to correlate the recording results with pain, which is the bottleneck in electrophysiological studies of visceral pain. To explore the relationship between neurons and visceral pain, two hypotheses must be made: first, that neurons studied are true injury-receptive neurons; and second, that the excitability of neuronal cells is indeed related to pain.

5.2.4 Response of the Model to Drug Disposition

Visceral pain can also be assessed by using strong analgesics such as morphine on models. The pain can be evaluated by measuring the animal's demand for drugs such as morphine or quantitatively assessed by the improvement of physiological indices by morphine, thus overcoming the limitations of electrophysiological methods. Dose-dependent inhibition experiments with morphine can successfully suppress the pain response of animals and thus better assess visceral pain. Moreover, Harada et al. showed that the mechanism of the dose-dependent inhibition effect of morphine on visceral pain differs between opioid receptors when using this assessment method, and they could inhibit the visceral pain response in a colonic dilatation model in a dose-dependent manner when intrathecal administration of μ receptor agonist (DAMGO) and δ receptor agonist (DPDPE), but the administration of κ receptor agonist (U50488) had no effect [2]. In contrast, κ receptor agonist dose-dependently inhibited the visceral pain response when administered systemically, suggesting that U50488 acts primarily on peripheral κ receptors. This was demonstrated in experiments by Gebhart et al., who used intrathecal injection of antisense oligonucleotides of the κ receptor into the sheath of rats, and proved successful reduction of κ receptor expression by antisense oligonucleotides using plantar injections of formalin. They conducted colonic dilatation experiments on the same rats and observed by pelvic nerve recordings [3]. The results manifested that systemic administration of κ agonists was able to inhibit the noxious stimuli response induced by the colonic dilatation assay in a dose-dependent manner. It was assumed that the κ receptor attenuates the noxious stimuli of colonic dilation mainly through peripheral receptor rather than central neurotransmitter receptors.

5.3 Assessment of Visceral Pain in Humans

5.3.1 Principles of Pain Assessment

Compared to animals, humans can in most cases actively express their subjective feelings, which is more conducive to the assessment of psychological factors of pain, but this also makes the assessment more complicated. Pain should be characterized by its location, duration, severity, aggravating and relieving factors, and associated symptoms. It is also important to note whether the patient has recurrent episodes of similar pain, as this can narrow the differential. The assessment of human pain has its own specific assessment principles.

1. Believing the patient's complaint is the key to assessing pain. Pain is a subjective feeling and the person who is experiencing pain is the most authoritative in expressing it. Therefore, it is important to trust the patient from the beginning to the end when evaluating the pain and encourage the patient to speak out the pain experience which should be referred as the most important assessment information.
2. Collect a comprehensive and detailed pain history. When pain is observed or is complained by the patient, a thorough physical examination should be performed to make a comprehensive assessment of pain and related factors. The comprehensive assessment includes a detailed description of the intensity, nature, location, onset and duration of the pain, and the factors that make it worse or relieved.
3. Pay attention to the assessment of the patient's psychosomatic condition. The patient's mental status and the analysis of relevant psychosocial factors should be observed when checking the patient's medical history in order to make the appropriate supportive treatment.
4. While treating, observe the therapeutic effect and evaluate dynamically. The evaluation is divided into the initial assessment and ongoing evaluation. Selecting an assessment tool that is simple and easy to use and suitable to conduct pain assessment dynamically is more conducive to the treatment plan and the evaluation of the effect.
5. Patient's age, gender, personality, and cultural background should also be noticed while evaluating. In general, elder patients have a higher pain tolerance than younger ones, males have a higher pain tolerance than females, and extroverts have a stronger response to pain than introverts. Factors such as fatigue, stress, anxiety, and terror can lower the pain threshold and strengthen the perception of pain. In addition, personal experience, religious beliefs, family, and cultural background can have an impact on the assessment of pain.

5.3.2 Pain Evaluation Approach

QUESTT is a commonly used pain evaluation approach. Q stands for "question the patient", U for "use pain rating scale", E for "evaluate behavior and physiologic signs", S for "secure family's involvement", T for "take cause of pain into account", and the last T for "take action and assess effectiveness". This process may better guide the practice of clinical pain assessment.

5.3.3 Determination of Location of Pain

Figuring out the location where pain derives from can help determine the cause of pain, and it has been reported in the literature that the 45 Body Areas Rating Scale (BARS-45) indicates both the range and degree of pain [4]. The BARS-45 divides the body surface into 45 zones, and each zone is labeled with a number. Similar to the method used to calculate burn area, patients are asked to mark their painful areas on the chart, and each colored zone is scored with 1 point. If patients get 0 point, it means they do not have pain. In the corresponding pain zone, green, red, blue, and black colors can be used to show different feeling like no pain, mild pain, moderate pain, and severe pain, respectively. This method also calculates the percentage of the patient's pain area to the body surface area.

5.3.4 Commonly Used Self-Report and Behavioral Analysis Methods for Evaluating Pain Level

1. Visual Analogue Scale (VAS)

   The VAS is a simple, validated, and minimally involved measure of pain intensity. It is highly correlated with quantitative scales indicated by pain measurement and has been widely used in clinical and research work to obtain rapid indicators of pain with designed quantitative values.

VAS has two versions of charts, namely, linear and facial ones, which is the most commonly used tool for pain assessment. The VAS card, supervised by the Chinese Association for the Study of Pain of the Chinese Medical Association, is a linear chart divided pain into ten levels, with larger numbers indicating greater pain intensity. The pain score is obtained by measuring the pain levels with a ruler. The other type is the face chart, which is based on the VAS ruler with a laughing or crying face next to it, so that it can be easily understood by children. It is mainly suitable for the assessment of pain of various nature in children over 7 years of age who are conscious. Preoperatively, the mechanism of pain onset, the method of describing pain and using the measuring scales should be explained to the patient. An accurate assessment of pain is the key to help the medical staffs understand the patient's pain level should be explicitly explained and appropriate measures should be taken to eliminate or reduce the pain in order to win the patient's cooperation.

2. Numerical Rating Scale (NRS)

   The NRS is composed of 11 numbers from 0 to 10 which represent the level of pain felt by patients. The larger the number is, the more severe the pain level is, and the scale is similar to the VAS. It has high reliability and validity, is easy to record, and is suitable for patients with relatively well educated. Yet for patients who are illiterate, it is abstract and difficult to explain to patients in clinical work.

3. Wong-Banker Faces Pain Scale-Revised (Fps-R)

   First used for clinical assessment in 1990, this scale uses six facial expressions ranging from smiling, sadness to painful crying to express the pain level. While evaluating, the patient is asked to choose a face that fit their pain experience best. This method was initially used for pain assessment in children, but it has been proven that this scale is suitable for any age, especially for patients above 3 years old, and there is no specific cultural background or gender requirement.

   Fps-R is simple, intuitive, visual and easy to grasp, does not require any additional equipment, and is especially suitable for people with acute pain, elders, pediatric patients, illiterate people, people without the ability to express, and people with cognitive dysfunction. It has been demonstrated that comparing with other assessment tools introduced above, namely, NRS and VAS, the FPS-R is the most suitable one for pain assessment in the elderly.

4. Verbal Rating Scale (VRS)

   There are two types of VRS, namely, 5-point verbal rating scale (VRS-5) and 4-point oral grading scale (VRS-4). VRS-5 is part of the Canadian McGill pain questionnaire, which is a specific grading of the pain level according to the degree of the impact of pain on the quality of life. Each pain level is illustrated, which objectively reflects the severity of pain and is also easy to be understood by both medical staff and patients. Specifically, it is divided into 6 levels, i.e., level 0, 1, 2, 3, 4, and 5. In VRS-4, pain is classified into level 0, 1, 2, and 3. It is the simplest scale to measure pain, but will be influenced by the patient's literacy level.

5. Verbal Description Scales (VDS)

   VDS consists of a series of adjectives describing pain, with the mildest pain being scored as 0 and each subsequent pain level increasing by 1 point, so that each adjective has a corresponding score. The patient's pain level is the number represented by the adjective most appropriate for that patient's pain. Melzeak used mild pain, severe pain, labor pain, terrible pain, and unbearable pain to define the level of pain. The words used in this method are easy to understand, can be verbalized at any time, so that it satisfies both communication requirement and the psychological needs of the patient, but the disadvantages are that the assessment will be severely influenced by subjective factors and is not suitable for patients with expressive language disorders.

6. Pain Questionnaires

   Pain questionnaires is designed to evaluate the intensity and nature of pain more accurately because it is based on various factors such as physical sensation, emotional factors, and perception of pain.

   (a) McGill Pain Questionnaire (MPQ)

      The MPQ was proposed by Melzack and Torgerson to assess the effectiveness of treatment for various types of pain. It is currently the most widely used pain assessment tool in English-speaking countries, and consists of 20 pain descriptors in four categories, providing a more comprehensive assessment of pain intensity in terms of four factors: sensory, affective, evaluative, and miscellaneous categories, as well as present pain intensity (PPI). Each group of words was arranged in increasing level of pain intensity, with groups 1–10 being sensory, 11–15 being affective, 16 being evaluation, and 17–20 being miscellaneous. Respondents choose one word in each group with the same level of pain as their own (no suitable one could be left out). Three important indices can be obtained from the MPQ: (1) Pain rating index (PRI), which is a value (ordinal number) based on the position of the word selected by the participant in the group. The sum of the values of all these selected words constitutes the PRI, which can be calculated as a total of four categories. The PRI can be used to calculate the total number of four categories, or as a classified counting; (2) Number of words chosen (NWC); (3) Present Pain Intensity is the combination of selected words and number of words, representing the total pain intensity, i.e., the pain intensity of 1–5.

   (b) Short-Form of McGill Pain Questionnaire (SF-MPQ)

      The MPQ is cumbersome and inconvenient to apply clinically. In 1987, Melzack proposed a simplified pain questionnaire based on the MPQ and added the visual simulation method to it, which became a simple and practical comprehensive questionnaire, called the short-form McGill Pain Questionnaire. The SF-MPQ consists of only 11 sensory and 4 affective pain descriptors as well as PPI and VAS. All the descriptors indicate different levels of pain as "absent", "mild", "moderate", and "severe" and label with 0–3 points respectively. Because the PPI or total PPI can be categorized, the SF-MPQ is suitable for the situation when testing time is limited and other pain intensity information, such as VAS scores, is available.

   (c) Brief Pain Questionnaire (BPQ)

      Also called brief pain inventory (BPI), BPQ is a separate quantification of the three factors of sensation, emotion, and evaluation. This questionnaire includes descriptors about the cause of pain, nature of pain, impact on life, and site of pain, as well as the use of NRS to reflect the degree of pain in a variety of ways. BPQ is a rapid multidimensional method of measuring and evaluating pain.

7. Quantitative Sensory Testing (QST)

   Questionnaires, however, may be unable to reflect the complexity of visceral pain, and studies have paid attention to identifying alternative methods for assessing pain and guiding treatment strategies [5]. QST can assist the assessment of visceral pain, characterizing sensory processing in peripheral and central pain pathways. It can be used as a means to depict a patient's nociceptive profile. In the QST, standardized stimuli to body and visceral tissues are used to explore different neural pathways and networks. This leads to responses that are quantified by psychophysical and/or objective methods [6]. Furthermore, when adding more specific examinations, such as the assessment of endogenous descending inhibition and temporal summation from brainstem centers, researchers can analyze whether pain processing in central pathways is abnormal. QST can serve as a biomarker to classify pain phenotypes according to the affected pain mechanisms [7].

8. Chinese Cancer Pain Assessment Tool (CCPAT)

   In 1996, Dr. Chung of the Department of Nursing and Medical Sciences of the Hong Kong Polytechnic University began to develop a culturally appropriate multifaceted pain assessment tool in China and launched CCPAT in 1998 [8]. The tool consists of 56 indicators in six areas: physical function, medication use, psychosocial, pain beliefs, emotion and pain severity, and each indicator is scored 5, 4, 3, 2, or 1. The higher the total score, the more severe the pain impact the patient suffers.

9. Prince-Henry Pain Scale

   The scale is mainly applicable to the determination of pain severity after open-heart and abdominal surgery and is relatively sensitive, but it is only applicable to patients over 7 years of age and may be greatly influenced by the patient's literacy level.

10. Color Analog Scale (CAS)

   CAS uses colors to represent pain, with red representing severe pain, yellow representing moderate pain, and green representing comfort. Patients were asked to mark the degree and location of pain on a pattern with a colored pen. The researchers suggested the validity and reliability of the facial expression scale and CAS to assess pain in pediatric patients in the emergency setting [9].

11. Pain Observation Scale for Young Children (POCIS)

   This scale was first proposed by Boelen and colleagues in 1998 and carried out at the University of Amsterdam in the Netherlands. It is used in children aged 1–4 years to assess postoperative pain, and transient acute or chronic pain as well. The main indicators include facial expression, crying, breathing, tension, tension in the arms and fingers, tension in the legs and toes, and arousal. The measurement can be done in less than 1 minute, but for chronic pain, the pain response is diminished when the child is fatigued [10].

   In addition to the above assessment instruments, there are the Modified Objective Pain Scale (MOPS), Modified Behavioral Pain Scale (MBPS), Newborn Acute Pain Scale (DAN), Children's Hospital of Eastern Ontario Pain Scale (CHEOPS), Riley Infant Pain Scale (RIPS), Neonatal Infant Pain Scale (NIPS), Premature Infant Pain Profile-Revised (PIPP-R), CRIES scale, Neonatal Facial Coding System (NFCS), Infant Body Coding System (IBCS), CHIPPS scale, etc. With various pain evaluating scales, a trained practitioner should select the most appropriate scales for patients. The requirement for using different tools is the consistency in the assessment results while observing by different assessors, because the dynamic and comprehensive assessment of pain in clinical practice is often completed by different assessors. Only when assessment methods meet this criterion can the reliability and accuracy of the assessment results be ensured.

5.4 Special Features of Visceral Pain Assessment

Due to the neuroanatomical characteristics of visceral pain, the assessment of visceral pain also has its special features.

5.4.1 True Visceral Pain and Pseudovisceral Pain

The priority of the visceral pain assessment is to distinguish between true visceral pain and pseudovisceral pain (mural visceral pain). Generally, pain caused by lesions occurred in the chest, abdomen, and pelvic viscera belongs to true visceral pain. One of the characteristics of this pain category is that the pain is widespread in the early stages of diseases, and the localization is uncertain, and it is mostly intermittent which may be related to the periodic contracture of smooth muscle and hyperperistalsis of the cavernous organs. It is in most cases accompanied by autonomic reflex symptoms such as nausea and vomiting, sweating, pallor, decreased blood pressure, and abortion. This may be due to the formation of a reflex arc between the visceral pain centripetal conduction pathway and the autonomic centrifugal conduction pathway. Visceral pain is often described by patients as being symmetrical on the body surface and deep in the midline of the body. In true visceral pain, the pain can sometimes be relieved by a change in posture; thus patients want to relieve their pain by changing position constantly. It is often accompanied by visceral referred pain which can be treated effectively with antispasmodic drugs.

Pseudovisceral pain is characterized as a painful sensation caused by physical and chemical factors such as stretching and inflammation of the thorax, peritoneal bilayer, mesentery, and diaphragm. It is a kind of intense, sharp, cut-like pain, often persistent for a long time, and the site of pain can be accurately identified. When the lesion involves the thorax and peritoneum, the pain is felt close to the diseased viscera. Such pain is only occasionally associated with autonomic symptoms such as nausea and vomiting, and the pain can be aggravated by a change in the body position, forcing patients to squat and stay still. Antispasmodics are not efficient in controlling the pain, while analgesic treatment is effective. After all, the nature of the pain should be distinguished first during pain assessment.

5.4.2 Visceral Referred Pain

Visceral pain can often spread to the skin of the body innervated by the same or adjacent spinal segments, which is known as visceral referred pain. Some features have been detected from clinical practices. For example, heartache usually springs out behind the sternum and involves the precordial region, the left shoulder, the ulnar side of the left arm or the neck, shoulder and back. The referred pain often conforms to the pattern of spinal nerve segments' innervation, manifesting as haphalgesia and hyperalgesia on the skin innervated by the same or adjacent spinal cord segments at the site of the lesion, often accompanied by muscle spasms. However, there are exceptional cases called habitual referred pain, in which pain occurs in certain parts of the body that has trauma or disease before when stimulated.

Referred pain is characterized by deep hyperalgesia and dull pain, such as renal colic in which the patient has abnormal testicular pain and tenderness. Referred pain often manifests with sympathetic or parasympathetic hyperfunction symptoms, such as elevated blood pressure, tachycardia, anxiety, arrector muscle spasm, epidermal vasoconstriction, or skin pallor. Involvement referred pain can be alleviated or relieved by injection of local anesthetics in the dermal area, such as procaine in the lower abdomen to reduce labor pain in the first stage of labor. Understanding these correlations benefits the diagnosis of the visceral lesion. The nature and location of visceral pain and referred pain should be considered during pain assessment.

5.5 Initial Diagnosis of Visceral Pain

5.5.1 Medical History

An accurate understanding of the factors contributing to visceral pain requires a sequential and systematic inquiry of patients' medical history, which is particularly important for the diagnosis of visceral pain. When possible, a history should be obtained from a conscious patient. The initial differential diagnosis can be determined by delineating the location, radiation, and movement of the pain. After determining the location, the physician should obtain general information about the onset, duration, severity and quality of pain, as well as aggravating and relieving factors. Associated symptoms often allow the physician to further define the focus of the differential diagnosis.

1. The outbreak of visceral pain goes through the process of being triggered, becoming

urgent, and the symptoms appearing. Factors involved may concern with the breathing, stimulations, diets, postures, movements, defecation and urination, etc.
2. The body parts where pain is felt include both the main part of pain occurrence and the part of referred pain. The sensitivity to pain varies from organs to organs, which must be taken into consideration when analyzing and diagnosing diseases.
3. The nature of visceral pain, which is similar to most types of pain, can be divided into three types. Understanding it has significant diagnostic meaning. (a) Persistent pain, which is mostly dull pain or vague pain; (b) Paroxysmal pain, which is rapid and cut-like, mostly caused by smooth muscle spasm of cavity organs; and (c) Persistent pain with paroxysmal intensification, which is a combined state of the above two types of abdominal pain, mostly characterized by pain complicated by inflammation and obstruction of cavity organs.
4. The pain level can reflect the pathological changes and the intensity of stimulations. Indeed, it may differ from person to person as the sensitivity to pain varies.
5. The pain ignited by visceral diseases is often accompanied by gastrointestinal symptoms such as nausea and vomiting, abdominal distension and diarrhea. These symptoms are also meaningful for the diagnosis of pain.

5.5.2 Physical Examination

Patients with chronic abdominal pain should have a thorough physical examination. All patients should have vital signs and an abdominal examination. The general appearance and vital signs of the patient can help narrow the differential diagnosis. Other physical examination will depend on the history. Patients with peritonitis tend to lie still, whereas patients with renal colic seem unable to remain stationary. Fever suggests infection; however, the absence of fever does not rule out infection, especially in older or immunocompromised patients. Tachycardia and upright hypotension suggest hypovolemia. The location of the pain guides the remainder of the physical examination. Physicians should pay close attention to cardiac and pulmonary examinations in patients with epigastric pain, as they may indicate pneumonia or cardiac ischemia [11].

There are several specialized methods to assess for signs associated with the cause of abdominal pain. When present, some signs can be highly predictive of certain diseases. These include Carnett's sign in patients with abdominal wall pain, such as pain that increases when a supine patient tenses the abdominal wall by lifting the head and shoulders off the examination table [12]; and Murphy's sign in patients with cholecystitis [13], although it is present in only 65% of adults with cholecystitis and is particularly unreliable in older patients [14].

The abdominal examination includes examination, auscultation, percussion, and palpation. In patients with suspected psychogenic abdominal pain, it is important to perform the abdominal examination with the patient distracted.

1. Inspection: General appearance and level of comfort or discomfort should be noted. Examination of the abdomen should include attention to the posture patients assumes in pain; strict immobility is typical of patients with peritonitis, whereas patients with biliary or renal colic wriggle in pain. Patients with peritonitis have pain that worsens when the examiner gently taps the stretcher.
2. Auscultation: The abdomen should be auscultated for bowel sounds. Auscultation is a useful physical finding, especially in detecting ileus. Abnormal bowel sounds are highly predictive of small bowel obstruction in patients with acute abdominal pain. Abnormally active high-pitched bowel sounds are a characteristic of early intestinal obstruction, while in patients with splenic infarction friction sounds may be heard at the appropriate site.
3. Percussion: Start with gentle percussion, not palpation. Patients with peritonitis will feel pain on gentle percussion. Percussion can also be used to identify ascites and liver enlargement. Tympany means that the bowel is

distended, while a dullness may mean that there is a mass. A metastatic dullness is a reliable and fairly accurate marker for detecting ascites.

4. Palpation: Palpation is used to assess tenderness in the abdomen, as well as to evaluate enlarged organs (such as an enlarged liver or enlarged spleen) or masses. Physicians begin by examining the quadrant of the abdomen where the patient has the least pain.

Muscle stiffness or a guarding posture (waist bowing) is an important early sign of peritoneal inflammation; it may be unilateral in patients with focal inflammatory masses (e.g., diverticular abscesses) and diffuse in peritonitis. Deeper sources of pain such as renal colic and pancreatitis are usually not with a guarding posture.

Rebound tenderness may reflect peritonitis. If testing for rebound tenderness is appropriate, physicians begin with gentle palpation and release. If the patient has no rebound pain on gentle palpation, physicians perform a harder palpation and release.

The patient should be examined for signs of nerve and muscle wall injury and herniation. Pain and hyperalgesia in the cortical distribution are signs of nerve involvement such as herpes zoster or nerve root impingement. Abdominal wall lesions can be detected by palpation or by noting increased pain when using the abdominal wall muscles such as sitting up.

Rectal and pelvic examinations are recommended for patients with lower abdominal and pelvic pain. Rectal examination may reveal fecal impaction, palpable masses, or occult blood in the stool. Tenderness and fullness on the right side of the rectum suggest a posterior cecum. Pelvic examination may reveal vaginal discharge, which may suggest vaginitis. The presence of active cervical pressure and peritoneal signs increases the likelihood of ectopic pregnancy or other gynecologic complications, such as tubal inflammation or tubal abscesses [15].

5.6 Diagnostic Testing

The initial workup focuses on distinguishing benign functional disease from organic lesions. Features suggestive of organic disease include weight loss, fever, hypovolemia, electrolyte abnormalities, signs or symptoms of gastrointestinal blood loss, anemia, or signs of malnutrition. Laboratory tests in patients with functional abdominal pain should be normal.

The following laboratory measurements should be performed in most patients with chronic abdominal pain:

1. Complete blood count and differential;
2. Electrolytes, blood urea nitrogen (BUN), creatinine, and glucose;
3. Calcium;
4. Transaminases, alkaline phosphatase, and bilirubin;
5. Lipase and/or amylase;
6. Serum iron, total iron binding capacity and ferritin;
7. Anti-tissue transglutaminase.

Further imaging evaluation will depend on the differential diagnosis based on history, physical and laboratory studies.

At the end of the initial workup, young patients without evidence of organic disease may receive symptomatic treatment. The use of further invasive tests should be done to rule out specific diseases and not as a general screening. However, in patients over 50 years of age, a diagnosis of new onset functional disease should only be made with great caution. These patients will likely require abdominal imaging based on their signs and symptoms due to the increased risk of malignancy. A further and detailed discussion of different types of diseases and their diagnosis and treatment will be provided in the following chapters.

5.7 Summary

Pain assessment is the first and also the most critical step in pain treatment and management [16]. Careful and accurate assessment of pain not only identifies the presence of pain, but also helps in the evaluation of pain treatment effects. In clinical work, appropriate and effective pain assessment methods should be selected according to the characteristics of different patients. Continuous and dynamic assessment should be performed. Diseases should be diagnosed in light of the characteristics of visceral pain. And effective analgesic measures should be taken to reduce or eliminate the pain, improving patients' quality of life and strengthening their confidence in overcoming the disease.

References

1. Sherrington C. The integrative activity of the nervous system. New York: Charles Scribner's Sons; 1906.
2. Harada Y, Nishioka K, Kitahata LM, Kishikawa K, Collins JG. Visceral antinociceptive effects of spinal clonidine combined with morphine, [D-Pen2, D-Pen5] enkephalin, or U50,488H. Anesthesiology. 1995;83(2):344–52. https://doi.org/10.1097/00000542-199508000-00015.
3. Sohn CI, Park HJ, Gebhart GF. Adenosine receptor agonists modulate visceral hyperalgesia in the rat. Gut Liver. 2008;2(1):39–46. https://doi.org/10.5009/gnl.2008.2.1.39. Epub 2008 Jun 30.
4. Liu Q, Wu X, Guo J, et al. Analgesic effect of electroacupuncture on postherpetic neuralgia: a trial protocol for a multicenter randomized controlled trial. Pain Ther. 2021;10:1755–71. https://doi.org/10.1007/s40122-021-00283-8.
5. Phillips AE, Faghih M, Kuhlmann L, Larsen IM, Drewes AM, Singh VK, et al. A clinically feasible method for the assessment and characterization of pain in patients with chronic pancreatitis. Pancreatology. 2020;20(1):25–34. https://doi.org/10.1016/j.pan.2019.11.007.
6. Olesen SS, van Goor H, Bouwense SAW, Wilder-Smith OHG, Drewes AM. Reliability of static and dynamic quantitative sensory testing in patients with painful chronic pancreatitis. Reg Anesth Pain Med. 2012;37(5):530–6. https://doi.org/10.1097/AAP.0b013e3182632c40.
7. Smith SM, Dworkin RH, Turk DC, Baron R, Polydefkis M, Tracey I, et al. The potential role of sensory testing, skin biopsy, and functional brain imaging as biomarkers in chronic pain clinical trials: iMMPACT considerations. J Pain. 2017;18(7):757–77. https://doi.org/10.1016/j.jpain.2017.02.429.
8. Chung JW, Wong TK, Yang JC. A preliminary report on the Chinese Cancer Pain Assessment Tool (CCPAT): reliability and validity. Acta Anaesthesiol Sin. 2001;39(1):33–40.
9. Bulloch B, Garcia-Filion P, Notricia D, Bryson M, McConahay T. Reliability of the color analog scale: repeatability of scores in traumatic and nontraumatic injuries. Acad Emerg Med. 2009;16(5):465–9. https://doi.org/10.1111/j.1553-2712.2009.00404.x.
10. Bai J, Jiang N. Where are we: a systematic evaluation of the psychometric properties of pain assessment scales for use in Chinese children. Pain Manag Nurs. 2015;16(4):617–31. https://doi.org/10.1016/j.pmn.2014.11.003.
11. Cartwright SL, Knudson MP. Evaluation of acute abdominal pain in adults. Am Fam Physician. 2008;77(7):971–8.
12. Srinivasan R, Greenbaum DS. Chronic abdominal wall pain: a frequently overlooked problem. Practical approach to diagnosis and management. Am J Gastroenterol. 2002;97(4):824–30.
13. Trowbridge RL, Rutkowski NK, Shojania KG. Does this patient have acute cholecystitis? JAMA. 2003;289(1):80–6.
14. Adedeji OA, McAdam WA. Murphy's sign, acute cholecystitis and elderly people. J R Coll Surg Edinb. 1996;41(2):88–9.
15. Buckley RG, King KJ, Disney JD, Gorman JD, Klausen JH. History and physical examination to estimate the risk of ectopic pregnancy: validation of a clinical prediction model. Ann Emerg Med. 1999;34(5):589–94.
16. Zhijie L. Visceral pain—basic and clinical. Beijing: Science Publishing House; 2018.

Medication Treatment for Visceral Pain

6

Bifa Fan

Treatments for visceral pain can be summarized as conventional drug therapy, non-conventional drug therapy, and non-drug therapy. Except for emergent cases, medication has always been the first-line treatment method for chronic and certain acute pains. In this chapter, detailed information about commonly used medication for visceral pain will be presented. Specifically, therapy targets visceral pain (opioid receptors and non-opioid receptors), and the current status of pharmacological treatment of visceral pain and commonly used drugs will be described. Conventional drug therapy includes opioids, non-opioids and non-steroidal anti-inflammatory drugs (NSAIDs), GABA and tricyclic antidepressants, combination therapy, traditional Chinese medicine, and so on. Non-conventional drug therapy mainly comprises TRPV1 receptor antagonists, ketamine, humanized anti-NGF monoclonal antibodies, and α2 adrenergic receptor antagonists, etc.

B. Fan (✉)
Department of Pain Medicine, China-Japan Friendship Hospital, Beijing, China

6.1 Current Status of Pharmacological Treatment of Visceral Pain and Commonly Used Drugs

Despite the discovery of numerous targets for pharmacological interventions for visceral pain, the development of current therapeutic methods for visceral pain is unsatisfactory.

With the continuous improvement of basic research and clinical translation of research results, the selective drug targets for visceral pain are gradually being improved. In the last few years, many new drugs for the treatment of visceral pain have entered clinical trials.

The main symptomatic treatment for visceral pain is opioid-based pharmacotherapy. Effective opioid therapy depends on the appropriate choice of drug and route of administration and dose and requires consideration of the so-called emergency dose for sudden onset pain and the side effects of common opioids. In addition, non-steroidal anti-inflammatory drugs (NSAIDs) may be helpful in opioid therapy, especially in some painful conditions, but the gastrointestinal, cardiovascular, and renal risks of these drugs should be weighed against their benefits when administered according to the status of the case. When opioid therapy is not effective, adjuvant analgesics such as glucocorticoids, antidepressants, and anticonvulsants can also be very helpful in relieving pain. In addition, besides cancer pain itself, the chemotherapeutic agents used,

M. Xia et al. (eds.), *Visceral Pain*, https://doi.org/10.1007/978-981-99-9167-9_6

radiation therapy and surgery may also aggravate pain.

Studies suggest that multiple mechanisms may be involved in the development and maintenance of visceral pain [1, 2]. Emerging therapeutic approaches can be located in: (1) dysfunction of visceral organs; (2) high sensitivity of afferent neurons; and (3) amplification of afferent information in the brain. Because sensory sensitization of afferent neurons induced by mechanical and chemical stimuli has been associated with many visceral pain syndromes, most studies have focused on the mechanisms of triggering and maintaining high afferent neuronal excitability. External stimuli elicit the release of the neurotransmitters glutamate, calcitonin gene-related peptide, and substance P from nociceptive receptors, which transmit signals to secondary neurons in the spinal cord. These secondary neurons pass to the cerebral spinal cord and up to the thalamus, where they pass to tertiary neurons that project to the sensory cortex and thus perceive pain. Pain signals are regulated by the release of endorphins and enkephalins in the midbrain. These neurotransmitters interact with specific opioid receptors on modulatory neurons and primarily complete pain transmission to secondary neurons. Although many relay levels of the brain-gut axis have been found to be altered in the pathogenesis of visceral pain, current novel therapies are still mainly focused on the sensory neuron level. In addition, it is generally believed that drugs targeted to injurious sensory afferent neurons do not enter the brain and therefore do not have adverse effects on central nervous system function. Selective sensory neuron targets can be classified as follows: (1) receptors at the terminals of peripheral afferent neurons associated with stimulus transduction; (2) ion channels that modulate excitability and conductivity of afferent neurons; and (3) transmitters and transmitter receptors that modulate the upstream or downstream conduction of central circuits of pain. The relationship between these targets needs to be evaluated by reasonable experimental models of visceral nociceptive hypersensitivity and clinical proof-of-concept study. Looking at all possible targets of nociceptive hypersensitivity, another question arises as to whether the desired therapeutic effect can be achieved by modulation of a single target.

6.2 Current Medications for Visceral Pain

Visceral pain is a complex condition that can be difficult to manage, and patients fear that their abdominal pain may be a more dangerous condition and visit their physicians frequently to seek the peace of mind and demand effective analgesics. However, there are no approved medications specifically for visceral pain, and patients often receive trial-and-error approaches to treating their pain.

6.2.1 Opioids

Opioids are the main choice of treatment for patients with severe visceral pain. Drugs in this class include morphine, oxycodone, and fentanyl. However, the use of these drugs is limited by many side effects, including nausea, constipation, respiratory depression, chronic analgesic tolerance, and drug dependence. The evidence further suggests that nociceptive sensitization and opioid-induced nociceptive hypersensitivity can progress as a result of long-term opioid use.

6.2.1.1 κ-Opioid Receptor Drugs

1. κ-opioid receptor agonists

   κ-opioid receptor agonists are one of the most promising drugs for visceral pain in recent days. κ-opioid receptors were discovered by chance during receptor subtype hybridization screening. The mouse κ receptor consists of 380 amino acid residues and shares >60% homology with the mouse δ receptor [3]. The homologous regions include the second, third, and seventh transmembrane regions and the second intracellular loop region, but all intracellular regions and the C-terminal homology are low. κ receptors have two N2 glycosylation sites in the N-terminal extracellular region as in the δ receptor. The first and second extracellular loop regions each contain one cysteine (Cys) that can form disulfide bonds with each other. A number of phosphorylation sites are present in the intracellular loop region and at the C-terminus. Genomic analysis revealed a 79-kb intron between the first transmembrane region and the first intracellular loop region, and a 3.2-kb intron after the fourth transmembrane region. Unlike the μ and δ receptors, the κ receptor has a negatively charged second extracellular loop region. From sequence analysis, it appears that this region can specifically interact with the biallelic residues in preprodynorphin-derived peptides, leading to the selective binding of opioid peptides to the κ receptor. κ receptor subtypes are more complex to classify, and initial analysis of κ receptor-enriched guinea pig brain and spinal cord with 3H-labeled ethylketocyclazocine (EKC) revealed the presence of different sources of this led to the proposal of κ receptor typing and the classification of κ receptors into κ_1 and κ_2 receptor subtypes based on different sensitivities to DADLE (an opioid receptor agonist). Later, the κ_1 receptor subtype was subdivided into κ_{1a} and κ_{1b} subtypes by replacing the prednisolone response with 3H-labeled EKC. The binding analysis of 3H-labeled bremazocine suggested that the κ_2 subtype could be subdivided into κ_{2a} and κ_{2b} subtypes. κ_{2b} has a high affinity for β-endorphins. So far, only the κ_1 isoform has been cloned in humans and rodents. The cloned κ_1 isoforms are pharmacologically identical to the natural κ_1 isoforms. The ligands of the currently documented selective κ-opioid receptor agonists are mostly 1-receptors with an agonistic potency of 0.1–10 nmol/L [4]. Representative agonists include U50488, enadoline, asimadoline, ADL10-0101, ADL10-0116, and peptide molecules (e.g., CR665, FE200665, and FE200666), U50488 and enadoline can cross the blood-brain barrier, while other κ-opioid receptor agonists are mostly peripherally selective, such as asimadoline, ADL10-0101, ADL10-0116, and CR665.

2. Therapeutic effects of κ-opioid receptor agonists on visceral pain

   Systemic administration of κ-opioid receptor agonists showed good analgesic effects on different types of visceral pain, with significant effects on visceral pain in the duodenum, colon, bladder, vagina, and uterus. κ-opioid receptor agonists can block pain due to peritoneal irritation, normalize intestinal peristalsis, and reverse intestinal obstruction caused by peritoneal irritation. This evidence suggests that κ-opioid receptor agonists are effective agents for the treatment of visceral pain.

   (a) Fedotozine: Clinical data on κ-opioid receptor agonists for visceral pain remain scarce. Fedotozine is the first κ-opioid receptor agonist used clinically for the treatment of visceral pain. Fedotozine is more effective than the usual placebo in relieving abdominal pain and flatulence caused by ulcer-free dyspepsia and irritable bowel syndrome (IBS). It can increase the pain threshold in patients with irritable bowel syndrome. Fedotozine is an atypical class of κ-opioid receptor agonists because it activates both κ- and μ-opioid receptors, and it has a high affinity for the κ_{1a} binding site and a relatively low affinity for the cloned κ_1 subtype.

   (b) ADL10-0101: The κ-opioid receptor agonist ADL10-0101 has been reported to have significant effects in relieving pain in patients with chronic pancreatitis. ADL10-0101 is a typical class of peripheral selective κ_1 receptor agonists. The analgesic effect is very pronounced and there are no central adverse effects, probably due to the compound's inability to cross the blood-brain barrier: this also confirms that ADL10-0101 acts peripherally. The onset of action of ADL10-0101 is particularly rapid, reaching its maximum effect within 60 min and maintaining it for about 4 h. During this time, the plasma concentration of the compound decreases, dropping to 100 nmol/L or less after 3–4 h [5]. Although the preliminary findings are encouraging today, more in-depth clinical evidence studies are needed to determine whether it can eventually be used as a suitable drug for the treatment of visceral pain and other related diseases.

(c) Asimadoline: Asimadoline is a potent κ-opioid receptor agonist with a diarylacetamide chemical structure. It has a high affinity to κ-opioid receptors, and the IC50 value in human recombinants is 1.2 nmol/L [6]. Asimadoline is a selective κ-opioid receptor agonist with a low rate of crossing the blood-brain barrier, it does not produce significant effects on central κ-opioid receptors, so the adverse effects (e.g., anxiety, hallucinations) produced by it can also be avoided. In addition, the distribution of acemadoline in central neurons is relatively low, and its dose that produces central adverse effects is 10 times its threshold dose for analgesic action. Opioid receptors produce analgesia by decreasing the excitability of injurious receptors in peripheral nerve endings, and this analgesic effect can be antagonized by systemic application of naloxone hydrochloride or by local application of κ-opioid receptor antagonists. Administration of high doses of acepromazoline (1–3 mg/kg) produces adverse effects such as anxiety, sedation, and polyuria, and this dose is 50–600 times its analgesic dose in rats and 30–100 times its analgesic dose in mice. In a study on post-extraction pain, acepromazine showed a bell-shaped dose-dependent curve (0.1–2.5 mg) and was most effective at 0.15 and 0.5 mg doses [7]. A total of 5 mg doses did not reduce pain. In human trials, 10 mg of acepromazine increased pain after knee injury, which may be related to NMDA-mediated nociceptive hypersensitivity and inflammatory effects. This result suggests that high doses (10 mg) of asimadoline are not beneficial for pain treatment in humans.

There was no cross-resistance between the analgesic effects of asimadoline and systemically applied morphine in rats, suggesting that asimadoline may be less resistant than morphine. These studies also suggest that neurotrophic (somatic) pain due to chronic constrictive injury in rats is more responsive to relatively small doses of peripheral selective κ-receptor agonists. The blood-brain barrier can restrict the passage of asimadoline due to the presence of P-glycoprotein (P-gp), whereas the intestinal P-gp barrier does not prevent intestinal uptake of asimadoline. κ-opioid receptors modulate vagally mediated visceral sensation in the gastrointestinal tract, and κ-opioid receptor expression is upregulated after colonic inflammation. Intestinal mechanical and thermal pain innervated by multiple pelvic nerve fibers can be antagonized by intestinal infusion of asimadoline, suggesting that its therapeutic effects are peripheral.

Asimadoline can exert a relaxed inhibition of the transient calcium-dependent chloride secretion in the colonic mucosal layer of rats activated by the muscarinic receptor agonist carbachol (100 μmol/L) or the purinergic receptor agonist ATP (100 μmol/L) [8], suggesting that asimadoline may be effective in diarrheal dysentery by inhibiting fluid and electrolyte secretion. In addition, asimadoline also increased substance P in the joint fluid, which mediated the peripheral anti-infective effect. This effect was more pronounced in female rats with arthritis than in male rats. Asimadoline was effective in reducing joint damage caused by Freund's adjuvant-induced arthritis in rats and showed analgesic effects on mechanical injury perception thresholds; however, its anti-infective effects in visceral sensation are still unknown.

No significant adverse effects were observed with the administration of target doses of asimadoline (0.5 or 1 mg twice daily) to patients with functional gastrointestinal disorders [9]. High doses of asimadoline can cause polyuria and other adverse effects, therefore, the clinical use of asimadoline should be particularly careful to control its dose in order to maximize its efficacy and minimize adverse effects.

6.2.1.2 μ-Opioid Receptor Class of Drugs

In addition to κ-opioid receptors, which are mainly involved in visceral pain, other opioid receptors such as μ-opioid receptors and δ-opioid receptors also play important roles in the occurrence and development of visceral pain and have achieved good results in the treatment of visceral pain. One important class of receptor agonists is the μ-opioid receptor agonists, and new opioid receptor agonists have been continuously applied in the clinical treatment of visceral pain in recent years with satisfactory results.

1. μ-opioid receptors

   The μ receptor has five N-terminal glycosylation sites in its chemical structure and phosphorylation sites for protein kinase A and protein kinase C in the C inner loop, which are functional sites for opioid receptor regulation. μ receptors are coupled to G proteins and act through second messengers, including inhibition of adenylate cyclase activity, inhibition of calcium channels, and activation of potassium channels. Compared to other G protein-coupled receptors, the μ-opioid receptor molecule has a smaller cytoplasmic loop and inner cytosolic core and a smaller hydrophobic group. Using radioligand studies, μ receptors are divided into two subtypes, μ_1 and μ_2. The selective receptor antagonist naloxazone selectively blocks morphine-induced anti-injurious effects, but not morphine-induced respiratory depression and morphine-dependent effects. Some studies have shown that there may also be novel μ receptors, and morphine-6-β-glucuronide, heroin, and 6-acetylmorphine are such novel receptor agonists with which morphine itself does not interact.
2. μ-opioid receptor agonists

   Traditional μ-opioid receptor agonists such as morphine, pethidine hydrochloride, and dihydroetorphine hydrochloride are now commercialized and widely used in clinical practice, which are very classical analgesic drugs and can achieve good analgesic effects. However, they are still not the most ideal drugs for the treatment of visceral pain because of the obvious adverse effects accompanying the administration of the drugs. The analgesic effect of these drugs is very precise. In the following, morphine and pethidine hydrochloride will be used as representatives to make an introduction.

   (a) Morphine: Morphine is an analgesic drug that acts on opioid receptors within the central nervous system. Its analgesic characteristics are wide range, strong and long-lasting effect, accompanied by sedative effect. Its mechanism of action: (1) Binding to opioid receptors (mainly μ receptors) in different regions of the central nervous system, producing opioid-mediated effects, reducing or blocking the central transmission of nociceptive impulses by inhibiting the release of substance P at the end of primary afferent fibers; changing the emotional response and thus improving the tolerance of pain. (2) Morphine can also inhibit respiration. It has an inhibitory effect on the respiratory center, slowing down the respiratory rate and reducing the tidal volume, mainly because it reduces the sensitivity of the respiratory center to CO_2, and it may also be the result of morphine's agonism on μ_2 receptors. (3) Excites smooth muscle, especially the smooth muscle and sphincter of gastrointestinal tract, so that the tension of intestinal smooth muscle increases and intestinal peristalsis slows down, which can cause constipation: increase the tension of smooth muscle of ureter and bladder; the therapeutic dose can prolong the labor process of maternity. (4) Excites the parasympathetic nerve innervating the pupil, causing pupillary constriction. (5) Dilates peripheral blood vessels, promotes histamine release, reduces peripheral resistance, and may reduce cardiac load. (6) Anti-cough effect: Inhibits the cough center and is associated with the medullary solitary bundle nucleus opioid receptors. It is not generally used as a cough suppressant because it is easily addictive.

Morphine is mainly used as a strong analgesic, and is effective for all kinds of pain. The treatment of visceral pain is an important part of its analgesic effect, but it is easily addictive. It is suitable for acute pain where other analgesics are ineffective, such as advanced cancer pain and myocardial infarction. In clinical practice, morphine is often associated with adverse effects, mainly dizziness, nausea, vomiting, respiratory depression, constipation, difficulty urinating, tachycardia, drowsiness, and itchy skin. In addition, morphine tends to cause psychological dependence and physical dependence (i.e., addiction), which are the most serious problems associated with morphine use. The general therapeutic dose of continuous use for 1 week is likely to become magic.

(b) Pethidine hydrochloride: Pethidine hydrochloride is a μ agonist, its action and mechanism of action is roughly the same as morphine, the analgesic strength is about 1/10 of morphine [10], but the excitation of the smooth muscle of the gastrointestinal tract is relatively weaker than morphine, so less likely to cause constipation and urinary retention. It has only a slight cough suppressant effect. Therapeutic doses have no significant effect on the cardiovascular system.

Pethidine hydrochloride is the most commonly used synthetic potent analgesic for severe pain, such as post-surgical pain, advanced cancer pain, traumatic pain, etc. It is also effective for visceral colic (biliary colic and renal colic): when used for labor analgesia, the drug's respiratory depressant effect on the newborn fetus should be monitored. Pethidine hydrochloride's adverse reactions are milder than morphine, but still accompanied by certain adverse reactions, mainly dizziness, nausea, vomiting, dry mouth, etc. In acute poisoning, respiratory depression, drowsiness, and then coma, blood pressure drop; after repeatedly giving large doses of pethidine for a short time, it can cause tremors, muscle convulsions, pupil dilation and convulsions, and other symptoms.

(c) Dihydroetorphine hydrochloride: Dihydroetorphine hydrochloride is a μ-opioid receptor agonist, and also has a very weak effect on δ and κ receptors. Its analgesic effect is stronger than morphine, and the analgesic dose is 1/1000 of morphine and 1/5000 of pethidine [11], which is by far the strongest drug in clinical application in terms of analgesic efficacy. The drug also has sedative and hypnotic effects, and has a relaxing effect on the smooth muscle of the gastrointestinal tract, and its dependence is mainly manifested as strong mental dependence. Dihydroetorphine hydrochloride is mainly used clinically for: (1) chronic intractable pain and advanced cancer pain where morphine and pethidine are not effective; (2) colic caused by smooth muscle spasm, such as acute attacks of pancreatitis; (3) it can also be used as anesthetic adjuvant. Like morphine and pethidine hydrochloride, dihydroetorphine hydrochloride also has adverse reactions, mainly including: (1) light adverse reactions at analgesic dose, some patients can see slower breathing and drowsiness, 0.2–0.3 μg/kg intravenous injection can show obvious respiratory depression, or even apnea; (2) there is a transient decrease in blood pressure with excessive dosage, but no change in heart rate; (3) it can cause nausea and vomiting; (4) repeated dosing can produce tolerance, addiction, and withdrawal symptoms.

In addition, other μ-opioid receptor agonists such as bupropion and isoproterenol are widely used in clinical treatment of different types of visceral pain, but they are accompanied by corresponding adverse effects and different contraindications, which limit the application of such drugs to some extent. Therefore, the development of new opioids with high efficiency and low adverse effects for the treatment of visceral pain remains one of the key medical challenges that need to be addressed urgently.

6.2.1.3 κ, μ Double Receptor Drugs: Oxycodone Hydrochloride

Oxycodone (oxycodone) is a pure opioid κ and μ receptor agonist extracted from the alkaloid thebaine, which is a non-selective opioid receptor agonist and acts by acting on opioid receptors to reduce or block transmission from somatic afferent fibers and postganglionic fibers of autonomic nerves to neurons in the dorsal horn of the spinal cord, preventing or delaying pain from blood. Oxycodone acts primarily on the central nervous system and organs composed of smooth muscle. Oxycodone acts similarly to morphine, with the main pharmacological effect being analgesia and other pharmacological effects including anxiolysis, cough suppression, and sedation. Oxycodone is widely used in clinical practice because of its high bioavailability, multiple routes of administration, rapid onset of action, strong analgesic effect, long-lasting effect, maintenance of hemodynamic stability, and low incidence of postoperative nausea and vomiting. However, it has been found that after continuous use of oxycodone at high doses, some patients have withdrawal syndrome when the dose is suddenly interrupted or reduced. This suggests that oxycodone has the same adverse effects common to other opioids. Oxycodone hydrochloride controlled-release tablets were approved by the U.S. Food and Drug Administration (FDA) in 1997 for the treatment of patients with moderate to severe pain who require several days of opioid analgesics [12].

6.2.2 Non-opioid Drugs

In recent years, the discovery of the many drawbacks of opioids (adverse effects, tolerability, dependence, and strict regulatory restrictions on their use) has stimulated the development of non-opioid therapeutic agents that are effective in the long-term treatment of chronic pain states. The classification of non-opioid analgesics covers a collection of compounds with analgesic effects, including NSAIDs, voltage-gated ion channel (VGIC) modulators, cannabinoids, antidepressants, and others. NSAIDs are recommended for patients with mild to moderate acute pain, and most are available over the counter or by prescription in hospitals or pharmacies. Also, NSAID treatment is associated with potentially serious side effects, where higher doses and long-term use increase these risks. Irritable bowel syndrome (IBS) is one of the most representative types of visceral pain, the mechanisms of which are not yet fully understood. In patients with IBS, abdominal pain is closely related to their quality of life; chronic visceral nociceptive hypersensitivity is an important manifestation of the pathophysiology of IBS, so it is urgent to address this issue. Experimental studies have shown some non-opioid agents' potential to treat IBS.

6.2.2.1 NSAID

NSAID relieves pain by indirectly inhibiting cyclic oxygenase activity, thereby preventing prostaglandin formation. The use of this compound should be carefully dose adhered to, which is essential to avoid gastric ulcer formation and harmful effects on renal function. Acetaminophen (alone or in combination with opiates) can be administered as an alternative therapy, but is potentially harmful. In patients with chronic abdominal pain associated with IBS, conventional treatment includes the use of anticholinergic/antispasmodic agents such as dicyclopamine and scopolamine as smooth muscle relaxants and antidepressants, neither of which has been shown to be effective for visceral pain. However, 5-hydroxytryptamine compounds (5-HT_3 antagonists) and tegaserod (5-HT_4 agonists) have been shown to be effective in the treatment of visceral pain caused by IBS. 5-HT$_3$ receptors are mainly expressed in intestinal tissues and the nervous system. Several 5-HT$_3$ receptor antagonists have been studied for the treatment of BS and abdominal pain with diarrhea as a prominent feature. However, the exact mechanism remains unclear and may be the result of action on peripheral 5-HT$_3$ receptors. The first 5-HT$_3$ receptor antagonists used in clinical trials for the treatment of visceral pain had to be prematurely discontinued because of serious adverse effects (ischemic colitis and severe constipation). Recently, two new selective 5-HT$_3$ receptor antagonists, DPP-733 and NARI, have been tested in small clinical trials for the treatment of IBS with good results. However, studies on the specific mechanisms by which 5-HT receptor antagonists cause the adverse effects of ischemic colitis and severe constipation, as well as the distribution of different 5-HT receptor subtypes in different sites and neurons in the intestine, are still in their early stages.

6.2.2.2 Beneficial Intestinal Bacteria

The role of beneficial bacteria in the function of the gastrointestinal tract is to influence the adhesion of pathogenic bacteria and to enhance the barrier effect of epithelial cells. *Escherichia coli* can reduce the level of trinitrobenzene sulfonic acid in rats and alleviate the visceral nociceptive hypersensitivity caused by colitis. Lactobacillus also reduced antibiotic-mediated visceral nociceptive hypersensitivity in inflamed mice. Clinically, although new data continue to show that beneficial bacteria have very good efficacy in the treatment of IBS, it is difficult to draw definite conclusions whether beneficial bacteria have therapeutic effects on human visceral pain due to inadequate test methods.

6.2.2.3 Corticotropin-Releasing Factor Receptor-1 (CRF1R) Antagonists

Studies have shown that the brain CRF-CRFIR signaling system modulates endocrine activity and stress pain, and in particular, CRF1R antagonists have significant analgesic effects on stress-induced visceral nociceptive hyperalgesia, suggesting that the CRF-CRFIR signaling system may play an important role in functional gastrointestinal disorders. In a recent human trial, Sagami et al. noted that intravenous administration of the CRF1R antagonist α-helical CRF9-41 significantly suppressed the extent of abdominal pain and anxiety index in patients with IBS. The state is that this compound does not cross the blood-brain barrier, so the therapeutic effect of CRF1R antagonists may act through the periphery. However, there are also clinical studies showing that female IBS patients did not feel a significant reduction in pain levels after treatment with the selective CRFIR antagonist Bms-562086. Therefore, stronger evidence is still needed to demonstrate the role of CRF1R antagonists in reversing stress-induced visceral nociceptive hyperalgesia.

6.2.2.4 Pregabalin

Pregabalin, a second-generation ligand for the $\alpha_2\delta$ subunit of the calcium channel, has been shown to be useful in the treatment of peripheral neuropathic pain, as well as in the adjunctive treatment of limited partial seizures. Although the mechanism of pain relief by pregabalin is not fully understood, it is currently believed to inhibit the $\alpha_2\delta$ subunit of voltage-dependent calcium channels in the central nervous system, reducing calcium inward flow and subsequently reducing the release of excitatory neurotransmitters such as glutamate, norepinephrine, and substance P, thus effectively controlling neuropathic pain, and also having anxiolytic and anticonvulsant effects. In animal models of visceral pain, pregabalin can effectively reduce visceral nociceptive hyperalgesia induced by trinitrobenzene sulfonic acid (TNBS) and lipopolysaccharide (LPS). A recent randomized double-blind clinical trial showed that continuous oral administration of pregabalin for 3 weeks significantly alleviated nociceptive hypersensitivity in patients with IBS [13].

6.2.2.5 TRP Ion Channel Orange Resistance Drug

Unlike other calcium channels such as voltage-gated and ligand-gated channels, which are involved in relatively specialized cellular functions, the transient receptor potential (TRP) family of ion channels is intriguing because of its potential universality and diversity of functions. Their tissue distribution is extremely broad, with distribution in the peripheral nervous system, sensory organs, and cardiovascular, gastrointestinal, respiratory, urinary, reproductive, hematopoietic, and immune systems, in addition to the central nervous system. Increasing evidence suggests that TRP proteins may be involved in mediating vision, hearing, taste, pain, touch, and neurotransmitter release; as well as in regulating blood pressure, intestinal motility, mineral absorption, fluid homeostasis, cell survival, growth, and death, and pheromane behavior in animals. This functional diversity may be related to its ability to sense numerous intra- and extracellular signals, such as cell membrane receptor stimulation, temperature, acidity, mechanical stress, redox status, etc.; it may also be related to the formation of homo or heterodimeric TRP channels and their involvement in the formation of complex signal transduction complexes. The main members of TRP family are TRPC, TRPM, TRPML, TRPA, TRPP, and TRPV, among which TRPV1 and TRPV4 are closely associated with chemical or mechanical stimulation-induced visceral pain. In a model of colonic pain sensitivity caused by stimulation of the neonatal rat colon, TRPV1 antagonists reduced pain induced by colonic dilation. Chen et al. showed that increased rectal sensitivity was associated with increased TRPV1 fibers in the intestinal wall [14]. Therefore, TRPV1 and TRPV4 can be used as targets for drug binding and design of new drugs for visceral pain.

6.3 Combination Therapy

An alternative treatment approach to visceral pain has emerged in recent years, which involves the combined use of two or more analgesic drug treatments without drug toxicity overlap. The use of drug combinations combining opioid-like substances and adjuvant medications is referred to as multimodal or balanced analgesia. Several combinations containing opioids and NSAIDs, several opioids in a single formulation or anti-inflammatory drugs plus gastroprotective agents are being developed. Fixed doses for the treatment of polymyalgia are described by Raffa et al. [15]. When the pathophysiology of a medical condition is multimodal, i.e., associated with multiple physiological causes or mediated by multiple pathways, the best strategy for treatment may be to use a single drug or a combination of drugs that provide multiple mechanisms for achieving the ultimate goal of treatment. In such cases, a rational multimodal approach may also lead to minimal disadvantages. Due to the anatomical and physiological characteristics of pain transmission, most pain is multifactorial. Therefore, further exploration of combined drug therapy for visceral pain is imminent.

6.4 Summary

With the continuous advancement of basic research and precision medicine, the concept of visceral pain has shifted from an organ-centered disease concept to one that integrates psychological and gender dimensions of pathophysiological mechanisms. Despite the growing body of literature on visceral pain, the exact mechanisms underlying visceral pain remain less clear compared to somatic pain. Research to understand the underlying mechanisms behind pain has made significant progress in the last few decades, but despite these significant advances to support it, pain still exists and occurs at a high rate.

Traditional opioid receptor drugs have been effective in the treatment of visceral pain, but are accompanied by non-negligible adverse effects, such as respiratory depression, euphoria, and addiction. These adverse effects may be caused by the fact that μ opioids can cross the blood-brain barrier, thus also limiting the clinical application of such drugs. In recent years, κ-opioid receptor drugs, which have a lower rate of crossing the blood-brain barrier (thus avoiding central adverse effects), have gained attention for acting mainly through the peripheral nervous system. κ-opioid receptor agonist pharmacology experiments for the treatment of visceral pain suggest that peripherally selective, opioid receptor agonists may be effective drugs for the treatment of different types of visceral pain. The development of κ-opioid receptor agonists with high peripheral hyperselectivity remains one of the current problems to be solved.

In addition to opioids used to treat visceral pain, non-opioid drugs have also been effective in the treatment of visceral pain, such as 5-HT_3 receptor antagonists and CRF1R antagonists. However, the research on most of the drugs is still in the primary stage and further in-depth studies are needed.

In addition, there are often significant differences between the results of animal experiments and clinical trials. There are many reasons for this discrepancy, one of which may be that although many drugs can significantly reduce injurious stimuli in rodents, this is not necessarily necessary for the normalization of visceral sensory signals in patients with visceral pain. Therefore, the differences between animal and human visceral pain mechanisms should be understood before developing drugs for visceral pain.

References

1. Farmer AD, Aziz Q. Mechanisms of visceral pain in health and functional gastrointestinal disorders. Scand J Pain. 2014;5(2):51–60.
2. Sengupta JN. Visceral pain: the neurophysiological mechanism. Sensory Nerves. 2009;194:31–74.
3. Yasuda K, Raynor K, Kong H, Breder CD, Takeda J, Reisine T, et al. Cloning and functional comparison of kappa and delta opioid receptors from mouse brain. Proc Natl Acad Sci. 1993;90(14):6736–40.
4. Zhang L-S, Wang J, Chen J-C, Tao Y-M, Wang Y-H, Xu X-J, et al. Novel κ-opioid receptor agonist MB-1C-OH produces potent analgesia with less depression and sedation. Acta Pharmacol Sin. 2015;36(5):565–71.
5. Gabrielsson J, Meibohm B, Weiner D. Pattern recognition in pharmacokinetic data analysis. AAPS J. 2015;18(1):47–63.
6. Camilleri M. Novel pharmacology: asimadoline, a κ-opioid agonist, and visceral sensation. Neurogastroenterol Motil. 2008;20(9):971–9.
7. Foley PL, Kendall LV, Turner PV. Clinical management of pain in rodents. Comp Med. 2019;69(6):468–89.
8. Zhou H, Kong D-H, Pan Q-W, Wang H-H. Sources of calcium in agonist-induced contraction of rat distal colon smooth muscle in vitro. World J Gastroenterol. 2008;14(7):1077.
9. Fikree A, Byrne P. Management of functional gastrointestinal disorders. Clin Med. 2021;21(1):44–52.
10. Drewes AM, Jensen RD, Nielsen LM, Droney J, Christrup LL, Arendt-Nielsen L, et al. Differences between opioids: pharmacological, experimental, clinical and economical perspectives. Br J Clin Pharmacol. 2012;75(1):60–78.
11. Hanna MH, Elliott KM, Stuart-Taylor ME, Roberts DR, Buggy D, Arthurs GJ. Comparative study of analgesic efficacy and morphine-sparing effect of intramuscular dexketoprofen trometamol with ketoprofen or placebo after major orthopaedic surgery. Br J Clin Pharmacol. 2003;55(2):126–33.
12. Center for Drug Evaluation and Research. Substance use and overdose prevention timeline. U.S. Food and Drug Administration [cited 2023 Apr 11]. Available from: https://www.fda.gov/drugs/information-drug-class/timeline-selected-fda-activities-and-significant-events-addressing-substance-use-and-overdose.
13. Ravnefjord A, Brusberg M, Larsson H, Lindström E, Martínez V. Effects of pregabalin on visceral pain responses and colonic compliance in rats. Br J Pharmacol. 2008;155(3):407–16.
14. Chen Y, Mu J, Zhu M, Mukherjee A, Zhang H. Transient receptor potential channels and inflammatory bowel disease. Front Immunol. 2020;11:180.
15. Raffa RB, Connelly CD, Martinez RP, Schupsky JJ, Argentieri DC, Singer MM, et al. Antinociceptive effects of a novel dual cyclooxygenase/5-lipoxygenase inhibitor (tepoxalin) and its primary (carboxylic acid) metabolite (RWJ 20142) in acute tests in mice and rats. Drug Dev Res. 1995;36(2):81–90.

Neuromodulation Therapy for Visceral Pain

7

Bifa Fan

When drugs fail to reduce or eliminate the pain feeling, patients may seek other therapies to treat their diseases. Under such circumstances, technologies such as neuromodulation therapy (nerve block) and neuroelectrical stimulation technique (spinal cord stimulation, peripheral nerve stimulation, transcutaneous electrical nerve stimulation, motor cortex stimulation, deep brain stimulation, and so on) are used to effectively control the pain.

Since the mechanism of visceral pain is not yet fully understood, the current treatment also lacks specificity, resulting in the poor effect of the commonly used analgesic drugs on the treatment of certain visceral pain, especially intractable visceral pain. The more common ones are cancerous visceral pain caused by tumors and visceral pain caused by chronic inflammation, postoperative adhesions, and so on. Its treatment requires the participation of multidisciplinary doctors from pain, neurology, neurosurgery, and orthopedics, as well as psychologists and physical therapists. In the treatment of visceral pain, the cause of the pain should be clarified. If the pain is caused by a tumor, tissue, or organ anatomical changes (e.g., herniated disc, etc.), the primary cause and the compression of the nerve by the anatomical changes should be treated first, and then the treatment should be directed to the pain. If non-surgical treatments such as medication, nerve block, physiotherapy, psychotherapy, acupuncture, etc. are ineffective or have intolerable adverse reactions, neuromodulation therapy (mainly including nerve block, neurolysis, electrical stimulation, etc.) or even surgical treatment can be used.

7.1 Nerve Block or Neurolysis

There are often many options for visceral pain treatment. Imaging-mediated diagnostic blocks at the target site, usually with local anesthetics, and once the target site has been identified, nerve disruption may also be used for the relief of underlying long-term pain. Nerve blocks/neurolysis are primarily used in patients with intractable visceral pain and some cancer pain.

Nerve block therapy is a class of methods in which local anesthetics, such as lidocaine and bupivacaine, are injected directly into and around ganglia, nerve trunks, or plexuses to block pain transmission. Neurolysis can be divided into the application of chemical and physical agents to a nerve to make it temporarily or permanently degenerated. Neurolysis with chemical agents provides long-term analgesia primarily through the damage of nerve structures by chemical agents. These techniques originated in the 1930s, and chemicals were initially used to treat severe malignant pain and other non-malignant chronic conditions [1]. The most commonly used agents

B. Fan (✉)
Department of Pain Medicine, China-Japan Friendship Hospital, Beijing, China

M. Xia et al. (eds.), *Visceral Pain*, https://doi.org/10.1007/978-981-99-9167-9_7

were phenol glycerin (phenol) and anhydrous ethanol. Neurolysis with physical agents is mainly radiofrequency treatment, including continuous radiofrequency ablation (CRFA) [2] and pulsed radiofrequency ablation (PRFA) [3], the principle of which is to denature the nerve tissue associated with pain and obtain a longer period of continuous analgesia. It also includes cryoablation and water-cooled RFA, which is a new radiofrequency technique used to treat various pain syndromes, with the principle of action similar to CRFA, in which the electrode is as close as possible to the target nerve to reduce pain by cutting off nerve conduction. Water-cooled RF ablation uses a special electrode that can be actively cooled by a continuous flow of water at ambient temperature. The main nerve block/neurolysis methods for the treatment of intractable visceral pain that have been reported more frequently in the literature in recent years are as follows.

7.1.1 Abdominal Plexus or Visceral Nerve Block/Neurolysis

The first historical neurolytic celiac plexus blockade (NCPB) was performed by Max Kappis in 1914 [4]. The celiac plexus is responsible for innervating the nerves of the gastrointestinal tract including the liver, bile duct, kidney, spleen, adrenal glands, and mesentery. Because it innervates the nerves of the gastrointestinal tract so extensively, a local anesthetic block of the celiac plexus is commonly used clinically to diagnostically treat some patients with visceral pain, including pancreatic cancer, upper abdominal malignancies, and chronic pancreatitis. If there is pain relief, nerve-destroying drugs may be injected around the celiac plexus or visceral nerves for neurolysis.

The celiac plexus, the largest autonomic plexus in the body, is generally located in the retroperitoneum and consists of two larger celiac ganglia surrounding the celiac artery or superior mesenteric artery, which are hidden medial to the adrenal glands and anterior to the pedicle of the diaphragm. A recent cadaveric study found that 94% of the celiac ganglia were at T_{12} or L_1 [5]. The celiac nerve consists of a reticular formation of sympathetic and parasympathetic fibers that receive fibers from three visceral nerves (visceral major, visceral minor, and visceral minor) that originate at the level of the T_{5-12} segment, and it also receives parasympathetic fibers from the vagus nerve. The celiac plexus is the origin of the distribution of nerves in the liver, pancreas, gallbladder, stomach, spleen, kidneys, intestines, adrenal glands, and blood vessels.

Percutaneous peritoneal plexus dissection is usually performed under CT, ultrasound, and X-ray fluoroscopic guidance, and can be divided into the following types of procedures according to the orientation of the blocking needle into the peritoneal plexus.

1. Anterior approach method

   When the anterior approach technique is applied, the patient is generally positioned in a supine position using transabdominal CT guidance, and the needle is punctured from 1 to 2 cm below the glabella slightly to the left, with a single needle puncture with a vertical approach. The drug is injected next to the abdominal trunk or between the abdominal trunk and the root of the superior mesenteric artery by passing above the lesser curvature of the stomach to reach the abdominal aorta and the diaphragmatic foot directly in front. In recent years, ultrasound-guided puncture techniques have also been carried out. Unlike CT, ultrasound has no radiological damage, does not require injection of contrast agent during operation, can guide the puncture needle in real-time and confirm the position of the needle tip in relation to the abdominal aorta, abdominal trunk, and superior mesenteric artery, and can dynamically observe the diffusion range of the drug, which has the advantages of real-time monitoring, no radiation, and relatively easy operation. For those patients with abdominal tumor compression who cannot be in a prone position for a long time, the anterior approach has certain advantages, allowing those patients who cannot easily be in a prone position to perform abdominal plexus puncture through the abdominal approach, while reducing the risk of puncture. However, in general, the anterior approach has the potential to cause gastric, intestinal, or pancreatic fistulas, and is not widely used.

2. Posterior approach via the intervertebral disc (anterior phrenic foot method)

   The skin puncture point is mostly chosen at the level of the T_{12}–L_1 intervertebral disc, and the needle is inserted dorsally along the outer edge of the vertebral body or disc, 5 cm from the midline or slightly anterior to the lateral side, or through the abdominal aorta to its anterior side if necessary. In this method, the puncture needle should penetrate the pedicle of the diaphragm from the posterior side to reach directly near the abdominal plexus, and the injected drug diffuses directly on the anterolateral side of the aorta. At the same time, due to the blocking effect of the diaphragm, the neurodestructive drug does not penetrate the nerve roots and spinal arteries near the vertebral body, avoiding accidental damage to adjacent tissue structures. Using the ipsilateral approach, i.e., if the skin puncture point is located on the right side of the midline, the needle tip is also located on the right side of the abdominal aorta after needle entry. Then inject the diluted contrast agent, observe the distribution of the contrast agent, and after the contrast agent diffusion range reaches the expected target, inject 1–2% lidocaine diagnostically, observe for 10–15 min, and if there is no numbness and motor impairment in both lower limbs and pain relief, inject the nerve-destroying drug ethanol or phenol via the puncture needle. It can also be punctured from the left side, and the needle tip should be directed toward the lower 1/3 of the L_1 vertebral body, penetrating the aorta until the blood flow through the needle stops, at which point the prediaphragmatic foot method is also known as the transaortic method. This method has gained much attention in recent years because of its simplicity and safety, as well as the advantages of good results and low adverse effects.

3. Posterior approach via the diaphragmatic foot method (posterior diaphragmatic foot method)

   The posterior method differs from the anterior method of the diaphragmatic foot in that the injected drug is mainly distributed between the diaphragmatic foot and the spine rather than near the abdominal plexus in front of the diaphragmatic foot, and the puncture needle should reach the anterior edge of the vertebral body and stop behind the diaphragmatic foot. Firstly, the abdominal plexus puncture channel is measured by CT, and then a suitable angle is selected for needle entry. The guidance method and the selection of the puncture point and the method of drug delivery are the same as the transvertebral disc method, but the needle entry requires that the needle tip should be directed toward L_1, the upper 1/3 of the vertebral body, reaching the anterolateral aspect of the T_{12} vertebral body, above the point of attachment of the diaphragm, medial to the mural pleura, and not beyond the anterior edge of the vertebral body by 0.5 cm. The purpose of this method is to block the large visceral nerves. It is suitable for those whose upper abdominal tumors involve the abdominal plexus or those who have difficulty destroying the abdominal plexus.

4. Posterior approach to continuous percutaneous neurolysis of the celiac plexus

   The abdominal plexus innervates almost all the internal organs of the abdominal cavity except the pelvic organs, and the pain of some patients cannot be completely relieved by conventional one-time injections of destructive drugs. In addition to changes in the patient's own condition, the main reason for the recent poor efficacy is that the dose of blocking drugs injected at once is relatively insufficient to fully infiltrate and block the entire abdominal plexus, and the residual nerve fibers cause the patient to still feel pain, or the neurolysis of the nerve is not complete, resulting in nerve repair and pain recurrence in a relatively short period of time. Therefore, percutaneous continuous abdominal plexus neurolysis can make up for the above deficiencies.

5. Transesophageal ultrasound endoscopic laparoscopic plexus dissection

   Ultrasound imaging offers unique advantages, including detailed soft tissue imaging and the ability to provide real-time tissue sampling. However, a limitation of ultrasound is its inability to visualize air-filled structures or extremely dense structures (e.g., calcifications). Transabdominal ultrasound usually does not adequately visualize all abdominal structures when there are large amounts of fat or air artifacts in the abdominal cavity. Esophageal ultrasonography (EUS) overcomes this limitation by endoscopically placing ultrasound probes under the stomach and duodenum, such that the ultrasound probe in contact with the duodenal wall is only 5 mm away from the common bile duct in the inner segment of the pancreas, making EUS a low-risk procedure similar to minimally invasive upper gastrointestinal endoscopy.

   Injection of nerve-disrupting agents into the abdominal ganglion region via EUS guidance is mostly used to treat severe abdominal pain caused by upper abdominal diseases such as pancreatic cancer and chronic pancreatitis. The abdominal ganglion is located anterolaterally to the abdominal aorta, and the relative relationship between the abdominal ganglion and the root of the abdominal trunk is relatively fixed and can be clearly displayed under EUS. The abdominal ganglion can be localized more accurately with EUS. Compared with the traditional percutaneous puncture method, the abdominal ganglion is separated from the gastric cavity by only one wall, the puncture distance is close and the localization is accurate, so the side effects and complications are greatly reduced.
6. Visceral nerve block

   At this stage, abdominal plexus block for the treatment of upper abdominal visceral pain, especially cancer pain, has been widely recognized. It should be noted that there are many factors affecting the efficacy of abdominal plexus block in patients with intermediate and advanced cancer pain, such as the anatomical location of the retroperitoneum changed by tumor spread and neurolysis of local structures, the invasion of the abdominal plexus and conduction channels by ascites or cancer foci, and the influence of peritoneal tissue on drug diffusion. Abdominal plexus block/neurolysis has a good analgesic effect in the early stage of upper abdominal cancer invasion of the abdominal plexus and when the metastases are small (this is because the gap around the abdominal plexus is still large and the destructive drugs can be easily diffused to achieve more extensive abdominal nerve degeneration, so satisfactory analgesic effect can be achieved); however, when cancer invades metastases extensively, the efficacy of abdominal plexus block is not satisfactory, which is mainly related to the degree of tumor invasion of the abdominal plexus. According to the visceral nociceptive pathway in the upper abdomen, it is known that pain in mid- to late-stage cancer is transmitted through nerve fibers to the celiac plexus and from the celiac plexus to the visceral nerves. The visceral size nerves leave the ventral plexus crossing the pedicle of the diaphragm and enter the nerve fibers along the surface of the vertebral body in the posterior hiatus of the pedicle to connect to the sympathetic chain. Therefore, in order to improve the efficacy, visceral nerve block, also known as splanchnic nerve block (SNB), has been tried to treat patients with mid- to late-stage cancer pain using ultrasound, CT, and other adjuvant means, and it has been found that SNB has better results both in terms of analgesic effect and improvement of quality of life. Since advanced malignant tumors often present with extensive abdominal and pelvic metastases, injurious nerve impulses often cannot be blocked by a single sympathetic plexus disruption. In this situation, it is also useful to try to combine multiple nerve blocks for the treatment of intractable visceral cancer pain. SNB is very similar to the posterior approach via the pedicle of the diaphragm, compared to the latter with a higher puncture position, when applying SNB, the needle tip is directed toward the T_{12} vertebral body, and the final radiographic image needle tip is located in the junctional area of the anterior 1/3 and inferior 1/3 of the T_{12} vertebral body. Both methods are essentially the same in that they block the visceral nerve by injecting drug diffusion toward the cephalic end of the guard. The operation is usually performed by bilateral puncture, with the puncture needle reaching the anterior part of the vertebral body as close to the midline as possible under X-ray fluoroscopy or CT guidance, followed by injection of destructive drugs.

There are some potential complications associated with abdominal plexus block, including hypotension after penetration of the dura, sympathetic chain block, localized low back pain after the puncture, retroperitoneal hematoma after injury to the vessels, diarrhea, pneumothorax, celiac disease, renal injury, dysuria, ejaculation disorder, and aortic entrapment caused by needle tip puncture. The occurrence of complications is related to the type of block used. Ischia et al. studied the effectiveness and complications in 61 patients with pancreatic cancer after the application of three techniques (anterior phrenic foot, posterior phrenic foot, and visceral nerve block) and they found a higher incidence of upright hypotension with the posterior phrenic foot or visceral nerve block, 50% and 52%, respectively, compared to 10% with the anterior phrenic foot method [6]. However, the incidence of diarrhea was 65% with the anterior diaphragmatic foot approach and only 25% and 5% with the posterior diaphragmatic foot approach and visceral nerve block, respectively, and there was no significant difference in the incidence of abnormal pain, hematuria, eructation, interscapular region pain, and reactive pleurisy between the three groups when evaluated.

7.1.2 Superior Hypogastric Plexus Block

The superior hypogastric plexus, like the ganglion impar is a retroperitoneal structure located between the lower 1/3 of L_5 and the upper 1/3 of S_1, distributed on both sides of the anterior border of the vertebral body, and located close to the bifurcation of the common iliac vessels on the left and right sides. The inferior epigastric plexus innervates the pelvic organs through the hypogastric nerve. The inferior epigastric plexus block can alleviate pelvic visceral pain caused by cancer or chronic non-cancerous diseases.

The operation is performed with the patient in a prone position with a pillow placed under the lower abdomen so that the lumbar spine is not too anteriorly convex, the lumbosacral region is routinely disinfected and prepared with towels, the $L_{4,5}$ intervertebral space is defined under anteroposterior fluoroscopic guidance, the skin, and subcutaneous tissues are local anesthetized with a 5–7 cm paracentesis from the midline bilaterally at the level of this intervertebral space, followed by an oblique medial puncture with two 18-cm-long 22G puncture needles with the needle tips adjusted to 45° medially and 30° caudally toward the anterolateral aspect of the L_5 vertebral body. During puncture, the L_5 transverse process and iliac crest can obstruct the course of the needle, at which point the entrance to the needle or the direction of needle entry must be slightly adjusted. Intermittent use of X-ray fluoroscopy is required during needle insertion. The needle tip is considered to reach the L_5 vertebral body if it is in contact with the bone during travel, and the needle tip should be located anterolaterally to the L_5 vertebral body under X-ray fluoroscopy. If the bone of the L_5 vertebral body is contacted, the needle tip should slide along the bone and reach the anterior edge of the vertebral body 1 cm forward, at which point there will be a falling sensation, signifying that the needle tip has penetrated the lumbaris major fascia and entered the retroperitoneal region, at which point the needle tip is located at the joint of the L_5–S_1 vertebral body in the anteroposterior X-ray visualization, and the needle tip should be just in front of the anterolateral edge of the L_5 vertebral body in the lateral visualization. Subsequently, negative pressure aspiration is performed and 3–4 mL of contrast agent is injected, and a smooth posterior margin is revealed under lateral fluoroscopy; this is the formation of the lumbaris major fascia, and the contrast agent for anterior-posterior imaging should be confined to the midline.

In the traditional operation, since the iliac crest, L_5 transverse process and L_5 nerve root can be an obstacle to puncture and may cause damage to the nerve root at the same time, in 2005 Turker et al. proposed a modified method in which the patient is placed in the lateral position, the L_5/S_1 gap is confirmed using X-ray imaging, the skin is disinfected and toweled and local anesthesia is administered, and a 15-cm-long 20G millipede needle is placed under fluoroscopic guidance toward the under lateral fluoroscopy, the needle should pass through the intrasheath capsule and continue through the disc until the tip of the needle breaks through the anterior edge of the disc, at which point contrast is injected and anteroposterior and lateral fluoroscopy is used to confirm the tip position [7].

When performing an inferior epigastric plexus block, a number of potential complications can occur in its adjacent anatomic tissues, the most significant of which include intravascular injection and/or hemorrhage and hematoma after penetrating a vessel due to the proximity of the common iliac vessel bifurcation. Second, intramuscular or intraperitoneal injections can occur if the depth of the needle tip is not anticipated, and some minor complications include epidural or intrathecal injections, L_5 nerve root injury, and renal ureteral injury. In addition to complications due to anatomic causes in the adjacent superior-inferior abdominal plexus, there are also complications inherent in the method of operation, and discitis may occur due to disruption of the integrity of the disc during transsphenoidal puncture, usually with prophylactic antibiotics, but there is still a risk of disc degeneration. If the anterior approach is used, complications include injury to the bladder, common iliac artery, and bowel.

7.1.3 Inferior Hypogastric Plexus Block

The inferior hypogastric plexus is a paravertebral network of paired sympathetic fibers that lie anterior to the sacrum, dorsally adjacent to the sacrum, and ventrally adjacent to the posterior rectum wall. Pain management of malignant and nonmalignant sympathetic persistent painful disorders, including the distal colon, bladder, penis, vagina, rectum, anus, and perineum regions, can generally be treated by interfering with the transmission of the inferior abdominal plexus.

A trans-sacral approach to block the lower abdominal hypogastric plexus is usually advocated. The patient is placed in a prone position, the location of the S_2 sacral foramen is determined by anteroposterior X-ray fluoroscopy, routine sterilization is performed, a subcutaneous local anesthetic injection is performed 1 cm lateral to the S_2 sacral foramen, a 22G lumbar anesthetic needle is used to penetrate the skin and puncture is performed lateral to the S_2 sacral foramen toward the sacrum, and the puncture needle is then entered into the lateral portion of the S_2 sacral foramen, gradually traveling ventrally and medially to avoid causing sensory abnormalities. The optimal trajectory is to have the needle in the sacral foramen with the tip facing the midline under X-ray fluoroscopy. If 1 mL of contrast is injected, the anterior sacral cephalocaudal spread can be seen under anteroposterior fluoroscopy. If unilateral diffusion is seen, the procedure can be repeated on the contralateral side. The block is usually treated with 5–15 mL of local anesthetic or with the addition of steroids. If a unilateral diagnostic block is causing contralateral spread, a bilateral block via the sacral foramen should be eliminated to avoid penetrating the disc and its resulting set of adverse consequences. If the S_2 sacral foramen is not particularly well defined or if the sacral foramen is narrow, then the needle can be accessed through S_1 or S_3. It is usually rare for a puncture to reach the S_2 nerve root and cause sensory abnormalities. If it does occur, the needle is withdrawn and reoriented within the sacral foramen. Since the rectum is located ventrally in the lower inferior abdominal plexus, it may lead to abdominal infection in the patient if the needle tip enters the cavernous organs of the abdomen.

7.1.4 Ganglion Impar Block

The ganglion impar, also known as the Walther ganglion or sacrococcygeal ganglion, is an isolated retroperitoneal structure located at the sacrococcygeal junction anterior to the sacrococcygeal joint, which marks the caudal termination of two paravertebral sympathetic nerve chains. The innervation of the ganglion impar includes the perineum, distal rectum, anal region, distal urethra, vulva, and outer 1/3 of the vagina. Blocking the ganglion impar allows for diagnosing and treating visceral or sympathetic persistent pain in these areas. The transsacrococcygeal approach described by Wemm and Semerski in 1995 [8] is still widely used. In this operation, the puncture needle is inserted directly into the retroperitoneal space through the sacrococcygeal junction. The sacrococcygeal junction is sometimes difficult to visualize during anterior-posterior fluoroscopy due to bowel distension or fecal matter, and Lin et al. successfully combined ultrasound guidance during fluoroscopy with good results [9]. Ultrasound guidance is mainly used to define the sacrococcygeal junction in combination with anterior-posterior and lateral visualization, the latter being used to define the depth of the needle tip and to observe the diffusion of the contrast medium. Another modified block method is designed to overcome patients who have difficulty penetrating or cannot perform transsacrococcygeal puncture due to calcification of the sacrococcygeal ligament. This operation is fluoroscopically guided, with the puncture needle pointing below the transverse process of the coccyx, and once it touches the bone it is considered to have touched the transverse process, at which point the needle tip continues to slide downwards, over the surface of the anterior border of the coccyx and towards the level of the sacrococcygeal junction. CT-guided ganglion impar block has also been reported.

To perform a transsacrococcygeal approach block, the patient is placed in a prone position, the position of the sacrococcygeal junction is confirmed using anterior-posterior fluoroscopic guidance, the skin, and subcutaneous tissue are locally anesthetized, a 22G, 9-cm lumbar puncture needle is applied and combined with anterior-posterior and lateral fluoroscopy, the posterior peritoneal space is punctured, and contrast is injected to determine the location of the needle tip. If nerve disruption is performed, phenol is injected.

Recent literature has reported possible complications arising from the above-mentioned operations. Tissue injury, infection due to rectal penetration, etc., bleeding due to vascular injury, and periosteal injection can occur using the curved needle technique. The transsacrococcygeal approach is more comfortable for the patient and is theoretically less traumatic for the patient because of the use of a straight needle. However, after multiple operations, the sclerosis of the sacrococcygeal disc, which prevents good visualization under fluoroscopy, can make the operation more difficult. Potential complications of the transcaudal block method are caused by penetration of the articular disc, including arthritis of the disc, fistula formation, and bleeding.

7.1.5 Intraspinal Infusion

In the 1980s, after the discovery of opioid receptors in the spinal cord, the administration of drugs, especially opioids, through the intraspinal route gained popularity. As patients with advanced cancer cannot tolerate the severe side effects associated with the systemic administration of opioids, they are usually adjusted to intraspinal administration, which can significantly reduce the dose of opioids. Today, the method of infusion has evolved from a simple percutaneous epidural catheter to a fully placed epidural or intrathecal infusion pump. Fully placed systems have a low risk of infection and low maintenance, but are longer and more costly to perform. Recent randomized controlled trials have shown that drug administration via the total placement system improves pain relief rates and drug-related side effects. The drug of choice is usually an opioid combined with a local anesthetic, in addition, morphine, the most commonly used and studied opioid, is often used in combination with bupivacaine. Patients with subarachnoid morphine infusion have fewer side effects compared to patients with systemic morphine infusion. Intrathecal administration also allows for the infusion of drugs such as colistin and ziconotide.

To perform traditional intrathecal administration, the patient is placed in the lateral position and saline and various concentrations of local anesthetics are given through a lumbar arachnoid puncture. This subarachnoid technique has certain drawbacks, and Raj proposed the epidural technique in 1977 [10] to avoid the headache problems caused by the subarachnoid puncture and to allow continuous injection of local anesthetics through an epidural catheter subcutaneously tunneled to an electronic micropump for the treatment of intractable advanced cancer pain for cancer pain in the spinal nerve distribution area from the neck to the sacrum. The treatment can be performed by puncture placement according to the midpoint of the corresponding spinal nerve innervation segment of the tumor site and pain area as the puncture point; 0.6–1.2 mL of local anesthetic is administered to each spinal nerve segment according to the patient's height, physical strength, nutritional status, and pain range. The excellent rate of analgesia was 97.87%, with more definite results. The epidural cavity technique also has complications such as nausea, vomiting, urinary retention, skin pruritus, motor block, and failed catheter placement, which can cause some distress to patients. Complications such as severe nerve injury, epidural hematoma, or abscess are less common. In a single epidural block, a local anesthetic is often injected to verify the correct puncture location, followed by the injection of a nerve-disrupting drug (e.g., ethanol) to achieve long-term analgesia. When injecting nerve-destroying drugs into the epidural cavity, it is necessary to both dehydrate and degenerate the sensory nerves or undergo demyelination changes, so that they lose their conduction function and achieve the purpose of analgesia, and to minimize the impact on motor nerve function to avoid the occurrence of adverse reactions such as motor nerve paralysis and bladder and rectal dysfunction that accompany sensory nerve block. Therefore, it is particularly important to select the appropriate drug concentration and dose.

Intrathecal drug infusion therapy is administered to the patient's subarachnoid space through a drug infusion pump buried in the patient's body, which acts on the corresponding spinal cord segments to block the transmission of pain signals to the brain through the spinal cord, thus achieving pain control. The intrathecal drug infusion system consists of two components: a catheter placed in the subarachnoid space of the patient's spinal cord and a drug infusion pump placed subcutaneously in the patient's abdomen. The patient's response to the medication and pain relief is observed by a preoperative drug test. If the test is good, the full infusion system is placed. The greatest advantage of intrathecal drug infusion is that the amount of drug used can be greatly reduced (about 1/300th of the oral dose), the adverse effects are small and mild, and the entire system is fully inserted into the patient without affecting the patient's quality of life. The intrathecal infusion system has a variety of adjustable modes that allow different infusion patterns to be given to patients depending on their pain conditions in order to obtain maximum pain relief using the smallest amount of medication. The disadvantage of intrathecal drug infusion therapy is that it is relatively expensive and requires replacement of the subcutaneously placed drug pump after 6–7 years of use.

7.2 Neuroelectrical Stimulation Techniques

Neuroelectrical stimulation techniques have been developed for 40–50 years, mainly targeting different nerve sites that conduct pain with electrical stimulation to reduce pain transmission and reception, thus relieving pain. In recent years, nerve electrical stimulation techniques have been increasingly used in the treatment of visceral pain. According to the site of stimulation, it can be divided into gastrointestinal electrical stimulation, peripheral nerve electrical stimulation, peripheral nerve regional electrical stimulation, spinal cord electrical stimulation, motor cortex electrical stimulation, deep brain electrical stimulation, and non-invasive transcranial electrical stimulation.

7.2.1 Gastrointestinal Electrical Stimulation Techniques and Gastrointestinal Tract Movement Disorders

1. Functional gastrointestinal disorders

   Functional gastrointestinal disorder (FGID), including functional dyspepsia (FD) and irritable bowel syndrome (IBS), usually manifests as abdominal pain and/or abdominal discomfort. FGID is a clinical diagnosis of a series of chronic or recurrent abdominal syndromes for which no clear etiology has been identified with current diagnostic techniques. The symptoms of FD and IBS are usually associated with eating and include flatulence, early satiety, bloating, belching, and nausea in addition to abdominal pain. The pathophysiological mechanisms of chronic visceral pain include hypersensitivity to dilatation, abnormal gastrointestinal motility, autonomic dysfunction, and central nervous function involvement. However, because the mechanisms of chronic visceral pain accompanying FGID are still unknown, there is a lack of still effective therapeutic measures. Pharmacological treatments for visceral pain include opioids, low-dose tricyclic antidepressants, and 5-HT reuptake inhibitors. However, these drugs are not effective in all patients and their long-term effects are uncertain. Other treatments include hypnosis, cognitive behavioral therapy, electroacupuncture, and biological agents, the efficacy of which needs further study. Therefore, new treatments are urgently needed to relieve visceral pain in patients with FGID.

   Abnormal gastric motility may be the cause of secondary abdominal discomfort or pain in patients with FGID. The main gastric motility dysfunctions in patients with FD include: (a) hypokinetic gastric sinus and delayed gastric emptying, but the asynchronous nature of this dysfunction and abdominal pain symptoms makes this causal relationship uncertain; (b) abnormal rhythm of gastric triggered electrical activity, which is demonstrated in 36% of patients with FD and 25% of patients with IBS [11], and is associated with delayed gastric emptying, but not with abdominal pain symptoms; and (c) abnormal gastric tone and adaptive diastole. It has been reported that dyspepsia is associated with abnormal gastric accommodative diastole in a proportion of FD patients.

   Only 20–75% of patients with IBS exhibit kinetic abnormalities [12]. Ileum, colon, and rectum of patients with IBS exhibit enhanced responses to stimuli such as feeding, dilation, stress, cholecystokinin, neostigmine, and adrenocorticotropin-releasing hormone injections; the stomach and proximal small intestine do not exhibit such enhanced responses.

   A common feature of patients with FGID is enhanced sensitivity to stimuli, i.e., visceral hypersensitivity. This may be associated with abnormal sensitization of sensory receptors, abnormal central pain transmission, and autonomic dysfunction. A subset of patients with FD and IBS have selective mechanical dilatation of visceral hypersensitivity and are associated with symptoms of belching, pain, and weight loss. However, some patients also have no hypersensitivity to dilation, suggesting that other important mechanisms are involved in the production of symptoms.

   Injurious stimuli prompt the release of peripheral inflammatory mediators, such as ATP, 5-HT, bradykinin, prostaglandins, capsaicin receptors 1 and 4, protease-activated receptor 2, nitric oxide (NO), and mast cells, which lower the conduction threshold of silent injurious receptors, thereby causing peripheral sensitization of injurious afferent nerves. The primary result of these inflammatory mediators is enhanced pain sensitivity at the site of injury, i.e., primary sensitization. Ion channels such as voltage-gated sodium channel (VGSC), neurotransmitter receptors, and trophic factors are also thought to be involved in the peripheral sensitization process.

It has been shown that prostaglandin E_2 (PGE_2) and NMDA receptors are the most important factors involved in the formation of central sensitization in the dorsal horn of the spinal cord, and the NMDA receptor antagonist ketamine can also reverse the already formed visceral sensitization. Central sensitization may also occur following distant injurious stimuli, such as esophageal sensitization following injurious stimulation of the duodenum and rectal sensitization following balloon dilation of the left hemicolectum. Central sensitization following repeated dilation of the sigmoid colon in IBS patients may be responsible for rectal sensitization.

Peripheral sensitization and central sensitization do not fully explain the mechanism of visceral hypersensitivity. The central processing of injurious afferents involves a range of cortical and subcortical brain structures. Functional neuroimaging, such as functional magnetic resonance imaging (fMRI), positron emission computed tomography (PET), magnetoencephalography (MEG), electroencephalography (EEG), and cortical-evoked potential (CEP), providing a convenient examination of central regions. The abnormal activation of the anterior cingulate gyrus, amygdala, and brainstem is also found in IBS patients, suggesting that part of the mechanism of abnormal visceral hurt feelings originates in the center.

The central information transmission with the gastrointestinal tract is carried out through the autonomic nervous system (ANS), including the parasympathetic nervous system (PNS) and sympathetic nervous system (SNS) pathways. An important approach to studying ANS is to look at heart rate variability (HRV). Most studies have shown no difference in HRV between IBS patients and healthy controls; however, differences in autonomic function were demonstrated when IBS were classified according to whether they had predominantly small bowel symptoms, degree of clinical symptoms, whether they had comorbid depressive manifestations, or whether they had a history of drug use.

2. Gastrointestinal electrical stimulation in patients with FGID

Gastrointestinal (GI) electrical stimulation consists of a series of pulsed stimuli, usually rectangular pulsed waves with constant current or voltage; the stimulation parameters include frequency, pulse width, and amplitude. Long-pulse stimulation, short-pulse stimulation, and cascade pulse stimulation. Depending on the number of stimulating electrodes, there are single-channel and multichannel GI electrical stimulation. Long pulse stimulation consists of a series of individual pulses of 10–600 ms in sequence, with a stimulation frequency similar to the physiological frequency of the gastric slow wave. Short pulse stimulation consists of a series of pulses of several hundred microseconds in sequence, and the stimulation frequency is usually several times higher than the physiological frequency of the gastric slow wave. Short pulse series stimulation consists of a sequence of short pulses that are jointly controlled by two signals: a continuous high-frequency short pulse (5–100 Hz) and a control signal to turn the pulse on or off.

Recently, new methods of GI stimulation have been developed, including synchronous electrical stimulation and double-pulse electrical stimulation. The electrical stimulation is synchronized with an intrinsic slow wave. The stimulation of double-pulse electrical stimulation consists of a short pulse (a few hundred microseconds) followed by a long pulse (a few hundred milliseconds) with two stimulation sites.

In normal dogs subjected to long-pulse electrical stimulation, gastrointestinal pacing or drive occurs in the stomach and small intestine, and the maximum drive frequency of the gastric and small intestinal slow waves is approximately 20% higher than the intrinsic frequency [13]. Slow-wave drive of gastrointestinal pacing is not modulated by vagal or sympathetic pathways, suggesting a purely peripheral or intramuscular effect. Other animal studies have shown that long-pulse/low-frequency gastric electrical stimulation (GES) corrects vasoconstrictor- or glucagon-induced gastric rhythm abnormalities and streptozotocin-induced diabetes mellitus. Transcutaneous GES also alters gastric slow waves and inhibits gastric motility, which may have therapeutic effects on eating disorders such as obesity. Long-pulse small bowel electrical stimulation (intestinalelectrical stimulation (IES)) has also been shown to drive small bowel slow waves and correct small bowel rhythm abnormalities.

Although long-pulse single-channel GES does not work on gastric emptying in healthy dogs, it improves gastric emptying in animals and patients with gastroparesis. The long-pulse four-channel GES improves gastric emptying in both healthy and diseased animals. A multi-channel microprocessor-controlled sequence of pulsed GES has a similar effect. Dual-channel, dual-pulse GES or synchronized GES has been shown to improve gastric sinus contraction via cholinergic channels, accelerate gastric emptying and improve abnormal rhythms and vomiting-like responses in diabetic patients. Low-stimulus microenergetic long-pulse GES can mildly alter gastric tone, which is beneficial in patients with abnormal gastric diastole. High stimulation energy GES inhibits gastric tone and leads to gastric dilation, which may benefit obese patients by producing early satiety.

IES may have multiple effects on gastrointestinal function, including gastric emptying, small bowel contraction, nutrient absorption, and satiety return to the central nervous system. IES has been shown to reduce gastric tone via the nitrogenergic pathway, inhibit sinus contraction, and prolong gastric emptying of fluid via the adrenergic pathway. High stimulation energy long-pulse ES may enhance small bowel contraction inhibition by 60–74% via sympathetic pathways, and this inhibition effect is dependent on pulse width and amplitude [14]. Short-pulse IES reduces nausea and vomiting in vasopressin animal models and ameliorates the delayed gastric emptying mediated by duodenal dilation; thus preventing nausea and vomiting symptoms caused by duodenal dilation. Synchronized IES (SIES) mediates intestinal contraction and accelerates small intestinal transit through a cholinergic pathway, and the site of action of IES has an important role in intestinal transit and absorption. IES electrodes placed in the terminal small intestine (backward IES) can delay intestinal transit and increase absorption in dogs with dissection and dumping syndrome. IES electrodes placed in the proximal small intestine (antegrade IES) can accelerate small intestinal transit that is slowed by ileal brake feedback mechanisms.

Colonic electrical stimulation (CES) has an excitatory effect on colonic transit, which may be achieved through the nitrogen energy pathway. However, CES inhibits gastric emptying and small bowel motility and inhibits gastric tone via the sympathetic pathway and rectal tone via the nitrogen pathway.

In the treatment of gastroparesis, gastrointestinal electrical stimulation is more effective in patients with comorbid diabetes than in those without diabetes; it is more effective in patients not taking opioid analgesia than in those taking opioids. Although gastrointestinal electrical stimulation relieves epigastric pain in 90% of patients with combined gastroparesis, a small percentage of patients fail to improve [15].

7.2.2 Spinal Cord Stimulation (SCS)

SCS is a neuromodulation method to relieve pain by implanting microelectrodes into the spinal canal and stimulating the sensory neurons in the posterior horn of the spinal cord and the transmission bundles in the posterior column with electrical pulses, thereby altering the transmission of pain signals.

1. Mechanism of action

   The gate control doctrine is the accepted mechanism of action of SCS, i.e., the current from the pulse generator reaches the electrode via the wire, and the electrical pulse signal blocks the pain signal before it reaches the brain so that the pain is replaced by a comfortable abnormal sensation. The mechanism of SCS for relieving chronic abdominal pain is not yet clear, and recent studies include activation of regulatory pathways above the spinal cord, the release of inhibitory neuromodulators (e.g., GABA), reverse activation followed by nerve conduction block, direct inhibition of the postsynaptic visceral dorsal column pathway and downregulation of sympathetic release at the segmental or supraspinal level.

The neuromodulatory system of gastrointestinal motility includes the intrinsic enteric nervous system (ENS) and the extrinsic vagal and visceral nerves, which are subdivided into afferent and efferent components loaded with information by parasympathetic and sympathetic bundles. Most parasympathetic and sympathetic efferent fibers terminate in the interosseous plexus of the gut, which is connected to the enteric ganglion; some sympathetic axons also terminate directly in the smooth muscle of the sphincter.

A variety of sensory receptors are present in the gastrointestinal tract and transmit information to afferent nerve fibers. Activated sensory receptors transmit information to the CNS via the vagus and visceral nerves. Visceral nerve-loaded spinal afferent fibers are present in the dorsal root ganglia and form synaptic connections with the dorsal horn spinal tract, activating second-level neurons that return information to the gut or up through the spinal cord to the center. Afferent fibers in six segments of the lower thoracic and three segments of the upper lumbar segments of the spinal cord may transmit pain signals from the viscera and may be the site of action of the SCS. It is well known that GI movements are enhanced by vagal activation and inhibited by sympathetic activation, which remain in relative balance. There is evidence that SCS decreases sympathetic tone and sympathetic vagal balance, which may account for its increased GI movement. It has also been shown that SCS acts by inhibiting spinal visceral afferent neurons within the DRG.

2. Clinical application

In 1967, Shealey first implanted stimulation electrodes into the spinal dorsal column for pain treatment and achieved success [16]. After that, SCS technology has been developed rapidly. It is now used not only for neuropathic pain, but also for the treatment of injurious pain such as intractable angina pectoris, ischemic limb pain, and peripheral vascular diseases.

The earliest report of the application of SCS technique for the treatment of chronic visceral pain was in 2000 in a 78-year-old male with chronic severe postprandial pain due to mesenteric ischemia, whose pain was completely relieved after epidural implantation of SCS electrodes at the T6 level. Case reports of SCS technique in other visceral pain applications have also yielded positive results, including esophageal dysmotility, irritable bowel syndrome (IBS), chronic pancreatitis, familial Mediterranean fever, post-traumatic splenectomy pain, general chronic abdominal pain, and chronic visceral pelvic pain.

To date, there are few studies on the effects of spinal cord stimulation in G-priming movements. An animal study after intestinal obstruction found that SCS placed at T_5 and T_8 normalized gastric emptying and improved upper gastrointestinal transit. Another systematic study of SCS in GI motility found that in healthy rats, SCS placed at T_9 and T_{10} showed an intensity-dependent increase in gastric tone, increased gastric fluid emptying, and accelerated small intestinal transit: SCS accelerated gastric solid emptying by 24% and 78% in healthy and diabetic rats, respectively [17].

Because patient selection, electrode placement, and type of instrumentation vary in these reports, it is difficult to extrapolate these positive findings to the long-term efficacy of SCS in patients with chronic visceral pain. In the year 2010, a retrospective study [18] examined the 1-year long-term efficacy of SCS after application in 35 patients with chronic abdominal pain. Consistent with most studies, electrodes were placed at the epidural T_5 or T_6 level. A total of 86% of patients had more than 50% pain relief at the end of testing, and 19 of 28 patients who received permanent implants completed 1-year follow-up with VAS scores remaining low [(3.8 ± 1.9) points]. Results of a prospective study of SCS in 32 patients with abdominal pain in the inguinal region last year showed that dorsal root ganglion electrical stimulation provided long-term relief of neuropathic inguinal region pain.

The protocol for the application of SCS techniques for the treatment of chronic visceral abdominal pain has not been standardized. It usually starts with a multidisciplinary evaluation and development of a treatment plan, which usually includes cognitive and behavioral management, pharmacotherapy, adjuvant therapy, interventional diagnostic blocks, and therapeutic blocks. The following points have been agreed upon: the use of reverse epidural block techniques to identify the nature of abdominal pain (visceral, somatic, or central); the application of SCS techniques usually only after failure of other conservative treatments; the need for a psychological evaluation and multidisciplinary discussion before permanent implantation of SCS; and a period of test treatment before permanent implantation of SCS, which is only considered in patients with >50% pain relief permanent implantation [19].

7.2.3 Peripheral Nerve Electrical Stimulation

Peripheral nerve stimulation (PNS) is an important method for the treatment of peripheral single neuropathy and sympathetic-mediated topical pain by directly stimulating peripheral nerves to suppress pain.

1. Mechanism of action

   Similar to SCS, the mechanism of action of PNS is not yet clear, and the theoretical basis may be the gate control theory that large peripheral nerve fiber stimulation inhibits C-fiber activity, thereby decreasing the response of spinal cord posterior horn neurons to injurious stimuli. This inhibition may be present in local tissues, the spinal cord, and the supraspinal pathway. The sensory abnormalities induced by peripheral nerve stimulation are mediated by Aβ fibers, which is consistent with the gate theory. Direct stimulation of peripheral nerves can lead to a decrease in their excitability, a temporary slowing of conduction velocity, and an increase in the electrical threshold. Experiments in rats have shown that low-frequency stimulation of Aδ fibers enhances the long-range inhibition of monosynaptic and polysynaptic excitatory postsynaptic potentials in spinal glia. Patients with chronic headaches showed increased blood flow in the dorsal anterior region of the pons, anterior cingulate gyrus, and cuneus lobe after application of occipital nerve stimulation.

   PNS may also have a role in injurious pain, and cases have been reported of its use in lower back pain and neck pain. In this regard, PNS is superior to SCS, which has a prominent effect on neuropathic pain and ischemic pain but very little effect on injurious pain. It is found that the infrared laser promoted the activation of Aδ and C fibers and that all volunteers receiving laser stimulation produced pinprick-like pain; compared to controls, superficial radial nerve stimulation greatly reduced the evoked potentials and shortened the latency period.

   However, whether these mechanisms can be extrapolated to the modulation of visceral pain by peripheral modulation remains to be further investigated. Qin et al. [20] observed that stimulation of somatic afferent fibers elicited a cardiovascular response to gastric dilation in previous experiments with animal models. They established a visceral pain model of gastric dilation in anesthetized rats by implanting two electrodes into the median nerve of the forelimb and the common peroneal nerve of the hindlimb, respectively, and giving electrical stimulation at a frequency of

50 Hz and an intensity of 0.5–2.0 mA. This stimulation usually activates both A and C fibers. They measured the extracellular potentials of T_9 and T_{10} by placing microelectrodes in the thoracic segment of the spinal cord to assess the modulatory effects of peripheral stimulation. The results showed that stimulation of somatic afferent fibers could influence the transmission of visceral injurious information. Stimulation of the median and common peroneal nerves altered the response of 63–67% T_9 and T_{10} level neurons to gastric dilation. This mechanism is thought to act through both intrinsic spinal pathways and supraspinal inhibitory pathways. Another possibility is that diffuse injurious inhibition controls the phenomenon of dorsal horn convergence neuron inhibition caused by widespread injurious stimulation of the soma and viscera.

2. Clinical applications

As early as the fifteenth century, Scribonius Lagus observed that a king's servant greatly relieved his gouty chronic foot pain after stepping on an electric ray. In 1887, Althaus documented a female patient with abdominal pain and epigastric edema who experienced complete pain relief and complete resolution of the edema after receiving electrical stimulation. In 1968, Sweet and Wepsic implanted a peripheral nerve stimulator in a 26-year-old patient with neuropathic hand pain and obtained significant pain relief [21]. Plexuses and single nerves that converge in injurious nerve pathways can be targets for peripheral nerve modulation, and the most commonly selected peripheral nerves currently include the ulnar, median, radial, posterior tibial, common peroneal, and greater occipital nerves.

The use of PNS in chronic visceral abdominal pain is not yet available, and only a few cases have been reported, but the results are positive. Injurious afferents from the gastrointestinal tract are usually thought to reach the spinal cord center at the T_5–L_2 level via the celiac plexus and visceral nerves. The vagus nerve is usually considered to transmit only functional and physiological information and is not involved in pain information transmission; however, recent studies suggest its involvement in the emotional effects of injurious sensations and in the autonomic component of gastric pain. The lumbar sympathetic chain is also an important target for peripheral stimulation and is commonly used to treat sympathetically mediated pain in the lower extremities and has recently been used for renal pain. Sacral nerve stimulation (SNS) is effective for IBS and bladder pain, and reduces visceral mechanical pain sensitivity in a cross-organ sensitization model.

The first visceral nerve stimulation was used in a 36-year-old patient with chronic pancreatitis with severe right upper abdominal pain [22]. She underwent endoscopic cholecystectomy, Oddi sphincterotomy, and Roux-en-Y gastric bypass, but the pain persisted and worsened with feeding. The patient underwent ethanol neurolysis of the abdominal plexus and was able to obtain pain relief for only 3 months, requiring large amounts of fentanyl daily for pain relief. Initially, abdominal plexus stimulation was administered to the patient, and after two 150-mm-long stimulation needles were placed at the location of the abdominal plexus at the L1 level and given for 5 min at 2 Hz, the patient felt well and the VAS decreased from 9 to 0 and was maintained for 48 h. Subsequently, two monopolar electrodes were implanted to the above location for test stimulation and complete pain relief was achieved, requiring stimulation for 10 min every 12 h. However, there were technical difficulties in implanting permanent multipolar electrodes in the same locations, thus the final electrodes were implanted in front of the T_{11} and T_{12} vertebrae, and the patient had satisfactory pain relief with <6 h of stimulation per day and a decrease in fentanyl requirement from 225 to 12.5 μg/h.

The clinical manifestations of loin pain hematuria syndrome (LPHS) are low back pain and hematuria of unknown etiology, renal function is usually unaffected, and the goal of treatment is symptom control. These patients tend to have more intense low back pain and do not respond well to conservative treatment modalities. Since most injurious afferent fibers are autonomic, the lumbar sympathetic chain is an ideal target for stimulation. In 2009, Goroszeniuk et al. reported that lumbar sympathetic chain stimulation at the L_3 level was used to predict the effectiveness of visceral nerve stimulation [22]. After five patients with visceral pain were maintained with 2-Hz low-frequency stimulation for 5 min, two patients obtained complete pain relief for 24 h. After placement of test monopolar electrodes at the anterior level of the L vertebral body in these five patients, complete pain relief was obtained in three patients. Two of the patients who had permanent multipolar electrodes implanted achieved long-term pain relief and required only 2–3 stimulations per day.

The target of action, technique, instrumentation, mode of action, and optimal frequency of PNS need to be further explored. Specialized stimulators for peripheral nerve stimulation, especially for the abdominal sympathetic chain, will soon be designed for clinical application.

The application of peripheral nerve electrical stimulation is subject to certain limitations, such as electrodes usually needing to be done by surgeons, and there is a risk of perineural fibrosis and direct nerve damage during implantation.

7.2.4 Transcutaneous Electrical Nerve Stimulation

Transcutaneous electrical nerve stimulation (TENS) is a method of treating pain through low-frequency pulsed electrical stimulation by implanting electrodes directly under the skin at the site of pain through a puncture technique, similar to the traditional acupuncture electrotherapy. Unlike PNS and SCS, this type of stimulation does not require the selection of a peripheral nerve or the region of the dorsal column of the spinal cord as the target site, and can be applied to pain in areas that do not present a nerve distribution, and the risk of complications is relatively low.

1. Mechanism of action

   The effect of the TENS technique depends on its frequency, and the mechanism of action differs between high-frequency (50–100 Hz) stimulation and low-frequency (<10 Hz) stimulation. Low-frequency TENS is antagonized by μ-opioid receptors, $GABA_A$ receptors, 5-hydroxytryptamine receptors and muscarinic M1 and M3 receptor blockers, and repeated stimulation produces tolerance, suggesting that low-frequency TENS may act through the downstream inhibitory pathway, μ-opioid, 5-hydroxytryptamine, and cholinergic neurotransmitters. The high-frequency TENS mechanism is related to the opioid pathway, which increases β-endorphin levels in the bloodstream and methionine enkephalin levels in the cerebrospinal fluid, and blocking δ-opioid receptors antagonizes its analgesic effects. The high-frequency TENS effect can be antagonized by GABA receptor antagonists, but not by 5-hydroxytryptamine receptor antagonists, which is different from low-frequency TENS.
2. Clinical application

   Weiner first successfully treated occipital neuropathic neuralgia by subcutaneous electrode implantation in 1999 [23]. TENS has been widely used for cervicogenic headache, infraorbital neuralgia, atypical facial pain, postherpetic neuralgia, ilioinguinal neuralgia, ulnar neuralgia, sciatica, and brachial plexus neuropathy. Targeted stimulation (STS)/regional stimulation techniques have been shown to be effective in many painful conditions (e.g., low back pain, costochondritis, intractable angina pectoris, and pelvic pain) and can be an alternative or combined application technique to SCS.

   Although the use of percutaneous peripheral neuromodulation in chronic abdominal pain is not yet widespread, with only a few case reports, the results are positive. Three patients with visceral pain treated with this technique were reported in 2006 [24]. All of these patients had mixed visceral and abdominal wall pain and the pain areas were not distributed in a dermatomal pattern. Since abdominal visceral pain may be associated with secondary somatic nociceptive sensitization of the abdominal wall, and targeting the abdominal wall may improve the corresponding visceral pain, the investigators concluded that the use of percutaneous stimulation was more appropriate than SCS. In the first case, a patient with chronic right lower abdominal pain after inguinal hernia repair, a permanent stimulator was implanted after successful subcutaneous stimulation testing, and the pain was completely relieved. The second case was a patient with right abdominal pain after liver transplantation with ventral hernia repair, and the pain was significantly improved after the implantation of three subcutaneous electrodes. The third case was a patient with right upper abdominal pain after modified Wipple surgery with chronic pancreatitis. Initially, two electrodes were placed parallel to the longitudinal axis of the spine with poor efficacy, and the pain relief was better when the electrodes were placed in a horizontal line at the follow-up visit. At the third follow-up, the efficacy was affected by the electrodes shifting into a deeper position, and the pain was relieved when the electrodes were adjusted to a more superficial position again. This shows that the orientation and depth of the electrodes are important factors in the application of TENS that affect efficacy.

The general approach to TENS application is to introduce the electrode via a modified 14G Tuohy puncture needle or catheter under blind or imaging guidance and then test stimulate it in situ. An important drawback of this method is that if the stimulation is incorrect, the electrodes need to be reintroduced, and this repeated puncture introduction may lead to damage to the surrounding tissue, patient discomfort, and increased operating time.

7.2.5 Non-invasive In Vitro Neuromodulation

Non-invasive extracorporeal neuromodulation is a technique that uses low-frequency stimulation with extracorporeal nerve mapping electrodes to achieve neuromodulation. The stimulation is usually performed at a low frequency of 2 Hz with spherical electrodes placed at the location of the nerve projection or the most painful part of the non-nerve distribution, and the intensity of stimulation is gradually increased until sensory abnormalities occur. This technique can be used in outpatients, and the machine can be provided to patients who have experienced prolonged pain relief after use and are instructed on how to use it. The technique is also used to screen patients for the suitability of other peripheral neuromodulation techniques.

While this extracorporeal stimulation has been successful in patients with intractable angina and pathological neuralgia, its diagnostic and therapeutic role in abdominal visceral pain needs to be further investigated.

A new noninvasive intraaural placement of transcutaneous electrical nerve area stimulation has been shown to modulate central pain pathways and reduce basal firing of amygdala and spinal cord neurons, thereby alleviating visceral and somatic hypersensitivity in animal models of postinflammatory pain.

7.2.6 Motor Cortex Stimulation

Motor cortex stimulation (MCS) is a method that uses neuronavigation techniques to determine the relationship between the central sulcus and precentral gyrus and the body surface of the skull and scalp, places electrodes on the surface of the precentral gyrus, and then stimulates with a temporary stimulator, and regulates the optimal voltage, frequency, and pulse width of the stimulator to deliver electrical stimulation to achieve the best effect for pain treatment. The optimal voltage, frequency, and pulse width of the stimulator are adjusted to achieve the best effect of pain treatment.

1. Mechanism of action

   The analgesic mechanism of MCS is still unclear and controversial. Some scholars believe that MCS activates the downstream pathway from the cortex to the thalamus or spinal cord and the upstream pathway from the thalamus to the cortex by stimulating the subcortical transverse fibers. It has also been suggested that MCS decreases the original hyperexcitability of the painful thalamus. A PET study showed that MCS could enhance the release of endogenous opioids from related structures in the brain and exert analgesic effects.

2. Clinical application

   The clinical application of MCS is based on the theory that electrical stimulation of the motor cortex in rats can significantly and temporarily inhibit the response of dorsal spinal cord neurons to strong mechanical stimuli without affecting their response to harmless stimuli, and MCS is currently used in clinical practice mainly for central and peripheral afferent nerve blocking pain, such as central pain after cerebral hemorrhage or infarction, stump pain after amputation, phantom limb pain and neuralgia after trigeminal nerve injury. These pains are difficult to improve by peripheral electrical stimulation, and electrical stimulation of the motor cortex can inhibit the perception of pain in adjacent areas of the cerebral cortex and, in patients with pain after stroke, can also improve motor function in the painful limb. The application of MCS in visceral pain has not been reported.

   The total implementation process of MCS usually takes about 1 week, starting with the surgical implantation of a pulse generator to which electrodes are connected with wires to measure the corresponding parameters; then a second adjustment is made according to the degree of improvement of the patient's symptoms, and the parameters are adjusted to achieve optimal clinical efficacy. The key to treatment lies in the precise localization of the central sulcus and the selection of the appropriate stimulation parameters. It has been suggested that stimulation of the motor cortex in the precentral gyrus is more effective in relieving pain than stimulation of the sensory cortex in the postcentral gyrus.

7.2.7 Deep Brain Stimulation

Deep brain stimulation (DBS) is a stereotactic method that precisely locates the treatment target according to MRI images, places electrodes in the motor nuclei in the deep brain, and stimulates the corresponding nuclei with high-frequency electrical pulses through a stimulator implanted in the chest to produce a series of biochemical and physical effects. The pain threshold is lowered to achieve the purpose of effective analgesia.

1. Mechanism of action

   Despite the profound understanding of pain, a variety of DBS therapeutic targets have been explored. The only certainty in the mechanism of DBS for chronic pain is that the stimulation electrodes need to be precisely implanted in the corresponding target sites to achieve good results. It has been shown that electrical stimulation of periaqueductal gray (PAG)/periventricular gray (PVG) targets in the midbrain conductance can cause an increase in endogenous opioid peptide release, and it has been shown that the opioid inhibitor naloxone can reverse this analgesic effect. However, this theory does not explain why some patients treated with PVG/PAG targets can have good analgesic effects without an increase in endogenous opioid peptides. This suggests that a non-opioid peptide-dependent mechanism may exist.

   Analgesia in the sensory thalamus may depend on a non-opioid peptide-dependent mechanism. The thalamus is the "relay" of the sensory transmission pathway, the main tissue structure for the integration and perception of injurious sensations, and it receives and transmits episodic sensory signals, including pain. Electrical stimulation can affect the integration of superior injurious sensations in the medial and lateral thalamic tracts, and can also affect the activity of neurons in the dorsal horn of the spinal cord along the neuromedial tract. On the other hand, the analgesic cause of DBS may also be its activation of long-loop polysynaptic transmission pathways between the sensorimotor cortex, basal ganglia, and medial thalamus. Adjusting the frequency and intensity of DBS electrical stimulation can have significantly different effects on patient analgesia. This also suggests that DBS may have an analgesic effect by affecting the rhythm of specific neural circuits.

The ACC/dACC area has important roles in human sensory, motor, and cognitive aspects, including visceral movement, skeletal muscle movement, endocrine activity, vocalization, concentration, anticipation of pain, and empathy. Electrical stimulation of this area may reduce negative feelings of anxiety and depression caused by chronic pain in order to improve quality of life. Therefore, dACC may achieve analgesia by improving the emotional experience of patients. Meanwhile, Mohseni et al. used voxel-based morphological analysis to find that pain caused a decrease in gray matter density in the ACC region. Subsequently, Rodriguez et al. further demonstrated that when patients underwent DBS surgery for pain relief, the gray matter density in the ACC area gradually increased compared to the preoperative period [25]. The change in cortical density may also explain the cause of ACC analgesia, but more in-depth studies are needed.

2. Clinical application

DBS has been used for the treatment of intractable pain since the 1950s, and many clinical cases have been reported so far. DBS has been effective in relieving many chronic intractable pains, including nerve injury pain, cluster headache, phantom limb pain, and low back pain due to failed surgical treatment, with an overall efficiency of 50–60% and some up to 80% [26]. The DBS in the ventral caudal nucleus of the thalamus and the PAG/PVG area was applied to treat 21 patients with chronic pain. Thirteen of them were treated with permanent stimulator implantation and five achieved long-term relief, and the target of implantation was subnucleus of the thalamus. Bitar et al. reported that DBS in the PAG/PVG area was very effective in treating phantom limb pain [27]. Leone et al. reported bilateral hypothalamic DBS for cluster headache with good long-term results [28]. Franzini et al. reported the efficacy of DBS in the posterior hypothalamus for neuropathic trigeminal neuralgia and trigeminal neuralgia due to multiple sclerosis, in which DBS was ineffective for neuropathic trigeminal neuralgia, while trigeminal neuralgia due to multiple sclerosis was significantly improved [29]. Walcott et al. reported significant relief in a patient with paroxysmal migraine treated with DBS in the posterior hypothalamus [30]. A larger survey [31] found that of 424 patients with chronic intractable pain treated with DBS, the immediate effectiveness was 70% and the long-term efficacy was 50%, with chronic low back pain being the most effective of all pain types, with 80% of patients achieving long-term relief.

Effective stimulation targets for DBS include the PAG, PVG, periglottis, hypothalamus, nucleus ventralis posterior lateralis (VPL) and ventralis posteromedialis (VPM), thalamic structures adjacent to the periventricular gray matter such as the dorsal medial thalamus, parabrachial nucleus, median thalamic nucleus and other sites such as the internal capsule, septum and caudate nucleus. The most commonly used stimulation targets are PAG/PVG, VPL/VPM, and hypothalamus.

The use of DBS in chronic abdominal pain has not been reported.

7.2.8 Non-invasive Transcranial Stimulation

Transcranial direct current stimulation (tDCS) is a non-invasive and relatively safe technique for applying electrical currents to modulate brain functions. tDCS is a relatively well-established technique that conducts low-amplitude electrical currents through scalp electrodes to specific sites such as the cortex. tDCS stimulation sites include motor cortex, dorsolateral prefrontal cortices, visual cortex, and somatosensory cortex.

The mechanism of action of tDCS may be through polarity-dependent migration of the resting membrane potential of neurons, resulting in changes in excitability of nerve cells at the stimulation site and in the connected area; however, the neuromolecular mechanism is not well understood.

tDCS has been used in several aspects of clinical treatment, including analgesia for neuropathic pain, treatment of depression, and analgesia for chronic abdominal pain caused by enterocolitis. A recent clinical study showed that tDCS treatment relieves visceral pain in patients with hepatocellular carcinomatosis. The results of a randomized controlled study [32] of 20 patients with chronic abdominal pain from Crohn's disease and ulcerative colitis showed that the relief of pain by tDCS did not correlate with inflammatory activity and that this mechanism of action may be central.

Transcranial magneticstimulation (tMS) is a brain stimulation based on temporal magnetic field alteration by applying a strong and rapidly varying current to the cerebral cortex through a coil. tMS modulation of cortical activity is dependent on the parameters of stimulation and can produce either inhibitory or euphoric effects. In general, low-frequency stimulation (1 Hz) suppresses the excitability of target cortical areas; high-frequency stimulation (20 Hz) does the opposite. Animal studies have shown that tMS is associated with NMDA binding sites and increases transient-early gene expression.

tMS has been used to treat several types of chronic visceral pain, including organic and functional pain syndromes. Recent findings suggest that tMS increases pain thresholds in response to mechanical and electrical stimulation of the colon and relieves clinical pain in patients with IBS. Results of a study [33] in which tMS was applied to five patients with pancreatitis showed excellent results in three patients, with a 59% pain relief rate.

References

1. Leite P. PAHO/WHO: Health indicators: conceptual and operational considerations (section 4). 2018 [cited 2023 May 22]. Available from: https://www3.paho.org/hq/index.php?option=com_content&view=article&id=14411%3Ahealth-indicators-conceptual-and-operational-considerations-section-4&Itemid=0&showall=1&lang=en.
2. Mermekli A, Reddy P, McKean D, Abdelsalam H, Teh J, Mansour R. Ultrasound-guided continuous radiofrequency ablation of the suprascapular nerve for chronic shoulder pain secondary to osteoarthritis: a retrospective cohort study. Eur Radiol. 2022;32(9):6230–7. https://doi.org/10.1007/s00330-022-08763-x.
3. Lee H, Cho HH, Nahm FS, Lee P, Choi E. Pulsed radiofrequency ablation of the C2 dorsal root ganglion using a posterior approach for treating cervicogenic headache: a retrospective chart review. Headache. 2020;60(10):2463–72. https://doi.org/10.1111/head.13759.
4. Hameed M, Hameed H, Erdek M. Pain management in pancreatic cancer. Cancers. 2010;3(1):43–60. https://doi.org/10.3390/cancers3010043.
5. Zhang XM, Zhao QH, Zeng NL, Cai CP, Xie XG, Li CJ, et al. The celiac ganglia: anatomic study using MRI in cadavers. Am J Roentgenol. 2006;186(6):1520–3. https://doi.org/10.2214/ajr.04.1765.
6. Ischia S, Ischia A, Polati E, Finco G. Three posterior percutaneous celiac plexus block techniques a prospective, randomized study in 61 patients with pancreatic cancer pain. Anesthesiology. 1992;76(4):534–40. https://doi.org/10.1097/00000542-199204000-00008.
7. Turker G, Basagan-Mogol E, Gurbet A, Ozturk C, Uckunkaya N, Sahin S. A new technique for superior hypogastric plexus block: the posteromedian transdiscal approach. Tohoku J Exp Med. 2005;206(3):277–81. https://doi.org/10.1620/tjem.206.277.
8. Cha YD, Yang CW, Han JU, Song JH, Na W, Oh S, et al. Transsacrococcygeal approach to ganglion impar block for treatment of chronic coccygodynia after spinal arachnoid cyst removal. Medicine. 2016;95(39):e5010. https://doi.org/10.1097/md.0000000000005010.
9. Lin M-C, Liu H-W, Su Y-K, Lo W-L, Lin C-M. Robot-guided versus freehand fluoroscopy-guided minimally invasive transforaminal lumbar interbody fusion: a single-institution, observational, case-control study. Neurosurg Focus. 2022;52(1):E9. https://doi.org/10.3171/2021.10.focus21514.
10. Raj PP, Rosenblatt R, Miller J, Katz RL, Carden E. Dynamics of local-anesthetic compounds in regional anesthesia. Anesth Analg. 1977;56(1):110. https://doi.org/10.1213/00000539-197701000-00025.
11. Yin J, Chen JD. Electrogastrography: methodology, validation and applications. J Neurogastroenterol Motil. 2013;19(1):5–17. https://doi.org/10.5056/jnm.2013.19.1.5.

12. Hadjivasilis A. New insights into irritable bowel syndrome: from pathophysiology to treatment. Ann Gastroenterol. 2019; https://doi.org/10.20524/aog.2019.0428.
13. Sun Y, Song G-Q, Yin J, Lei Y, Chen JD. Effects and mechanisms of gastrointestinal electrical stimulation on SLOW WAVES: a systematic canine study. Am J Physiol Regul Integr Comp Physiol. 2009;297(5):R1392. https://doi.org/10.1152/ajpregu.00006.2009.
14. Li S, Chen JD. Pulse width-dependent effects of intestinal electrical stimulation for obesity: role of gastrointestinal motility and hormones. Obes Surg. 2016;27(1):70–7. https://doi.org/10.1007/s11695-016-2238-5.
15. Soffer EE. Gastric electrical stimulation for gastroparesis. J Neurogastroenterol Motil. 2012;18(2):131–7. https://doi.org/10.5056/jnm.2012.18.2.131.
16. Shealy CN, Mortimer JT, Reswick JB. Electrical inhibition of pain by stimulation of the dorsal columns. Anesth Analg. 1967;46(4):489. https://doi.org/10.1213/00000539-196707000-00025.
17. Song G-Q, Sun Y, Foreman RD, Chen JD. Therapeutic potential of spinal cord stimulation for gastrointestinal motility disorders: a preliminary rodent study. Neurogastroenterol Motil. 2013;26(3):377–84. https://doi.org/10.1111/nmo.12273.
18. Kapural L, Nagem H, Tlucek H, Sessler DI. Spinal cord stimulation for chronic visceral abdominal pain. Pain Med. 2010;11(3):347–55. https://doi.org/10.1111/j.1526-4637.2009.00785.x.
19. Eldabe S, Duarte RV, Gulve A, Thomson S, Baranidharan G, Houten R, et al. Does a screening trial for spinal cord stimulation in patients with chronic pain of neuropathic origin have clinical utility and cost-effectiveness (trial-stim): a randomised controlled trial. Pain. 2020;161(12):2820–9. https://doi.org/10.1097/j.pain.0000000000001977.
20. Qin Y, Liu X, Guo X, Liu M, Li H, Xu S. Low-frequency repetitive transcranial magnetic stimulation restores dynamic functional connectivity in subcortical stroke. Front Neurol. 2021;12:771034. https://doi.org/10.3389/fneur.2021.771034.
21. Gildenberg PL. History of electrical neuromodulation for chronic pain. Oxford University Press; 2006 [cited 2023 May 22]. Available from: https://academic.oup.com/painmedicine/article/7/suppl_1/S7/1819491.
22. Goroszeniuk T, Khan R. Permanent percutaneous splanchnic nerve neuromodulation for management of pain due to chronic pancreatitis: a case report. Neuromodulation. 2011;14(3):253–7. https://doi.org/10.1111/j.1525-1403.2011.00347.x.
23. Weiner RL, Reed KL. Peripheral neurostimulation for control of intractable occipital neuralgia. Neuromodulation. 1999;2(3):217–21. https://doi.org/10.1046/j.1525-1403.1999.00217.x.
24. Hingne PM, Sluka KA. Differences in waveform characteristics have no effect on the anti-hyperalgesia produced by transcutaneous electrical nerve stimulation (TENS) in rats with joint inflammation. J Pain. 2007;8(3):251–5. https://doi.org/10.1016/j.jpain.2006.08.008.
25. Rodriguez RL, Fernandez HH, Haq I, Okun MS. Pearls in patient selection for deep brain stimulation. Neurologist. 2007;13(5):253–60. https://doi.org/10.1097/nrl.0b013e318095a4d5.
26. Falowski SM. Deep brain stimulation for chronic pain. Curr Pain Headache Rep. 2015;19(7) https://doi.org/10.1007/s11916-015-0504-1.
27. Bitar R, Leung G, Perng R, Tadros S, Moody AR, Sarrazin J, et al. Mr pulse sequences: what every radiologist wants to know but is afraid to ask. Radiographics. 2006;26(2):513–37. https://doi.org/10.1148/rg.262055063.
28. Leone M, May A, Franzini A, Broggi G, Dodick D, Rapoport A, et al. Deep brain stimulation for intractable chronic cluster headache: proposals for patient selection. Cephalalgia. 2004;24(11):934–7. https://doi.org/10.1111/j.1468-2982.2004.00742.x.
29. Franzini A, Broggi G, Cordella R, Dones I, Messina G. Deep-brain stimulation for aggressive and disruptive behavior. World Neurosurg. 2013;80(3–4):S29.e11. https://doi.org/10.1016/j.wneu.2012.06.038.
30. Walcott BP, Nahed BV, Kahle KT, Duhaime A-C, Sharma N, Eskandar EN. Deep brain stimulation for medically refractory life-threatening status dystonicus in children. J Neurosurg Pediatr. 2012;9(1):99–102. https://doi.org/10.3171/2011.10.peds11360.
31. Stinca S, Andersson M, Erhardt J, Zimmermann MB. Development and validation of a new low-cost enzyme-linked immunoassay for serum and dried blood spot thyroglobulin. Thyroid. 2015;25(12):1297–305. https://doi.org/10.1089/thy.2015.0428.
32. Yanai H, Levine A, Hirsch A, Boneh RS, Kopylov U, Eran HB, et al. The crohn's disease exclusion diet for induction and maintenance of remission in adults with mild-to-moderate crohn's disease (cded-AD): an open-label, pilot, randomised trial. Lancet Gastroenterol Hepatol. 2022;7(1):49–59. https://doi.org/10.1016/s2468-1253(21)00299-5.
33. Drewes AM, Bouwense SAW, Campbell CM, Ceyhan GO, Delhaye M, Demir IE, et al. Guidelines for the understanding and management of pain in chronic pancreatitis. Pancreatology. 2017;17(5):720–31. https://doi.org/10.1016/j.pan.2017.07.006.

8 Traditional Chinese Medicine for Visceral Pain

Haipeng Liu

8.1 Introduction

Visceral pain is a common clinical condition that may be induced by stimuli such as mechanical stretching, spasm, ischemia, and inflammation. Compared with somatic pain, the mechanisms of generation, maintenance, and regulation of visceral pain are more complex, and therefore it is one of the key points and difficulties in the field of basic pain research at present. Visceral pain exhibits the following clinical characteristics: (1) vague location; (2) often accompanied by referred pain; (3) usually with reflex behaviors such as muscle contraction; (4) not exclusively caused by injury to internal organs; (5) insensitive to distending and pulling stimuli; (6) slow onset and lasting for a long time, that is, chronic pain with progressive intensification, but sometimes rapidly progressing to severe pain; and (7) particularly prone to ignite unpleasant emotions and accompanied by nausea, vomiting, and cardiovascular and respiratory changes.

Visceral pain is a complex and heterogeneous disease. According to statistics, over 20% of the world's population experienced visceral pain, which brings great pain to people's lives and causes serious mental and economic burden to patients [1].

H. Liu (✉)
Department of Pain Medicine, Gansu Provincial Hospital, Lanzhou, Gansu, China

8.1.1 Pathogenesis and Etiology of Visceral Pain

Visceral pain has not been widely studied due to the lack of reliable research models. With the increased availability of visceral pain models in recent years, it has been further studied. The etiologies of visceral pain are diverse and cover extremely wide ranges, which cannot be summarized with one concept, and the mechanisms of the pain are hard to describe in a clear and organized manner. Generally speaking, the visceral nerve centers are located in the spinal cord, brainstem, diencephalon, and cerebral cortex. Typical visceral pain usually refers to the transmission of visceral signaling impulses to the brain to produce sensory awareness. The peripheral nerves are mainly located in the visceral, cardiovascular, and glandular areas. The visceral nerves are divided into sensory and motor fibers, similar to the somatic nerves. Peripheral receptors receive certain stimulus signals, which are transmitted to centers at all levels and also to the cerebral cortex, where they are integrated to regulate the corresponding organ activities through motor nerves, leading to different clinical features. In recent years, the search for a single biological cause has been expanded to explain visceral pain symptoms in terms of physiological alterations (e.g., altered kinetics, visceral sensory hypersensitivity, dysfunction of brain–gut axis), as well as recognizing

M. Xia et al. (eds.), *Visceral Pain*, https://doi.org/10.1007/978-981-99-9167-9_8

the sociocultural and psychological influence, and progress has been made in pathogenesis and other aspects.

8.1.2 Classification of Visceral Pain

Due to the multiorigin, diversity, and complexity of its manifestations, there is no recognized classification of visceral pain. Generally speaking, the pain can be classified into acute and chronic visceral pain according to the duration of the pain; and functional and organic visceral pain according to the presence or absence of substantial lesions. Patients with clear causes of visceral pain, such as infection, occupying, injury, and obstruction, can often obtain symptomatic relief after the causes are treated; however, a considerable number of patients without obvious organic lesions, such as irritable bowel syndrome, can be classified as functional visceral pain. According to the location of pain, it can be divided into chest pain, abdominal pain, pelvic pain, low back pain, etc. In this chapter, visceral pain is classified into cancerous visceral pain and noncancerous visceral pain. Cancerous visceral pain, as the name suggests, is the visceral pain associated with various types of malignant tumors. As for noncancerous visceral pain, clinically common ones include functional abdominal pain syndrome (FAPS), inflammatory visceral pain (such as biliary colic, chronic pancreatitis pain, stomach pain, and irritable bowel syndrome), pain related to gynecological diseases (such as chronic pelvic inflammatory disease and dysmenorrhea), testicular pain, interstitial cystitis, ulcerative colitis, Crohn's disease, pelvic pain syndromes, mechanical visceral pain and visceral pain of vascular origin, postoperative visceral pain, etc.

At present, the Western medicine treatments of visceral pain mainly include (1) treatment of primary diseases, including surgery, anti-inflammatory, and antitumor; (2) symptomatic pain relief, including various types of pain medications and nerve block; and (3) adjuvant treatments such as tricyclic antidepressants and other psychiatric treatment, and symptomatic treatment for the complications of visceral pain. However, visceral pain is mostly chronic, prone to recur, and with unknown etiology, resulting in limitations of Western medicine treatment. TCM has gradually become a popular topic for research as a powerful supplement or even an alternative to Western medicine. The integration of traditional Chinese and Western medicine has become a trend in the treatment of visceral pain. In this chapter, the author introduces the use of TCM for cancerous visceral and noncancerous visceral pain.

8.2 TCM for Visceral Cancer Pain

Visceral cancer pain is one of the common symptoms of cancer and has a significant impact on patients' quality of life. At present, the main management method of visceral cancer pain in Western medicine is antitumor treatment combining the three-step analgesic ladder, biological therapy, nerve blocks, and other surgical means to achieve the purpose of pain relief. Comprehensive treatments, including the management of adverse reactions to medications and psychotherapy, are also adopted. However, after accepting the above treatments, 36–50% of patients with cancer still endured much pain in that their daily life was influenced [2]. On the other hand, cancer pain prolongs the time of hospitalization and increases medical expenses, which adds to the economic burden of the country and individuals. Therefore, it has become a trend to explore TCM for the treatment of cancer pain. A large number of experimental studies have shown that TCM combined with modern medical treatments, together with different degrees of pharmacological or nonpharmacological psycho-emotional interventions, can achieve the goals of overcoming or delaying the analgesic resistance, reducing the dosage of Western drugs, preventing and managing constipation and other adverse effects, and improving patients' quality of life. TCM has unique advantages and prospects in the treatment of cancer pain with remarkable clinical efficacy and various treatment choices. Clinical practice shows that the use of TCM and the combination of TCM and Western medicine in the treatment of visceral cancer pain in China have borne remarkable and fruitful results.

8.2.1 Perception of Visceral Cancer Pain in TCM

Western medicine believes that the pathogenesis of cancer pain is complex and can be broadly summarized from the following three aspects: (1) the cancer tumor compresses the adjacent nerves and tissues, causing ischemia and necrosis, and the tumor cells infiltrate into lymphatic tissues, releasing chemical algogenic substances and inflammatory mediators; (2) cancer pain is related to the cancer treatment process, such as tissue reaction caused by chemotherapy drugs and skin mucosal damage caused by radiotherapy; and (3) cancer pain is caused by cancer concomitant diseases. In recent years, progress has been made in the shift of the analgesia concept, the application of analgesic drugs and treatment techniques, which have played a positive role in relieving the pain symptoms of patients with cancer. This has been discussed in detail in other chapters.

TCM has formed its own perception of pain for a long time. As described in the *Jue Monograph* of *Miraculous Pivot* of *Huangdi Neijing* (*Yellow Emperor's Inner Canon*), "a true headache, a severe pain throughout the brain, feeling cold from hands up to the elbows and from feet up to the knees, is an incurable disease," the pain is similar to the headache caused by brain tumor. There are also descriptions of bone tumor pain in the *Cijie Zhen Xie Monograph* of *Miraculous Pivot*, "Pain in bone and atrophy in muscle, and the internal injury to the bone leads to osteolysis, all of which are caused by a malignant tumor that is hard when pressed by hands. The disease is agglomerated, penetrating deeper and hurting the bones, and the pathogen is attached to and merged with the bones and grows larger day by day, resulting in bone necrosis." When discussing lung mass (lung cancer) in *General Treatise on the Causes and Symptoms of Diseases*, it is mentioned that "a patient with lung mass has a floating pulse which disappears when it is pressed hard, with symptoms of reversed flow of *Qi* under the rib-side, pain in the back, and deficiency of *Qi*," which is very similar to the chest pain caused by lung cancer. In the same book, it liver mass (liver cancer) is discussed as "liver mass ...... is due to conflicts of *Qi* which accumulates and does not flow smoothly, so the pain is severe under the rib-side." These statements have laid a solid theoretical foundation for the treatment of cancer pain with modern TCM [3].

TCM does not grant diseases with the name cancer, but according to different parts of visceral cancer pain, they are classified as pain of corresponding parts, such as pain caused by esophageal cancer and lung cancer is defined as "chest pain," pain caused by gastric cancer as "stomach pain," pain caused by liver cancer as "hypochondriac pain," and pain caused by pancreatic cancer and colorectal cancer as "abdominal pain."

In terms of the nature of cancer pain, TCM divides cancer pain into two categories: repletion and deficiency. The repletion pain is caused by the invasion of pathogen (pathogenic factors) that results in "blood stasis, coagulated phlegm, and congestion of pathogen," which accumulate in the internal organs and meridians and cause "pain of congestion." The deficiency pain is caused by the deficiency of the body, damage to the internal organs, insufficiency of *Qi* and blood, and lack of nourishment of the meridians, which is called "pain of lacking spirit." Therefore, the pathogenesis of pain is summarized in TCM as "pain of congestion" and "pain of lacking spirit" [4]. By analyzing the orally taken prescriptions, Wang Yanling concluded that "overall lacking spirit and partially being congested" is the main pathogenesis of cancer pain [5]. The pathogenesis of cancer pain is complex and cannot be explained simply by "repletion" or "deficiency." Most of the advanced cancer pain is characterized by deficient diseases and repletion symptoms, including deficiency of *Qi*, deficiency of *Yin*, coagulated phlegm, *Qi* stagnation, and blood stasis. In clinical practice, sheer repletion or deficiency of cancer pain is less common. Mostly, the disease is caused by deficiency and the pain is caused by repletion, which is a kind of disease with general deficiency and local repletion.

The etiology of visceral cancer pain is restricted to six exogenous pathogenic factors, internal emotional trauma, and deficiency of healthy *Qi*, which lead to the dysfunction of visceral organs, the disharmony of *Qi* and blood, and phlegm besieged in the interior, all of which constitute the cancerous toxin. Cancerous toxin, phlegm condensation, and blood stasis intertwine to form a cancer tumor, which leads to stagnation of meridians and channels and pain, which is called "pain of congestion"; cancer toxin injures healthy *Qi* over time, resulting in dysfunction of visceral organs and insufficient *Qi* and blood that cannot provide nourishment to the visceral organs and meridians, which ignites "pain of lacking spirit." For exogenous pathogenic factors, pathogenic cold is the primary one. In the *Plain Questions* of *Miraculous Pivot* of *Huangdi Neijing*, it is described that "those who suffer from pain have much pathogenic cold in their body and cold causes pain." The *Causes of Diseases Monograph of Miraculous Pivot* says that "the formation of mass starts from cold." Cancer is related to exogenous pathogenic factors, especially cold, because it leads to contraction and stagnation, which can easily cause cold accumulation, blood stasis, and poor circulation of *Qi* and blood, and in return, the congestion brings pain. For internal emotional trauma, TCM believes that patients with cancer pain are often worried, frightened, and depressed. Seven emotions are too intensified to hurt five organs. "Anger hurts the liver, thought over depression hurts the spleen, and sadness hurts the lungs …… All diseases are generated from *Qi*." When *Qi* is not smooth, it leads to *Qi* stagnation and blood stasis; thus, pain of congestion occurs. It is no coincidence that the disease caused by emotions is similar to the disease caused by psychological factors in modern medicine. For deficiency of healthy *Qi*, it means that if the body is weak or has been sick for a long time, there is a deficiency of *Qi* and blood, *Yin* and *Yang*; thus, cancerous toxins will easily invade the body and stay there for a long time. Li Zhongzi discussed the cause of "mass" that "those who have mass in their bodies are lack of healthy *Qi* and their bodies are occupied by unhealthy *Qi*." Also, Zhang Jingyue pointed out that "people who have deficiencies in the spleen and kidneys and who are weak and have disorders often have masses in their visceral organs." Insufficient healthy *Qi* and deficiency of internal organs are prone to incur pathological changes such as stagnation of *Qi*, blood stasis, phlegm coagulation, and toxic accumulation, thereby forming cancer tumors. Zhang Yuansu suggested that "a healthy person has no mass in the body, but masses may form in the body of a weak person due to weak spleen and stomach, weak *Qi* and blood in different seasons, all of which can lead to masses," indicating that cancer is closely associated with the weakness of human internal organs, insufficient *Qi* and blood, and the sensation of pathogenic factors.

Although there is a consensus on the etiology and pathogenesis of cancer pain, it is still difficult to agree on its syndrome differentiation. At present, the syndrome of cancer pain is mostly differentiated based on etiologies, pathogenesis, and symptoms. For example, according to *Qi* stagnation, blood stasis, and phlegm dampness, which are regarded as the pathological factors of cancer pain, Li Hangsen divided cancer pain into three syndromes, namely, *Qi* stagnation and blood stasis, phlegm condensation and dampness, and *Qi* and blood deficiency. Li Huibo classified visceral cancer pain into the syndrome of cold-invading meridians, the syndrome of accumulation of pathogenic cold causing *Qi* stagnation and blood stasis, the syndrome of *Yang* deficiency and pathogenic cold accumulation causing phlegm obstruction, and the syndrome of *Qi* and blood deficiency. By analyzing the clinical symptoms of 100 cases of visceral cancer pain through factor analysis and other statistical methods, Che Yong et al. classified the syndromes into eight types—deficiency of *Qi* and blood, deficiency of lung *Qi*, endogenous heat due to *Yin* deficiency, *Yang* deficiency of the spleen and kidney, internal obstruction due to blood stasis, stagnation of liver *Qi*, *Yin* deficiency of stomach, and phlegm obstruction and dampness—among which the most common type is the deficiency of *Qi* and blood. Wu Dengbin et al. classified visceral cancer pain into six major syndrome types—vital *Qi* deficiency and binding of static blood, *Qi* stagnation, blood stasis and obstruction, phlegm dampness and condensation, damp and heat accumulation, and *Qi* and blood deficiency—and found that vital *Qi* deficiency and binding of static blood is the most commonly seen, followed by *Qi* and blood deficiency syndrome according to the frequency of related symptoms.

8.2.2 TCM in the Treatment of Visceral Cancer Pain

8.2.2.1 Internal Treatment Methods

At present, there is no uniformity in the classifications and treatments of visceral cancer pain. Most scholars agree that the internal treatment of visceral cancer pain should follow the principles of abiding by the disease pathogenesis, treating both symptoms and root causes, and eradicating pathogeny and nourishing the body at the same time to achieve the purpose of treating cancer pain by supporting the vital *Qi* and eliminating the pathogenic factors, and regulating the *Yin* and *Yang*, organs and meridians, and *Qi* and blood of human body.

The internal treatment method means that patients with visceral cancer pain can take oral Chinese medicine to relieve the pain and adopt different treatments and medicine formulas according to the etiology and pathogenesis of their cancer pain and the classification of syndromes. Examples are listed as follows.

1. Relieving pain by dispelling pathogenic cold and regulating the function of meridians

   The *Huangdi Neijing* said that "if the pathogenic cold invades the meridians, the circulation of *Qi* and blood in the meridians is stagnant, coagulated and do not flow smoothly." Clinical cancer pain is mostly the type of accumulation of pathogenic cold causing blood stasis. The pain is fixed to a region and mostly of stabbing characteristics. It is intense but will be relieved when the pain region is warmed. Patients' tongues are dark and the coating on the tongue is white and moist, while veins under the tongue are cyanosis. Their pulses are unsmooth or tight. Under such circumstances, the pain should be relieved by dispelling pathogenic cold and regulating the function of meridians. Herbal products that can warm the meridians and disperse cold such as Fu Zi (Aconiti Lateralis Radix Praeparata), Rou Gui (cinnamon), and Wu Tou (the rhizome of Chinese monkshood) are frequently used. Cui Hao conducted a study in which 40 patients with cancer pain belonging to the type of accumulation of pathogenic cold causing blood stasis were randomly divided into two groups. In the control group, opioids were given, and in the observation group, apart from opioids, Yuan Hu Analgesic Formula, which consists of Yanhusuo (Rhizoma Corydalis), Bing Pian (Borneol), Chuan Wu (Radix Aconiti), Ru Xiang (Boswellia), Mo Yao (Myrrh), Rou Gui, Zi Cao (Radix Lithospermi), and Chuan Xiong (*Ligusticum wallichii*), was added. The pain intensity score and pain relief rate were compared before and after treatment, and it was concluded that the Yuan Hu Analgesic Formula has significant analgesic and synergistic effects with opioids.
2. Relieving pain by warming *Yang Qi* to dispel the pathogenic cold

   In the late stage of cancer, *Yang Qi* is insufficient, cold is generated from it, and the body is deprived of warmth, manifesting as *Yang* deficiency and pathogenic cold accumulation. The pain is mostly of cold nature; thus, patients like warmth and being pressed. They are fatigued, with poor appetite, diarrhea, pale tongue, white and moist coating, and weak pulses. Such symptoms should be treated by warming *Yang* to dispel the pathogenic cold. Guo Qingwei et al. considered that in the late stage of cancer, there is deficiency and cold in the spleen and stomach, with *Yang* deficiency as the root cause and cold condensation as the symptom. The Da Jianzhong Decoction should be prescribed to warm and invigorate the spleen and disperse pathogenic cold. Li Yanping et al. believed that patients with advanced cancer mostly have weak *Yang Qi* and strong *Yin Qi* and cold inside, so they should take Jia Wei Wu Tou Decoction to warm the meridians to disperse cold, regulate the meridians, and relieve pain.
3. Relieving pain by warming *Yang Qi* to remove blood stasis

Yang Qi has the function of warming the body and promoting blood flow. When the *Yang Qi* is in deficiency, the blood circulation would be impaired. Therefore, cancer pain is present as accumulation of pathogenic cold and blood stasis. The pain is mostly stabbing and decreases with warmth. Patients are fatigued, with dark purple tongue, and white and thin tongue coating. Their pulses are unsmooth and rough. Zhang Ying et al. reckoned that cancer pain in the early stage is either of repletion or deficiency characteristic, but as the disease progresses and prolongs, combined with the effects of surgery, radiotherapy, and chemotherapy, the human body is deficient in *Qi* and blood, and phlegm and stasis are intertwined, leading to *Yang* deficiency and stasis, so the treatment of warming *Yang Qi* to remove stasis will be effective.

4. Relieving pain by eliminating phlegm and resolving turbidity

   "All diseases are mostly caused by phlegm." Phlegm is everywhere with the ascending and descending of *Qi*, but patients with visceral cancer pain suffer from deficiency of internal organs for a long time, so the deficient spleen function and internally generated phlegm and turbidity lead to abnormal ascending and descending of *Qi*, with lucid *Yang* not ascending and turbid *Qi* not descending. The symptoms are pain and stuffiness, accompanied by nausea and vomiting, plenty of phlegm and sputum, dizziness, fatigue and weakness, obesity, sleepiness and heaviness, drowsiness, and shapeless stools. Patients have fat tongue with teeth marks, dark tongue, white and smooth coating, and smooth or unhurried pulse. The symptoms can be relieved by eliminating phlegm and resolving turbidity. Zhang Liping and others used Decoction for Clearing Away Gallbladder-Heat to treat severe cancer pain of the phlegm dampness and obstruction type, which can reduce the adverse effects such as nausea and vomiting after taking analgesics. Liu Weisheng assumed that the phlegm dampness and accumulation type is commonly seen in lung cancer, intestinal cancer, thyroid cancer, etc., and can be treated with Decoction of Four Noble Drugs, which can be added with Sha Ren (Fructus Amomi) and Dafupi (Areca Peel) to treat abdominal distension; or with fried Gu Ya (rice-grain sprout) and fried Mai Ya (malt) to treat anorexia.

5. Relieving pain by invigorating *Yang Qi* to remove phlegm

   "Patients with phlegm and mucus should be treated with warm medicines." *Yang* deficiency negatively influences diuresis, so mucus is collected and accumulated internally to form phlegm, which is condensed to obstruct *Qi*. Consequently, cancer pain of congestion is caused. If *Yang Qi* is sufficient, phlegm will be dissolved into mucus, which will be excreted with urination. When the phlegm is removed, the pain will be relieved. Patients with cancer pain of the *Yang* deficiency and phlegm condensation type mostly have symptoms of suffocation, chest tightness, vomiting, fatigue, and weakness. Their tongues are pale, white, and fatty, with smooth or greasy white coating. Their pulses are unhurried and thin. By randomly dividing 72 patients with the *Yang* deficiency and phlegm coagulation-type cancer pain into the observation group and control group, Xiang Juhua et al. compared the degree of pain relief and quality-of-life scores before and after treatment between the two groups, and proved the efficacy of modified Aconite and Rice Decoction in treating patients of this type.

6. Relieving pain by activating *Qi* for removing blood stasis

   Patients with tumor are normally depressed, which leads to the liver *Qi* stagnation, *Qi* and blood obstruction and meridians stagnation, and finally experience the pain of congestion. In the book *Yixue Faming* (*Medical Inventions*), it is said that "when all the systems of the body circulate smoothly, one will not feel pain, but if one feels pain, it indicates that his or her body has congestions. If the pain can be relieved by purgation, then the meridians should be regulated to eliminate the pain." In the treatment of cancer pain of the *Qi* stagnation and blood stasis type, formulas or modified formulas of Bupleurum Decoction for Relieving Liver-*Qi*, Tao Hong Si Wu Decoction, Didang Decoction for Removing Phlegm-heat from Chest, and Decoction for Removing Blood Stasis are always used. The symptoms of *Qi* stagnation and blood stasis include distension or pain (more distension and pain in the *Qi* branch, more stabbing pain in the blood branch). Patients resist being pressed, have gloomy or darkish complexion, feel distension and pain in the chest, and prefer to sigh. Their tongues are dark purple or have petechia and ecchymosis, and the veins under the tongue are thick. Also, their pulses are rough. Zhou Zhongying first proposed the theory of "diseases are caused by cancerous cells." While treating lung cancer pain, he emphasized the "examination of the syndromes and exploring the mechanisms." He summarized the disease mechanisms as phlegm, stasis, depression, toxin, and deficiency. In the early stage of lung cancer, *Qi* stagnation prevails; while in the late stage of lung cancer, the blood stasis prevails. Therefore, the modified formula of Tao Hong Si Wu Decoction in combination with Wonderful Powder for Relieving Blood Stagnation can be used to activate *Qi* for removing blood stasis and disperse mass to relieve pain by making good use of special herbal medicines such as Jixueteng (Caulis Spatholobi), Jiang Huang (turmeric), Nan Xing (Rhizoma Arisaematis), and Donglingcao (*Rabdosia rubescens*).

7. Relieving pain by invigorating *Qi* for removing blood stasis

   For patients who suffer from cancer pain for a long time, their *Qi* is in deficiency, which leads to weak and poor blood circulation and flow and blocked meridians. Such a syndrome is called *Qi* deficiency and blood stasis. The symptoms of this syndrome are mainly stabbing pain fixed in one region, accompanied by fatigue, being listless and reticent. Their tongues are dark, with a thin and pale coating. Their pulses are weak or rough. Wu Wenzhuo et al. added the formula of Invigorating *Qi* for Removing Blood Stasis, which consists of 40 g Huang *Qi* (*Astragalus membranaceus*), 20 g Dang Shen (Radix Codonopsis Pilosulae), 20 g Chai Hu (Radix Bupleurum), 20 g Sheng Ma (Bugbane), 20 g San Leng (Rhizoma Sparganii), 20 g E Shu (Rhizoma Curcumae), 15 g Chuan Xiong, 15 g Quan Xie (dried body of scorpion), 30 g Hong Hua (Rhizoma Safflower), 30 g Tao Ren (Semen Persicae), 30 g Chaobaizhu (fried Rhizoma Atractylodis Macrocephalae), and a centipede to treat patients with primary hepatic carcinoma pain on the basis of oral MS Contin. After receiving the combined treatment for 14 days, patients' pain level and quality of life have been improved significantly through the evaluation of Numeric Rating Scale and QOL.

8. Relieving pain by benefiting *Qi* and nourishing blood

   The condition of patients with cancer pain deteriorates in the late stage. Because of the long torment of cancer pain, their spleen and stomach are in deficiency, being unable to generate new *Qi* and blood and muscles being weak, leading to weakened visceral organs. The symptoms of cancer pain include dull pain, dizziness, pale complexion, body being thin and weak, shortness of breath, poor appetite, poor bowel movement, poor sleep, pale tongue with white coating, and weak pulse. The *Golden Mirror of Medicine* goes like "with the symptoms of getting injured, the pain is caused by blood deficiency." Ouyang Xuenong et al. considered that high doses of Bai Shao (root of herbaceous peony) and prepared Gan Cao (liquorice root) can effectively relieve pain. They randomly divided 85 patients with cancer pain into the control group (tramadol capsule) and the treatment group (tramadol in combination with Shao Yao and Gan Cao Decoction consisting of 80 g Bai Shao and 30 g prepared Gan Cao), and found that the level of pain in the treatment group was relieved by 95.2%, which was significantly higher than that of 76.7% in the control group, indicating that Shao Yao and Gan Cao Decoction can be used in combination with tramadol to treat moderate-to-severe cancer pain. Sun Jing et al. assumed that advanced cancer pain is due to a deficiency of *Qi* and blood, and loss of nourishment of the body; thus, Decoction of Ten Powerful Tonics should be prescribed to relieve the pain, benefit *Qi*, and nourish the blood.

9. Relieving pain by benefiting *Qi* and nourishing *Yin*

   Patients with advanced cancer pain have deficiency in the liver and kidney and disharmonious meridians, with symptoms of vague pain, accompanied by dry mouth and throat, emaciation, weakness of waist and knees, dizziness and tinnitus, dry stools, red tongue with little coating and weak or light pulse, and should be treated by benefiting *Qi* and nourishing *Yin*. In a study evaluating the efficacy of Sha Shen and Mai Dong Decoction in the treatment of advanced lung cancer, Zha Hongqun et al. randomly grouped 70 patients with advanced lung cancer into the control group in which patients were treated with the GP regimen and the study group in which patients were treated with modified Sha Shen and Mai Dong Decoction in combination with GP regimen. By comparing the pain scores and quality of life of the two groups ($P < 0.05$), it was shown that modified Sha Shen and Mai Dong Decoction could relieve advanced lung cancer pain.

10. Relieving pain by removing cancer and toxic substances

    Cancer is caused by *Qi* stagnation, blood stasis, phlegm condensation, and toxic aggregation. The stagnation of *Qi* and blood leads to pain of congestion. Yang Xiangdong reckoned that the root cause of cancer pain is "tumor toxicity." Therefore, detoxification is indispensable in the treatment of cancer pain. Detoxification is not just about purgation. In the treatment of colorectal cancer pain, it is recommended that the Ji Chuan Zao Yan Powder consisting of Chuanbeimu (*Fritillaria cirrhosa*), Jiuhuanglian (prepared Rhizoma Coptidis with Vino), *Andrographis paniculata*, Hong Hua, Pao Jiang (prepared dried ginger), Rou Gui, Fabanxia (Rhizoma Pinellinae Praeparata), Dang Shen, Fu Ling (*Poria cocos*), prepared Gan Cao, Dang Gui (*Angelica sinensis*), Jiuchuanxiong (prepared Ligusticum Wallichii with Vino), Shudihuang (prepared Rehmannia root), Bai Shao, Banzhilian (*Scutellaria barbata*), and Baihuasheshe grass (*Oldenlandia diffusa*) could be the main formula. In addition, TCM inclines us to use empirical and special medicines to treat cancer pain according to the characteristics of cancer patients' pathologies, and results are proven to be ideal. In Li Shizhen's *Compendium of Materia Medica*, it says that Yanhusuo "can invigorate the stagnant *Qi* in the blood and the stagnant blood in the *Qi*, so it is able to relieve all the pains throughout the body." Li Hangsen is good at prescribing the basic formula of Yanhusuo with the addition of Chi Shao (red peony root) and Bai Shao (white peony root) to treat cancer pain. Yanhusuo in combination with Chi Shao can clear heat to relieve pain, and with Bai Shao can soften the liver to relieve pain. In addition, some TCM doctors are also good at using worm medicines to treat cancer pain. The *Prescriptions for Fifty-Two Diseases* is the earliest work that recorded worm medicines [6].

11. Summary

    Among the internal treatment methods, treatment based on syndrome differentiation is the main concept of perceiving and treating diseases in TCM, which is also its strength. The four diagnostic methods and eight principal syndromes are used to comprehensively analyze and determine the location, nature, and mechanism of diseases, as well as the prognosis of diseases, and then formulate treatment methods and prescriptions. In the treatment of cancer pain in TCM, besides paying attention to the characteristics of various tumors, the treatment should be based on the differences of patients' physique and symptoms, and the corresponding TCM decoction or Chinese medicines should be selected. When treating cancer pain, doctors should not simply aim at controlling the pain symptoms, but also take into account the individual physique, disease development stages, psychological and emotional conditions of patients with cancer pain, and according to the situation of healthy and unhealthy *Qi* in the body, the strategies of "eradicating pathogeny first and nourishing the body later," "nourishing the body first and eradicating pathogeny later," or "eradicating pathogeny and nourishing the body at the same time" should be adopted. This makes it possible to eliminate the unhealthy *Qi* without overlooking the health condition of the body, and to empower the healthy *Qi* without restraining the eradication of unhealthy *Qi*. The *Required Readings for Medical Professionals—Mass* written by Li Zhongzhi goes like this, "In the beginning, when the disease just develops, the healthy *Qi* is still strong and the unhealthy *Qi* is weak, then the main task is to eradicate pathogeny; in the middle stage, when the disease lingers for a long time, the unhealthy *Qi* grows stronger and the healthy *Qi* is weaker, then the main task is to eradicate pathogeny and nourish the body at the same time; in the late stage, as the disease continues to progress, the unhealthy *Qi* is invasive and the healthy *Qi* is dissipated, then the main task is to nourish the body." In other words, doctors should grasp the right opportunity to remove phlegm, stagnation, and cancer toxicity, regulate *Qi*, blood, *Yin* and *Yang*, and invigorate *Qi* flow to relieve the patient's pain and improve their quality of life.

8.2.2.2 External Treatment Methods

Orally taking Chinese medicines still has some limitations for those who lose swallowing function and refuse to accept them. Thus, the external treatment methods of TCM to control cancer pain have precise efficacy and mild adverse effects. It is more advantageous to patients with advanced cancer pain who are already deficient in vital energy and are not tolerant to aggressive treatment; whose spleen and stomach have weakened absorption function; to patients where the internal medication is not effective; or those who cannot take medication orally. External treatment is an indispensable method of TCM. In the *Plain Questions* of *Miraculous Pivot* of *Huangdi Neijing*, it is said that "internal treatment for internal diseases and external treatment for external diseases." In the *Li Lun Pian Wen* published in Qing Dynasty, it is said that "the principles of external treatment are the same as that of the internal treatment, and the external treatment medicine is the same as the internal treatment medicine; the only difference lies in the routes of administration." The external treatment methods of TCM mainly include application, patches, fumigation, washing, acupuncture, moxibustion, and other methods. Herbal preparations are applied to the body surface or treatments are applied externally. Medicines or drugs are absorbed directly through the skin, mucous membrane, acupuncture points, orifices, and other parts while they play overall as well as local regulating roles. The external treatment is one of the most common methods of TCM used in treating visceral cancer pain. It is characterized by rapid pain relief, safety in use, and minimal toxic adverse effects.

There are various external treatment methods for visceral cancer pain, such as TCM external application, TCM inunction, TCM nasal mucous membrane inhalation, TCM fumigation, TCM coloclysis, acupuncture, electroacupuncture, cupping therapy, and acupoint injection therapy.

1. TCM external application therapy

   The external application therapy makes the medicine penetrate through the skin mucous membrane into the grain of skin and the texture of the subcutaneous flesh to invigorate the meridians, work on the lesions directly, and eradicate or disperse the toxin. There are a large number of clinical studies proving its effectiveness [7]. Tang Shusheng et al. used Paste for Detumescence consisting of 20 Chinese medicines, including Xiong Huang (Realgar) (2.5%), Ru Xiang (3.5%), Mo Yao (3.5%), Ba Dou (Fructus Crotonis) (0.5%), Zhang Nao (Cinnamomum Camphora) (1.5%), Bai Fan (Alum) (5%), Mubiezi (*Momordica cochinchinensis*) (6%),

Maqianzi (prepared Semen Strychni) (2.5%), Chuan Wu (2.5%), Ban Mou (prepared cantharides) (0.5%), etc., which are finely processed into powder and mixed with alcohol (9.5%) and honey (11%). The 71 patients with advanced malignant tumors were divided and treated in two groups: 35 cases with tumor reduction and 36 cases with cancer pain management. In the cancer pain management group, the paste was applied to the area with intensive cancer pain and changed once in 3 days. The results showed that the efficiency of treating cancer pain mainly with external application was 89.7%. Yang Chenguang used Cancer Pain Relief Paste made of Maqianzi, Wushaoshe (Zaocys), Ru Xiang, Mo Yao, and Bing Pian on the painful area of 30 patients with cancer pain, and changed it once a day for 7 days as a course of treatment, with an overall efficiency of 96.7%, an average onset time of 1.5 h, and an average duration of 25 h.

2. Acupoint application therapy

   The acupoint application therapy refers to applying traditional Chinese herbs on the surface of acupuncture points to treat cancer pain. On the one hand, herbs directly work on the point; on the other hand, with the transmission effect of meridians, herbs can work on all parts of the body, raising the pain threshold and regulating the function of nerve and fluid systems to enhance the pain-relieving effect of traditional Chinese medicines [8]. Zhao Yuxiang et al. used Paste for Clearing Meridians consisting of Xi Xin (the root of Chinese wild ginger), Baijiezi (Semen Sinapis), Yanhusu, She Xiang (Moschus), Gan Sui (Radix Kansui), and Shengjiangzhi (*Zingiber officinale* Rosc.) externally on acupuncture points.

   The principles of selecting acupuncture points are as follows. For patients with primary liver cancer and liver metastasis, select Qi Men, Liver Shu, and Gallbladder Shu as the main acupuncture points, and Tsusanli and Quan Xi as adjunct points; for patients with lung cancer, select Lung Shu and Yunmen as the main acupuncture points, and Quan Xi and Large Intestine Shu as adjunct points; for patients with bone metastasis, osteosarcoma, and multiple myeloma, select acupuncture points according to the location of pain; and for patients with carcinoma of the head of the pancreas, select Pancreas Shu and Zhong Wan as the main acupuncture points, and Tsusanli and He Gu as adjunct points. The selection of acupoints can vary depending on the disease, and the total effective rate of 80 cases is 88.75%.

3. TCM inunction therapy

   TCM inunction is a therapy of pain relief by applying decoctions of Chinese herbal medicines to a specific area. Guo Jun et al. used the Tincture of Chinese Herbal Medicine for Relieving Pain to rub the painful area directly. The tincture is made by finely ground herbal medicine of Yanhusuo, Hong Hua, Baiqucai (*Chelidonium majus*), Chen Pi (Pericarpium Citri Reticulatae), Huangyaozi (*Dioscorea bulbifera* L.), Difuzi (Fructus Kochiae), Xue Jie (Sanguis Draxonisb), Ru Xiang, Mo Yao, and Bing Pian, with the powder being soaked in 75% ethanol for 1 week. It should be used at least three times a day without a limited course of treatment. The results showed that the total effective rate is 95.1%. Wang Weidong rubbed the skin or pain area with the Wu Bing Tincture for Relieving Pain made of raw Chuan Wu, raw Cao Wu, Xi Xin, raw Nan Xing, Bing Pian, Chan Su (*Venenum bufonis*), and Da Huang (Radix Et Rhizoma Rhei) soaked in 1000 mL 75% alcohol for 1 week. The tincture is applied three times a day for 14 days. The tincture is used externally in the first stage of cancer pain and in combination with analgesics in the second and third stages. In the control group, the WHO three-step analgesic ladder was adopted. The results showed that the total effective rate of the treatment group is 86.95%, while the total effective rate of the control group is 63.04%. Kou Shengling et al. treated 38 cases of tumor bone metastases with Yuan She Pain Relieving Liquid (soaking Yanhusuo, Chan Su, Cha Xiang, Niu Huang, and Bing Pian in 75% ethanol for 1 week), which is applied externally to the corresponding body surface of cancer pain several times a day. The total effective rate is 86.84%.

4. TCM nasal mucous membrane inhalation therapy

   Administering drugs through the nasal cavity for therapeutic purposes is not a common clinical practice in TCM, but there are many clinical trials associated with it. Niu Hongmei applied the nasal drop made of Xi Xin, Bing Pian, Fang Feng (Radix Saposhnikoviae), Jing Jie (Herba Schizonepetae), Ge Gen (Radix Puerariae), Baihuasheshe Grass, Wuweizi (Fructus Schisandrae Chinensis), Gou Qi (*F. lycii*), etc., containing 4 g of raw herbs per mL to treat 41 patients with cancer pain. The drop is used with two drops once every 6 h for 7 days. The total effective rate is 92.68%, with no significant adverse effects. Zhang Lipei et al. treated 31 cases of cancer pain with the nasal mucosal administration of Laugh and Cry Powder, which is made of Xiong Huang, Xi Xin, Chuan Xiong, Huo Xiao (saltpetre), and Ru Xiang. When the powder was inhaled into the nasal cavity, cancer pain was relieved immediately in most cases. There were 18 cases with significant effects, 10 cases with normal effects, and 3 cases with no effects.

5. TCM coloclysis therapy

   TCM coloclysis therapy is a frequently used treatment method, which is easy to practice and takes effect quickly. Shi Rongkang et al. treated 47 patients with cancer pain with oral mescaline for 24 h followed by coloclysis with an analgesic solution made of Shu Fu (*Porcellio scaber* Latreille), raw Maqianzi, raw Nan Xing, Zao Xiu (*Paris polyphylla*), Wu Gong (*Scolopendra*), Yanhusuo, Ru Xiang, and Mo Yao. The total effective rate is 83%. Liu Ruhan treated 47 cases of cancer pain with Shou Nian Powder (10 g Yanhusuo, 10 g Xiang Fu or Rhizoma Cyperi, 10 g Mo Yao, 10 g Wulingzhi or *Trogopterus xanthipes* Milne-Edwards) in combination with enema. The results proved that 10 cases achieved significant effects, 17 cases achieved normal effects, and 3 cases had no effects, with an overall efficiency of 90%.

6. Acupuncture therapy

   Acupuncture is an effective method for treating visceral cancer pain. Xu Shuying et al. treated 92 cases of cancer abdominal pain by performing acupuncture at the point of Tsusanli. During the treatment, all analgesics were stopped, and Tsusanli of both feet were acupunctured once a day, and 15 times for a course of treatment. The total effective rate is 88.04%, while the effective rate for mild pain is 100%, moderate pain is 97.6%, and severe pain is 72.33%. Dan Yu et al. treated 113 patients with cancer with different levels of pain with acupuncture therapy, the WHO three-step analgesic ladder and acupuncture, respectively, in combination with medicinal herbs. The main acupoints selected are He Gu, Nei Guan, and Zhi Gou, together with the Back Shu point. The acupuncture needles were kept for 0.5–1.5 h, 1–2 times a day, with 10 days as a course. The results showed a significant difference between the drug group (20.59%) and the acupuncture group (48.65%); the total effective rate was significantly different between the drug group (50.00%) and the acupuncture group (72.97%), and the differences were more significant when comparing these two groups with the acupuncture and herb group (95.24%). Zuo Xiuling et al. treated chest pain and upper extremity pain in patients with lung cancer by performing acupuncture at the Kong Zui point, with additional acupuncturing at the Ashi point, and then the adjunct points Chi Ze or Tai Yuan were also selected according to the characteristic of lung cancer. The needle tip was in the direction of meridian circulation and stimulated rapidly and strongly, and the needles were retained for 30–60 min to achieve satisfactory pain relief.

7. Electroacupuncture therapy

   Xu Jinhua et al. used the before-and-after self-control method to observe the efficacy of electroacupuncture in combination with the three-step analgesic ladder on 15 patients with cancer pain. The acupuncture points are

He Gu, Nei Guan, Xue Hai, Tsusanli, and Sanyinjiao. After needling, the acupuncture needles were connected to a G6805 electro-acupuncture instrument with high frequency (30 mW) and moderate stimulation and retained for 30 min, twice a day, for 14 days. At the same time, analgesics were administered twice a day according to the patient's needs. The total effective rate of treatment was 92.86%, and the duration of pain relief after each electroacupuncture treatment was 11 h average. The results demonstrated that electroacupuncture with the three-step analgesic ladder could better control cancer pain, reduce the dosage of analgesic drugs used, and improve the systemic symptoms and the survival quality of patients.

8. Moxibustion therapy

   Currently, the most commonly used moxibustion therapy is Herbs-partitioned Moxibustion. Because of the dual effect of herbs and moxa sticks, the efficacy is significant. Cai Shengchao et al. treated 31 cases of cancer pain with Herbs-partitioned Moxibustion. On the basis of oral paracetamol and codeine, they applied Pain Relieving Paste on the skin of the pain area and smoked the area with moxa stick. Two other control groups were set up, one treated by Pain Relieving Paste and the other administered oral paracetamol and codeine. The results showed that the treatment of 29 cases in the treatment group was effective and two were ineffective. There is a significant difference ($P < 0.01$) compared with both the Pain-Relieving Paste group and the oral paracetamol and codeine group. Gao Zhan et al. used acupuncture and moxibustion plus topical application of self-prescribed cancer pain relief solution to treat 50 patients with mid- to late-stage pain from malignant tumors. They first used moxa sticks to smoke Feng Fu, Da Zhi, and Wei Lu acupoints, and then acupunctured He Gu, Nei Guan, Tsusanli, and Ashi points. The results showed that the pain in 28 cases was completely relieved and in 20 cases was partially relieved, the treatment of 2 cases was ineffective, and the total effective rate of pain relief was 96%.

9. Iontophoresis of Chinese herbal medicine

   Wan Donggui et al. treated 18 cases of cancer pain with iontophoresis of Chinese herbal medicine. They soaked 100 g each of Yanhusuo, Ru Xiang, Mo Yao, and Dan Shen (Radix Salvia Miltiorrhiza), and 150 g Xuchangqing (Radix Cynanchi Paniculati) in 75% alcohol. Then, they added a small amount of Bing Pian and dimethylsulfoxide in the solution to moisten the electrode case of BG Electronic Pain Relief Therapy Instrument, and placed the electrode (copper plate) in the case. And then they put it on the selected acupuncture points for iontophoresis. The selected acupoints are Nei Guan, Tan Zhong, and Ah Yes points for chest pain; Huan Tiao, Kidney Shu, Yanglingquan, and Kun Lun points for low back and leg pain; Tian Zong, Shoulder Du, and Ashi points for shoulder and back pain; Shu, Mu, and Yuan points of corresponding organs for visceral pain. If the blood stasis is obvious, Xue Hai and Diaphragm Shu are selected as adjunct points. If there is phlegm coagulation, choose Feng Long as the adjunct points. And if there is *Qi* stagnation, select Xing Jian or Tai Chong points. In the treatment of 18 cases of cancer pain, 3 cases achieved complete relief, 12 cases acquired moderate relief, and 3 cases had no effects, with an efficiency of 84%.

10. Acupoint injection therapy

    Dang Wen et al. treated 48 patients with stomach cancer pain. After 2 months of treatment, the long-term analgesic efficacy of the filiform needle acupuncture group and the acupoint injection group (injection of lyophilized human transfer factor twice a week) was similar to that of the Western Medicine group, while the long-term efficacy was better. The two groups were able to counteract the toxic adverse effects caused by chemotherapy. Tao Min et al. used hydro-acupuncture technique to treat cancer pain and set up a control group of Western medicine bucinperazine. Different acupuncture points were taken according to the type of disease and pain area, and the main and adjunct acupuncture points were acupunctured together or alternately. The injected drugs were 30 mg bucinperazine, 0.5 mg dexamethasone, and 0.25 g vitamin B. Each acupuncture point was injected with 0.5–1 mL. The results showed that 45 patients in the group treated with hydro-acupuncture had obvious pain relief, among which 15 patients with moderate persistent pain were completely relieved; and among 30 patients with severe pain, 25 were completely relieved, and 5 achieved significant effects, with a total efficacy of 100%. The onset time was significantly shorter among patients in the hydro-acupuncture group (3.21 ± 1.28 min), compared with that of the control group (29.79 ± 5.40 min). Moreover, the maintenance time of pain relief in the hydro-acupuncture group was 25.03 ± 11.57 h, which was significantly longer than that of the control group, which was 8.29 ± 2.26 h.

11. Acupoint-medicated thread embedding therapy

    For all kinds of pain that are effectively treated by acupuncture and whose effects are difficult to maintain after removal of needles, acupoint-medicated thread embedding therapy can be considered to prolong the analgesic effect. Dong Zibin treated 320 cases of sciatica by embedding medicated catgut into Huan Tiao, Zhi Bian, Yin Men, and Yanglingquan points once every 15 days, with four times as a course of treatment, obtaining a total efficacy of 98.75%.

12. Cupping therapy

    Cupping therapy is a TCM external treatment method, the principle of which is to use mechanical or heating methods to vacuumize the jar and make the jar attach to the skin by negative pressure, bringing small subcutaneous stasis in the local area that can stimulate the body's own functions (such as the nervous system and endocrine system) to achieve the effect of pain relief. Cupping therapy is easy to perform and widely accessible without emphasizing the selection of precise points and can achieve satisfactory effects without causing extra pain; thus, patients are willing to accept it. The main treating acupoint is Back Shu as it is close to the visceral organs. From the perspective of anatomy, the back is innervated by the branch of the spinal cord. By taking the therapy of cupping, the nerve transmission may be blocked to realize the purpose of pain relief. According to the theory of TCM, cupping has the effect and benefit of warming the meridians, dispersing dampness and cold, invigorating *Qi* and blood, and harmonizing the *Qi* of the visceral organs, so that it can reduce the pain of patients with cancer, improve their quality of life, and prolong survival.

13. Muscle regions acupuncture therapy

    (a) Definition of muscle regions

        The earliest record of muscle regions in China was in the *Jingjin Monograph* of *Miraculous Pivot* of *Huangdi Neijing*, which discusses the circulation and disease symptoms of each fascia. There are different views on the essence of muscle regions. In the *Shuowen Jiezi* (*Analytical Dictionary of Characters*), it is said that "muscle regions are the strength of the muscle; tendons are the essence of muscle regions and are attached to the bone." The *Lei Jing* (*Category Canon*) proposed that muscle regions are tissues that "connect all the bones" and "maintain the body," "meet in the joints," "with no space in the middle," and "each with its own position." According to Liu Tao, Huang Jingwei, and Yang Shifang, muscle regions are the tissues of the body that "connect all the bones" and form the body shape with the bones, surround the joints, and control the body movement. The function of muscle regions is similar to that of the skeletal muscle and its auxiliary structures in modern anatomy, including the sarcolemma, tendons, fasciae, ligaments, and connective tissues of the joints, which is a huge organ of the body dominating biological activity. Through a comparative analysis of acupoint anatomy, acupoint location, symptoms of muscle regions disease, and clinical applications of muscle regions, Qin Yuge proposed that the substance of muscle regions in the *Huangdi Neijing* is dominated by the somatic nerves of the peripheral nerves, and partially innervated by central nerves and autonomic nerves. Wang Yu reckoned that muscle regions are similar to fasciae (mainly tendons and ligaments) and peripheral nerves. According to the *Soft Tissue Injury in TCM*, "muscle regions" are equivalent to the soft tissues of the extremities and trunk. Wu Jinpeng believed that muscle regions are homologous with the membrane as well as the various forms of fasciae, and that the integration of the anatomical substance of muscle regions with the membrane is an independent functional system composed of fascial tissues, which is distinct from the other nine systems of the body and is closely linked to the other systems to maintain the normal function of the body.

(b) Distribution pattern of 12 muscle regions

Yang Shangshan in the *Taisu* of *Huangdi Neijing* pointed out that "twelve meridians refer to three *Yin* meridians and three *Yang* meridians in hands and feet respectively. But twelve meridians dominate *Qi* and blood and run internally through viscera organs and externally through the head and body. Twelve muscle regions operate in the chest and abdomen, but not into visceral organs." Twelve muscle regions go parallel with meridians but not into visceral organs; thus, they do not have visceral affiliations and streaming, and only rely on the nourishment from the *Qi* and blood of meridians. They start from the end of limbs toward the head and body, directing toward the heart without differentiation of forward or backward, the distribution pattern of which is similar to that of 12 meridians. That is, six *Yin* muscle regions of hands and feet lie on the inner side, following the sequence of Tai Yin, Jue Yin, and Shao Yin. Correspondingly, six *Yang* muscle regions of hands and feet lie on the outside, following the sequence of Yang Ming, Shao Yang, and Tai Yang. In addition, the circulation and distribution of muscle regions have the characteristics of "assembling" and "convergence." For example, three *Yang* muscle regions of feet assemble at the "Tian" (face), three *Yin* muscle regions of feet assemble at the "Yinqi" (abdomen), three *Yang* muscle regions of hands assemble at the "Jiao" (head), and three *Yin* muscle regions of hands assemble at the "Ben" (chest), which is called "assembling." In the joints of the limbs and thickly muscled regions, such as the ankles, diaphragm, knees, femurs, thighs, arms, wrists, elbows, armpits, shoulders, and necks, the neighboring muscle regions assemble and converge, which is called "convergence."

(c) Physiological function of 12 muscle regions

The *Meridian Wing of Miraculous Pivot* says, "When a person is born, he or she first only has a spirit, and then the brain is formed; bones for skeletons, meridians for management, muscle regions for strength, muscles for protection, skin for protection and hair growing long and when grains are swallowed and fulfill the stomach, *Qi* and blood are invigorated." According to this text, Yang Shifang explained the role of muscle regions. First, they connect the limbs and bones and maintain the body by the assembling and convergence of muscle regions. Twelve muscle regions have the functions of muscles, tendons, fascia, and membranes. "Muscle regions for strength" means that the muscles and tendons attached to the bones and joints can enable the human body to stand, walk, and carry out normal flexion and extension movement and other activities, showing the strength and power of muscle regions. Second, they protect the tissues and visceral organs of the body, which is the meaning of "…… muscles for protection ……" In other words, muscles cover the body and limbs and form a peripheral tissue system that can resist external evils and protect the tissues and visceral organs of the body. *Wei Monograph* of *Plain Questions* provides the simplest summarization of the physiological function of muscle regions as "restraining the bones and joints and making the joints move flexibly."

(d) Twelve muscle regions and visceral cancer pain

Cancer pain is mostly caused by exogenous pathogenic factors, improper diet, internal emotional trauma, and over-exertion. *Yingyang Yingxiang Monographs of Plain Questions* says that "wind injures muscle regions." The liver governs muscle regions and the wind stirs the liver, so the disease caused by wind is often manifested through muscle regions. Cold and heat pathogenic factors can also lead to muscle regions lesions as described by *Pibu Monographs* of *Plain Questions*: "they (pathogenic factors) stay between the bones and muscle regions; when the cold is overwhelming, there is spasm and pain in the bones; when the heat is overwhelming, the muscle regions are flabby and the bones wither away." In the *Bi Monographs* of *Plain Questions*, it is said that "arthralgias are acute when they are caused by cold and are chronic when they are caused by heat." Cold induces involuntary muscular contraction, so when influenced by cold, muscle regions suffer from contracture and spasm. On the other hand, heat leads to expansion, and when influenced by heat, muscle regions tend to be relaxed and flabby. The *Xuanji Yuanbing Monographs* of *Plain Questions* says, "When patients who suffer from wind develop into muscular atonia in October, the reason lies in the overwhelming dryness." The *Zhizhenyao Monographs* of *Plain Questions* says, "The spasm and stiff neck muscles and tendons are all induced by dampness." This shows that dryness and dampness may lead to tendon lesions. In the Five Elements, liver corresponds to sour flavor, and gold corresponds to pungent flavor, which overwhelms the sour flavor of wood; thus, if sour flavor and pungent flavor are properly utilized, they can nourish muscle regions; otherwise, they will harm muscle regions. The *Five Flavors Monographs* of *Plain Questions* says, "Sour goes along the muscle regions, and taking too much sour food may cause infirmity." The *Jingui Yaolue* (*Synopsis of Prescriptions of the Golden Chamber*) says that "sour flavor is harmful to muscle regions and the injury of muscle regions leads to sluggish, which is called flabby." That is to say, eating too much sour food can damage the human tendon so that the body movement becomes slow. The *Shengqi Tongtian Monographs* of *Plain Questions* says, "Eating too much pungent food can lead to the gradual weakness of muscle regions and loss of spirit." Pungent flavor can disperse *Qi* and taking too much spicy food will hurt the tendons, manifested as tendon relaxation and weakness. Besides, the *Jiuzhen Monographs* of *Plain Questions* says, "For people who are repeatedly frightened, their meridians do not flow smoothly due to disturbances of *Qi*, and are mostly numb." Frequently feeling terrified can disturb the circulation of meridians and muscle regions, leading to loss of nourishment in *Qi* and blood, numb, and insensitive symptoms. In addition, *Xuanming Wuqi* of *Plain Questions* says, "Walking too much hurts the tendons." Fatigue originates from the liver and muscle regions that govern movements; thus, overwork injuries muscle regions [9]. Wei Shimin et al. observed the therapeutic effect of muscle regions acupuncture on pharmacogenic constipation in patients with cancer pain. Fifty-two cases of patients with lung cancer with moderate-to-severe pain and constipation were randomly divided into treatment group and control group, with 26 patients in each group. On the basis of routine nursing care, the control group was treated with Western drugs [10], and the treatment group was treated with Western drugs in combination with the muscle regions acupuncture. The defecation, pain score, and quality of life of the two groups were recorded before and after treatment. The total points of constipation symptoms and NRS scores of both groups decreased after treatment, and the scores of quality of life increased ($P<0.05$). Overall, the constipation symptoms, NRS scores, and quality of life improved significantly in the treatment group compared with that in the control group.

14. Summary

    TCM external treatment of visceral cancer pain embodies the holistic view and the spirit of diagnosis and treatment of TCM, its therapeutic effect is precise and rapid, with little adverse effects, and it is easy to apply and control. It is especially desirable for those who are not suitable for taking medicines orally or those whose stomach cannot tolerate the medicines for a long time, and it can also reduce the adverse reactions and effects caused by some oral medicines. For example, because the external therapies do not need to be taken orally and absorbed gastrointestinally, they prevent gastrointestinal side effects in patients with dyspepsia, and the withdrawal of the medicine is also more convenient.

According to TCM, the pathogenesis of cancer pain is mainly due to the internal invasion of pathogenic factors such as *Qi* stagnation, blood stasis, dryness of body fluid, and blockage of meridians that induce pain of congestion. The lack of healthy *Qi* and deficiency of *Qi* and blood over a long period of time cause pain of lacking spirit. Fortunately, external treatment has the efficacy of removing obstructions in the meridians, harmonizing *Qi* and blood, balancing *Yin* and *Yang*, and relieving pain, and thus is widely used in the clinical treatment of pain caused by various cancers.

Although external treatment methods have good pain-relieving effects, there is also the problem of incomplete analgesia when they are applied alone in treating cancer pain, especially when the cancer is in the middle to advanced stage when opioid analgesics represented by morphine are required, which has achieved satisfactory effect in managing cancer pain. Obviously, the adverse outcomes of using morphine are astonishing. It often produces drug dependence, tolerance, addiction, and adverse effects such as nausea, vomiting, and mental disorders, which greatly impact the patients' quality of life. Therefore, a combination of external therapeutic methods and medicines with the effect of improving immunity and analgesia should be recommended, so the risk of opioid addiction can be reduced by replacing certain dosage of opioids with acupuncture. The significance of cancer pain treatment goes far beyond pain relief itself; it also aims to improve the patients' quality of life, ability to work, and enjoyment of recreation, and enable them to perform normal functions in the family and society.

8.2.2.3 A Combination of Internal and External Treatment Methods

Wu Jian treated 42 cases of patients with different cancer pain in late stage with an analgesic capsule consisting of raw Nan Xing, raw Ban Xia (Rhizoma Pinelliae), prepared Maqianzi, Tulip, and Wulingzhi internally, and an analgesic cream consisting of raw Nan Xing, raw Fu Zi, raw Chuan Wu, Maqianzi, Huangyaozi (*Dioscorea bulbifera* L.), Chuanshanjia (Squama Manis), Ru Xiang, Mo Yao, Chan Su, Bing Pian, and externally. The results showed that 15 cases achieved significant effects of pain relieving, 8 cases achieved normal effects, while the treatment of 4 cases was ineffective, with a total effective rate of 90.48% [11].

8.2.3 Integration and Complementation of TCM with Western Medicine Treatments

8.2.3.1 Opioid-Induced Constipation

According to the statistics released by WHO, by 2020, there were about 10 million new patients with cancer worldwide each year [12]. The prevalence of pain in patients who were first diagnosed with cancer is 25%; one-third of the patients with advanced cancer suffer severe pain. Based on the three-step analgesic ladder for cancer pain, opioids are recommended for managing moderate-to-severe cancer pain. The side effects of opioids should not be ignored despite their effective analgesic role. And constipation is one of the most intolerable and severe adverse effects of opioids. Modern medicine focuses on symptomatic treatment, yet the efficacy of which is unstable. TCM, on the other hand, treats opioid-associated constipation in various ways and has obvious advantages. Opioid-induced constipation (OIC) refers to the change in bowel habits due to receiving opioid treatments for more than 1 week, with manifestations of weakening of intestinal peristalsis leading to spontaneous defecation less than three times per week, laborious defecation, poor stool output, and hard stools. In recent years, many clinical studies have shown that clinical constipation is more common in patients with cancer pain who have been using opioids in high doses for a long period of time. OIC can occur at the initial stage of administering opioids and persist throughout the whole process of using the medication. Patients cannot become tolerant to OIC as the treatment is prolonged. In contrast, OIC will be aggravated progressively and even lead to intestinal obstruction.

1. How does modern medicine perceive the pathogenesis of OIC?

   As for the main mechanism and etiology of OIC, Western medicine believes that the main cause is that opioids increase intestinal sphincter tone and segmental motor function throughout the human body as opioid receptors are closely related to the μ-opioid receptor, which is mainly distributed in the intestinal nerves. Research results show that opioids have a significant inhibitory response to μ receptor, inhibiting the production of second messengers (cAMP and PKA) and Ca^{2+} channels, which in turn reduces the release of acetylcholine, and continues to activate K^+ channels to the hyperpolarization state [3]. The receptor in combination with opioids can markedly inhibit the relaxation of the smooth muscles of the gastrointestinal tract and delay gastric emptying, which contributes to the slowdown of bowel movement and the delay of defecation. Secondly, opioids greatly weaken the secretory function of the intestinal tract, which stimulates the reabsorption of water, making the feces become dry and hard and resulting in constipation.

2. Etiology and pathogenesis of opioid associated constipation in TCM

   TCM first proposed the etiology of constipation in the *Huangdi Neijing*: "The five viscera store *Qi* instead of send it outward, so it is often full of spirit. The six viscera transmit and transform water and grain rather than store them, so it sometimes appears to be full, but it cannot remain full forever," "the large intestine conducts unclean dross and turns the dross into tangible feces." The large intestine is where the main lesion develops and leads to constipation. Constipation is the result of the large intestine conductivity malfunction, and its pathogenesis may include visceral dysfunction, *Qi*, blood and fluid deficiency, and *Yin* and *Yang* imbalance. Currently, patients with cancer may first consider whether they can undergo radiotherapy or not, and most of the patients with cancer have already received radiotherapy in the early stage. Whereas, according to TCM, chemotherapy drugs or radiotherapy are considered to have fire toxin, which can burn the human body's fluids, and make the body deficient in *Qi* and blood. Therefore, deficiency of vital energy has always been an important internal mechanism to be considered while planning the treatment of patients with cancer pain. According to the viewpoint of TCM, the vital energy of patients with cancer is greatly damaged, and the deficiency of *Qi* cannot promote the flow of blood in the human body, and the flow of *Qi* is not smooth, which makes the meridians stagnant and blocked, or the *Qi* of internal organs do not move downward smoothly, which makes the function of the gastrointestinal movement impaired and movement of gastrointestinal tract inhibited, which makes the release of *Qi* and stool cease. Opium tastes pungent, bitter, sour, and astringent, with characteristics of warm, dry, and poisonous. It is good at moving around, so it may disrupt the circulation of the body's *Yang Qi*, deplete the spleen and stomach, affect the *Qi*, blood and fluid generation, especially the *Qi* of large and small intestinal tracts, and lead to difficulty in defecation. After *Huangdi Neijing*, later generations of medical practitioners have summarized and absorbed the experience of their predecessors, while giving full play to the advantages of each doctor to develop their unique insights into the theory of constipation.

3. TCM treatment for opioid-associated constipation
   (a) Internal treatment

   Gao Yinli et al. divided the patients into two groups and gave Chinese medicines for invigorating *Qi* and moisturizing bowel (basic formula: 20 g Dang Shen, 20 g raw Di Huang, 20 g Xuan Shen, 20 g Gou Qi, 20 g raw Bai Zhu or Bighead Atractylodes, 20 g prepared Heshouwu, 20 g Huomaren, 10 g Zhi Ke or *Fructus aurantii*, 15 g Wu Yao, 10 g Rou Gui, 10 g Roucongrong, and 6 g Xing Ren) and oral liquid of lactulose, respectively. The observational results showed that the Chinese herbs are more effective than lactulose in stimulating the first bowel movement and relieving the concomitant symptoms [13]. Moreover, Li Jun used an oral solution of Simo Decoction for the treatment of opioid-associated constipation and concluded that the effective rate of constipation relief in the treatment group was higher than that in the lactulose group, and the level of pain was reduced in the treatment group.

   (b) External treatment
   - Acupuncture therapy

     Xu Haiyan et al. randomly selected 72 patients receiving opioids for constipation and divided them into control group and observation group. The observation group was treated with acupuncture simultaneously at Tian Shu, Large Intestine Shu, Shangjuxu, Zhi Gou, and Zhao Hai points; while the control group was given Ma Ren Intestinal Pills orally. The results showed that acupuncture treatment for OIC has significant efficacy and can effectively relieve the pain of constipation patients, and improve their quality of daily life and work [13]. Zhou Yu et al. conducted a clinical study on the prevention and treatment of opioid-induced constipation by acupuncture. They chose eight acupuncture points, including Tian Shu (bilateral), Shen Que., Tsusanli (bilateral), Shangjuxu (bilateral), and Yin Men (left side) points. Among 25 cases, 64% of them displayed clinical efficacy.

     Acupoint paste therapy

     Zheng Chao et al. observed the efficacy of TCM acupoint pastes in the treatment of opioid-induced constipation. The paste is made of Xuan Shen, Mai Dong, raw Di Huang, Da Huang, Mang Xiao, and a small amount of honey. It is applied with a sterile gauze. The treatment group received acupoint paste with enema therapy, while the control group was treated simply with enema. The results proved that the treatment group achieved an effective rate of 71% and the control group 33%, manifesting that the treatment of the treatment group was more efficient. Deng Haiyan et al., through the experimental observation, concluded that applying Laxative TCM Paste on the Shen Que. point can effectively treat the constipation caused by opioids, with minimum adverse effects and convenient administration.

4. Summary

Treatment of OIC with Western medicine methods and drugs is often of limited choice. Commonly used laxatives are osmotic laxatives (polyethylene glycol, lactulose, sorbitol), stimulant laxatives (Da Huang, senna, aloe vera), and lubricating laxatives (liquid paraffin, glycerol, docusate, polyaldehydes, and other vegetable oils), etc. Long-term use of laxatives will directly cause severe diarrhea and electrolyte disturbance, affect the normal digestion and absorption of vitamins and microelements, and even damage the intestinal nerves, leading to drug dependence.

TCM treatment of opioid-associated constipation emphasizes treatment based on syndrome differentiation, the holistic view of TCM. Many studies have shown that when oral opioids are given for pain relief, relevant interventions based on TCM syndrome differentiation can effectively alleviate the symptoms of drug-induced constipation in patients with cancer pain, and at the same time improve their quality of life. Furthermore, TCM not only has various methods for treating OIC, but is also easy to operate, with remarkable efficacy and reliable safety, which makes it easier to be accepted by patients. At present, most of the clinical studies on the treatment of OIC with TCM are restrained to short-term efficacy assessment and with small sample sizes. Whether there are obvious side effects after long-term use of these Chinese medicines needs to be further explored.

8.2.3.2 Combination of TCM and Three-Step Analgesic Ladder

For patients with cancer, the fear of tumor pain is often greater than the disease itself, which is a serious challenge for the patient's psychology. Long-term pain often brings a series of negative psychological changes, such as fear and despair, which leads to intensified sensitivity to pain and even deterioration of the patient's condition. The three-step analgesic ladder is a commonly used clinical method for treating cancer pain, that is, nonsteroidal anti-inflammatory analgesics (NSAIDs), weak opioid analgesics, and strong opioid analgesics. However, the above drugs are almost invariably associated to potential toxic side effects of varying degrees, such as constipation, nausea, vomiting, respiratory depression, drug dependence, and drug addiction at a later stage. Studies have found that long-term use of anesthetics may accelerate tumor angiogenesis, tumor growth, the spread of cancer cells, and the recurrence of tumors [14, 15]. The combination of TCM with the three-step analgesic ladder for cancer pain can not only reduce the dose and toxic side effects of drugs, but also slow down the occurrence of opioid resistance.

8.2.3.3 TCM in Three-Step Analgesic Ladder

1. First step of analgesic ladder: non-narcotics

   NSAIDs are the major drugs used in this category. Represented by aspirin, paracetamol, ibuprofen, etc., NSAIDs have functions of antipyretic, analgesic and anti-inflammatory, acting on the periphery, with moderate analgesic effect. They work effectively on headache, toothache, neuralgia, muscle pain, joint pain, and inflammatory pain. They are also applicable for mild cancer pain and serve as the basic drugs for medical treatment of cancer, with no tolerance or addiction in long-term application. However, these kinds of drugs have dose limits (ceiling effect), so they should not be blindly applied to liver and kidney toxicity, leukocyte decline, platelet dysfunction, etc. Patients who overdose often first manifest digestive symptoms, such as epigastric discomfort, nausea, vomiting, and even perforation and other emergencies. Therefore, the Decoction of Cyperus and Amomum with Six Noble Ingredients can be used as the base formula for the addition and reduction of herbs to warm the spleen and stomach, regulate *Qi* and relieve pain, using herbs such as Sha Ren, Xiang Fu, Bai Zhu, Dang Shen, Fu Ling, raw Gan Cao, Chen Pi, Ban Xia, Zhi Ke, Yanhusuo, and Bai Shao. If patients have ulcer bleeding and the stool is black, Bai Ji and Heidiyu should be added. If patients are depressed, Bupleurum Powder for Relieving Liver-*Qi* can be used in combination to disperse stagnated liver *Qi*. For patients with stomach distention, Jiaosanxian should be added.

2. Second step of analgesic ladder: weak opioids

   The representative drug is codeine, and the main drugs are dihydrocodeine, dextropropoxyphene, propooxyphene, tramadol, and bucinnazine. When NSAIDs are administered, weak opioid analgesics are supplemented. In order to strengthen the efficacy of pain relief in clinical practice, the first- and second steps of analgesics are often made into compound products such as Galake and Propooxyphene.

3. Third step of analgesic ladder: strong opioids

   The representative drug is morphine, and the main drugs are morphine controlled-release tablets, dolantin, buprenorphine, etc. Morphine can be applied to all kinds of pain, especially to pain that is ineffectively treated with other analgesics, such as post-surgical wound pain, bone fracture, severe trauma, and advanced malignant tumor pain. The sedative and euphoric effects it produces can significantly help patients with cancer fall asleep and improve psychological tolerance to illness and pain. It is applicable to severe cancer pain and is an essential drug for the treatment of advanced cancer pain. The maximum dose ranges of this category of drugs are 330–1200 mg/day, with no dose limit, and high-dose opioids for the treatment of patients with advanced cancer with severe pain are safe and effective. The most common side effects are constipation and nausea. Other side effects include respiratory depression, confusion, and addiction.

8.2.3.4 TCM for Cancer Pain Relief

TCM internal and external treatments often use aromatic, strong-smelling, and penetrating mineral medicines. Most of the formulas used are "removing obstruction to relieve pain," "treating deficient pain with tonifying method," "regulating meridians to relieve pain," "removing toxin to relieve pain," "activating blood circulation to relieve pain," etc. Chinese patent medicines include Pill of Cow-bezoare, Cinobufotalin, Aidi Injection, Kang'ai Injection, etc. Clinical acupuncture is effective for treating both the tumor itself and the pain. Acupuncture for pain relief should target on the relationship between the pain sites and the meridians. Pain in the forehead belongs to the *Yang* Ming meridian, in the back of the head and neck belongs to the Tai *Yang* meridian, on both sides of the head belongs to the Shao *Yang* meridian, over the head belongs to the Que. *Yin* meridian. The heart and lungs belong to the Shang Jiao (upper visceral organs); the spleen, stomach, liver, and gallbladder belong to the Zhong Jiao (middle visceral organs); and the kidney and bladder belong to the Xia Jiao (lower visceral organs). Pain in both sides of the ribs belongs to the liver and gallbladder meridians, in the shoulder and back belongs to the heart and lungs meridians, and in the breast belongs to the liver and stomach meridians. The points selected are He Gu, Nei Guan, Zhi Gou points together with Feng Long and Shao Fu for chest pain, Tai Chong and Qiu Xu for pain in ribs, and Tsusanli and Sanyinjiao for abdominal pain. The 113 cases were divided into the drug group, the acupuncture group, and the combination of acupuncture and drug group, and the results showed that acupuncture achieved better analgesia outcomes than drugs. In addition, Luo Zhenghui et al. took the most sensitive point of radial of the second metacarpal bone as the Quan Xi acupoint and carried out acupuncture treatment for 33 cases of patients with advanced cancer with severe pain. They also set up another group with 40 cases of patients with advanced cancer with severe pain who were treated with muscular injection of analgesics. The results showed that the analgesic effect of the acupuncture group was significantly better than that of the control group.

8.2.3.5 TCM with Chemotherapy

In the clinical treatment of cancer pain, Dong Sheng Yun et al. treated 30 cases with chemotherapy combined with pain-eliminating decoction in the experimental group, and 30 cases with simple chemotherapy in the control group, and the results showed that the therapeutic effect of the experimental group was better than that of the control group. There was no significant adverse reaction in the experimental group [16]. Besides, Sun Fuxiang et al. observed bone metastatic cancer clinically and proposed that chemotherapy was the first choice for treating tumor proliferation, but the effect of a comprehensive therapy consisting of chemotherapy and TCM was more outstanding in terms of analgesia. Specifically, the Odynolysis Cataplasm was applied to the painful region, and the pain-relieving efficacy could be maintained for 18 h.

8.2.3.6 TCM with Radiotherapy

Radiotherapy is also a commonly used method in the clinical treatment of cancer. Whereas radiotherapy often kills normal cells and jeopardizes the immune function when eliminating cancerous factors, and is often accompanied by inflammation of the lungs, bladder and spinal cord, and oral ulcers. Fortunately, if radiotherapy is combined with TCM, it will be more effective in relieving pain. Liu Zhaoling et al. randomized 40 cases of patients with pain complicated by bone metastatic cancer. The experimental group used tincture of TCM on the pain area at the same time of radiotherapy, and the control group received radiotherapy alone. Comparing the effect of pain relief after 1 week of medication, the efficiency of the experimental group was 60% and that of the control group was 10%, indicating that the former was significantly superior to that of the latter. After 4 weeks of medication, the efficiency of the experimental group reached 90% and that of the control group was 60%, and the difference between the two groups was significant ($P<0.05$).

8.2.4 TCM Five-Element Emotional Therapy in Visceral Pain

Modern medicine believes that every pain experience has psychological aspects. Pain is the patient's subjective response to an adverse stimulus. It can be caused by organic lesions and is often influenced by mental factors. Pain is a major concern for patients, but most patients may have severe psychological problems that make them more vulnerable to harm and more likely to experience discomfort during any disease process. Psychological treatment may reduce the harm and loss of function in chronic pelvic pain, which is a valuable treatment method. Therefore, it is necessary to pay attention to the treatment of organic lesions while observing whether the patient has psychopathological symptoms and providing psychological treatment. However, many patients are unable to bear or unwilling to accept the diagnosis and treatment of psychologists or psychiatrists, making psychological evaluation and treatment sometimes difficult to carry out.

After numerous years of research, Western medicine psychotherapy has developed its own system, content, and methods, with both experimental and theoretical research being relatively well established. Its clinical efficacy is widely recognized, and it finds broad applications in clinical settings. However, substantial differences between China and the West in cultural tradition, social structure, economic conditions, values, and lifestyle customs contribute to significant variations. The personality traits and mental states of Chinese individuals markedly differ from those of Westerners. This disparity makes it challenging to adapt Western theories and models to Chinese psychological characteristics without considering the cultural nuances.

TCM emotional therapy involves the treatment of mental and psychosomatic disorders by healthcare professionals or psychologists using theories and methods from TCM emotional theory or psychological behavior theory. The goal is to enhance patients' psychosomatic conditions. As one of the traditional Chinese medical therapies, TCM emotional therapy boasts a rich history. It not only possesses profound medical philosophy and scientific underpinnings but also stands out for being "simple, safe, and effective." These attributes have garnered favor among a majority of patients and provided relief for countless individuals suffering both physically and psychologically.

TCM places significant emphasis on psychological therapy, specifically emotional therapy. *Tangye Laoli Monographs of Plain Questions* highlights that acupuncture and herbal medicine are ineffective in treating emotional diseases since "the spirit is passive, and the will is not treated, so the disease cannot be cured." TCM has long acknowledged the role of emotional therapy in disease prevention and treatment, with ongoing enrichment and improvement in both theory and clinical research. For instance, *Wuyun Xingda Monographs of Plain Questions* introduces the restraining relations among five emotions that "anger hurts the liver, sadness restrains anger," "joy hurts heart, fear restrains joy," and so on. These texts advocate that a competent clinician must first address the mental illness and then attend to the body, emphasizing the holistic treatment of both body and mind. Research on sequelae of pelvic inflammatory disease (SPID) indicates lower SAS and SDS scores in the study group after five-element emotional therapy, suggesting that TCM emotional nursing can provide targeted regulation based on patients' psychological and emotional characteristics [17]. Similarly, a clinical study on pelvic stasis syndrome (PCS) reached the conclusion that TCM emotional nursing, including the playing of music, regulating emotions, and exchanging emotions, can effectively improve negative emotions in patients [18]. PCS, characterized by chronic pelvic pain, is closely linked to neuropsychiatric factors, highlighting the importance of addressing mental and psychological aspects in treatment. Patients with PCS often experience long-term incurable pain, leading to mental burdens such as depression and irritability. Given the challenges of long-term treatment, building trust and effective communication between clinicians and patients is crucial. Verbal communication serves as a powerful tool, acting as an antidote to doubt and a key to resolving confusion. Clinicians should engage in real communication with patients to remove worries, instill confidence in recovery, and mobilize the patient's potential to resist the disease. Positive psychological hints during communication contribute to a patient's overall well-being.

Throughout ancient and modern times, the specific methods of emotional therapy have been subject to diverse opinions, representing a multitude of schools of thought. However, the general principles remain consistent. These methods have been synthesized later and several effective approaches have been identified, which are illustrated as follows [19, 20].

8.2.4.1 Music Delighting Emotions

Playing music based on the patient's personal preferences allows them to lie quietly in bed while listening to music to relax. Music can stimulate the patient's hypothalamus cortex and brain, regulating their nervous state, sleep quality, and pain levels.

8.2.4.2 Following Desires with Understanding

Healthcare professionals should strive to fulfill patients' wishes to the greatest extent, accommodating their psychological needs to further alleviate anxiety and depression. Simultaneously, instructing family members to meet patients' needs to the fullest extent possible helps improve the patient's overall mood. Subsequently, instruct patients in implementing the tranquillization method, encouraging them to maintain stillness, lie quietly, and practice controlled breathing.

8.2.4.3 Comfort and Uplift Emotions

Healthcare professionals should try to grasp the patient's work experience, family roles, work environment, disease occurrence, and social status, engaging in targeted communication. They should explain to the patients the treatment techniques and process, thereby enhancing patients' confidence and self-care abilities, and alleviating psychological stress.

8.2.4.4 Providing Comfortable Environment

Create a clean, quiet, and comfortable treatment environment for patients, minimizing the impact of the surroundings on mood and sleep quality. Encourage patients to engage in physical activities, such as *Tai Ji* or *Qi Gong*, which can effectively promote prognosis and recovery.

8.2.4.5 Exchanging Feelings and Experience

Medical staff should divert the patient's attention from the disease to other things and invite patients who have successfully recovered from visceral pain to share their experiences, enhancing the patient's self-care ability and rehabilitation confidence.

8.2.4.6 Elimination of Psychogenic Factors

Elimination of psychogenic factors involves adopting various means and methods to address pathogenic psychological factors based on individual patient characteristics. It can be further categorized into two types: expressing and solving the mental discomforts and persuasion. Expressing and solving the mental discomforts refer to using diverse approaches, including language, behavior, and medications, to help patients consciously or unconsciously escape from unhealthy situations and emotions. This method is particularly effective for individuals suffering from illnesses rooted in doubts, panic, anger, jealousy, and other adverse emotional activities. Just as mental disease requires psychological treatment, language serves as the antidote to doubt and the key to resolving confusion. In *Spiritual Pivot* of *Ling Shu*, it is introduced that "inform patients about what is harmful to their bodies and what is beneficial, guide patients to do appropriate things, cite the suffering of the sick to advise and admonish them. In this way, even those who are unreasonable will be more likely to take the advice."

8.2.4.7 Suggestion Therapy

Suggestion therapy, involving the use of language, behavior, and other subtle, indirect methods by clinicians to influence a patient's psychological state, enables patients to inadvertently accept hints and achieve a therapeutic effect. This includes both language-based indications and indications by objects or medications to address patients' psychological issues.

8.2.4.8 Overcoming One Emotion by Another Emotion

This method entails consciously inducing or arousing a new, temporary, and intense emotional reaction in patients to counteract or alleviate the original, persistent, and strong pathological emotional activity. Two specific approaches are "Yin and Yang Balance Therapy" and "Five Elements Counterbalance Therapy" rooted in the idea that sorrow overcomes anger, fear overcomes joy, and so on, which are described in *Canon of Internal Medicine*. Historical examples, such as Fan Jin's restoration to normalcy through intimidation in *The Scholars*, highlight the effectiveness of overcoming one emotion by another emotion.

8.2.4.9 Emotion Activation Method

This method involves consciously inducing a patient's passion and leveraging the strong behavioral response that accompanies passion to correct or improve the original pathological state, thereby achieving the treatment goal.

In conclusion, TCM is not merely a natural science; it encompasses cultural, philosophical, sociological, and humanistic dimensions. Physicians should avoid complex medical terminology and instead use plain language to elucidate the causes of diseases and actively address patients' psychological disturbance, to foster patients' collaboration with treatment and positive psychological expectations and enhance treatment outcomes. Establishing a strong doctor-patient relationship is crucial. This connection often allows physicians to uncover information about the disease that patients may not have disclosed before. Leveraging this information to assist patients in resolving their issues can lead to rapid improvements in their conditions.

8.3 TCM in Noncancer Visceral Pain

At present, the application of TCM in the clinical treatment of visceral pain is common, especially in the case of ineffective Western medicine treatment of pain, where TCM shows better results. Because of its diverse, flexible, and convenient application methods, safety, and reliability, it is often used as a complementary to Western medical treatment. In the previous section, the use of TCM in visceral cancer pain was listed and introduced in detail, including the existing methods of TCM treatment of visceral pain, which will not be repeated in this section. This section will enumerate the typical ways of treating noncancer visceral pain with TCM.

8.3.1 Functional Abdominal Pain Syndrome

Functional abdominal pain syndrome (FAPS) refers to persistent or recurrent abdominal pain that has a long course and is a class of functional diseases that have no or little relationship with the gastrointestinal tract. Clinical manifestations include recurrent abdominal distension, abdominal pain, nausea, constipation or diarrhea, etc. Patients often experience other generalized discomfort and may even suffer from psychological disorders such as depression and anxiety. At present, the etiology and pathogenesis of FAPS are not clear, and studies suggest that it is related to increased visceral sensitivity, brain–gut interaction, and psychosocial factors. Clinical treatment is mainly antispasmodic and analgesic, together with gastric dynamics, acid suppression, protection of gastric mucosa, and other symptomatic treatments, but the effect is not significant, and symptoms are prone to recur.

FAPS belongs to the category of abdominal pain in TCM. The ancient TCM doctors have their own theories on its etiology and pathogenesis, the earliest records of which were found in the *Ju Tong Monographs* of *Plain Questions*, which believed that the occurrence of abdominal pain is related to viscera organs such as stomach and intestines, and that the pathogenesis is related to changes of cold, heat, deficiency, and repletion. It is said that "cold resides as a guest in the large intestines, the small intestines, and the stomach, underneath the membrane, where the blood cannot be dispersed, and the small meridians, because of the rapidity of the circulation, provoke a feeling of pain. ...... Heat will be retained in the small intestines and feelings of pain, hot, damp, and dry are generated in the bowels, leading to hard, dry, and difficulty in stools, so the body feels painful and congested rather than circulates smoothly." Some TCM experts summarized the etiology of FAPS as weakness of the spleen and stomach, emotional upset, exogenous toxins, and dietary irregularities.

The main pathogenesis is the deficiency in visceral organs and repletion of *Qi* and blood. On the one hand, the deficiency in visceral organs is due to spleen and stomach weakness or the *Qi* deficiency of the spleen and stomach that leads to transportation and transformation disorder, abnormal ascending and descending of *Qi* in the spleen and stomach, or due to the lack of the spleen *Yang* that leads to cold and dampness stagnation and loss of warmth and nourishment. As a result, abdominal pain with the characteristic of lacking spirit occurred. The weakness of the spleen and stomach, therefore, is the pathological basis of the FAPS. On the other hand, the repletion of *Qi* and blood is often a result of a direct attack of the pathogenic cold that causes stagnation of *Qi* and blockage of meridians, or emotional upset, depression, or anger that harms the liver and leads to the liver and spleen disharmony, stagnation of *Qi*, and blood stasis. Or the repletion of *Qi* and blood is caused by dietary irregularities and eating too much spicy food, which stimulate the internal generation of dampness and heat, congestion of the stomach and intestines, and dysfunction of the stomach and spleen to carry and digest food, that is, "pain of congestion." Therefore, liver depression, pathogenic cold coagulation, and heat contribute to the disease. In other words, the etiology and pathogenesis of FAPS are complex as the cold and heat, the deficiency and repletion, can not only be transformed into each other, but also accompany each other. As a result, the disease lasts long and is difficult to treat. The clinical use of medication should be careful and based on the etiology and pathogenesis of the disease.

TCM treatment of FAPS emphasizes treatment based on syndrome differentiation in the prescription and use of medicines. Treatment based on syndrome differentiation is the basic principle of recognizing and treating diseases in TCM, which is also the essence of TCM. The syndromes of FAPS can be divided into four major types: spleen and stomach weakness, liver depression and *Qi* stagnation, cold accumulation and *Qi* stagnation, and indigestion and heat accumulation. The clinical treatment of the disease is mostly aimed at "circulating smoothly," but "circulating smoothly" is not just about purgation. The clinical diagnosis should differentiate deficiency and repletion, cold and heat, in light of which arranging the appropriate treatment for both causes and symptoms. As indicated in the *Yixue Zhenzhuan* (*True Biography of Medicine*), "It is reasonable to say that when all the systems of the body circulate smoothly, one will not feel pain, but methods for achieving smooth circulation can be various. Regulating *Qi*-flowing for harmonizing blood or vice versa is a kind of smooth circulation. Nourishing deficient patients, warming cold patients, all of which are methods for circulating smoothly." The prescription and medication need to be decided after reasonable differentiation, depending on the main symptoms to add or reduce herbs, in order to complement each other [21].

8.3.1.1 Spleen and Stomach Weakness Type

For FAPS patients who belong to the spleen and stomach weakness type, the priority is to strengthen the spleen. The *Zhongman Fuzhang* (abdominal distension) of *Lanshi Micang* (*Secret Book of Orchid Chamber*) says that "people who have eaten too much cold food, or those whose spleen and stomach are in deficiency for a long time, have a stomach invaded by pathogenic cold, which leads to a feeling of fullness in the stomach, or their internal organs are of cold characteristic, resulting in abdominal distension." Weakness of the spleen and stomach is often associated with uncontrolled diet, overexertion, and depletion of *Qi* due to prolonged illness. Transportation and transformation failure due to spleen deficiency, and unsmooth *Qi*, or the lack of *Yang* in the spleen and cold and deficiency in the spleen lead to abdominal pain. Symptoms of abdominal pain include the extended course, predilection for warmth and being pressed, pain of varying intensity, abdominal distension after eating food, loose stools and diarrhea, tired and taciturn, pale red tongue with thin white coating or teeth marks, and light and weak pulse. To strengthen the spleen and replenish the *Qi* and stomach, Powder of Dang Shen, Fu Ling, and Bai Zhu should be used with the addition or reduction of herbs. The formula of the powder consists of Dang Shen, Fu Ling, and Bai Zhu 15 g each; Baibiandou (Semen Lablab Album), Yiyiren (Semen Coicis), and Shan Yao 12 g each; 9 g Chen Pi; Sha Ren (adding later), Ju Geng (Radix Platycodonis) 6 g each. This formula is derived from the *Taiping Huimin Heji Jufang* (*Prescription of Peaceful Benevolent Dispensary*) and is modified from the classic formula Decoction of Four Noble Drugs for promoting *Qi* and strengthening the spleen. Modern pharmacological studies have found that this formula can regulate gastrointestinal motility, improve metabolism, and enhance immunity. The main herbs for invigorating and strengthening the spleen and stomach are Dang Shen, Fu Ling, and Bai Zhu; Baibiandou, Yiyiren, and Shan Yao taste sweet, and Lian Zi tastes bitter, serving as assistant drugs for diffusing dampness. Chen Pi can regulate *Qi* while strengthening the spleen. Sha Ren can invigorate the spleen to stop diarrhea. Ju Geng is a channel guiding herb, and when it is used in the formula, other drugs will be carried upward toward Shang Jiao to benefit the *Qi* activity in the lungs. Prepared Gan Cao strengthens the spleen and harmonize Zhong Jiao and reconciles other herbs, serving as the envoy drug.

The *Piwei Lun* (*Treatise on the Spleen and Stomach*) records that "all diseases derive from the spleen and stomach." The spleen is in charge of transportation and transformation, while the stomach is in charge of accommodation and digestion. The water and grain essence the human body needs are accommodated and digested through the stomach and then transformed and transported by the spleen to all parts of the body. If the spleen and stomach are weak, it will lead to the abnormal ascending of lucid *Yang* and abnormal descending of turbid *Yin*. Consequently, the water and grain essence is distributed disorderly, which is prone to cause dampness and phlegm, and the entire internal organs' functions will inevitably be affected, giving rise to exogenous pathogenic factor invasion and diseases.

In sum, strengthening the spleen and replenishing the Zhong Jiao is the fundamental treatment method of FAPS. The abovementioned formula not only strengthens the spleen and replenishes the Zhong Jiao, but also diffuses dampness and removes turbidity. When the dampness is diffused, the spleen *Qi* is invigorated and harmonized, which in turn enables the stomach *Qi* to digest. When the spleen and stomach are strengthened, the symptoms will be eliminated.

8.3.1.2 Liver Depression and *Qi* Stagnation Type

Liver depression and *Qi* stagnation is the most common clinical syndrome of FAPS, and it is more prevalent in middle-aged women. FAPS is mostly due to emotional stimulation, which leads to liver *Qi* stagnation and disorder of *Qi* in the internal organs and affects the spleen and stomach. The spleen and stomach are the foundation of the human body, and the spleen and stomach *Qi* are the hub of all *Qi*. When *Qi* is not smooth and dispersed, the spleen and stomach *Qi*'s ascending and descending will be disturbed, and thus, a series of symptoms occur such as liver and stomach disharmony. *Danxi Xinfa* said that "when the *Qi* and blood are in harmony, no disease exists; yet once depression arises, all diseases might show up." Abdominal pain of this type is clinically characterized by pain in variable locations, sometimes concentrated, sometimes scattered, relieved by belching, accompanied by a feeling of fullness and stuffiness between the chest and under the ribs, dry and bitter in the mouth, lack of sleep or dreaminess, with indigestion and loose stools, red tongue with thin coating, and taut pulse. Female patients may also experience premenstrual breast swelling and irregular menstruation.

Liver depression and *Qi* stagnation should be treated by regulating and dispersing stagnated liver *Qi*. Bupleurum Powder for Relieving Liver-*Qi* is a classic formula to disperse the liver and regulate *Qi*. Recent studies showed that the powder is effective in treating abdominal pain of liver depression and *Qi* stagnation type, which helps improve the quality of life of patients. The formula is composed of 12 g Chai Hu, 12 g Chen Pi, 10 g Chuan Xiong, 10 g Shao Yao, 10 g Xiang Fu, 10 g Zhi Ke, 10 g Bai Shu, 10 g Shan Yao 10 g Yu Jin (Radix Curcumae), and 6 g prepared Gan Cao. Emotional upset will negatively affect the liver's ability to regulate the flow of *Qi*, resulting in the imbalance of *Yin* and *Yang*, *Qi* and blood, and pain. In this formula, Chai Hu is good at regulating liver *Qi* and relieving depression, so it is used as the main ingredient; Xiang Fu regulates *Qi* and relieves liver pain, and Chuan Xiong invigorates blood and promotes *Qi* to relieve pain, so they are the secondary ingredients of the formula; Chen Pi regulates *Qi*, removes stagnation, and reconciles the stomach; Bai Shu and Shan Yao strengthen the spleen and stomach; Zhi Ke and Yu Jin promote *Qi* and relieve depression and pain in order to disperse the liver; Shao Yao nourishes blood and softens the liver to alleviate the acute pain, which is the adjuvant of the formula; and Gan Cao regulates and unites all the medicines to regulate the liver, relieve depression, and promote the movement of *Qi* to achieve the goal of mitigating pain. Moreover, modern pharmacology found that the saponin and volatile oil in Chai Hu has sedative, analgesic, and choleretic effects; the volatile oil contained in Chen Pi can relax the smooth muscle; Shao Yao has an inhibitory effect on the central nervous system and can relax the smooth muscle; Xiang Fu contains volatile oil and sugar, which have the effect of stomachic and elimination of pneumoperitoneum; and Gan Cao can relieve gastric and intestinal spasm, etc. Above all, the treatment of liver depression and *Qi* stagnation-type abdominal pain with Bupleurum Powder for Relieving Liver-*Qi* is clinically effective, economical, and safe, and helps improve the quality of life of patients.

The abovementioned formula can be modified to tackle specific symptoms. If a long-term liver stagnation is transformed into heat, Dan Pi and Shanzhizi can be added to clear the liver and heat. If *Qi* stagnation and distention pain are severe, Yanhuisuo can be added to regulate *Qi* and relieve pain. If there is liver and stomach stagnation and heat, Huang Lian and Wuzhuyu can be added to disperse stagnated liver *Qi* for regulating the stomach. If there is stagnation of *Qi* and blood stasis, Pu Huang and Wulingzhi can be added to promote blood circulation for removing blood stasis. If there exists abdominal pain and borborygmi, *Qi* stagnation and diarrhea, Fang Feng and Chen Pi can be used to harmonize the liver and spleen, invigorate the spleen, and soften the liver. More importantly, offering patients psychological counseling is indispensable. Communication with patients, providing spiritual encouragement, and making them pay attention to emotional self-management may help achieve the purpose of both physical and mental treatments.

8.3.1.3 Cold Accumulation and *Qi* Stagnation Type

For this type, it is important to activate *Qi* for warming the spleen and stomach.

According to the *General Treatise on the Causes and Symptoms of Diseases*: "Due to the weakness of the internal organs, the cold *Qi* gathers between the intestinal and gastric membranes, the healthy *Qi* and the unhealthy *Qi* combat with each other, triggering the pain." This type of pain occurs when pathogenic cold invades the meridians, leading to cold and *Qi* condensation, obstruction of meridians, and stomach *Qi* distention and fullness, thereby producing pain of congestion. Common symptoms are abdominal pain that stretches for a long time, severe diarrhea, vomiting of water, tastelessness, abdominal distension, clear white urine, pale red tongue with white coating, and dull and slow pulse. It should be treated with Liang Fu Wan (*Alpinia-cyperus* Pill) in combination with Zhengqi Tianxiang Powder to activate *Qi* for warming the spleen and stomach, and dispel cold for relieving pain. The formula contains 15 g Gaoliangjiang (Rhizoma *Alpiniae officinarum*) and Xiang Fu each, and 10 g dry Jiang (ginger), Zi Su (*Perilla*), Wu Yao, and Chen Pi each. In the formula, Gaoliangjiang warms the Zhong Jiao and disperses cold, and Xiang Fu regulates *Qi* and relieves pain, so they are the main ingredients; dry Jiang warms the Zhong Jiao and restores *Yang*, Zi Su promotes *Qi* and harmonizes the stomach, Wu yao disperses cold, and Chen Pi regulates *Qi* and strengthens the spleen, serving as the secondary ingredients. Herbs for activating *Qi* and warming the visceral organs are paired with each other to play the role of dispersing cold and relieving pain together. Additionally, modern pharmacological research showed that the main component of herbs for warming visceral organs such as Gaoliangjiang, Fu Zi, and dry Jiang is volatile oil, which has anti-inflammatory and analgesic effects and can regulate gastrointestinal motility and control diarrhea. Paired with Chen Pi and other herbs activating *Qi*, which are resuscitation-inducing aromatic herbs, the effect of the main ingredients will be enhanced to dispel cold and activate *Qi*, so that the *Qi* of visceral organs will be smooth and abdominal pain will be mitigated. In addition, clinically, in cases of thundering and cutting pain in the abdomen, fullness in the chest and under the ribs, and vomiting, herbs such as Gan Cao, Ban Xia, and Zao (jujube) can be added to warm the Zhong Jiao and lower adverse *Qi*; in cases of cold pain in the abdomen and pain in the whole body, add Wu Tou and Gui Zhi to warm the visceral organs and dispel cold; in cases of constriction and cold pain in the abdomen and cold stagnation in the liver veins, add Dang Gui, Gou *Qi*, and Hui Xiang (Fennel Fruit) to warm up the liver and disperse cold; and in cases of constriction abdominal pain, constipation, and cold accumulation, add Da Huang to enable purgation.

8.3.1.4 Indigestion and Heat Accumulation Type

Indigestion and heat accumulation should be treated by clearing heat for resolving food stagnation.

Consuming too much spicy and heavy taste food causes dampness and heat in the body, which gathers in the stomach and intestines, or overeating results in too much food accumulating in the stomach. All these lead to insufficient digestive capacity of the spleen, and the accumulation of food turns into heat and causes pathogenic factors to invade the Zhong Jiao, triggering abdominal pain. Common symptoms are abdominal distension and pain, which can be exacerbated by pressing, anorexia, halitosis, hiccups, acid reflux, foul-smelling stools or painful diarrhea, and a red tongue with a thick coating. As stated in the *Yixue Zhenzhuan*, "Most of diseases are caused by dietary indulgence, preference for spicy and sour foods, and wanton drinking … The toxins accumulate day by day and ultimately penetrate deeper into the body … and hence the stomach is painful and uncomfortable …." The main treatment for this type of pain is to clear away heat and stagnation, and harmonize the stomach to relieve pain. The Powder of Agastachis for Restoring Health is often used. The formula contains 15 g Huo Xiang (*Agastache rugosus*); 12 g Hou Pu (Cortex *Magnoliae officinalis*), Yu Jin, Bai Shu, and Fu Ling each; 10 g Chai Hu, Ke Zhi, Jiang Ban Xia, and Chen Pi each; and 6 g prepared Gan Cao. Experiments showed that the volatile oil of Huo Xiang and Chen Pi in the formula can stimulate the gastrointestinal mucosa, promote the secretion of digestive juices, expel stagnant *Qi* in the intestinal tract, and help digestion; Zi Su and Fu Ling can promote the motility of small intestines; Ban Xia can inhibit vomiting; Bai Shu has a bidirectional regulating effect on the intestinal tract; and prepared Gan Cao can promote the proliferation of digestive epithelial cells and protect the gastric mucosa. Therefore, this formula can relieve abdominal pain caused by smooth muscle spasms and is often used in the treatment of digestive diseases. When using this formula, Huo Xiang is the main herb, using its aroma to remove dampness and turbidity and its effect to harmonize the stomach and spleen; supplementary ingredients are Hou Pu, which can promote the ascending of clear *Qi* and descending of turbidity *Qi*, and resolve fullness, Yu Jin, which can resolve the depression and clear the heart heat, and Bai Shu, which can strengthen the spleen to help transportation and control diarrhea, all of them serving as the secondary ingredients. Moreover, Chai Hu can clear away the heat and promote the ascending of clear *Qi*; Zhi Ke can resolve food stagnation; Chen Pi and Jiang Bian Xia can activate *Qi* to remove dampness, and harmonize the Zhong Jiao to resolve food stagnation; and Fu Ling has the effect of strengthening the spleen and eliminating dampness. Importantly, prepared Gan Cao can harmonize the medicinal properties of all herbs in the formula. All medicines are used together to strengthen the spleen and eliminate dampness, regulate *Qi* and stomach, so that *Qi* can be cleared, the spleen and stomach can be harmonized, clear *Qi* can be raised, and turbid *Qi* can be lowered. In the end, abdominal pain and other symptoms can be eliminated.

The pathogenesis of FAPS is complex as most of the symptoms are mixed, so in diagnosis and treatment, it is necessary to distinguish the pathogenesis of the disease, grasp the main symptoms, and at the same time take into account the secondary symptoms. Based on this, doctors should insist on the combination of diagnosis and treatment, adjustment, and care in order to improve the overall efficacy of the clinical treatment of FAPS.

8.3.1.5 Summary

"As the disease varies, so does the treating formulas." When treating FAPS, doctors should delve into the pathogenesis and assess changes accordingly. The flavor and dosage of medicines should not be confined to the formula. Meanwhile, the dosage of medicines should not be carefully determined as an overdose would harm the gastrointestinal functions. Furthermore, FAPS is closely associated with diet and emotion, indicating that while considering the medical treatment, patients' mental health and diet should also be regulated.

8.3.2 Biliary Colic

Biliary colic is often caused by the stimulation of choledochus by gallstones, infections, roundworms, etc., which induces the strong spasm of the Oddi's sphincter, increases the pressure of the bile duct, and finally results in paroxysmal severe abdominal pain. Although surgical treatment is the first choice, for patients with clear clinical symptoms who do not have the indication of surgery, or surgery is a contraindication, TCM treatment may be a more appropriate choice. In TCM, biliary colic caused by acute cholecystitis is categorized as "rib pain," while biliary colic caused by chronic cholecystitis is categorized as "distended gallbladder." The earliest record of biliary colic was in the *Miu Ci Monograph* of *Plain Questions*, "Unhealthy *Qi* invades the foot Shao *Yang* meridian, causing rib pain and dyspnea." The causes of biliary colic are emotional upset, dietary irregularities, invasion of exogenous pathogenic factors, obstruction of gallstone, and excessive labor.

Dampness and heat in the liver and gallbladder, and blockage of *Qi* are the main causes. Clearing the liver and gallbladder and regulating

Qi are the key treatment methods. Accordingly, the treatment should be clearing the liver and gallbladder for easing the pain, dispersing stagnated liver *Qi* for relieving *Qi* stagnation, and resolving food stagnation. The liver is one of the five internal organs with the characteristics and functions of ascending and dispersing, regulating and invigorating, while gallbladder belongs to the six hollow organs with the characteristics and functions of smooth circulation and descending. Therefore, the prescription should follow the physiological characteristics of the liver and gallbladder, with clearing heat and dampness as the main target. The formula selected is Si Jin Decoction consisting of Jinqiancao (Herba Lysimachiae), Haijinsha (Spora Lygodii), and Yu Jin and Jineijin (the membrane of a chicken's gizzard). In the formula, Jinqiancao is sweet, salty, and cold, penetrating to the liver, gallbladder, kidney, and bladder meridians; Haijinsha is sweet, salty, and cold, penetrating to the bladder and small intestine meridians. They are the main ingredients. The sweet flavor eases the urgency, the salty flavor softens the hard, and the cold clears the heat, so when they are combined, they have the effect of clearing the heat and dampness and relieving the pain. Yu Jin is pungent, bitter, and cold, penetrating to the liver, heart, and lung meridians. The pungency is used to disperse dampness, the bitterness and cold can remove dampness and heat. When they are combined, they can disperse stagnated liver *Qi* for removing the depression and promoting bile flow. Yu Jin, thus, serves as the secondary ingredients. Jineijin is sweet and balanced, penetrating to the spleen, stomach, small intestine, and bladder meridians. The *Records of Traditional Chinese and Western Medicine in Combination* says that Jineijin is "the chicken's spleen and stomach, which originally contains dilute hydrochloric acid, so its taste is acid and its nature is slightly warm. It can digest ceramics, stone, copper and iron, showing that it is good at resolving food stagnation." Therefore, it is used for its digestive functions and the ability to strengthen the stomach as the adjuvant ingredient. Modern pharmacological research suggests that Jinqiancao has the pharmacological effect of promoting gallbladder contraction and regulating bile salt metabolism, which enables the discharge of stones and helps prevent the formation of stones; Haijinsha, Yu Jin, and Jineijin can inhibit the activation of the inflammatory pathway and the production of pro-inflammatory transmitters and have anti-inflammatory function. At the same time, Yu Jin has an analgesic effect, and Jineijin has the effect of regulating lipid metabolism and can alleviate inflammatory reaction and pain brought by stones and prevent stone formation. If the pain is severe, Shao Yao and Gan Cao can be used to relieve acute pain, Yanhusuo can activate *Qi* for eliminating pain, and Baiqucai (Celandine) in combination with Yuzhengu (auricular bones in fish head) can help remove the stone and relieve pain. Noticeably, although Baiqucai has good anti-inflammatory and peripheral analgesic effects, it has a certain degree of toxicity. Therefore, when it is applied, the dosage and dose time should be carefully measured and liver and kidney function should be monitored.

In addition, the combined use of external therapies such as acupuncture and auricular point pressing therapy should be advocated, which achieve good efficacy of relieving pain. Wai Qiu is a *Xi* point of the foot Shao Yang bile meridian, which has a very good effect of controlling acute and painful conditions. Besides, Yanglingquan and gallbladder point are also commonly used pain relief points. Many clinical trials have shown that acupuncture treatment of biliary colic can relieve pain effectively and cause few side effects. Yanglingquan, gallbladder point, and gallbladder Shu are mostly selected points in modern clinical treatment of biliary colic. The gallbladder meridian of foot Shao Yang, bladder meridian of foot Tai Yang, and liver meridian of foot Jue Yin are selected. Specific acupoints selected are Wu Shu point, Xia He point, and Ba Hui point. Contemporary TCM doctors prefer selecting meridian acupoints together with specific acupoints, especially the stomach channel of foot Yang Ming, as the disease is always accompanied by nausea and vomiting, abdominal distension, etc. Modern research has found that needling Yanglingquan and gallbladder point can stimulate the release of analgesic substances, such as the expression of endorphins and the brain–gut peptides, both belonging to the neuropeptide active substances, which play an important role in the analgesic process. Also, it was found that acupuncture can achieve spasmolytic effects by promoting tensional vasomotor activity and promoting gallbladder expansion, which is conducive to the discharge of biliary inflammatory secretions and stones, thus relieving pain. External therapies can realize the clinical compound effects of pain relief, stone dissolution, and stone discharge.

In conclusion, due to the various symptoms and complications of gallbladder stones, dietary adjustments, drugs, endoscopy, surgery, and other treatment methods may all be effective in different stages of the development of this disease. The timing of applying different therapeutic modalities should be carefully measured. When choosing conservative treatments, the progress of the disease should be monitored. TCM internal and external combination treatments have the characteristics of multitargets and multipathways and will play a comprehensive role in alleviating the pain, dissolving the stone, and accelerating the stone discharge, which is beneficial to the clinical diagnosis and treatment of the disease, and worthwhile to be explored further.

8.3.3 Chronic Pancreatitis Pain

Chronic pancreatitis refers to repeated episodes of pancreatic or persistent inflammatory lesions of the pancreatic acinar cells gradually replaced by fibrous tissues, resulting in serious damage to the pancreatic function, so that the digestion of food becomes difficult. Patients with acute pancreatitis recurrent or persistent episodes of chronic pancreatic duct obstruction caused by chronic alcoholism are often accompanied by epigastric pain, nausea, and vomiting, and upper abdominal distension and diarrhea after eating greasy food. Due to a reduced diet, they lose weight gradually. Chronic pancreatitis pain belongs to the category of gastric and epigastric pain, and abdominal and rib pain in TCM.

8.3.3.1 Treatment Based on Syndrome Differentiation

1. Syndrome of heat in intestines and stomach

   Etiology and pathogenesis: external pathogenic factors transforming into the heat; overeating spicy and heavy taste food leading to dampness, heat, food stagnation in the interior; *Qi* inharmonious, and *Qi* deficiency in internal organs.

   Clinical symptoms: abdominal distension and pain, resistance to pressure, nausea and vomiting, dry mouth, constipation, red tongue with yellow and dry coating, and slippery pulse.

   Treatment: clearing away dampness and heat, and activating the stomach by purgation.

   Formula: Qing Yi Decoction combined with Potent Purgative Decoction.
2. Syndrome of dampness and heat in the liver and gallbladder

   Etiology and pathogenesis: external pathogenic factors invading the liver and gallbladder or the accumulation of dampness and heat in the liver and gallbladder due to dietary irregularities, being unable to detoxify.

   Clinical symptoms: pain in the stomach and ribs, anorexia of greasy food, fever, nausea, fatigue, jaundice, yellow and oily tongue coating, and slippery pulse.

   Treatment: purging liver and gallbladder, and clearing heat dampness.

   Formula: Qing Yi Decoction combined with Decoction of Gentiana for Purging Liver-fire.
3. Syndrome of food retention due to spleen deficiency

   Etiology and pathogenesis: weakness of the spleen and stomach, coupled with overeating, the spleen being unable to transport, the intestines and stomach getting injured, resulting in food and *Qi* stagnation.

   Clinical symptoms: fullness and discomfort in the epigastric region after eating, diarrhea, sour stool with undigested food, yellow face, thinness, lassitude, pale and puffy tongue with white coating, and weak pulse.

   Treatment: strengthening spleen for resolving food stagnation and regulating *Qi*.

   Formula: Qing Yi Decoction combined with Pill of Immature Bitter Orange for Removing Stagnancy.
4. Syndrome of blood stasis

Etiology and pathogenesis: prolonged illness invading the meridians, resulting in blood stasis and internal stagnation, and *Qi* stagnation.

Clinical symptoms: intensified pain in the epigastric region with a fixed location, and a lump formed in the abdomen or under the left rib.

Treatment: promoting blood circulation for removing blood stasis and regulating *Qi*-flowing for relieving pain.

Formula: Shaofu Zhuyu Decoction.

8.3.3.2 Precautions

If the following conditions are encountered, patients should be hospitalized in time for surgery: (1) acute attack with severe intractable pain; and (2) ineffective treatment by internal medicine (combined with large bile duct stones, biliary tract stenosis, and pancreatic pseudocysts; when the patient loses weight in a short period of time, and pancreatic cancer is suspected).

8.3.4 Stomach Pain

Stomach pain, also known as epigastralgia, is a condition in which pain appears in the stomach and epigastric region below the heart and above the umbilicus as the main symptom, accompanied by symptoms such as epigastric distension, nausea, acidity, noise, and vomiting. Acute and chronic gastritis, peptic ulcer, functional dyspepsia, gastric ptosis, gastric cancer, chronic pancreatitis, and cholecystitis in Western medicine can be treated with reference to this section when stomach pain is the main symptom. The main pathogenesis of stomach pain is "pain of congestion." However, it has a close relationship with the liver and spleen, as recorded in *Jingmai Bielun* of *Plain Questions*: "After the water flows into the stomach, the overflow spreads its essence upward to the spleen by which the essence is transferred up to the lungs which is in charge of the clearing and regulating *Qi* and waterway, down to the bladder. In this way, the water essence is spread in all directions, externally to the skin and hair, and internally in the meridians of the five organs." The movement of the spleen *Qi* is predominantly ascending, while the flow of stomach *Qi* is predominantly descending. These two organs are the pivots of *Qi*'s ascending and descending in the body. As Ye Tianshi said, if the ascending spleen *Qi* is smooth, then the spleen is strong; if the descending stomach *Qi* is smooth, then the stomach is harmonious. As for the methods of flowing and descending, they are different, as stated in the *Yixue Zhenzhuan* (*True Biography of Medicine*), "Regulating *Qi*-flowing for harmonizing blood or vice versa is a kind of smooth circulation. Nourishing patients with deficiency, warming patients with cold, all of which are methods for circulating smoothly." Clinical symptoms can be treated with 10 methods of treating stomach pain, which are warming, clearing, nourishing, eliminating, removing, purging, astringing, lowering, harmonizing, and producing.

Firstly, for pain that is of cold nature, patients should be warmed. Medicines or formulas commonly used to eliminate dampness are of pungent and warm nature, such as Liang Fu Wan, Jiang Fu Decoction, and Li Zhong Decoction. Besides, Bi Ba (Fructus Piperis Longi), Wuzhuyu (Fructus Evodiae), Fu Zi, Rou Gui, Shu Jiao (*Piperitum*), and Caodoukou (Semen Alpiniae Katsumadai) are often prescribed as well.

Secondly, for pain that is of deficient nature, patients should be nourished. The commonly used formulas or medicines to strengthen the spleen and replenish the kidney are Decoction of Four Noble Drugs, Dang Shen, Huang Qi, Lian Rou (edible lotus seed), Qian Shi, Yiyiren, and Bian Dou.

Thirdly, for pain that is of repletion nature, patients should be helped to promote digestion. If food accumulation is beyond the capacity of digestion, then formulas or medicines must be prescribed to help digestion, such as Lenitive Pill, Zhi Shi (Fructus Aurantii Immaturus), Zhi Ke, Bin Lang (Semen Arecae), Shen Qu (Medicated Leaven), Chenxiangqu (Aquilaria Leaven), Jineijin, Hou Pu, Chen Pi, Shan Zha, fried Gu Ya, and fried Mai Ya.

Fourthly, for pain that is due to the unobstructed flow of *Qi* and blood, the obstruction should be removed. The obstructed *Qi* should be regulated with Mu Xiang (Radix Aucklandiae), Tan Xiang (Lignum Santali Albi), Huo Xiang,

Chen Xiang, Wu Yao, Qing Pi (Pericarpium Citri Reticulatae Viride), Chen Pi, Hou Pu, Sha Ren, Dou Kou (Fructus Amomi Rotundus), etc., and Xiaodao Kuanzhong Decoction, Chenxiang Shengjiang Powder, etc. The obstructed blood should be regulated with Yuan Hu, Dan Shen, Wulingzhi, Jiangzhenxiang (*Acronychia pedunculata*), Ru Xiang, Mo Yao, Xue Xie, Tao Ren, Hong Hua, San Qi (*Pseudo-ginseng*), Pu Huang (Pollen Typhae), Yu Jin, San Leng (Rhizoma Sparganii), E Shu, Xiang Fu, etc., and Shou Nian Powder and Jiuqi Niantong Powder.

Fifthly, if the internal organs are solid, diarrhea is helpful. All kinds of Potent Purgative Decoction or Fanxieye (Folium Sennae) can be used. But for patients whose bodies are weak and stools are dry as a result of constipation, medicines with the effect of moistening dryness should be used, such as Yuliren (Semen Pruni), Huomaren (Fructus Cannabis), Gua Wei (Fructus Trichosanthis), Xing Ren, Roucongrong (Herba Cistanches), Xie Bai (Bulbus Allii Macrostemonis), and Zaojiazi (seed of Chinese Honeylocust).

Sixthly, if the gut is weak and slippery, it should be astringed. Commonly used medicines are Chishizhi (Halloysitum Rubrum), Lian Rou, He Zi (Fructus Chebulae), Cang Shu (Rhizoma Atractylodis), Yingsuke (Pericarpium Papaveris), Wubeizi (Galla Chinensis), Jinyingzi (Fructus Rosae Laevigatae), Baitouweng (Radix Pulsatillae), Qin Pi (Cortex Fraxini), etc.

Seventhly, if there is retching and vomiting, converse *Qi* should be lowered. The stomach *Qi* should go descending, and when it is ascending, it will induce hiccupping and vomiting. Cloves and Kaki Calyx Decoction, Tangerine Peel and Bamboo Shavings Decoction, and Decoction of Inula and Hematitum could be used. Also, aromatic medicines eliminating turbid pathogen can stop hiccupping and vomiting, such as Zi Su, Foshouhua (Flower of Fleshfingered Citron), Huo Xiang, Biandouhua (Flower of Hyacinth Dolichos), and Peilanye (Herba Eupatorii leaves).

Eighthly, if there is gastric and stomach discomfort, the stomach should be regulated. Wu Yu and Huang Lian, Gan Jiang and Huang Lian, Huang Qin (Radix Scutellariae) and Ban Xia have the characteristics of both cold and warm and could be used to regulate the stomach. When the stomach is harmonized, the discomfort could be eliminated.

Ninthly, if there is a lack of body fluid, fluid production should be promoted. When the spleen and stomach are weak, the fluids are withered, and the appetite is poor, it is advisable to nourish the spleen and stomach *Yin* to produce fluids. Medicines used are Xiyangshen (Radix Panacis Quinquefolii), Shi Hu (Herba Dendrobii), raw Gu Ya, raw Jineijin, He Ye (Folium Nelumbinis), Sha Shen (Adenophora Tetraphylla), Mai Dong (Radix Ophiopogonis), Yuan Shen, etc.

Finally, the emetic method is rarely used now. As a supplement, dampness and heat should be removed by using medicines such as Fu Ling, Yiyiren, Huo Xiang, and Pei Lan; hyperchlorhydria should be treated with Wanglengzi (Concha Arcae), Haipiaoshao (Endoconcha Sepiae), Mu Li (Concha Ostreae), and Hongdoukou; recurrent dysentery should be treated with Baitouweng, Ku Shen; for promoting *Yang* and strengthening stomach, Chai Hu and Sheng Ma should be used [22].

Whenever there is pain in the stomach and epigastric region, the above 10 methods can be applied, but accurate differentiation must be made. Only when the diagnosis is accurate can the treatment be appropriate. When recognizing the symptoms, doctors should pay attention to both the main symptoms and the concurrent symptoms; when discussing the treatment, doctors should apply the common methods as well as their variations. Only by applying them flexibly can better therapeutic effects be achieved.

8.3.5 Irritable Bowel Syndrome

Irritable bowel syndrome (IBS) is a functional intestinal disorder characterized by abdominal pain or discomfort, accompanied by changes in bowel habits. The etiology and pathogenesis of IBS have not been fully elucidated. Clinically, IBS can be divided into diarrhea, constipation, mixed and indeterminate types, of which diarrhea is the main clinical type. Gastrointestinal symptoms are the main clinical manifestations of IBS patients, and patients have many clinical symptoms that cannot be eliminated in a timely manner, which will have a serious impact on their quality of life. Therefore, it is necessary to notice the diarrhea-type IBS to understand the changes in the gastrointestinal symptoms and adopt active and effective treatments to promote the prognosis of the disease. For the treatment of this disease, Western medicine prefers to use antispasmodic drugs, osmotic laxatives, pro-secretory agents, but the overall effect is not ideal, and the symptoms are easy to recur. With the increasing research interest in the treatment of IBS-C by TCM, the TCM external treatment method has received higher attention in the clinical practice because of its convenient operation, acceptable to patients, safety, and efficacy.

8.3.5.1 External Treatment Methods in TCM Ancient Classics

According to the clinical symptoms of IBS-C, TCM categorized it as "constipation" and "abdominal pain." The *Zhenjiu Jiayi Jing* (*A-B Classic of Acupuncture and Moxibustion*) says: "For difficulty in bowel movement and distension, Cheng Shan point is the dominant acupoint." The *Zhenjiu Dacheng* (*Compendium of Acupuncture and Moxibustion*) says: "Bladder Shu is the main acupoint for treating abdominal fullness and difficult defecation." The *Qianjin Fang* (*Thousand Pieces of Precious Formulae*) says: "Shi Guan is the main acupoint for treating constipation, cold coagulation and heart fullness." Statistical analysis of the literature reveals that acupuncture is the most commonly used treatment method for this disease, and the meridian points are mostly taken from the bladder meridian (commonly used points are the Large Intestine Shu, Cheng Shan, Bladder Shu, and Zhong Liao), the kidney meridian (commonly used points are Zhao Hai, Tai Xi, Da Zhong, and Yong Quan), and the Three Jiao meridians (commonly used points are Zhi Gou), while acupoints are often taken from Ren Mai point (commonly used points are Shen Que., Zhong Wan, and Qi Hai) and points of the spleen, stomach, and liver meridians (commonly used points are Tai Bai, Sanyinjiao, Shang Qiu; Tsusanli, Nei Ting, Feng Long; Zhang Men, Tai Chong, Da Dun). Branch points are mostly taken from the foot Yin point, abdominal points, lower back points, and leg Yang points. The *Shi Yi De Xiao Fang* (*Effective Formulae Handed Down for Generations*), *Shou Shi Bao Yuan, and Zazheng Fang Shu* (*Book of Miscellaneous Syndrome Formulae*) suggest using application on the navel to treat constipation and abdominal pain through the infiltration of medication into the abdomen. The *Sha Jing He Bi* (*Skin Scraping*) suggests that if the disease is related to blood problems, then it can be treated with skin scraping therapy. *Shou Shi Bao Yuan* proposes suction method to regulate meridians for facilitating defecation. The *Ji Sheng Ba Cui* put forward acupuncture assisted by rubbing the stomach meridian to treat constipation.

8.3.5.2 Clinical External Treatment Methods of TCM

1. Acupuncture therapy

   Studies have shown that acupuncture can promote gastrointestinal peristalsis and significantly improve the symptoms of abdominal pain, abdominal distension, and constipation. Zhang Aijun et al. treated IBS-C with shallow needling of liver meridian, stomach meridian, and spleen meridian, together with the quivering method, which was based on the principle of treating by regulating the liver and the *Qi* for relieving pain, and the clinical effect was remarkable [23]. He Lei and others directly needled the Tian Shu, the Large Intestine Shu, Tsusanli, Shangjuxu, Gong Sun, and Nei Guan points, with normal reinforcement and normal reduction maneuver, to smooth intestinal and bowel *Qi*, and the symptoms were significantly improved. Han Feng practiced the acupuncture method of "soothing the liver, strengthening the spleen and regulating the spirit," which was superior in treating abdominal pain, distention, and constipation and improving neurological symptoms. Wang Jin also used a similar acupuncture method to improve the symptoms of constipation and depression. Moreover, the plasma 5-HT level was reduced, the sensitivity of the internal organs was decreased, while the gastrointestinal dynamics and secretion of body fluids were reinforced. Wang Cailing needled Tian Shu (bilateral), Nei Guan and Wai Guan (bilateral), Tsusanli (bilateral), Tai Chong (bilateral), Shangjuxu (bilateral), Yinlingquan (bilateral), Sanyinjiao (bilateral), and Yin Tang and Bai Hui points with normal reinforcement and normal reduction maneuver, which significantly improved the clinical symptoms and reduced the scores of visual analog scale (VAS) for pain. Zhu Li [16] adopted acupuncture treatment, taking Tian Shu (bilateral), Tsusanli (bilateral), Shangjuxu (bilateral), Tai Chong (bilateral), Sanyinjiao (bilateral), Shen Que. and Bai hui points to reduce plasma 5-HT level, neuropeptide Y (NPY), and Calcitonin gene-related peptide (CGRP), and the total score of the IBS Quality of Life Scale (IBS-QOL) in the follow-up after 2 months was higher than that of the control group, which indicated that the long-term efficacy of acupuncture was better than the control group.

2. Moxibustion therapy

   Moxibustion has the function of warming the vital *Qi*, dispersing cold and dampness, and activating blood circulation, so it can treat diseases caused by deficiency, cold, and stagnation. Shu Xiang Moxibustion, Lei Huo Moxibustion, Herbs-partitioned Moxibustion, and Zheng Qi Moxibustion are commonly used moxibustion therapies. Luo Sha et al. selected IBS-C patients with liver depression and *Qi* stagnation type and applied Shu Xiang Moxibustion (Chai Hu, Zhi Ke, Qing Pi, Huomaren, Gu Ya, Shao Yao, and Laifuzi or Semen Raphani dried and powdered, and mixed into a herbal cake with ginger juice) on the Tsusanli, Tian Shu, Large Intestine Shu, Shangjuxu, and Zhong Wan and other acupoints, which can disperse stagnated liver *Qi*, relieve the pain of the internal organs, and significantly improve the clinical symptoms of patients by reducing the levels of 5-HT, NPY, and vasoactive intestinal peptide (VIP), with an overall effective rate of 97.22%. Elevated levels of 5-HT, NPY, and VIP cause constipation, abdominal pain, and distention as gastrointestinal peristalsis and secretion of intestinal fluids will be inhibited.

3. Electroacupuncture therapy

   In electroacupuncture therapy, acupoints are stimulated by micro low-frequency pulsed currents, which regulate meridians for relieving pain, and regulate the internal organs. Peng Suifeng et al. used electroacupuncture to stimulate the Tsusanli point and Tian Shu point, which reduces scores of the Self-Rating Depression Scale (SDS) and Self-Rating Anxiety Scale (SAS), increases the total score of the 36-Item Short Form Survey (SF-36), and improves the patients' quality of life. Pan Chen et al. used electroacupuncture to stimulate bilateral Tsusanli with a current of 0.5–2 mA, and found that the total effective rate of the treatment group was 85%, which improved the score of the Bristol Stool Form Scale.

4. Massage therapy

   The Huangdi Neijing says: "For those who have been subjected to repeated terrors their meridians do not flow smoothly due to disorganized *Qi* and are mostly numb and insensitive, so massage and medicinal wines are appropriate for treating such symptoms." Massage has the effect of dredging the meridians and regulating *Qi* and blood. Zhang Fengjun treated IBS-C with massage therapy of regulating *Qi* and visceral organs, which was able to significantly relieve symptoms, and the total effective rate was higher than that of the control group ($P < 0.05$), indicating that the massage therapy was more effective. Sun Guozheng applied massage therapy on the abdomen and waist to stimulate purgation, together with whole-body relaxation manual therapy to treat IBS-C, which can effectively restore clinical symptoms such as abdominal pain, distention, and constipation, and the recurrence rate was lower than that of the Western medicine group at the 3-month follow-up ($P < 0.05$). Wang Jingui et al. compared abdominal massage therapy (pressing, kneading, and pushing the abdomen) with traditional massage therapy (according to the textbook), and the total effective rate of the abdominal massage group was higher than that of the control group ($P < 0.05$). Pei Xuhai compared one-thumb massage technique with oral cisapride tablets and found that the recurrence rate of patients in the one-thumb massage technique group (12.5%) was lower than that of the control group in the long-term effect at the 6-month follow-up.

5. Combination therapies

   (a) Acupuncture combined with moxibustion

      Liang Xiaoling et al. performed warm acupuncture combined with moxibustion treatment, the total effective rate of which was 96.9%, which was superior to acupuncture or moxibustion treatment alone. Xu Fu gave acupuncture combined with Wen He moxibustion treatment, taking acupuncture points of the Zhong Wan, Tian Shu, Da Heng, Qi Hai, Tsusanli, Shangjuxu, Xiajuxu, and Sanyinjiao to regulate intestinal stagnation and purgation. The effective rate of the treatment group was 97.4% and 94.9% at a 1-month follow-up visit, manifesting that the combination of acupuncture with Wen He moxibustion has stable long-term effects on the treatment of IBS-C.

(b) Acupoint application therapy combined with other treatments

Hua Hanbing et al. performed acupoint application therapy combined with TDP therapy (bilateral Tian Shu, bilateral Fu Jie, Qi Hai, and Guan Yuan were the acupoints selected), achieving a total effective rate of 93.3%, and at the same time, TCM symptom score was reduced and clinical symptoms were alleviated. Liu Fei treated patients with auricular point sticking therapy (taking the points of stomach, large intestine, small intestine, rectum, spleen, lung, kidney, sympathetic, and San Jiao) and acupoint application therapy (self-made application of Zhi Ke, Hou Pu, Da Huang, and Mang Xiao was pasted on bilateral Tian Shu and Shen Que. points), and the total efficiency was 90.5%, which was higher than that in the group treated with Western medicines alone ($P < 0.05$). Fan Chunhua et al. also gave auricular point sticking therapy combined with acupoint application therapy and found that it could significantly reduce the serum 5-HT level.

(c) Enema therapy combined with other treatments

Hu Tuanmin randomly divided the patients into three groups: treatment group 1 received retention enema of the TCM prescription (Huang Qi, Da Huang, Huang Qin, Huang Lian, Bai Shu), treatment group 2 was treated with colon hydrotherapy combined with retention enema, and the control group received oral phenolphthalein tablets. The results demonstrated that the effective rates of treatment groups 1 and 2 were higher than that of the control group, and the recurrence rate of the retention enema combined with colon hydrotherapy was lower, indicating a better long-term therapeutic efficacy. Zhang Bo et al. treated the control group with forlax and oryzanol and added tranquilizer for anxious patients, and the treatment group was given retention enema of the self-prescribed herbal medicine to regulate *Qi*-flowing for purgation (Da Huang, Zhi Shi, Bin Lang, Mu Xiang, Wu Yao, Bai Shao) and moxibustion (taking the Tsusanli, Sanyinjiao, Shangjuxu, Guan Yuan, Shen Que., Tian Shu, Zhong Wan points) treatments. The results showed that in the treatment group patients' symptoms of constipation, abdominal pain, and abdominal distension were significantly improved and the effective rate reached 94.1%.

8.3.5.3 Summary

In recent years, TCM external treatment methods have made great progress in the treatment of gastrointestinal functional disorders represented by IBS-C. Acupuncture, moxibustion, acupoint application, and herbal enemas have achieved good clinical efficacy when they are applied alone or in combination, and have the advantages of being convenient to perform, reliable safety, and few side effects. Whereas the efficacy of external treatment methods was obtained mainly through clinical observations, instead of basic or clinical research, and the procedures were not standardized. Accordingly, the combination of clinical observation and research, and the standardization of operation procedures are important aspects of future research.

8.3.6 Chronic Pelvic Inflammatory Disease

Chronic pelvic inflammatory disease is an inflammatory lesion arising from the female internal reproductive organs and the surrounding connective tissues, and pelvic adnexa. It is also a common gynecological disease. As the disease is prone to recur and even cause infertility, ectopic pregnancy, and a series of other problems, it will have a serious impact on the patient's life and social functions. Therefore, it is crucial to find an effective treatment method. Conventional treatment methods include orally taking Western drugs, but due to the limited effect of the drugs, a multitarget or multipathway integrated treatment method is required.

Chronic pelvic inflammatory disease is caused by the proliferation of fibrous connective tissues in the reproductive organs and the inability of medication to work directly on the blood circulation. For women, "blood is the essence." When they are influenced by troubles in work, family, and other aspects, "unsmooth *Qi*," "blood stasis," and other signs may occur. In addition, menstruation, production, or various types of surgeries may lead to "internal invasion of dampness and heat," which deteriorates the disease. Clinical treatment generally regulates *Qi* and activates blood stasis, focusing on the regulation of the overall body function through TCM treatments to obtain a good therapeutic effect.

Since chronic pelvic inflammatory disease is prone to recur and the proliferation of fibrous connective tissue is relatively significant, the therapeutic effect of Western medicine alone is very limited. It is necessary to take comprehensive measures to treat the disease. The value of comprehensive therapy has been testified in previous studies [24], and TCM comprehensive therapy is proposed accordingly. Specifically, different herbs have their own efficacy. For example, Dan Shen can activate blood circulation to remove blood stasis and regulate menstruation to relieve pain; Gan Cao can harmonize all the herbs; Bai Shao can nourish *Yin* and replenish blood; Chai Hu can clear away heat and inflammation; and Wu Yao can resolve stagnation and disperse cold. When different herds are applied in combination, the simultaneous treatment of *Qi* and blood can be realized, and the healing process of the disease can be accelerated.

Enema is a part of the comprehensive therapy. The proliferation of inflammatory fibrous connective tissues of chronic pelvic inflammatory disease slows down the blood flow, and even if systemic medication is taken, the normal blood circulation will be affected and so will the curative effect. TCM enema may shorten the onset time than that of pills, tablets, and suppositories and keep the characteristics of traditional decoction in line with the requirements of TCM syndrome differentiation treatment. The external application of ground herbs can stimulate meridians and skin as the herbs infiltrate into the body and work on the lesions directly.

The combination of acupuncture and acupoint injection can also directly work on the disease and achieve good treatment and analgesic effect. When they are in combination with the oral administration of Western drugs, a comprehensive therapy is realized.

8.3.7 Dysmenorrhea

Dysmenorrhea refers to different degrees of pain experienced by women in the lower abdomen before and after menstruation or when menstruation begins, and the pain is periodic and may even lead to fainting. Dysmenorrhea is a common disease among women in China whose daily life may be affected by severe pain. Dysmenorrhea is divided into primary dysmenorrhea and secondary dysmenorrhea. Primary dysmenorrhea refers to dysmenorrhea without reproductive organic lesions, which is more common in adolescent women, accounting for more than 90% of dysmenorrhea. Secondary dysmenorrhea refers to dysmenorrhea caused by pelvic organic diseases, such as adenomyosis. In Western medicine, dysmenorrhea is treated mainly through oral prostaglandin synthase inhibitors (commonly used drug is ibuprofen) and oral contraceptives. These drugs are able to reduce prostaglandin production and relieve or eliminate pain. In some cases, dolantin is needed to alleviate the pain. However, such drugs can only temporarily relieve pain rather than eliminate it radically, and the pain may come back again, not to mention the side effects. In recent years, with the continuous development of TCM, the TCM treatment of dysmenorrhea has shown a great vitality. It has become popular with its diverse, effective, safe, and no side effect characteristics.

8.3.7.1 TCM Treatment

1. Oral herbs

   In TCM, oral administration of traditional Chinese herbs is the first and most common choice for treating dysmenorrhea. Through syndrome differentiation, herbs can regulate viscera, meridians, *Qi* and blood, cold, and heat, etc., showing a remarkable effect. Studies have shown that for primary dysmenorrhea of the cold and blood stasis type, TCM sequential therapy can effectively relieve patients' pain symptoms, improve uterine blood perfusion, and reduce the ratio of serum PGF2α/PGE2, the effect of which is stable and long-lasting. Besides, TCM combined with analgesics has better effects on treating primary dysmenorrhea than that of analgesics alone, which can effectively relieve the symptoms of abdominal pain. A satisfactory outcome can be achieved through the method of warming channels for dispelling cold and promoting blood circulation for removing blood stasis by orally taking Gui Zhi, Gan Jiang, Ai Ye, Wu Yao, Wansizi, Pu Huang, Dang Gui, Yanhusuo, Chi Shao, and prepared Gan Cao. Other researchers used the decoction to treat primary dysmenorrhea, with Dang Gui, Bai Shao, Gan Cao, Hui Xiang (Szechwan Chinaberry Fruit), raw Pu Huang, Wulingzhi, Gui Zhi, Yuan Hu, and Chuanlianzi (Szechwan Chinaberry Fruit) as the main drugs. The results showed that the decoction protected and regulated the patient's estrogen level and improved the hemodynamics.
2. TCM external treatment

   As introduced in the previous sections, TCM external treatment methods mainly include hot compress, application, fumigation, and enemas. By using these methods, the meridians, acupoints, skin, and visceral organs can be stimulated to relieve the symptoms. The external therapies are diversified with multipathways of drug delivery, such as located drug delivery through which drugs can be delivered directly to lesions, avoiding the side effects of oral administration on the stomach, intestines, liver, etc., and guarantee the safety. Firstly, acupoint application is efficient in treating dysmenorrhea. Studies used TCM application with Decoction for Warming Channels as the basic formula to apply on the acupoints of Sanyinjiao, Guan Yuan, Gui Lai, and Ming Men to treat primary dysmenorrhea of the cold and blood stasis type, which greatly relieves the pain during the menstruation, and the efficacy of the treatment is remarkable. Secondly, TCM hot compress is applied to the patient's abdomen after heating and achieves the effects of removing stagnation for activating meridians and invigorating blood circulation and *Qi*, through hot steam and permeation of Chinese herbs, which shortens the period of dysmenorrhea and alleviates the pain. Thirdly, the TCM fumigation treats pain with fumigation instrument where steam from decocting herbs is absorbed by the skin. In the *Yi Lin Gaicuo* (*Correction on Errors in Medical Classics*), fumigation using the Gexia Zhuyu Decoction can treat primary dysmenorrhea of the *Qi* stagnation and blood stasis type and achieve the effect of activating *Qi* and blood, resolving stasis and alleviating pain, especially the mild to moderate dysmenorrhea, without obvious adverse reactions. Lastly, the TCM enema is mainly the local filling of Chinese medicine liquid in the intestines and achieves treatment effect through the absorption of herbs by the intestinal walls. It is particularly effective in treating pelvic and abdominal diseases in proximity to the intestinal tracts. Some researchers used enema with Yiwei Tongjingling (endometriosis and dysmenorrhea granules) to treat endometriosis and dysmenorrhea patients, and found that enema can eliminate or reduce the patient's clinical pain symptoms. Moreover, it is convenient and easy to operate and will not cause any harm to the human body.

8.3.7.2 Acupuncture Therapy

Acupuncture therapy is effective in treating primary dysmenorrhea, which has been recognized by many doctors and patients. By applying acupuncture on Sanyinjiao, Tsusanli, Tai Chong, the primary dysmenorrhea of the cold stagnation and blood stasis type can be relieved significantly, and the symptoms of dysmenorrhea and the levels of PGE2 and PGF2α can be improved and regulated. Tang Xiaomin and others needled points of Master Tung's Acupuncture such as

Men Jin, Shui Qu, first San Cha, and third San Cha to treat primary dysmenorrhea, which obtained obvious short- and long-term analgesia efficacy with a low recurrence rate. Shiqizhui (17 vertebra) point is an extra-meridian point, also known as "Yao Kong," which is the point under the spinous process of the fifth lumbar vertebrae. A large number of researchers have proved that acupuncture on 17 vertebrae alone has the effect of relieving spasms of the uterine smooth muscle. Therefore, the point can be acupunctured to treat dysmenorrhea effectively.

8.3.7.3 Massage Therapy

Massage therapy for primary dysmenorrhea is effective as it improves blood circulation and reduces the production of prostaglandins, thus relieving dysmenorrhea caused by uterine smooth muscle contraction. Chen Ruyong et al. treated dysmenorrhea of the cold-dampness type through massage to disperse dampness, warm meridians, and dissipate cold, as well as guide blood flow downward, tonify the body, and enhance purgation, which could weaken the uterine contraction and alleviate the pain safely without side effects. In other cases, Wu Yan used TCM balanced massage techniques to treat dysmenorrhea, which not only treat local symptoms directly, but also have the characteristics of indirect and holistic treatment that balances the body's overall *Qi*, blood, *Yin* and *Yang*, so that the body is in dynamic balance and can resist the invasion of pathogenic factors.

8.3.7.4 Moxibustion Therapy

In moxibustion therapy, moxa sticks are used as the main medium for treating dysmenorrhea, and other mediums such as ginger and Chinese herbs also have good effects. Liu Yinghua et al. used old moxa sticks to fumigate the points of Shen Que. and Guan Yuan for the treatment of primary dysmenorrhea due to cold condensation and blood stasis. The results revealed that the pain of the patients was significantly alleviated. Moxibustion could help relieve pain by regulating the abnormal levels of PGF2α and argininopressin, inhibiting spastic contraction of the uterine smooth muscle, and triggering changes in the function of several brain regions related to pain. The use of ginger moxibustion on Qi Hai, Guan Yuan, Zhong Ji, and uterus points for the treatment of primary dysmenorrhea can inhibit inflammatory factors, regulate the level of prostaglandins, inhibit uterine contraction, and improve local ischemia and hypoxia to achieve the effects of relieving dysmenorrhea.

8.3.7.5 Acupoint Injection Therapy

Acupoint injection treats dysmenorrhea through the dual action of acupuncture and drugs. The commonly used acupoint is Sanyinjiao, and the drugs used can be either Western drugs or Chinese medicines. Yang Haixia injected dezocine at the Sanyinjiao point to treat primary dysmenorrhea. The analgesic effect can be improved and prolonged by pre-regulating physiological responses and blocking the input of pain signals, and at the same time stimulating the central nervous system to produce endorphins and other analgesic substances and activating the endogenous analgesic system. The administration of Gang Gui Injection at the Ci Liao point can treat dysmenorrhea by rapidly stimulating the meridian *Qi*, smoothing meridians, and activating collaterals. Likewise, the administration of vitamin B12 and compound Dang Gui Injection at the Tsusanli point is effective and convenient.

8.3.7.6 Auricular Point Pressing Therapy

Wei Bo et al. took four auricular points, namely, Shen Men, endocrine, liver, and internal genitalia organs, for the treatment of primary dysmenorrhea, which could effectively relieve smooth muscle spasms and inhibit the production of excessive PGF2α. Meanwhile, through the stimulation of the auricular points and the conduction of meridians, the excitability of the cerebral cortex could be suppressed, and the endocrine system could be regulated to alleviate the pain in the long term. Li Yingming et al. chose five auricular points for the treatment of dysmenorrhea, including the internal genitalia organs (uterus), Shen Men, sympathetic, endocrine, and subcortical points, which had the effect of smoothing the meridians, activating the collaterals, tranquilizing the mind, and controlling the pain. Its pain-relieving effect was much greater than that of oral ibuprofen, indicating that the therapy has advantages in relieving or preventing pain.

8.3.7.7 Other Treatments

Other TCM treatments have also been used in managing dysmenorrhea. Gao Yan and others used cupping therapy to treat dysmenorrhea and obtained significant clinical effects in relieving pain symptoms and improving the quality of life. Li Laiqiang et al. used three-edged needle bloodletting therapy combined with multidirection needling to treat primary dysmenorrhea and achieved remarkable pain-relieving efficacy with few adverse effects and a low recurrence rate [25].

8.3.7.8 Summary

The earliest record of dysmenorrhea in TCM is found in the book *Jingui Yaolue: Treatment of Pulses and Syndromes of Gynecological Diseases*. The pathogenesis of dysmenorrhea is mainly the pain caused by deficiency or repletion. The repletion syndromes are *Qi* stagnation, blood stasis, cold, dampness, heat, etc., while the deficient syndromes are weakness of *Qi* and blood, and kidney deficiency. The most primitive and common method of treating dysmenorrhea in TCM is orally taking Chinese medicines. Whereas the gradual integration of TCM with modern medical techniques further diversifies the methods of treating dysmenorrhea. At present, dysmenorrhea is often treated with a combination of at least two therapeutic methods, mostly traditional Chinese herbs and appropriate TCM therapies. The therapeutic efficacy of TCM in dysmenorrhea has been examined in clinical studies and recognized by patients. However, the mechanism behind the TCM treatment of dysmenorrhea has not been fully clarified, and it is anticipated that in the future more research on the mechanism will be conducted and more TCM treatment methods will be developed.

8.3.8 Testicular Pain

Among patients presenting in the department of urology, approximately 2.5% are with testicular pain. The clinical presentations of patients with chronic testicular pain are characterized by intermittent or persistent pain in one or both testicles. The pain is actually a squeezing pain deep in the testicle and usually lasts for more than 3 months. In some cases, the pain may refer to the groin, perineum, and lower back. If the pain is not relieved in a timely manner, it may lead to anxiety and depression, which will impact patients' quality of life.

Chronic testicular pain may be induced by diseases related to testicles and epididymis, including chronic orchiepididymitis, epididymal cysts, testicular tumors, testicular ischemia, hydrocele, chronic prostatitis, varicocele, and inguinal hernia. However, the etiologies of patients with chronic testicular pain may not be identified. For the treatment of pain, Western medicine usually uses antibiotics, antidepressants, and selective nerve block agents. When these drugs fail, patients may receive epididymis and testicular resections.

On the other hand, TCM categorizes chronic testicular pain as "nephralgia" and "scrotum and testicular pain." The etiology of chronic testicular pain has been documented in classical TCM books. In the *Miu Ci Monographs* of *Plain Questions*, it is recorded that "Evil *Qi* attacks the collaterals of the foot Que *Yin*, causing a sudden hernia with severe pain." The *Rumen Shiqin* (*Confucian's Duties to Their Parents*) by Zhang Congzheng says that "cold pain in two testicles may be caused by foot Yang Ming meridians and *Qi* …… evil *Qi* invades the middle Jue Yin meridians, inducing sudden hernia in the middle of the syncope Yin meridian, so the disease leads to testicular pain." These records displayed that chronic testicular pain is closely associated with the liver channel of foot Jue Yin. The liver meridians surround external genitals and also dominate purgation. Therefore, when patients suffer from emotional discomforts, dietary disorders, external pathogenic factors, or trauma, they may have liver *Qi* stagnation, blood stasis, and phlegm condensation. The unsmooth meridians damage the kidney blood flows, which is called nephralgia. Therefore, the principle of treating chronic testicular pain is dissipating nodules and swellings, resolving blood stasis, and relieving pain. Xiao Jin Wan (a pill), originally named Xiao Jin Dan, first appeared in Wang Hongxu's *Waike Quansheng Ji* (*The Complete Works of Surgery*) in the Qing Dynasty. Later, its current name was recorded in the *Chinese Pharmacopoeia* and was produced as a drug. The main ingredients of Xiao Jin Wan are artificial She Xiang, Mubiezi, prepared Wu Zi, Fengxiangzhi (Resina Liquidambaris), Ru Xiang, Mo Yao, Wulingzhi, Dang Gui, Di Long, and Xiang Mo. The prepared Cao Wu in this formula has the efficacy of warming meridians, dispersing cold, and removing dampness, while Fengxiangzhi, Ru Xiang, Mo Yao, and Dang Gui have the efficacy of activating blood circulation, regulating *Qi*, and relieving pain. Di Long has the efficacy of activating meridians and collaterals. She Xiang has the efficacy of resuscitation, activating blood circulation, resolving mass, and relieving pain. Mubiezi has the efficacy of resolving mass and swellings. Xiang Mo has the efficacy of stopping bleeding and detumescence. Wulingzhi has the efficacy of activating blood circulation and dispersing stasis. These herbs applied together can dissipate masses and swellings, dissolve blood stasis, and relieve pain.

In conclusion, testicular pain is also known as "nephralgia" and "scrotum and testicular pain" in TCM, the etiology and pathogenesis of which are external cold and dampness or dampness and heat invading the external genitals, resulting in stagnation of *Qi* and blood, and the accumulation of toxins; or dampness and toxicity descending to the liver meridians; or testicular blood stasis and stagnation of *Qi* due to injuries. Patients with testicular pain, regardless of its etiology being clear or not, can hardly be cured by a single therapy of antibiotics. TCM believes that the liver dominates the urogenital region and the liver meridians surround external genitals, including the testicles and scrotum. Testicular pain is mostly due to the liver meridian *Qi* and blood blockage, and the treatment should be promote *Qi* and blood and smooth the meridians.

8.3.9 Interstitial Cystitis

Interstitial cystitis (IC), also known as "bladder pain syndrome," is a chronic nonbacterial inflammatory lesion of the bladder. It is currently recognized as a chronic visceral pain syndrome with pain in the genitourinary and rectal regions. Its course is long with recurrent symptoms. Patients of all ages may be victims of this disease, but women in middle ages are more likely to be affected. The main clinical manifestations are frequent urination, urinary urgency, increased nocturia, and pain with full bladder (pain in the bladder or lower abdomen, suprapubic area, combined with pain in the perineal area), which is alleviated after urination, and some patients may have difficulty in urination, hematuria, and other symptoms. Its symptoms are similar to those of urinary tract infections, thus are often misdiagnosed, but the results of routine urine test and urine culture of IC are normal and cannot be relieved by anti-infective treatment. The diagnosis of IC is mainly a diagnosis by exclusion, relying on typical symptoms, routine urinalysis, urine culture, cystoscopy, and pathological examinations. At present, its etiology and pathogenesis have not been fully clarified, and many scholars believe that it may be related to autoimmunity, obstruction of blood-lymphatic reflux, endocrine factors, genetic factors, psychological factors, etc. So far there is no specific treatment for IC, and clinical treatments are mostly aimed at relieving symptoms and improving quality of life, with the use of oral medication, bladder perfusion, bladder water dilatation, surgery, and psychotherapy. There is no description of IC in TCM, but from its symptomatic characteristics and the evolution of the disease, it can be categorized as "stranguria" in TCM.

8.3.9.1 Etiology and Pathogenesis of Interstitial Cystitis [26]

1. Damp heat in urinary bladder

   According to Zhang Zhongjing in the *Symptoms and Treatment of Stranguria Caused by Thirst and Difficult Urination* of *Jingui Yaolue*, "Symptoms of stranguria include millet-like urine coming out in drips, constricted tense pain in the abdomen, and pain pulling into the umbilicus." This means that stranguria manifests as frequent urination, painful urination, and pain and discomfort in the abdomen, the symptoms of which are consistent with IC in modern medicine. Conventionally, stranguria is mostly caused by dampness and heat. For example, the *General Treatise on the Causes and Symptoms of Diseases* records that "the strangury disease is mainly due to kidney deficiency and heat in the bladder. Kidney deficiency leads to dripping of urine, while heat in the bladder leads to urination difficulty. Dripping urine and difficult urination, together with urinary incontinence, it is thus called stranguria." Therefore, kidney deficiency is the root cause and dampness heat in the bladder is the symptom, which are the major pathogenesis of IC.

2. *Qi* stagnation and blood stasis

   Patients with IC often present with pain and discomfort in the suprapubic bladder area. As mentioned earlier, in TCM, pain can be divided into two types, namely, pain of congestion and pain of lacking spirit. In the early stage of IC, blood stasis forms in the bladder as the circulation of blood and *Qi* is obstructed by external pathogenic factors, leading to pain of congestion. As the disease progresses, the stasis damages the body and blocks the nourishment of blood, leading to pain of lacking spirit. All these problems contribute to the discomfort of patients. Furthermore, when receiving cystoscopy, IC patients have been found to have punctate hemorrhage in the bladder mucosa and at the same time, the prolonged course of the disease and other aspects reflect the characteristics of stasis, which further proves that *Qi* stagnation and blood stasis are the pathogenesis of IC.

3. Deficiency and injury of visceral organs

   Due to the recurrent feature of IC, patients have to take Chinese medicines of bitter, cold, and Qingli (clearing away the damp heat) or a variety of antibiotics. As a result, their *Yang Qi* may be injured and visceral organs are in deficiency. The *Xuanming Five Qi Monographs* of *Plain Questions* says that "the cause of incontinence is the inability of the bladder to restrain urine." According to this, frequent urination is the result of the inability of the bladder to restrain urine, which is caused by the kidney *Qi* deficiency and cold, and loss of functions of warm and *Qi*. Therefore, stubborn frequent urinary can be treated with Decoction for Reinforcing the Middle-Jiao and Replenishing *Qi*, which showed good clinical efficacy. To summarize, IC is due to external pathogenic factors invading the body, dampness, and heat accumulation and unsmooth circulation of *Qi* and blood, resulting in visceral and warming function failure and inducing the symptoms of frequent urination, urinary urgency, and suprapubic bladder pain and discomfort. This disease contains both deficiency and repletion syndromes, so the treatment should be clearly differentiated, in order to better improve clinical efficacy.

8.3.9.2 Prescriptions for Treating Interstitial Cystitis

As a long-course disease, IC is characterized by the syndrome of kidney *Yang* deficiency and blood stasis, so the treatment should target on warming the kidneys to disperse cold, activating blood circulation to remove blood stasis. In the stage when no co-infection conditions occur, Chinese medicines of bitter, cold, and Qingli nature should not be used since such kinds of medicines are harmful to *Yang Qi* and healthy *Qi*, and may induce kidney *Yang* deficiency and injury, and deteriorate the cold condensation. Zhu Danxi wrote in the *Ge Zhi Yu Lun* (*Further Treatises on the Properties of Things*) that "dietary disorders and inappropriate medicines may all damage the body." Treating cold symptoms with cold medicines is fruitless, and may even damage *Yang Qi* and make *Yin Qi* and cold more prevalent, resulting in coldness of limbs and cold pain in the abdomen. However, if there is a stage of co-infection, medicines for warming the kidney should be temporarily suspended to prevent aggravation and lingering of the disease. Under such circumstances, the disease should be treated with the method of activating blood circulation, removing blood stasis, and freeing strangury. Medicines such as amber powder can be used, but still the use of medicines should be appropriate and medicines of cold and bitter nature should be used with caution as they may damage kidney *Yang*. If it is determined that no co-infection occurs, the methods of activating blood circulation to eliminate blood stasis and warming the kidney to disperse cold can be adopted to alleviate the symptoms and restore the function of the bladder. "Smooth flow of *Qi* and blood is a way of tonifying *Qi* and blood; thus, activation of blood is critical." Whereas medicines with the nature of activating blood and *Qi* overly should not be abused as they may damage the healthy *Qi*. The author of this chapter often chooses to use the Shaofu Zhuyu Decoction to warm meridians and blood. With the addition of Tao Ren and Hong Hua (Flos Carthami), the decoction helps promote blood circulation; by adding Ru Xiang and Mo Yao, the formula can activate blood circulation to relieve pain and promote detumescence and granulation to restore the contracture function of the bladder; if the disease lasts too long and induces kidney injury, then Yinyanghuo (Herba Epimedii), Tusizi (Semen Cuscutae), Gou Qi, and Buguzhi (Fructus Psoraleae) should be added to help the kidney *Qi* and avoid attacking and damaging the healthy *Qi*. If there are other concurrent symptoms, other herbs can also be added or the original herbs can be subtracted accordingly.

8.3.9.3 Summary

IC is different from general stranguria in terms of etiology, pathogenesis, and clinical manifestations, and is prone to misdiagnosis and mismanagement. Being recurrent and difficult to cure, the disease can lead to kidney *Yang* deficiency, blood stasis, and internal obstruction and contracture of bladder, which should attract the attention of clinicians. For patients who are not co-infected, bitter and cold medicines should not be used, and trying the method of warming the kidney to disperse cold and activating blood circulation to remove blood stasis may be effective. This disease has both characteristics of deficiency and repletion, and the clinical manifestations are complicated; thus, it should be further studied in order to accurately diagnose and treat it.

8.3.10 Ulcerative Colitis

Ulcerative colitis (UC) is a chronic nonspecific intestinal inflammatory disease triggered by a combination of environmental, genetic, intestinal microecological, and immunological factors. The active UC is characterized by diarrhea, mucus, and blood in stools and abdominal pain, and some patients may have extra-intestinal manifestations such as arthralgia and fatigue. The modernization and industrialization of the society boost the intake of refined food, and consequently raise the incidence of UC. In terms of Western medical treatment, mesalazine preparations, glucocorticoids, and immunosuppressants are often used to control the inflammatory response, relieve clinical symptoms, and promote mucosal healing under colonoscopy. In recent years, biological agents with new targets are also entering the stage of clinical trials. However, some patients experience drug nonresponse or relapse after stopping the administration of drugs, which is related to individual differences and environmental factors. Noticeably, TCM herb therapy has unique advantages for this disease, and it is of great clinical significance to explore the etiology and treatment of this disease. UC belongs to the categories of "prolonged dysentery" and "diarrhea" in TCM. Chao Yuanfang first proposed the name "dysentery" in the *General Treatise on the Causes and Symptoms of Diseases*, in which he illustrated that patients may have symptoms of stools in red and white, or stools covered with pus and mixed with blood and the intermittent characteristics are also recorded. The book also describes the concept of "prolonged dysentery," which means dysentery may not be improved over a long period of time. Prolonged dysentery will result in complications such as mucosal damage and even anal fistula. All these descriptions are similar to the symptoms, course, and onset of UC. In conclusion, this disease is located in the intestines, related to the spleen and stomach, and can refer to the kidney. The mechanism of UC may be lurking of pathogenic factors in the intestines, stagnation of *Qi*, blood stasis, conduction failure, and intestinal panniculitis.

8.3.10.1 Etiology and Pathogenesis

UC often has both deficiency and repletion, and cold and heat symptoms. The active UC mainly presents with repletion symptoms, manifested as dampness and heat, while in the relief period, the symptoms present with the characteristics of deficiency in the spleen and stomach and repletion in *Qi* and blood. Yang Yitian et al. reckoned that, caused by the invasion of external pathogenic factors and deficiency in healthy *Qi*, the beginning of UC or the acute attack of UC is related to external pathogenic factors and irregularity of diet, giving birth to the accumulation of dampness and heat in the intestines. Pathogenic heat damages mucosa and results in ulcer when pus and blood in stools can be observed. Or the lung heat descends to the intestines and leads to mucus and blood in stools. In the relief period, UC presents as the deficiency in the spleen and kidney type. The long course of diarrhea disease damages the healthy *Qi* and the spleen and stomach function. The inability to transport and transform water and grain essence to nourish the limbs and bones results in fatigue, lack of appetite, emaciation, and prolonged illness further deteriorating the digestive function of the spleen, making it unable to nourish the kidneys, so that the kidney *Yang* is in deficiency and diarrhea is difficult to be cured. Zhang Hui et al. believed that the onset of UC is similar to the disease of collaterals, and that prolonged diseases will invade the collaterals and cause other localized lesions, such as loss of appetite, skin and mucous membrane lesions, arthritis, and other systemic symptoms.

8.3.10.2 Treatment Based on Syndrome Differentiation

UC patients have different symptoms such as diarrhea, abdominal pain, and pus and blood in the stools, and need to be diagnosed and treated according to the main symptoms. In the acute stage of the disease, abdominal pain and blood in stools should be treated by clearing heat and removing toxins; if timely treatment is provided, the blood in stools will be reduced. For symptoms of thin sloppy stools, and blood and mucus in stools, the treatment should be to strengthen the spleen to remove dampness and also to clear away the residual toxins. In the stable stage of the disease when clinical symptoms are relieved, then it is necessary to warm up the kidneys and strengthen the spleen. At the same time, macroscopic symptoms and microscopic endoscopic manifestations should be combined. If mucosal erosion and edema are seen, then the blood should be cooled to stop bleeding; if it is accompanied by ulcers, then the methods of detoxification and promoting wound healing should be applied; if the mucosa is granular or manifested as polypoid hyperplasia, then the *Qi* should be activated to enhance the blood flow, and phlegm should be cleared to dissolve the masses.

8.3.10.3 Treatment Methods

1. Oral Chinese medicines

   Decoction of *Pueraria*, *Scutellaria*, and *Coptis*, recorded in the *Treatise on Febrile and Miscellaneous Diseases* written by Zhang Zhongjing, is effective in treating diarrhea caused by dampness and heat. Shao Yao Decoction can clear away heat and dampness and harmonize *Qi* and blood, and is widely used in the treatment of damp-heat dysentery. The combination of these two formulas can be modified into a formula for clearing intestines and removing dampness, which consists of Huang Lian, Huang Qin, Baijiangcao (Dahurian Patrinia Herb), Dang Gui, Bai Shao, Sheng Di (Drying Rehmannia Root), Zi Cao, Qian Cao (Radix Rubiae), Bai Shu, Mu Xiang, and Gan Cao. When the formula is orally taken by patients, symptoms such as diarrhea and blood in stools are rapidly relieved. The total efficacy rate of symptom relief is higher than that in the group of oral mesalazine granule. Dai Qiuying et al. believed that spleen deficiency and dampness are the key etiologies of UC, so they formulated a formula for dispelling wind and dampness, which was found to be safe and effective. The formula can lower the Geboes score and the disease activity index, reduce mucosal destruction, and repair the damaged colon mucosa [27].

2. Acupuncture and moxibustion

   Acupuncture and moxibustion therapies have unique advantages such as economic, safety, ease of operation, and minimal side effects, and are widely used in clinical practice. Wen Yong et al. compared the sequential therapy combining acupuncture (Tian Shu, Shangjiuxu, Qu Chi points) and catgut implantation at acupoint (spleen Shu, Tsusanli, Guan Yuan points) with oral mesalazine granule and found that the long-term efficacy of acupuncture therapy was obvious as the TCM symptom score of the patients with UC was lowered, the recurrence rate of the disease was reduced, the rate of the colon mucosal healing was promoted, and the expenses were cut down. The herbal cake-separated moxibustion promotes local blood circulation and mucosal repair through stimulations of acupoints, warmth, and medicines.

3. Combined treatment of TCM and western medicine

Aminosalicylic acids are the first choice for the treatment of mild-to-moderate UC, but the use of Western drugs alone has a long treatment period and a heavy financial burden, so a combination therapy has aroused the interest of researchers. Zeng Wumiao et al. administered mesalazine and probiotics orally in the control group, while the treatment group received oral mesalazine and probiotics in combination with oral Chinese medicines (fried Bai Shu, Bai Shao, Dang Shen, Yiyiren, Fu Ling, Huaishanyao or Rhizoma Dioscoreae, Chi Shao, Fang Feng, Qing Pi, Chai Hu, Chen Pi, prepared Gan Cao). The results showed that the addition of traditional Chinese medicines significantly improved the therapeutic efficacy and the abundance of *Lactobacillus* and *Bifidobacterium*, regulated the intestinal flora, and maintained the intestinal homeostasis. Wang Ye et al. gave oral mesalazine to patients in the control group, and in the treatment group, patients received oral mesalazine in combination with oral Decoction of Four Noble Drugs and Bai Shao and TCM enema. The results showed that the combined medication could alleviate the symptoms of abdominal pain, loose stools, urgency, mucus–pus–blood in stools, fatigue, and poor appetite, and reduce the levels of IL-17 and TNF-0t, which was conducive to the repair of the intestinal mucosa, increase of the hormone withdrawal rate, and improvement of the hormone dependence.

8.3.10.4 Summary

The symptoms of UC may occur repeatedly. With TCM, the disease can be transformed from the active stage into the remission stage and has the characteristics of minimal side effects, low recurrence rate, and small economic burdens, playing an irreplaceable role in the treatment of the disease. However, TCM also has deficiencies in the clinical research and treatment of UC. Firstly, the inclusion and selection of subjects in clinical trials lack the concept of combining diseases and syndromes, which cannot reflect the characteristics of TCM's treatment based on syndrome differentiation. Secondly, the TCM treatment of UC lacks a unified assessment system of therapeutic effect, and there is inconsistency between TCM syndrome-based remission and endoscopic mucosa repair. Thirdly, the mechanism of TCM in preventing and treating UC is unclear, and most of the studies have focused on inflammation and immunomodulation, while trials on the association between the intestinal flora and the disease are inadequate. Lastly, UC may lead to colorectal cancer if the course is long, and the evidence of the long-term efficacy of TCM treatment on the disease in clinical studies is inadequate as well. Therefore, it is necessary to develop safe and effective therapies based on the essence of TCM. At the same time, the clinical trials of the treatment of UC with the combination of TCM diseases and syndromes should be conducted to provide data support for TCM therapies.

8.3.11 Chronic Pelvic Pain Syndrome

Chronic pelvic inflammatory disease refers to the chronic inflammatory changes in the female reproductive organs and surrounding connective tissues and pelvic peritoneum, including salpingo oophoritis, hydrosalpinx, chronic salpingitis, endometritis, and chronic pelvic connective tissue inflammation. The disease is mainly caused by the incomplete treatment of acute pelvic inflammatory disease or the patient's weakness and the pathogen's insensitivity to drugs. Currently, Western antibiotics are the main drugs for treating chronic pelvic inflammatory disease in Western medicine, but the increasing drug resistance brings about a certain impact on the effectiveness and safety of clinical medication. Therefore, it is necessary to explore new therapies to relieve the clinical symptoms of patients with chronic pelvic inflammatory disease and ensure the therapeutic effect of the disease. TCM has unique characteristics in the treatment of chronic pelvic inflammatory disease and a variety of treatment methods, including internal treatment, external application, acupuncture, herbal enemas, and placement of medications in the vagina.

8.3.11.1 Etiology and Pathogenesis

According to TCM, chronic pelvic inflammatory disease belongs to the category of "women's abdominal pain," "menstrual pain," "leucorrhea," and "heat invading the blood chamber." It is related to phlegm dampness, dampness toxicity, dampness heat, etc., with the main manifestation of prosperous pathogen and asthenia healthy *Qi*. Its pathogenesis mainly consists of *Qi* and blood disorders, stagnation of *Qi* and blood, and deficiency of the spleen and prevailing dampness. In recent years, scholars have analyzed the etiology and pathogenesis of chronic pelvic inflammatory disease from different aspects and found that the disease originates from the Chong and Ren Vessel, Conception Vessel, and uterus, and its onset is related to the kidney, namely, kidney *Yin* deficiency, kidney *Yang* insufficiency, combined with dampness, heat, and stagnation. At the same time, it is also associate

d with the liver and spleen as *Qi* stagnation, dampness, heat, blood stasis, and other repletion pathogenic factors lurking in the uterus, resulting in the depletion of *Qi* and blood, mixed syndromes of deficiency and repletion, and difficulty of the treatment of the disease.

8.3.11.2 TCM Internal Treatment

From the perspective of TCM, the internal treatment of chronic pelvic inflammatory disease is mainly clearing heat and promoting warming, strengthening vital *Qi* to eliminate pathogenic factors, and promoting blood circulation for removing blood stasis [28].

The syndrome of *Qi* stagnation and blood stasis is mainly treated by regulating *Qi* to relieve pain and activating blood circulation to remove blood stasis. He Xiaoli et al. treated 58 patients with chronic pelvic inflammatory disease based on syndrome differentiation of supplementing and supporting healthy *Qi* and activating blood to remove blood stasis, and the results showed that the total effective rate of this group (98.3%) was higher than that of the conventional Western medicine group (84.5%). Consequently, they believed that the method could effectively improve the clinical symptoms and the quality of life of patients.

The syndrome of stagnation of cold and dampness should be treated by activating blood circulation to remove blood stasis and dispelling cold and dampness. He Changmin chose 58 cases of chronic pelvic inflammation patients with stagnation of cold and dampness as the research subjects, of which 29 cases in the control group were treated with antibiotics and 29 cases in the treatment group were treated with antibiotics in combination with Shaofu Zhuyu Decoction. The results showed that the total effective rate of the treatment group was higher than that of the control group, and the recovery time of menstruation, pelvic mass reduction, pelvic pain duration, and action time is shorter in the control group than that in the control group, which indicates that Shaofu Zhuyu Decoction can effectively accelerate the relief of symptoms and promote menstruation recovery.

The syndrome of stagnation of heat and dampness should be treated by activating blood circulation to remove blood stasis and relieve pain, clearing heat and promoting diuresis. Yinjia Pill or Danggui Shaoyao Powder can be used.

8.3.11.3 TCM External Application

Chronic pelvic inflammatory disease is a local lesion, so Chinese medicine applications for dispersing cold to warm meridians and activating blood circulation to remove blood stasis can be used on the outer part of the lower abdomen to accelerate the local blood circulation, promote the smooth circulation of blood, alleviate the local tissue adhesions, and then accelerate the subsiding speed of inflammatory factors and eliminate the clinical symptoms. Fang Guoping et al. treated patients with chronic pelvic inflammatory disease using TCM hot compresses in combination with acupoint application. The results showed that the total effective rate of the treatment group was 95.2%, and the recurrence rate was only 4.8%, suggesting that the treatment has a significant therapeutic effect on chronic pelvic inflammatory disease and reduces the risk of recurrence.

8.3.11.4 Acupuncture

For chronic pelvic inflammatory disease, acupuncture has the efficacy of dissolving masses to eliminate swelling, warming meridians to promote diuresis, and clearing away heat. Moreover, from the point of view of modern medicine, acupuncture can accelerate the body's blood circulation, promote the metabolism of the tissue cells, and reduce the adhesion of tissues. At the same time, on the basis of traditional acupuncture,

TCM scholars continued to develop acupuncture point injection therapy and achieved remarkable effects. Wu Chunling used the randomized number table to treat 43 cases of chronic pelvic inflammatory disease patients with warm needling, herbal enema, and acupoint injection. The results showed that the total effective rate of the treatment group was as high as 97.7%, which proved that the combination of acupoint injection, warm needling, and herbal enema can effectively improve the blood microcirculation, inhibit inflammatory cytokines, and improve the therapeutic effect.

8.3.11.5 TCM Retention Enema

In light of female physiological anatomy, the rectum and uterus are in the same pelvic cavity and adjacent to each other, and the uterus is located in front of the rectum. Through TCM retention enema, medicines can be absorbed through the rectal mucosa and take effect directly on the lesion site, avoiding the first-pass effect of the liver and directly entering the pelvic blood circulation. Above all, TCM retention enema not only has a direct effect, but also reduces adverse reactions of the digestive tract.

8.3.11.6 Summary

Chronic pelvic inflammatory disease is a common and frequent disease in gynecology, which is characterized by long-course, prolonged, and difficult-to-cure, and high recurrence rates, bringing serious impacts on the health and quality of life of patients. TCM has unique insights into the diagnosis and treatment of chronic pelvic inflammatory disease. In TCM, oral Chinese medicines, acupuncture, external application of Chinese medicines, TCM enema, etc., can not only be used alone, but also be used in combination, which has the effect of simultaneous treatment of the internal and external, and taking into account both the symptoms and the root causes of the disease. At the same time, according to the different syndromes of chronic pelvic inflammatory patients, TCM proposed specific treatment strategies, making the treatment more precise, reliable, and safe. Modern research has concluded that TCM treatments that activate blood circulation to eliminate blood stasis can improve local pelvic microcirculation, promote the absorption and elimination of inflammatory substances, regulate metabolism, and strengthen the immune function of the body. It should be noted that, although an in-depth study on TCM treatment of chronic pelvic inflammatory disease has been carried on, unified standards in the syndrome differentiation, treatment plan, therapy evaluation, etc., are still lacking and the mechanism of the Chinese medicines has not been completely clarified, requiring further studies referring to these aspects.

8.3.12 Postoperative Pain

Surgery has also been a way to mitigate pain, and, in most cases, surgery is the ultimate choice for patients whose pain cannot be relieved by other therapies, but unfortunately, chronic visceral pain after surgery is not uncommon. One of the most common examples is prostate-related postoperative pain.

8.3.12.1 Prostate-Related Postoperative Pain

Prostatic hyperplasia is a common disease in middle-aged and old-aged men, and the main symptoms include poor urination, urine dripping, or even unable to urinate. For the disease, prostate removal has been the most satisfactory, reliable, and effective treatment, but bladder spasms may occur after the surgery. Bladder spasmodic pain aggravates hematuria. The pain is paroxysmal, may last for severe hours or even has multiple episodes per hour in severe cases, or lasts for over 10 days in certain cases. Such circumstances greatly affect the recovery after surgery, prolonging the course of the disease and intensifying the pain. Generally, bladder spasms are considered to be induced by intraoperative and postoperative irritation of the bladder neck.

In TCM, prostate hyperplasia belongs to the category of "retention of urine." It is mainly due to a deficiency of kidney *Qi* and obstruction of unhealthy *Qi*. The kidney is in charge of urination and the division of the two *Yin*. The elderly's kidney deficiency weakens the spleen and stomach, which over time results in dampness, heat, and blood stasis, finally resulting in difficulty and dripping of urine. The commonly seen clinical syndrome of the disease is spleen and kidney *Yang* deficiency. The treatment is warming the kidneys, tonifying the spleen, and activating blood circulation to promote diuresis. For the treatment of bladder spasms after prostatectomy in Western medicine, conventional methods are applying antispasmodic and analgesic drugs and adding procaine to the rinse solution. In recent years, epidural analgesia pump was applied to relieve the postoperative pain of prostatectomy, yet the clinical observation of its effect is unsatisfactory and there were related complications. Whereas the effects of acupuncture and oral TCM decoctions are remarkable in treating postoperative pain, with no complications and side effects. "Retention of urine" is mostly caused by the deficiency of the spleen and kidney *Yang* in the elderly. When patients receive the prostatectomy, the syndrome of deficient healthy *Qi* and blood stasis is aggravated, and the bladder is out of control. Accordingly, the treatment of prostate hyperplasia should aim at both symptoms and root causes, and the symptoms should be treated first in urgent cases. To be specific, warming and tonifying the kidney *Yang* can strengthen the spleen *Yang*, and when the spleen and kidney *Yang* are strengthened, the healthy *Qi* can be supported, the blood flow can be facilitated to promote diuresis, and blood stasis can be resolved. As a result, "pain is released when the congestion is resolved" and the functions of the spleen and kidney are restored. Acupuncture and moxibustion activate blood circulation to eliminate blood stasis and relieve pain, while benefiting *Qi* and warming *Yang*. Decoction for Strengthening the Spleen-*Yang* warms kidneys to induce diuresis. The clinical application of these therapies can be modified based on the different conditions of patients.

8.3.12.2 TCM External Treatment

Acupuncture and moxibustion are effective therapies to treat the disease. For acupuncture, the Guan Yuan, Zhong Ji, Ci Qia, Yi Bian, Yanglingquan, and Sanyinjiao points are taken. Zhi bian point should be needled inwardly and downwardly, while other points are needle regularly, with intermittent strong wave stimulation of electroacupuncture for about 20–30 min, primarily in the reducing method. Acupuncture is performed once or twice a day. For moxibustion, Guan Yuan and Tsusanli points are taken. Use 7–20 moxa cones to conduct direct moxibustion on Guan Yuan point and 5–9 cones on Tsusanli point. Moxibustion on each point lasts for 10–20 min once a day.

8.3.12.3 TCM Internal Treatment

The Decoction for Strengthening the Spleen-*Yang* is prescribed, consisting of 15 g of Fu Zi, Bai Shao, Huang Bo (Cortex Phellodendri), Fu Ling, Ze Xie, Gouqizi, Shan Yao, Tao Ren, Chi Shao, and Zhi Mu (Rhizoma Anemarrhenae); 30 g Bai Shu; 9 g Chia Hu; 10 g of Sheng Ma, Rou Gui, and Da Huang; 6 g Jie Geng; and 12 g Yuan Hu. The above medicines are decocted twice in water, and 600 mL of juice is extracted and taken in the morning and evening separately, one dose a day. When the spasmodic pain of the bladder is relieved, the rinse solution becomes clear without blood clots and drainage tube obstruction. The urinary catheter is removed 10 days after the surgery, and the urination recovers, which is satisfactory to patients.

8.4 Summary

At present, the clinical treatment of visceral pain with TCM is widely used and shows better results in the case of ineffective treatment with conventional Western drugs. It has the advantages of diverse methods, being flexible, and convenient to use; rapid onset and extended maintenance of analgesic effect; being safe and reliable, almost without adverse reactions; and not easy to induce drug resistance and addiction. Thus, it not only relieves the symptoms, but also strengthens the body's immunity, improves the quality of life of patients, and prolongs the patient's life. With the rapid development of medical science, especially with the continuous progress of TCM diagnosis and treatment methods, the role of TCM in the treatment of visceral pain is inestimable and the diagnosis and treatment of visceral pain become more efficient, convenient, and individualized. TCM doctors should seek common ground while reserving differences, so that they can learn from others. Under the guidance of TCM theories, the excellent concepts, techniques, and methods from other disciplines should be introduced and learned to combine TCM and Western medicine to pave the way for the development of the discipline's inheritance and benefit patients.

References

1. Sharma GS, Tillisch K. Chapter 4—Visceral pain: mechanisms, syndromes, and treatment. In: Pangarkar S, Pham QG, Eapen BC, editors. Pain care essentials and innovations. Elsevier; 2021. p. 45–58. ISBN: 9780323722162. https://doi.org/10.1016/B978-0-323-72216-2.00004-1.
2. Wang JY, Xu L, Zhang RX, Lao L. Traditional Chinese medicine for cancer pain. J Chin Integr Med. 2011;9(2):129–34.
3. Wu XJ, Lan RJ, Lu M. Progress of traditional Chinese medicine for cancer pain. Xinjiang J Tradit Chin Med. 2021;39(2):98–100.
4. Liu YJ, Yang YQ. Present situation and prospect of TCM medicine for cancer pain. Clin J Chin Med. 2014;8:147–8.
5. Wang ZQ, Huang RJ, An K, Sun YC, Yuan XK. The new Progress of traditional Chinese medicine in the treatment of cancer pain. Chin Med Modern Dist Educ China. 2017;15(1):148–50, 143.
6. Wang X, Wang Y. Brief analysis of the clinical experience of insect medicine in the treatment of tumors. Anti-tumor Pharm. 2014;4:309–13.
7. Zhou Y, Cai A. Progress of clinical research on external treatment of cancer pain in traditional Chinese medicine. Nei Mongol J Tradit Chin Med. 2012;31(10):102–4.
8. Han ZY, Zhou YQ. Progress in the treatment of cancer pain by external treatment of traditional Chinese medicine acupoints. Chin J Manag Chin Med. 2007;2:142–6.
9. Wei SM, Dong BQ, Fu Y, Shi FY, Yang ZJ, Wang LC. Clinical study on treatment of cancer pain in patients with lung cancer of Yang deficiency type by combination of needling tendon method and moxibustion. Liaoning J Tradit Chin Med. 2020;47(2):169–71.
10. Cao B, Wang HW. Traditional Chinese medicine with the three step therapy analgesia treatment cancer pain. J Pract Tradit Chin Internal Med. 2010;24(3):50–1.
11. Wu HH, Shen WY. Clinical treatment of cancer pain with traditional Chinese medicine. Chin Tradit Herb Drug. 2004;35(9):1087–8.
12. World Health Organization. Cancer. 3 Feb 2022. Retrieved from https://www.who.int/news-room/fact-sheets/detail/cancer. Accessed 10 Aug 2023.
13. Wu YS, Shi L. Introduction to traditional Chinese medicine treatment of constipation due to opioid application in patients with cancer pain. Health Guide. 2021;47:154–5.
14. Brogi E, Forfori F. Anesthesia and cancer recurrence: an overview. J Anesth Analg Crit Care. 2022;2:33. https://doi.org/10.1186/s44158-022-00060-9.
15. Liu X, Wang Q. Application of anesthetics in cancer patients: reviewing current existing link with tumor recurrence. Front Oncol. 2022;12:759057. https://doi.org/10.3389/fonc.2022.759057.
16. Lai YW, Feng Z. Research progress of traditional Chinese medicine in the treatment of cancer pain. Popular Sci Technol. 2019;21(5):100–2.
17. Jianhong Y, Caixing X, Keru L. Effect of traditional Chinese medicine emotional regulation combined with hot compress on lower abdominal pain in patients with sequelae of pelvic inflammatory disease. Hebei Tradit Chin Med. 2023;45(10):1659–62.
18. Mingming Y, Khalizati B. The application of traditional Chinese medicine emotional therapy in pelvic stasis syndrome. Xinjiang J Tradit Chin Med. 2006;24(4):7–9.
19. Zhang Yirong: The effect of traditional Chinese medicine emotional therapy on the quality of life of cancer patients. 2009.
20. Qiuyue Y. The effect of TCM emotional therapy on the perioperative period of patients undergoing hysteroscopic surgery. Chin J Med. 2023;13(23):138–41. 190
21. Zhang JH, Xiao TG, Yuan AH, Que RH, Wang XY, Fu ZQ. Prof. Fu Zhiquan's experience on the treatment of functional abdominal pain syndrome. Shaanxi J Tradit Chin Med. 2019;40(12):1755–8.
22. Li TA. Introduction to ten methods of traditional Chinese medicine treatment of stomach pain. Guang Ming Zhong Yi. 2012;27(4):790–1.
23. Li H, Xu YS. Research progress of Chinese medicine external treatment of constipation predominant irritable bowel syndrome. J China Prescr Drug. 2022;20(12):187–90.
24. Hu DZ. A study on the clinical value of comprehensive treatment of chronic pelvic inflammatory disease by traditional Chinese medicine. Women's Health Res. 2023;1:85–7.
25. Yang JY, Zhao YQ, Jiang SS. Progress of traditional Chinese medicine treatment of dysmenorrhea. Women's Health Res. 2022;7:29–30, 37.
26. Yu SM, Liu YH, Guo DD, Zhang DX. Discussion on some points of traditional Chinese medicine diagnosis and treatment of interstitial cystitis. Jiangsu J Tradit Chin Med. 2018;50(5):12–3.
27. Fu J, Wang YY, Zhang YY, Lin M. Progress of clinical research on the treatment of ulcerative colitis with traditional Chinese medicine. Bachu Med J. 2023;6(1):108–11.
28. Wang Y. Analysis of research progress of traditional Chinese medicine in the treatment of chronic pelvic inflammatory disease. Nei Mongol J Tradit Chin Med. 2023;42(3):167–8.

Other Treatments for Visceral Pain

9

Ming Xia

As visceral pain may bring tremendous and persistent suffering for patients, researchers have paid great attention to the study and development of various treatments for resolving the torment. In the previous chapter, technologies such as neuroregulation therapy (nerve block) and neuroelectrical stimulation technique (spinal cord stimulation, peripheral nerve stimulation, transcutaneous electrical nerve stimulation, motor cortex stimulation, deep brain stimulation, etc.) were introduced in detail as effective treatment methods for visceral pain that cannot be managed by medical treatments. Apart from these, for patients with intractable visceral pain who did not benefit from conservative treatment and whose quality of life is seriously affected, surgical therapy (anterolateral cordotomy, anterior commissurotomy) may also be effective, and psychotherapy has become popular in treating visceral pain as more attention has been paid to the psychological factors of patients. In this chapter, surgical therapy and psychological mechanisms and treatment of visceral pain will be introduced.

M. Xia (✉)
Department of Anesthesiology, Shanghai Ninth People's Hospital Affiliated to Shanghai Jiao Tong University School of Medicine, Shanghai, China
e-mail: xiaming1980@xzhmu.edu.cn

9.1 Surgical Treatment

In general, surgical treatment of pain can be considered for patients for whom conservative treatment is not effective. The principle of surgical analgesia is to block the pathway of nociceptive conduction from peripheral receptors to the nociceptive center of the cerebral cortex.

9.1.1 Anterolateral Cordotomy

In 1912, Spiller and Martin were the first to carry out anterolateral cordotomy, which was used to treat intractable pain and achieved good results [1]. In 1963, Mullan and colleagues inserted strontium pins into the lateral tract of the spinal thalamus [2]. Since the 1960s, radiofrequency thermal coagulation destruction of the anterolateral spinal cord bundle by percutaneous lateral puncture has been advocated and performed. Compared to open surgery, it retains the advantages of anterolateral bundle dissection and allows the extent of destruction to be controlled by adjusting time and temperature, and can be performed while the patient is awake, thus avoiding the risks associated with general anesthesia. The analgesic effect is similar to that of open surgery but with fewer complications. In recent years, with the development of CT and other diagnostic imaging techniques and the continuous progress of destruction methods, percutaneous surgery has been improved and perfected.

M. Xia et al. (eds.), *Visceral Pain*, https://doi.org/10.1007/978-981-99-9167-9_9

The anterolateral tract of the spinal cord is mainly the lateral thalamic tract of the spinal cord, located in the anterolateral 1/4 quadrant of the spinal cord, and is the main afferent pathway for nociception and temperature sensation. Cutting the anterolateral tract of the spinal cord can block both the secondary conduction pathway of nociception and the nonspecific nociceptive conduction pathway, and the efficacy is more certain and long-lasting.

1. Indications

   Patients suffering from severe pain due to cancer, involving pelvic, leg, hip, and lower trunk pain, are the best indications for anterolateral spinal cordotomy. For pain in the upper limbs, upper abdomen, and chest, the anterolateral bundle of the spinal cord at the C_2 level is generally performed; for pain in the lower abdomen, perineum, and lower limbs, the anterolateral bundle of the spinal cord at the T_2 level should be performed: for pain in the midline or on both sides, the anterolateral bundle of the spinal cord can be cut on both sides, but in the high cervical medulla it is not advisable to perform bilateral cutting to avoid respiratory muscle paralysis.
2. Surgical methods

   Open anterolateral spinal cord bundle cut: Open anterolateral spinal cord bundle cut can be performed under general anesthesia, but more local anesthesia plus intravenous anesthesia, and local anesthesia surgery is conducive to intraoperative observation of changes in the plane of nociceptive loss and motor function of the limbs, to avoid injury to the corticospinal tract of the spinal cord. The patient is usually placed in the lateral or prone position, and a straight posterior median incision is made to remove the spinous processes and laminae of $C_{2,3}$ or $T_{1,2}$, and the dura is incised longitudinally. The dentate ligament is found between the superior and inferior nerve roots of the spinal cord, and its base should be located at the midpoint between the anterior and posterior roots of the spinal nerve. Anterior to the dentate ligament is the anterolateral bundle of the spinal cord (lateral bundle of the spinal thalamus) and posteriorly is the pyramidal bundle. In front of the dentate ligament, the spinal cord is incised to the medial aspect of the anterior root with a sharp pointed blade, the depth of the incision should not exceed 4.5 mm, and the incision can be repeated 2–3 times.

   During surgery, the dentate ligament can be clamped with a mosquito-type vascular clamp and the spinal cord can be pulled and rotated 45° backward to fully expose the anterolateral aspect of the spinal cord and facilitate surgical cutting of the anterolateral bundle of the spinal cord. There may be a small amount of bleeding, which is stopped by conventional hemostatic methods. The dura and soft membranes of the spinal cord are closed to reduce cerebrospinal fluid leakage. When performing bilateral anterolateral spinal cord cordotomy, the incisions on both sides of the spinal cord should not be on the same segment, but at least 1–2 segments apart, otherwise the blood supply to the spinal cord will be affected, leading to serious complications. It is best to complete the anterolateral spinal cord bundle dissection on both sides in two sessions, with an interval of more than 2 weeks.

   Percutaneous anterolateral spinal cord cordotomy: Percutaneous anterolateral spinal cord cordotomy is often performed under X-ray and CT guidance using a radiofrequency system for destruction. $C_{1,2}$-level anterolateral spinal cord cordotomy is performed using a lateral approach, while C_{4-7}-level anterolateral spinal cord cordotomy is performed using an anterior approach. The patient is placed in the supine position, and after local anesthesia, a puncture needle with electrodes is inserted percutaneously under X-ray and CT guidance. Clear visualization of the dentate ligament is essential for the success of the procedure, and the dentate ligament can be visualized using a water-soluble contrast agent (e.g., iohexol) or a small amount of air. The needle can be inserted into the spinal cord when the puncture needle is located just anterior to the dentate ligament.

Localization can be performed by impedance and neurophysiology. Impedance in the cerebrospinal fluid is approximately 400 Ω and in the spinal cord often exceeds 1000 Ω. Insertion of the puncture needle usually results in a temporary increase in local pain. Electrode location can be observed by X-ray or CT images, and localization can be performed using electrical stimulation.

Using low-frequency stimulation (2–5 Hz) and low-stimulation intensity, muscle twitching in the neck on the ipsilateral side of the body indicates that the tip of the puncture needle is located anteriorly or near the anterior root. Twitching of the muscles of the arm, shoulder, trunk, or leg ipsilateral to the body using low-stimulation intensity indicates that the head end of the puncture needle is near the corticospinal tract and the needle should be repositioned more anteriorly. The stimulation level is increased to a higher intensity (approximately 100 Hz) to induce the best stimulation effect. A warm or cold sensation is usually produced on the contralateral trunk or lower extremity of the stimulus, indicating that the electrode is positioned close to the painful area. If the patient complains of abnormal sensation in the ipsilateral arm or the back of the head, the electrodes are positioned too far back, dorsal to the dentate ligament. If the contralateral hand produces an abnormal sensation, the electrode is correctly placed.

A 2-mm bare end at the head end of the electrode can create a localized disruption in the spinal cord. The disruption temperature is usually 70–80 °C, and the duration is about 60 s (30–40 mA for 30–60 s), which can be disrupted 2–3 times. The patient should be checked for signs of motor weakness during and after performing the disruption procedure. Once the disruption is completed, the degree of nociceptive deficit should be recorded. Needle sensory reduction should cover the entire painful area, and if the degree of nociceptive deficit is not sufficient, the electrode position can be slightly adjusted and the same parameters used for disruption. If bilateral anterolateral spinal cord cordotomy needs to be performed, an interval of at least 1 week is required during this period to minimize adverse effects of the procedure.

3. Treatment results

Efficacy of open anterolateral spinal cord cordotomy: Almost all anterolateral spinal cord cordotomies are used for the treatment of cancer pain, usually lung cancer or gastrointestinal tumors. Few long-term follow-up studies beyond 2 years have been performed in this patient population because of the typically short survival period.

Most patients (77% as reported by White and Sweet) have immediate relief of cancer pain, and 1/4 patients have partial relief of cancer pain [3]. Some patients may be ineffective and even cause neurological dysfunction. At 6 months, more than half of the patients reappear with pain. In a review of the literature by Cowie and Hitchcock [4], the cases in the study of Piscol (1385 patients) [5] and Mansuy et al. (124 patients) [6] showed a decrease in pain relief 1 year after anterolateral cervical cord cordotomy or anterolateral thoracic cord cordotomy; however, patients are rarely put on secondary disruption.

With the exception of cancer pain, there are very few reports in the literature on the use of this procedure to treat lumbar radiculopathy or peripheral neuropathy. Approximately 23 patients have areas of pain in the lower part of the torso rather than the upper part of the torso. Immediate pain relief after unilateral anterolateral spinal cord cordotomy was seen in 70–90% of patients, while only 40–78% of patients had immediate pain relief after bilateral anterolateral spinal cordotomy [7].

The incidence of complications from unilateral open anterolateral spinal cord cordotomy is 3% compared with 20% for bilateral surgery [8]. The incidence of mild paralysis and urinary complications is higher (10–20%), especially in patients undergoing bilateral dissection. Complications such as sexual dysfunction may also occur with bilateral dissection, especially with bilateral anterolateral cervical medullary bundle dissection, which is more likely to cause respiratory muscle paralysis and respiratory dysfunction, which can lead to death in severe cases. Therefore, bilateral dissection should be done with caution.

Efficacy of percutaneous anterolateral cervical cord fasciculotomy: Most of the faithful can have immediate pain relief after undergoing the procedure, and the percentage of pain relief can reach 90%.

In general, only 50–60% of patients experienced sustained pain relief within 1 year, making percutaneous anterolateral spinal cord fasciculotomy indicated for the relief of severe pain due to malignancy. Other literature also reports that percutaneous anterolateral spinal cord fasciculotomy for noncancerous pain is not particularly effective. Lahuerta et al. reported in 1985 that the efficacy of percutaneous anterolateral spinal cord fasciculotomy in noncancerous pain was suboptimal in pain caused by benign tumors compared with pain caused by malignant tumors, with only 20% of patients experiencing complete pain relief (66% for malignant tumor pain) and 40% of patients experiencing no pain relief at all. Forty percent of patients had no pain relief at all (12% of malignancy patients) [9].

Although long-term pain relief is not possible after percutaneous anterolateral spinal cord cordotomy in cancer patients, most patients experience significant pain relief within 1 year after surgery. In a follow-up study of a large sample of cases, the majority of patients who required opioids or other analgesic medications before surgery no longer required analgesic medications within 6 months after surgery. In total, 789 patients were included in the study by Rosomoff and colleagues, and 84% of these patients no longer required analgesic medications within 3 months after percutaneous anterolateral spinal cordotomy. Percutaneous anterolateral spinal cord cordotomy resulted in a significant improvement in the quality of life of the patients at 2 years postoperatively.

4. Complications

(a) Complications of open anterolateral spinal cord fasciculotomy

Urinary retention or incontinence are the two most common complications, with an incidence of 11–33%. In addition, permanent sensory dullness (7–11%), transient mild hemiparesis (3.5–22%), and respiratory distress or respiratory depression (3.5–4%) from anterolateral cervical spinal cord fasciculotomy were also included. Patients with cancer may also develop mirror image pain after open anterolateral thoracic spinal cord dissection (7–11%), which presents as similar pain on the opposite side of the original painful area after the patient has undergone an anterolateral spinal cord dissection, usually lasting several weeks to months [10].

Complications resulting from dural dissection with laminectomy include spinal instability, cerebrospinal fluid leakage, and meningitis.

(b) Complications of percutaneous anterolateral spinal cord cordotomy

Similar to open anterolateral spinal cord cordotomy, percutaneous anterolateral spinal cord cordotomy can accidentally injure the spinal cord beyond the thalamus tract. Death due to percutaneous anterolateral fasciculotomy (mean mortality rate of 3%) may be related to respiratory depression and usually occurs after bilateral percutaneous anterolateral fasciculotomy. Other common complications include bladder dysfunction (7.6%), transient ipsilateral body weakness (7.6%), ataxia (4.0%), respiratory dysfunction (3.5%), and permanent ipsilateral body weakness (1.0%) [11].

9.1.2 Dorsal Root Entry Zone Dissection

In the 1960s, the dorsal root entry zone (DREZ) of the spinal cord was discovered to be associated with nociceptive transmission and began to be explored as a target for the surgical treatment of pain. The first dorsal root entry zone lesioning of the spinal cord was performed in a patient with Pancoast syndrome. In the same year, several other patients with cancer pain underwent the same procedure with satisfactory postoperative pain relief. Since then, several other patients with chronic neurogenic pain (including pain in the affected limb and pain after brachial plexus avulsion injury) have undergone the procedure. In 1979, Nashold et al. first reported microcoagulation of the dorsal root of the spinal cord into the medullary region in patients with painful brachial plexus avulsion injuries, with good results [12]. Subsequently, they performed microcoagulation of the dorsal root of the spinal cord into the medullary region in patients with spinal cord injuries. With the development of electrophysiological monitoring of the spinal cord, the complications of the procedure have decreased significantly, which has led to some promotion of the destruction of the dorsal root-into-myelination zone of the spinal cord.

The dorsal root entry zone of the spinal cord includes the dorsal root branches, the posterior lateral fasciculus, and laminae I–V of the posterior horn of the spinal cord. Each posterior root divides into 4–10 branch roots of 0.25–1.5 mm in diameter into the posterior horn of the spinal cord. Depending on the thickness and destination of the dorsal root afferent nerve fibers, they are rearranged in the dorsal root entry area of the spinal cord, with the fine fibers that transmit nociception located around the thick fibers that transmit touch. The posterior lateral tract, located posteriorly to the posterior horn, plays an important role in the modulation of afferent fibers for pain stimulation, with its medial portion transmitting excitatory impulses from the dorsal roots to adjacent segments and its lateral portion transmitting inhibitory influences from the central glial form to the proximal segments. The posterior horn is the site of the first synaptic transmission in the sensory system, with coarse afferent fibers projecting to laminae III and IV and fine afferent fibers projecting to laminae I and II and V. Injurious afferent signals are modulated in the posterior horn by interneuronal and downward connections.

The dorsal roots of the spinal cord into the medullary region are incised in the following areas: (1) small injurious fibers (fine fibers) in the part around the dorsal root branches: (2) the excitatory medial part of the posterior lateral fasciculus; and (3) the outermost layer of the posterior horn (laminae I–V of the Rexed laminae). The inhibitory structures in the dorsal root entry zone of the spinal cord, that is, the thalamic fibers (thick fibers) that reach the posterior horn and the intrinsic contact fibers of the spinal cord within the central colliculus that travels in the lateral part of the posterior lateral bundle, should be preserved. Dissection of the dorsal root of the spinal cord into the medullary region permanently destroys secondary neurons of the injurious afferent pathway, that is, it disrupts the normal injurious conduction pathway to relieve pain due to injurious stimuli. At the same time, some scholars have found that nociception is associated with the spontaneous firing of neurons within the central nervous system in addition to the response to injurious stimulus afferents. In some patients with afferent nerve block pain, the electrophysiological activity in the posterior horn of the spinal cord is abnormally active. Disruption of the dorsal root of the spinal cord into the medullary region can simultaneously eliminate the abnormal electrophysiological activity in the posterior horn of the spinal cord and provide pain relief.

1. Indications
   (a) Patients with cancer pain who have a long survival period are in good general condition, can tolerate open surgery under general anesthesia, and have limited pain sites. For example, Pancoast syndrome, neuropathic pain caused by tumor invasion of lumbosacral plexus, neuropathic pain caused by peripheral nerve, plexus, and nerve root tumor.
   (b) Pain after avulsion of the brachial plexus nerve is a better indication of spinal cord dorsal root into the medullary area dissection. The extent of spinal cord dorsal root

human medullary zone dissection should not be limited to the injured segment only, but should be extended to the adjacent nerve roots, especially when the level of injury coincides with the painful area.

(c) Pain after spinal cord or cauda equina injury. Most of these patients have a history of spinal trauma, and surgery is only effective if the patient's pain is segmental and the area of pain is consistent with the level and extent of the spinal cord injury. Spinal trauma below T_{10} (spinal cone), especially when the pain is located in the lower extremity rather than the perineum, is a better indication of spinal dorsal root entrapment myelotomy.

(d) Pain after peripheral nerve injury. If the pain manifests as paroxysmal lightning-like pain, abnormal nociception, or nociceptive hypersensitivity (such as residual limb pain, phantom limb pain, intercostal neuralgia after thoracotomy), the results of dorsal spinal root entrapment myelotomy are better.

(e) Postherpetic neuralgia. The efficacy of dorsal spinal root entrapment myelotomy for postherpetic neuralgia has been debated. Some scholars believe that spinal dorsal root entrapment myelotomy can only relieve superficial pain in the skin (e.g., abnormal nociception and nociceptive hypersensitivity), and some patients can develop new tightness after surgery. Therefore, caution must be exercised when deciding to use dorsal spinal root entrapment myelotomy for postherpetic neuralgia.

(f) Spasticity combined with pain. The dorsal spinal root medullary incision can also block the afferent signal of muscle extension reflex, reduce muscle tone, and improve spasticity.

2. Surgical method

The patient is placed under general anesthesia in the prone position, and the surgery is performed under a microscope. Patients undergoing neck surgery should be fixed in a head frame to keep the neck flexed. A hemilaminectomy or total laminectomy is performed at the corresponding painful segment, and the dura mater is incised longitudinally to reveal the posterior lateral aspect of the corresponding spinal cord segment on the affected side. Localization of the spinal cord segment is performed according to anatomy or with the aid of electrophysiological monitoring (electromyography). Along the selected spinal cord surgical area, the soft spinal membrane is incised ventral–lateral to the entrance of the small root branch into the posterior lateral sulcus longitudinally, and a microdissection instrument is used to bluntly separate along the dorsal root of the spinal cord into the medullary area to the posterior horn, which can be identified by its color change to gray. The posterior lateral spinal artery travels in the posterior lateral sulcus and has a diameter of 0.1–0.5 mm, emanating from the posterior root artery, and anastomoses caudally with the anterior descending branch of the Adamkiewicz artery through the Lazorthes spinal cone anastomosis ring.

In addition to the microsurgical technique of incising the dorsal root entry zone of the spinal cord, the dorsal root entry zone of the spinal cord can be destroyed by a specific radiofrequency electrode. The diameter of the electrode is 0.25 mm and the exposed tip is 2 mm long. The temperature and duration of the disruption determine the size of the disruption foci, usually 75 °C for 15 s, with disruption foci at 1 mm intervals.

In 1972, Sindou conducted an extensive study on the destruction and dissection of the dorsal root of the spinal cord into the medullary region [13]. The advantage of radiofrequency disruption is that the area of disruption is usually about 1 mm^2 and is reproducible. In addition, the Nashold RF electrode is used in the dorsal heel of the spinal cord to ensure a 2.5-mm depth of destruction, equally spaced with the electrode head. The disadvantage of RF destruction is that the actual extent of destruction within the spinal cord cannot be seen. There may be areas of jumping at the site of destruction, resulting in unsatisfactory results, and deviations from the line of destruction of the dorsal root of the spinal cord into the medullary region, which may increase the incidence of complications.

3. Efficacy of treatment

   In recent years, the success rate of radiofrequency disruption of the human medullary region of the dorsal spinal cord root has improved. Patients with brachial plexus avulsion injuries have had better surgical outcomes. One retrospective study reported that the pain relief rate for brachial plexus avulsion injuries has increased from 54% to 91%, with a 5-year pain relief rate of more than 50% [14]. Patients with terminal site pain rather than diffuse distal pain (associated with spinal cord injury) had better outcomes (78% and 20% relief rates, respectively). A study by Tomas and Haninec showed that intraoperative electrophysiological monitoring of the dorsal angle of the spinal cord improved the efficacy of the procedure and reduced the incidence of complications [15]. Surgical results are often less satisfactory in patients with dull, aching, and burning pain distal to the area of spinal cord injury (similar to phantom limb pain). These data suggest that the dorsal root entry area of the spinal cord may not contain the nociceptive pathways that regulate such pain. Autonomic pathways external to the spinal cord may be involved in modulating intractable pain that cannot be cured by dorsal root dissection of the spinal cord.

   The efficacy of spinal cord dorsal root entrapment dissection for limb pain after spinal cord injury is more satisfactory. Falci et al. reviewed 105 patients with pain after spinal cord injury and 83% of them had satisfactory pain relief. Seventy-four percent satisfaction rate of pain relief was reported [16].

   The efficacy of dorsal root dissection of the spinal cord into the medullary region for postherpetic neuralgia is not very conclusive. Friedman and Bullitt reported that 29 of 32 patients had pain relief several months after surgery, but only 8 patients had better pain relief after 1 year [17]. At Duke Hospital, 96 disruptions of the dorsal root of the spinal cord into the medullary region were performed in 86 patients with postherpetic pain. Early after surgery, 53% of patients had complete and 33% had partial pain relief. After 3 months, 47% of patients had complete and 28% had partial pain relief. Considering the high risk of impaired motor function associated with dorsal root dissection in the chest, caution should be exercised when performing dorsal root dissection in patients with postherpetic neuralgia.

   There is a paucity of information on the efficacy of dorsal root dissection in post-amputation pain (residual limb pain and phantom limb pain). Satisfactory pain relief has been reported in 6 of 9 patients with phantom limb pain and 5 of 6 patients with amputation-related nerve root avulsion injury. The efficacy of spinal cord dorsal root dissection into the medullary region is less satisfactory in patients with residual limb pain only.

4. Complications

   The phasic sensory loss or deficit corresponding to the disrupted segment is a side effect rather than a complication of spinal dorsal root entrapment myelotomy, and the side effect has little impact on the quality of life of the faithful because the majority of patients already had sensory loss or deficit before surgery.

   Complications of dorsal spinal root entrapment myelotomy are mainly spinal cord injuries, most commonly ipsilateral proprioceptive deficits due to ipsilateral posterior column injuries or ipsilateral limb weakness due to corticospinal tract injuries.

   The complication rate ranges from 3% to 14%. Injuries caused by disruption of the thoracic dorsal spinal cord roots into the medullary region are most common because the dorsal horn of the spinal cord is thinnest here, and the injury can manifest as permanent sensory loss below the disrupted area, that is, loss of proprioception and mild hypoesthesia on the ipsilateral side of the body, with an incidence of 2–70%. The incidence of this complication can be reduced by using smaller electrodes and improving surgical experience.

9.1.3 Anterior Commissurotomy

The indications for anterior commissurotomy are similar to those for anterolateral spinal cord bundle dissection. In 1927, Armour first reported anterior commissurotomy of the spinal cord, which was performed by cutting the secondary crossed fibers of nociceptive transmission on both sides, effectively relieving pain in the bilateral or midline areas, with less risk of motor nerve bundle injury than two unilateral disruptions of the spinal thalamic tract, and preserving tactile and motor sensation, with less impact on motor and autonomic functions. The surgery severed the connecting fibers that crossed the anterior part of the central canal, thus also blocking the thalamic tract of the spinal cord bilaterally. Viswanathan and colleagues performed an anterior spinal cord dissection of the thoracic segment for severe cancer pain in the lower abdomen, pelvis, or legs in LL patients. In 1997, Nauta and colleagues proposed that anterior spinal cord dissection should be performed purely for the purpose of relieving visceral pain and that the dissection should include the visceral pain pathways of the spinal cord, so that the dissection site should not be lower than the T_8 level of the upper thoracic segment [18].

1. Indications

   Anterior spinal cord commissurotomy is indicated for chronic pain in the thoracic, abdominal, pelvic, perineal, or lower extremities, and also for intractable pain due to spinal arachnoiditis, trauma, radiculitis, etc.

   The procedure is well suited for patients suffering from severe somatic and/or bilateral lower extremity pain. Patients suffering from abdominal or pelvic organ and bilateral lower extremity pain are better suited to undergo anterior spinal cord commissurotomy than anterolateral spinal cord fasciculotomy.

2. Surgical method

   The patient is placed under general anesthesia in the prone position and the target spinal cord segment (T_{10} ~ L_1 in most patients) is located. The dura mater is incised along the midline to expose the spinal cord. The midpoint between the dorsal roots of the spinal cord into the medullary region on both sides is found under the microscope. Then, using an arachnoid knife or microsurgical blade, the soft spinal membrane and spinal cord are incised longitudinally along the midline until the soft spinal membrane can be seen through the anterior sulcus.

   Similar to the anterolateral spinal cord bundle dissection, the key to avoiding complications when performing an anterior spinal cord commissurotomy is to clarify the location of the anterior spinal artery. Dexamethasone may be given postoperatively to reduce edema. If the surgical result is definitive, the patient can significantly reduce the use of analgesic drugs in the days after surgery.

3. Efficacy

   Most patients had good or better pain relief. The main difference between anterior commissurotomy and the limited midline spinal cord dissection is that anterior spinal cord dissection relieves the body of bilateral lower extremity pain and visceral pain. In contrast, a limited midline spinal cord dissection has a better outcome for simple visceral pain. Good or better relief of visceral pain has been reported in more than 50% of patients who underwent limited midline spinal cord dissection.

4. Complications

   Patients undergoing this type of surgery are usually in the advanced stages of cancer and thus have a high number of complications that can directly affect the patient's prognosis. In general, leg weakness (bilateral or unilateral) is the more serious complication, with an incidence of approximately 27%, and may be related to damage to the dorsal microstructure of the spinal cord, which can cause an abnormal sensation, sensory dullness or gait disturbance, or even severe burning sensation in the legs.

9.1.4 Posterior Median Spinal Cord Punctal Dissection

For a long time, there has been a lack of a safe and effective minimally invasive surgical method for intractable visceral pain. Traditional procedures such as anterolateral cordotomy, dorsal root entry zone dissection, and anterior commissurotomy are more effective in the treatment of trunk and extremity pain, but the results for visceral pain are mostly unsatisfactory. In the 1990s, Al-Chaer and Willis et al. [19–23] showed that visceral nociceptive conduction was mainly through the middle of the dorsal column (DC) of the ipsilateral spinal cord to the nucleus accumbens, and then through the nucleus tractus solitarius. The contralateral posterior lateral thalamic nucleus projects to the postcentral gyrus of the cerebral cortex. For visceral nociceptive transmission in the pelvis and lower abdomen, the role of the dorsal column of the spinal cord is even greater than that of the thalamic tract. Based on this theory, Nauta et al. in the United States in 1997 first reported a posterior median spinal cord punctate midline myelotomy [18], which was performed at the level of T_8 of the spinal cord to treat pelvic visceral pain caused by cervical cancer, and the procedure achieved more satisfactory results without other serious complications, except for transient lower limb numbness after surgery. This procedure selectively cut the middle part of the dorsal column of the spinal cord, blocking the conduction of visceral pain without damaging other important structures such as the thalamic tract of the spinal cord. The operation is operated under microscope, with high precision, less trauma, easy operation, more certain efficacy, and fewer complications, which can effectively control pain symptoms, reduce the dosage of analgesic drugs, significantly improve patients' quality of life, and create conditions for other treatments such as radiotherapy, immunotherapy, and biological therapy for tumor patients, and is an effective method for treating various intractable visceral pains.

1. Indications

   It is suitable for the treatment of cancerous visceral pain caused by various pelvic, abdominal, and thoracic organ tumors in the advanced stage; it is also suitable for stubborn visceral pain caused by chronic inflammation, radiotherapy, chemotherapy, and other reasons. However, it is not suitable for patients with severe dysfunction of multiple organs in the advanced stage of the tumor, severe bleeding tendency, or patients with tumor metastasis or infiltration near the operation site, local infection, ulcer, or necrosis.
2. Surgical method

   The operation is performed under general anesthesia, with the patient in pronc position. According to the location and extent of pain, the surgical segments for posterior median spinal cord dissection are determined; $T_{7,8}$ for pelvic pain, $T_{4,5}$ for lower abdominal pain, and $T_{2,3}$ for upper abdominal pain. For thoracic pain, surgery may cause serious complications such as respiratory muscle paralysis because the corresponding spinal cord segment is in the high cervical medulla, so surgery is generally performed with caution. The spinal processes of the corresponding vertebrae are occluded, a window (approximately 2 cm × 3 cm) is opened in the middle of the vertebral plate, and the dura is incised longitudinally along the midline. Under the operating microscope, a sharp-tipped blade is used to make a punctate incision approximately 2 mm wide and 5 mm deep on each side of the posterior median sulcus of the spinal cord to sever the visceral pain-conducting fibers in the middle part of the dorsal column of the spinal cord. During the operation, care should be taken to protect the posterior median spinal cord vein, which needs to be separated and pulled to one side before incising the posterior median spinal cord. The angle of the spinal cord incision should be perpendicular to the spinal cord surface, and care should be taken not to deviate too much from the midline or cut too deeply to avoid damaging other important structures of the spinal cord.

3. Efficacy

   In 1999, Becker et al. in Germany reported a patient with epigastric and mid-abdominal pain after lung cancer surgery, and the pain was significantly relieved after T_4 posterior median spinal cord dissection. Visceral pain is caused by gastric cancer, and 63% of the patients had satisfactory pain relief. In 2001, Villela-Filho et al. successfully treated two cases of intractable pelvic pain by using a CT-guided percutaneous puncture technique for posterior median spinal cord dissection.

4. Complications

   Transient lower limb numbness and deep sensory loss mostly occur after surgery and will gradually recover after a period of time, which may be related to surgical stimulation of the spinal cord, injury to the thin bundle, or postoperative edema involving the thin bundle, without any serious complications in general.

9.2 Psychological Treatment

Pain is one of the main clinical manifestations of visceral pain as a group of diseases. Psychological factors play an important role in pain perception and pain response, such as stress and emotions, which can influence the pathological development and outcome of visceral pain. Pain experience encompasses multiple dimensions such as sensory, emotional, cognitive, and behavioral. Pain therapies that focus only on a single dimension of the pain experience are doomed to failure. Instead, interventions that address multiple dimensions of pain, such as reducing the patient's physiological burden and alleviating negative emotions to change negative cognitions, will benefit the patient's recovery. Verbal guidance, distraction, re-empowering interpretation of situations, and a sense of self-control can all have a dramatic impact on the pain experience. Based on this evidence, psychologists and psychiatrists have developed a range of psychotherapeutic approaches to pain management. A growing number of studies have now demonstrated that psychotherapy can enhance the prognosis of patients with visceral pain, particularly in patients with moderate-to-severe pain symptoms, those who have had poor results with conventional medications, or those whose pain symptoms are exaggerated by psychogenic factors (stress, emotions, etc.). Psychotherapy can help control pain by improving the patient's self-efficacy. Having a high sense of self-efficacy regarding pain control can reduce psychological stress in daily life, reduce pain interference, and thus improve the patient's quality of life. These are made possible by the fact that psychotherapy can help patients acquire daily life skills to combat persistent pain, such as coping with increased pain, managing various negative emotions induced by pain (anxiety, fear, depression, etc.), and maintaining a positive and optimistic outlook. In addition, individualized psychotherapy may synergistically enhance with pharmacological treatment of pain, resulting in effective analgesia and facilitating clinical recovery. However, in order to achieve this goal, it is difficult to achieve it with a single pharmacological treatment alone. In developing an individualized psychotherapy program, it is particularly important to consider individual patient factors, such as the patient's personality traits, current situation (relevant life events, reasons for engaging in psychotherapy), the meaning the patient attributes to the illness (punishment or guilt), the patient's coping mechanisms for pain, and consistent behavior patterns. All of these factors can be used as predictors of psychotherapy efficacy and patient prognosis.

9.2.1 Relaxation Therapy

As a fundamental component of most pain psychotherapy, relaxation is effective in reducing the activity of the sympathetic and motor nervous systems. In a competitive situation, the body is often in a state of tension and stress, always ready for a possible sudden emergency, that is, the "fight-flight response." This psychological stress response will accelerate the body's adrenaline secretion, resulting in muscle tension, increased blood pressure, heart rate, and respiratory speed. This series of physiological activities will eventually feed back to the nervous system, producing a sense of tension and excitement, and may even directly trigger pain (such as tension headaches and low back pain), or indirectly affect the neuronal activity associated with projecting pain signals to the brain.

Benson et al. suggested that the "relaxation response" is the basis for all medical interventions. Based on their theory of the relaxation response, Benson developed a set of simple and easy-to-use relaxation techniques designed to guide individuals through progressive training to gradually relax various muscle groups in the body. The specific steps are as follows.

1. Sit quietly in a comfortable position and close your eyes.
2. Deeply relax the body muscles from the bottom up.
3. Breathe through the nose and pay attention to the rhythm of one exhale and one inhale. Whisper the word "one" with each exhalation. Repeat this step for up to 20 min. When you have completed this 20-min exercise, keep your eyes closed for a few minutes, and then slowly open them again.
4. Throughout the process, do not worry about whether or not you have successfully achieved a state of deep relaxation. Maintain a passive experience and let the relaxation happen naturally. When other distracting thoughts intrude, ignore them as much as possible and practice step 3 repeatedly. Practice this 1–2 times a day. Because the digestive process can affect this change in subjective experience, relaxation training should be avoided within 2 h of a meal.

This simple relaxation technique described above has been shown to affect physiological signs and produce deep relaxation effects such as lower metabolic rate, blood pressure, and respiratory rate. Compared to placebo, relaxation is effective in relieving tension headaches. Although there are no studies on the efficacy of relaxation for visceral pain, this technique has been used in the treatment of a range of clinical pathologies of pain and has been included in the treatment protocol for severe chronic pain, with further clinical applications of this technique to be pursued in the future.

9.2.2 Biofeedback

Biofeedback is to detect and amplify various information generated by human physiological activities, including brain waves, heart function, respiration, muscle activity, and skin temperature, with the help of sophisticated tools, and transform the information into easy-to-understand signals through display systems, so that individuals can learn to use the signals from their own physiological activities to consciously control various physiological processes in the body and promote the recovery of physiological functions, thus achieving the purpose of treating diseases. Often, biofeedback training can be combined with relaxation exercises to achieve better therapeutic results.

Research on the efficacy of biofeedback applied to chronic abdominal pain is very limited, with only a few results from studies of irritable bowel syndrome. Most current literature reviews point to the lack of evidence-based medicine for the clinical treatment of biofeedback applications in gastrointestinal disorders. There are still many questions regarding the effectiveness of biofeedback in the treatment of constipation, fecal incontinence, and abdominal pain. Nevertheless, some studies have confirmed the effectiveness of biofeedback in the treatment of visceral pain. Among them, thermal biofeedback combined with dietary therapy can be an effective treatment for recurrent abdominal pain: forehead EMG biofeedback and thermal biofeedback can relieve stress in patients with irritable bowel syndrome; EMG biofeedback can also significantly reduce the occurrence of constipation; biofeedback-guided relaxation exercises, including progressive muscle relaxation, thermal biofeedback, and cognitive therapy, can effectively reduce the gastrointestinal contractile function of the body by only 4 h of biofeedback training to control heart rate. However, these studies may have overstated the therapeutic effects of biofeedback because they used a randomized clinical control design and failed to effectively control for the desired effect of the control group (placebo). In addition, studies of biofeedback combined with breathing exercises in patients with functional dyspepsia have shown significant improvements in patients' tolerance of water intake and quality-of-life scores, but this study lacked observations on the long-term prognosis of patients and the efficacy of the control treatment group.

From the above clinical studies on biofeedback, it can be seen that biofeedback is a promising technique for clinical application, which can effectively distract patients, assist in relaxation exercises, and help patients gain a sense of self-control over their pain. The combination of biofeedback and other psychotherapeutic methods can significantly enhance the analgesic effect.

9.2.3 Hypnotherapy

Hypnosis (hypnosis) is a subconscious state of high internal concentration and self-focus. The intervention procedure of analgesia through hypnosis includes the induction of a relaxed state, guiding the individual to focus attention and inward focus, relatively suppressing the individual's awareness of the surrounding environment, and combining it with verbal guidance for analgesia.

Hypnosis has a therapeutic effect. Several independent randomized clinical controlled trials have demonstrated that hypnotherapy is an effective psychological treatment for irritable bowel syndrome, providing symptom relief and improving quality of life. In a systematic review, one investigator noted that hypnotherapy provides lasting improvements in patient symptoms, significantly affects colorectal sensitivity and motor function, and relieves psychological stress (e.g., anxiety, depression, nonadaptive cognitions) triggered by chronic bowel symptoms. After systematic hypnotherapy, 81% of patients maintained symptom improvement for 5 years, which shows that the effect of hypnotherapy is long-lasting and solid. In addition, hypnotherapy is not only effective in relieving the major symptom clusters of most patients with irritable bowel syndrome, but also positively affects noncolorectal classes of symptoms. For example, hypnotherapy can restore patients' visceral pain thresholds to normal, and changes in pain thresholds are significantly associated with improvements in clinical symptoms; the sensory and motor-related components of patients' gastrointestinal responses can also be significantly reduced by hypnotherapy.

Despite the success of hypnotherapy in the adjuvant treatment of irritable bowel syndrome, the analgesic mechanism of hypnosis remains unclear. The efficacy of hypnotherapy for other types of visceral pain also needs further validation. In addition, since hypnosis is indicated for those groups with high suggestibility characteristics, and less than 15% of people have such hypnotic susceptibility, hypnotherapy may have many difficulties in using it for nonhypnotic susceptible people, and it may even be difficult to be truly hypnotized, so the scope of hypnotherapy is somewhat limited.

9.2.4 Psychological Counseling

Psychological counseling aims to understand the patient's current situation and the unspeakable problems they face through a series of intervention strategies with a unified goal, and to alleviate or even solve the patient's psychological problems and eventually achieve a state of psychological balance through various modalities such as individual therapy, group therapy, or family therapy. Currently, there are several different therapeutic orientations for psychological counseling of pain patients, and the efficacy studies with more sufficient evidence of evidence-based medicine focus on psychodynamic and cognitive-behavioral orientations of treatment. Only through a comprehensive assessment of the patient's physiological and psychological status and the selection of appropriate psychological counseling methods can ideal treatment results be achieved.

1. Psychodynamic therapy
   Psychodynamic-oriented counseling emphasizes the differences in individual development, internal psychological conflicts, interpersonal relationships and the ability to adapt to chronic diseases, and searches for subconscious conflicts that lead to the occurrence of psychological problems, and the elimination of subconscious conflicts is the key to treatment. Psychodynamic therapy has achieved very significant efficacy in the treatment of cancer pain, relieving the symptoms of cancer pain patients, reducing the psychological distress caused by the disease, and improving the overall survival quality of patients. This suggests that psychodynamic therapy may also have significant efficacy on visceral pain.
2. Cognitive-behavioral therapy
   Cognitive-behavioral therapy (CBT) is widely used to control chronic pain symptoms, especially in the treatment of irritable bowel syndrome, chronic pelvic pain (CPP), and noncardiogenic chest pain (NCCP). The therapy combines specific skills training (e.g., relaxation, pain coping skills) and cognitive therapy (restructuring of negative cognitions, e.g., catastrophizing) to relieve pain, pain-induced disability, and stress, while enhancing the patient's sense of self-efficacy.

   In irritable bowel syndrome, both progressive muscle relaxation training and cognitive therapy are effective in reducing gastrointestinal reactions compared to self-help control interventions. In addition, the implementation of multivariate behavioral therapy (extended progressive muscle relaxation training with the addition of coping strategies and problem-solving skills) in addition to conventional treatment can greatly alleviate the abdominal pain symptoms of irritable bowel syndrome and improve patients' quality of life, despite the absence of any improvement in sensory allergy to rectal bladder dilation. Group cognitive-behavioral therapy also relieves pain and gastrointestinal reactions, increases patients' use of positive coping strategies, and reduces withdrawal behaviors, and these effects persist for up to 4 years as treatment progresses. A recent multisite trial of cognitive-behavioral therapy for severe functional bowel disorders showed that cognitive-behavioral therapy was more effective than verbal instruction alone in reducing symptoms in all subtypes of irritable bowel syndrome, whereas desipramine was more effective than placebo only for specific clinical subtypes, suggesting that psycho-behavioral interventions have broad application in the treatment of irritable bowel syndrome.

   Recently, researchers have modified the standardized cognitive-behavioral treatment protocol for irritable bowel syndrome to shorten the length of the intervention and make this therapy more practical for large-scale clinical application. For example, cognitive-behavioral therapy divided into eight sessions compared to usual care and a single long session of cognitive-behavioral therapy both improved patients' quality of life, but the former produced more solid treatment effects, reduced gastrointestinal reactions, and relieved psychological stress, suggesting that brief and efficient cognitive-behavioral therapy maintains long-term efficacy. In addition, patients' psychological distress varied along with their gastrointestinal response during the treatment. Patients with irritable bowel syndrome who successfully received cognitive-behavioral therapy showed fewer symptoms of depression and anxiety, while those whose gastrointestinal response did not improve failed to have their depression and anxiety symptoms relieved. Direct pharmacological treatment of psychiatric disorders in patients with irritable bowel syndrome was effective in improving both their gastrointestinal response and psychiatric symptoms. It is worth mentioning that the benefits from psychotherapy may have a cumulative effect over time, that is, they increase gradually over time. During the follow-up of up to 3–12 months after cognitive-behavioral therapy, the improvement in gastrointestinal symptoms was maintained and sustained, and their pain and bloating symptoms gradually decreased. In addition, patients also showed a reduction in depression and anxiety symptoms, and the reduction in gastrointestinal responses was significantly associated with an increase in positive automatic thinking and a decrease in negative automatic thinking.

In a series of 138 men with chronic pelvic pain, the researchers combined a technique called paradoxical relaxation training with myofascial trigger-point release therapy. Patients were guided by a psychologist for eight sessions and then began a 6-month period of home training. Patients continued to learn chest breathing and gradually accepted that muscle tension was also a form of muscle relaxation training. Overall, 72% of the patients showed a significant reduction in pain and urinary symptoms scores during the treatment. Although not technically a cognitive-behavioral intervention, a recent randomized controlled clinical trial of written emotional disclosure has shown that it is also effective in reducing evaluative pain in patients with chronic pelvic pain syndrome. Written emotional disclosure requires patients to spend 20 min a day writing about the impact of chronic pelvic pain syndrome on their lives and to practice this written expression for 3 days. This simple intervention has now been shown in several studies to be effective in relieving pain in patients with rheumatoid arthritis and fibromyalgia, although there are still some studies that have produced inconsistent results. It is worth pointing out that the efficacy of the emotional exposure approach may be modulated by factors related to mood and emotional expression.

Currently, researchers have developed a diverse array of interventions that combine exercise, biofeedback, and cognitive-behavioral therapy, operationalizing these interventions with relaxation tapes, electrodermal response biofeedback devices, and rapid relaxation exercises prompted by alarm watches, including verbal instruction, respiratory maintenance training (hyperventilation), physiological exercise, graded exposure, cognitive restructuring, and relaxation exercises. Small, uncontrolled studies have shown that this range of interventions significantly reduces the frequency of chest pain and depression, anxiety, and disability scores in patients with noncardiac chest pain, while enhancing exercise tolerance, and that these effects are maintained for up to 6 months. This result was validated in a randomized controlled trial of cognitive-behavioral therapy, and one study even further suggested that in addition to improving quality of life and mental status in patients with noncardiac chest pain, cognitive-behavioral therapy increased the likelihood that the pain would disappear after 6 months of treatment.

9.2.5 Mind–Body Intervention

In recent years, mind–body intervention has received much clinical and academic attention. Several studies have explored the efficacy of this therapy as an adjunctive clinical treatment for various types of pain. There is no doubt that stress can accumulate and exacerbate pain, and chronic pain is itself a form of intense stress. Therefore, treatments that relieve stress, promote relaxation, and enhance well-being have a wide range of clinical applications in visceral pain syndromes. A growing number of clinical studies suggest that combining mind–body therapies with existing treatments is particularly necessary.

If mind–body therapy can be used to relieve cancer pain, then it has high credibility for the treatment of visceral pain. Mind–body therapy is safe, inexpensive, and easy to administer. It can be done individually or in groups, and patients can often quickly master simple or even complex techniques. By maintaining a regular mind–body practice, patients can not only achieve improvement in their symptoms, but also increase their sense of self-efficacy and control over their current state.

Biofeedback in dysfunction aims to normalize the abnormal physiological functions whose changes are thought to underlie the symptoms of the disease. Nonadaptive thinking and perceptual biases can affect symptom severity and the interference of symptoms in the patient's life, and cognitive and cognitive-behavioral therapies can help identify such thinking patterns. Psychodynamic and interpersonal therapies aim to improve symptoms resulting from interpersonal difficulties. Stress management training (e.g., progressive muscle relaxation) is often combined with other specific interventions, such as biofeedback, hypnosis, and cognitive therapy, and these combined treatments help suppress sympathetic nervous system excitatory activity that may exacerbate or trigger disease symptoms and enhance overall health.

Several randomized controlled trials have shown significant efficacy of multimodal mind–body therapies for the treatment of a variety of visceral pain disorders, particularly in the treatment of pediatric patients with irritable bowel syndrome and recurrent abdominal pain. A recent review noted that mind–body therapies are effective in relieving the discomfort of gastrointestinal reactions. For example, biofeedback combined with cognitive therapy, stress management, and progressive muscle relaxation training reduces the occurrence of physical symptoms of irritable bowel syndrome as a whole, but only biofeedback and relaxation therapy can alleviate psychological symptom clusters.

9.2.6 Multidisciplinary Integrated Therapy

A growing body of research has demonstrated that multidisciplinary therapy can successfully treat chronic pain and has been further modified for the treatment of chronic pelvic pain syndrome. This intervention was initially tried by Rapkin and Kames and has been shown to be more effective than conventional treatment in a randomized controlled clinical trial [24]. Peter et al. further found that the overall pain, impairment in daily life, and other symptoms associated with chronic pelvic pain syndrome were significantly improved in women who received comprehensive treatment (including clinical consultation, psychotherapy, and physical therapy) compared to conventional treatment. Surprisingly, although many current reviews and commentaries highly tout the effectiveness of multidisciplinary integrative interventions (including cognitive-behavioral therapy, physical therapy), randomized controlled clinical trials are still lacking to further define the necessary components of this integrative approach.

References

1. Spiller WG. The treatment of persistent pain of organic origin in the lower part of the body by division of the anterolateral column of the spinal cord. JAMA J Am Med Assoc. 1912;LVIII(20):1489. https://doi.org/10.1001/jama.1912.04260050165001.
2. Mullan S, Harper PV, Hekmatpanah J, Torres H, Dobbin G. Percutaneous interruption of spinal-pain tracts by means of a Strontium90 needle. J Neurosurg. 1963;20(11):931–9. https://doi.org/10.3171/jns.1963.20.11.0931.
3. Dalal S, Hui D, Nguyen L, Chacko R, Scott C, Roberts L, et al. Achievement of personalized pain goal in cancer patients referred to a supportive care clinic at a comprehensive cancer center. Cancer. 2011;118(15):3869–77. https://doi.org/10.1002/cncr.26694.
4. Cowie RA, Hitchcock ER. The late results of antero-lateral cordotomy for pain relief. Acta Neurochir. 1982;64(1–2):39–50. https://doi.org/10.1007/bf01405617.
5. Piscol K. Open spinal surgery for (intractable) pain. Brain Hypoxia. 1975:157–69. https://doi.org/10.1007/978-3-642-66239-3_21.
6. Mansuy L, Sindou M, Fischer G, Brunon J. La cordotomie spino-thalamique dans les douleurs cancéreuses. Résultats d'une série de 124 malades opérés par abord direct postérieur [Spino-thalamic cordotomy in cancerous pain. Results of a series of 124 patients operated on by the direct posterior approach]. Neurochirurgie. 1976;22(5):437–44. French.
7. Lahuerta J, Bowsher D, Lipton S, Buxton PH. Percutaneous cervical cordotomy: a review of 181 operations on 146 patients with a study on the location of "pain fibers" in the C-2 spinal cord segment of 29 cases. J Neurosurg. 1994;80(6):975–85. https://doi.org/10.3171/jns.1994.80.6.0975.

8. Seba MC, Bernardo HN, Sarturi NM, Rossi TG, Oliveira NM, Aguiar PH. Cervical cordotomy in terminal cancer: pain relieving in oncological treatment. Arquivos Brasileiros de Neurocirurgia (Braz Neurosurg). 2020;40(01):071–7. https://doi.org/10.1055/s-0040-1718425.
9. Lahuerta J, Lipton S, Miles J. Percutaneous radio frequency gangliolysis in the treatment of trigeminal neuralgia. Eur Neurol. 1985;24(4):272–5. https://doi.org/10.1159/000115806.
10. 27th Annual meeting Chicago, Illinois, May 12–15, 2004. J Gen Intern Med. 2004;19(S1):23–241. https://doi.org/10.1111/j.1525-1497.2004.s1006_1.x.
11. Fox LM, Hoffman RS, Vlahov D, Manini AF. Risk factors for severe respiratory depression from prescription opioid overdose. Addiction. 2017;113(1):59–66. https://doi.org/10.1111/add.13925.
12. Nashold BS, Ostdahl RH. Dorsal root entry zone lesions for pain relief. J Neurosurg. 1979;51(1):59–69. https://doi.org/10.3171/jns.1979.51.1.0059.
13. Sindou M, Peronnet F, Laviron A, Quoex F, Gerin P, Courjon J. Étude comparative des Données électroencéphalographiques, transcorticographiques et straticorticographiques. Revue Electroencéphalographie et de Neurophysiologie Clinique. 1972;2(2):183–8. https://doi.org/10.1016/s0370-4475(72)80064-9.
14. Saiz-Sapena N, Vanaclocha-Vanaclocha V, María Ortiz-Criado J, Vanaclocha L, Vanaclocha N. Treatment of neuropathic pain in brachial plexus injuries. In: Treatment of brachial plexus injuries. InTech Open; 2019. https://doi.org/10.5772/intechopen.82084.
15. Tomáš R, Haninec P. Dorsal root entry zone (drez) localization using direct spinal cord stimulation can improve results of the drez thermocoagulation procedure for intractable pain relief. Pain. 2005;116(1):159–63. https://doi.org/10.1016/j.pain.2005.03.015.
16. Falci S, Best L, Bayles R, Lammertse D, Starnes C. Dorsal root entry zone microcoagulation for spinal cord injury—related central pain: operative intramedullary electrophysiological guidance and clinical outcome. J Neurosurg Spine. 2002;97(2):193–200. https://doi.org/10.3171/spi.2002.97.2.0193.
17. Friedman AH, Bullitt E. Dorsal root entry zone lesions in the treatment of pain following brachial plexus avulsion, spinal cord injury and herpes zoster. Stereotact Funct Neurosurg. 1988;51(2–5):164–9. https://doi.org/10.1159/000099959.
18. Nauta HJ, Hewitt E, Westlund KN, Willis WD. Surgical interruption of a midline dorsal column visceral pain pathway. J Neurosurg. 1997;86(3):538–42. https://doi.org/10.3171/jns.1997.86.3.0538.
19. Al-Chaer ED, Lawand NB, Westlund KN, Willis WD. Pelvic visceral input into the nucleus gracilis is largely mediated by the postsynaptic dorsal column pathway. J Neurophysiol. 1996;76(4):2675–90. https://doi.org/10.1152/jn.1996.76.4.2675.
20. Al-Chaer ED, Lawand NB, Westlund KN, Willis WD. Visceral nociceptive input into the ventral posterolateral nucleus of the thalamus: a new function for the dorsal column pathway. J Neurophysiol. 1996;76(4):2661–74. https://doi.org/10.1152/jn.1996.76.4.2661.
21. Al-Chaer ED, Westlund KN, Willis WD. Sensitization of postsynaptic dorsal column neuronal responses by colon inflammation. Neuroreport. 1997;8(15):3267–73. https://doi.org/10.1097/00001756-199710200-00016.
22. Al-Chaer ED, Feng Y, Willis WD. A role for the dorsal column in nociceptive visceral input into the thalamus of primates. J Neurophysiol. 1998;79(6):3143–50. https://doi.org/10.1152/jn.1998.79.6.3143.
23. Al-Chaer ED, Feng Y, Willis WD. Comparative study of viscerosomatic input onto postsynaptic dorsal column and spinothalamic tract neurons in the primate. J Neurophysiol. 1999;82(4):1876–82. https://doi.org/10.1152/jn.1999.82.4.1876.
24. Kames LD, Rapkin AJ, Naliboff BD, Afifi S, Ferrer-Brechner T. Effectiveness of an interdisciplinary pain management program for the treatment of chronic pelvic pain. Pain. 1990;41(1):41–6. https://doi.org/10.1016/0304-3959(90)91107-t.

Chest Pain

10

Ningning Ji

10.1 Introduction

Acute chest pain is one of the most common reasons for visits to the hospital, particularly the emergency department (ED). The annual incidence of chest pain in the primary care population is approximately 15.5%, with 20–40% of patients having a lifetime complaint. The prevalence is high in the elderly population, with men predominating. Among the 1,869,010 chest pain patients recorded by the China Chest Pain Center in 2020, 647,472 patients (33.57%) had acute coronary syndrome (ACS), 498,705 patients (26.68%) had non-ACS cardiogenic chest pain, 27,957 patients (1.5%) had non-ACS vascular emergencies, and 714,876 patients (38.25%) had chest pain with other causes [1].

A Chinese domestic clinical study of ACS reported that up to 20% of patients had a discharge diagnosis that did not match the objective findings, which may have been missed and misdiagnosed, suggesting the need to improve the accuracy of prehospital diagnosis [1]. The difficulty lies in differentiating patients with ACS or other life-threatening conditions from those with noncardiovascular, nonlife-threatening chest pain. ACS is missed in about 2% of patients, leading to serious consequences. For example, wrongly discharging patients with acute myocardial infarction (AMI) from the ED has a short-term mortality rate that is twice as high as the expected mortality rate of admitted patients. However, for patients at low risk for complications, these concerns must be balanced against the cost and inconvenience of hospital admission and the risk of complications from tests and procedures that have a lower probability of improving patient prognosis. Several recent advances have improved the accuracy and efficiency of the evaluation of patients with acute chest pain, including better cardiovascular markers of myocardial injury, decision aids to stratify patients according to risk of complications, early or even immediate exercise testing, and radionuclide scans for a subset of patients at lower risk. For example, multilayer computed tomography for anatomic evaluation of coronary artery disease, pulmonary embolism and aortic coarctation, and effective and rapid evaluation of low-risk patients using chest pain units and critical pathways [2].

10.2 Causes of Acute Chest Pain

Approximately 15–25% of the typical population evaluated in the emergency room for acute chest pain has an acute MI or unstable angina. A small percentage have other life-threatening problems, such as pulmonary embolism or acute aortic coarctation, but most are discharged without a diagnosis of cardiac disease or with a diagnosis of noncardiac disease. These noncardiac condi-

N. Ji (✉)
Department of Anesthesiology, Shanghai Ninth People's Hospital Affiliated to Shanghai Jiao Tong University School of Medicine, Shanghai, China

M. Xia et al. (eds.), *Visceral Pain*, https://doi.org/10.1007/978-981-99-9167-9_10

tions include musculoskeletal syndromes, abdominal visceral diseases (including gastroesophageal reflux disease), and psychological disorders [2, 3].

10.2.1 Myocardial Ischemia (MI)

The most common cause of acute chest discomfort is myocardial ischemia or infarction, which occurs when the supply of myocardial oxygen is inadequate compared to the demand. Myocardial ischemia usually occurs in the setting of coronary atherosclerosis, but it may also reflect a dynamic component of coronary vascular resistance. Coronary artery spasm can occur in normal coronary arteries or, in patients with coronary artery disease, in the vicinity of atherosclerotic plaques and in smaller coronary arteries. Other less common causes of impaired coronary blood flow include syndromes that damage the coronary artery orifice or lumen, such as coronary arteritis, proximal aortitis, spontaneous coronary artery entrapment, proximal aortic entrapment, infectious or noninfectious endocarditis or coronary embolism due to left atrial or left ventricular thrombus, myocardial bridges, or congenital anomalies of the coronary arteries [2].

The typical manifestation of ischemia is angina pectoris, often described as a heavy pressure or squeezing sensation in the chest, a burning sensation, or difficulty in breathing. This discomfort often radiates to the left shoulder, neck, or arm. It usually increases gradually over a few minutes. Pain may begin with exercise or psychological stress, but ACS most often occurs without an obvious precipitating factor.

The atypical description of chest pain reduces the likelihood that these symptoms represent myocardial ischemia or injury. The American College of Cardiology (ACC) and American Heart Association (AHA) guidelines list the following pain descriptions that are not characteristic of myocardial ischemia [4]:

1. Chest pain (i.e., sharp or knife-like pain brought on by breathing movements or coughing)
2. The main or only site of discomfort is in the mid- or lower abdominal region
3. The pain may be localized to one fingertip, especially at the apex of the left ventricle
4. Pain recurs with movement or palpation of the chest wall or arm
5. Pain that lasts for several hours
6. Very brief episodes of pain lasting a few seconds or less
7. Pain that radiates to the lower extremities

Data from a large number of patients with acute chest pain suggest that ACS occurs with such frequency in patients with atypical symptoms that a single factor should not be used to exclude the diagnosis of acute ischemic heart disease. In particular, women, the elderly, and diabetic patients may be more likely to report atypical symptoms of myocardial ischemia or infarction [2].

10.2.2 Pericardial Disease

The visceral surface of the pericardium is insensitive to pain, as is most of the parietal surface. As a result, noninfectious pericarditis usually involves little or no pain. In contrast, infectious pericarditis almost always involves the surrounding pleura, and, as a result, patients usually experience pleuritic pain when breathing, coughing, and changing position. Pain may be induced by swallowing because of the proximity of the esophagus to the posterior part of the heart. Because the central diaphragm receives sensory supply from the phrenic nerve, which arises from the third through fifth cervical segments of the spinal cord, pain in infectious pericarditis is often felt in the shoulder and neck. More lateral involvement of the diaphragm can lead to symptoms in the upper abdomen and back that are confused with pancreatitis or cholecystitis. Pericarditis occasionally causes steady, compressive subxiphoid pain, similar to acute MI.

10.2.3 Vascular Disease

Acute aortic segmentation usually causes sudden onset of severe tearing pain, the location of which reflects the site and progression of the dissection.

Ascending aortic entrapment tends to present as pain in the anterior midline of the chest, while posterior descending aortic entrapment tends to present as pain in the posterior chest. Aortic dissection is rare, with an estimated incidence of 3/100,000 per year, and usually occurs in the presence of risk factors, including Marfan and Ehlers–Danlos syndrome, aortic mitral valve, pregnancy (for proximal dissection), and hypertension (for distal dissection).

Pulmonary embolisms often lead to sudden onset of dyspnea and chest pain, although they may be asymptomatic. The incidence rate is about 1 in 1000 per year, but this number may be underestimated. Large pulmonary emboli often cause severe, persistent substernal pain, which is caused by the expansion of the pulmonary arteries. Smaller emboli causing pulmonary infarction can cause lateral pleuritic chest pain. Pulmonary emboli in the hemodynamic sense may cause hypotension, syncope, and symptoms of right heart failure. Pulmonary hypertension may cause chest pain similar to angina pectoris, possibly due to right heart hypertrophy and ischemia.

10.2.4 Pulmonary Disease

Pulmonary diseases that cause chest pain usually produce dyspnea and pleurisy symptoms, the location of which reveals the site of the lung disease. Tracheobronchitis is often associated with midline burning pain, while pneumonia produces pain in the affected lung. Pain in a pneumothorax occurs suddenly and is usually accompanied by dyspnea. Primary pneumothorax usually occurs in tall, thin young men; secondary pneumothorax occurs in the presence of lung diseases such as chronic obstructive pulmonary disease, asthma, or cystic fibrosis. Chest discomfort, typically characterized by constriction, can occur with exacerbations of asthma.

10.2.5 Gastrointestinal Disorders

Irritation of the esophagus by acid reflux produces a burning discomfort that is exacerbated by alcohol, aspirin, and some foods. Symptoms are often exacerbated by recumbent position and relieved by upright sitting position and acid reduction therapy. Esophageal spasm can produce a squeezing chest discomfort similar to angina pectoris. Mallory–Weiss tears of the esophagus can occur in patients who have been vomiting for a long time. Severe vomiting can also cause esophageal rupture, that is, Boerhaave's syndrome, with mediastinitis. Chest pain due to peptic ulcer disease often occurs 60–90 min after a meal and is usually rapidly relieved by acid reduction therapy. This pain normally presents in the upper abdomen, but can radiate to the chest and shoulders. Cholecystitis produces a widespread pain syndrome that usually causes right upper abdominal pain, but chest and back pain caused by this disease is not uncommon. The pain is described as vague or colicky. Pancreatitis frequently causes intense, vague epigastric pain that may radiate to the back. Relief through acid reduction therapy is limited.

10.2.6 Musculoskeletal and Other Causes

Chest pain can be caused by musculoskeletal disorders involving the chest wall such as costochondritis, disorders affecting the nerves in the chest wall such as cervical disc disease, herpes zoster, or after strenuous exercise. Musculoskeletal syndromes that bring chest pain are usually the result of direct pressure on the affected area or by the patient's neck movements. The pain itself may be brief or a dull ache that lasts for several hours. Panic syndrome is a major cause of chest discomfort in ED patients. Symptoms include chest tightness, often accompanied by shortness of breath and feelings of anxiety, and typically last 30 min or longer.

10.3 Classifications of Chest Pain

There are various types of chest pain. In general, according to its cause, it can be divided into two categories: noncardiac chest pain (NCCP) and cardiogenic chest pain. The previous section also introduced how chest pain is generated due to different conditions related to or irrelevant to cardio conditions. In this section, classifying them enables the recognition of diseases causing chest pain.

10.3.1 Noncardiac Chest Pain (NCCP)

NCCP is an angina-type discomfort without signs of ischemia. Because of its heterogeneity, diagnosis can be difficult. Classification varies among specialties; gastroenterology uses the terminology related to gastroesophageal reflux disease versus non-gastroesophageal reflux disease. Other disciplines consider NCCP to have an underlying gastrointestinal, musculoskeletal, psychiatric, or pulmonary/other etiology. Diagnosis yields a specific etiology for effective treatment, which aims to identify the underlying cause, but this is not always possible. Some patients with NCCP have comorbidities and persistent pain that result in decreased quality of life and continued use of healthcare services.

NCCP is often described as a burning, angina-like pain located in the sternal region with no evidence of ischemic disease. It is also known as atypical chest pain, effort syndrome, soldier's heart, irritable heart, DaCosta syndrome, unexplained chest pain, neurocirculatory debility, cardiac syndrome X, Gorlin–Likoff syndrome unexplained chest pain, and functional chest pain. There is inconsistency in the literature, especially among specialties, regarding the underlying etiology and how to classify it. Gastrointestinal specialties consider NCCP as a unique diagnosis that can be distinguished as gastroesophageal reflux disease (GERD)-related or non-GERD-related. Other specialties define NCCP more broadly.

The classification of NCCP varies by specialty. Its causes are broadly classified as gastrointestinal, musculoskeletal, psychiatric, and pulmonary/other.

The sheer number of conditions that cause NCCP and the variety of definitions and terminology make the understanding of the conditions challenging. NCCP occurs in approximately 13–25% of the general population, men and women alike [5]. However, women are more likely to present with symptoms of anxiety. Compared to patients with ischemic chest pain, patients with NCCP tend to be younger, have greater anxiety, drink more alcohol, and smoke more.

NCCP is a challenge to the healthcare system. Chest pain is the second most common cause of ED visits. NCCP results in frequent and repeated hospitalizations or outpatient visits. For example, in the United States, evaluation of nonspecific chest pain accounted for 233,200 ED visits among patients aged 45–64 years in 2011 [6]. Evaluation of chest pain typically involves electrocardiogram (ECG), monitoring, serial laboratory studies, cardiac stress testing, and various imaging modalities for intermediate care.

In addition to the healthcare system, there is a burden on the patients themselves. Persistent chest pain interferes with the daily life of these patients and leads to a reduced quality of life. In addition, NCCP can lead to mental stress, employment difficulties, family stress, and disability [7].

10.3.1.1 Etiologies of NCCP

Life-threatening conditions should be evaluated first. Cardiac events requiring rapid recognition and treatment are not limited but include acute coronary syndromes, aortic dissection, aortic stenosis, pericarditis, and pericardial tamponade. Extracardiac conditions may include tension pneumothorax, pulmonary embolism, or esophageal rupture.

Some forms of NCCP have a specific underlying condition, and some have features similar to other unexplained physical symptoms. The three main categories of NCCP identified include musculoskeletal, upper gastrointestinal, and disorders with a psychological component.

Gastrointestinal disorders causing chest pain can generally be traced to the esophagus, allergic disorders, or movement disorders. Among the gastrointestinal disorders, GERD is the most likely cause of NCCP.

Musculoskeletal chest wall pain can be induced by diseases that cause isolated pain, rheumatic diseases, or other systemic disorders.

Costochondritis is the most common cause of musculoskeletal chest pain.

Psychological disorders, such as anxiety and depression, may also lead to chest pain. Panic attacks may play a role in NCCP as well.

Given its complexity, the pathophysiology of NCCP has not been clearly defined. This is partly due to the large number of conditions that induce NCCP, leading to multiple potential mechanism changes. For example, gastroesophageal NCCP may be secondary to reflux, receptor changes, or altered sensory or processing of neural stimuli. In addition, NCCP patients may present with abnormal chest breathing, that is, hyperventilation. To escalate the complexity, patients may have more than one physiological cause. Husser and colleagues reviewed 37 patients with NCCP and found that approximately 16% had more than one diagnosis [8]. Another example is that fibromyalgia is associated with NCCP.

Psychological conditions are noted as a potential etiology. In some patients, psychological conditions may coexist with NCCP. Patients with NCCP may suffer from both psychiatric conditions and asthma, pneumonia, musculoskeletal, or other painful conditions. Depression and anxiety disorders are particularly associated with NCCP and can affect pain. Moreover, patients with NCCP are prone to do more self-monitoring and have poorer coping skills.

Lifestyle choices are also a potential factor contributing to the development of chest pain and need to be investigated for cardiac versus noncardiac origins. Food choices such as greasy/rich foods, spicy foods, acidic foods such as tomatoes and citrus fruits, mint, and overeating are suspected to be risk factors for NCCP. Beverages, such as alcohol and carbonated beverages, are also risk factors. Apart from being a risk factor for coronary artery disease, smoking also plays a role in causing GERD. Furthermore, there are connections between anxiety and smoking [9]. Cocaine may cause chest pain due to its effects on the sympathetic nervous system, myocytes, and blood vessels.

10.3.1.2 Evaluation of NCCP

Although life- and limb-threatening conditions should be ruled out first, Morrow summarized the approach to be considered after an urgent, life-threatening diagnosis has been ruled out: (1) Did a complication of a chronic disease cause the pain? (2) Did the acute illness cause the pain? (3) Is the pain secondary to another condition? Given the many different conditions in patients with chest pain symptoms, it is not possible to review all potential tests; therefore, gastroesophageal reflux disease, costochondritis, and anxiety are used as exemplars of potential etiologies of NCCP [10].

A thorough consultation of medical history should provide useful information about the chest pain. There are several ways to assess pain. For example, pain can be assessed with OPQRST (onset/duration, irritation or relief, quality, area or size of symptoms, severity, temporal pattern) or OLDCARTS (onset, location, duration, characteristics, exacerbation, relieving factors, treatment, or temporality). Pain assessment tools such as the McGill Pain Assessment Questionnaire, numeric rating scales, or visual analog scales are also convenient and effective. Associated symptoms such as nausea, diaphoresis, dyspnea, neurological symptoms, or palpitations should be considered.

History and physical examination are important for the diagnosis of NCCP. Apart from pain, a review of systems includes chief complaint, current symptoms, medical history (past medical, family, personal, social), perceived health status, functional status, and medication use should be taken into consideration as significant reference. The review of symptoms may include constitutional, cardiac, pulmonary, gastrointestinal, musculoskeletal, and psychiatric. The medical history taken should cover both patients' medical history and their family's history. After consulting the history, physical examination should be arranged accordingly. Specifically, the examinations may encompass hemodynamic stability, neurological, cardiac, pulmonary, abdominal musculoskeletal, and integumentary functions.

After cardiovascular disease has been excluded, gastroesophageal disease, primarily GERD, may be considered if the pain is associated with dysphagia, heartburn, and/or odynophagia, together with a pain lasting for at least an hour. Other symptoms may include pain associated with meals and a nonsmoker's cough that persists for more than 3 weeks. The GerdQ and Reflux Disease Questionnaire are tools that can be used to assess GERD. A clinical history is generally not sufficient, and additional testing should be supplemented. Some advocate that if an esophageal cause is suspected, the diagnosis is first made by a proton pump inhibitor (PPI) test. Evaluation of symptoms may suggest red flags such as anemia, loss of appetite, dysphagia, unintentional weight loss, dysphagia, or hematemesis, for which an upper gastrointestinal microscopy may be completed. If the results of the PPI test and/or endoscopy are inadequate, then additional testing, such as a wireless pH capsule, may be considered.

Chest pain that is reproducible with movement, such as manipulation or palpation, and supporting evidence of trauma or infection suggests a musculoskeletal etiology. Costochondritis may be described as a painful, compressive, or sharp pain that may worsen with deep breathing or exercise and is best evaluated with radiographs, computed tomography, or bone scans.

Psychiatric conditions such as anxiety may contribute to NCCP. Patients complaining of acute coronary syndrome-type symptoms lasting at least half an hour may be experiencing anxiety or panic attacks. Psychological assessment should include knowledge and perception of the cause of their chest pain and adherence to treatment. Psychological risk factors should be considered, as well as functional behavioral analysis and behavioral responses to pain. Evidence-based care includes the use of screening and assessment tools. Workup should be based on signs and symptoms, laboratory tests and imaging studies, and the use of assessment tools, which may include Generalized Anxiety Disorder (GAD)2, Generalized Anxiety Disorder (GAD)7, and/or the Hospital Anxiety and Depression Scale [11–13].

10.3.1.3 Summary

For healthcare providers, NCCP is a challenging condition given its heterogeneity. The term NCCP is generally understood to mean angina pectoris without evidence of ischemia, but otherwise there is a lack of consensus across specialties. The lack of understanding of pathophysiology and the coexistence of multiple etiologies in some patients add to its complexity. Comprehensive evaluation is often insufficient to diagnose or identify the underlying etiology. Treatment can be complex and needs to address multiple factors such as comorbidities and psychosocial conditions.

From the patient's perspective, the experience of chest pain can be frightening. Persistent chest pain can prompt dramatic changes in daily life and ongoing interactions with the healthcare system. NCCP can have financial implications and reduce quality of life. It is critical that healthcare providers understand the impact of NCCP on patient well-being, even if it is not caused by a life-threatening condition.

10.3.2 Cardiac Chest Pain

Chest pain has long been one of the most common complaints in the ED. Traditionally, due to concerns about missed MI, the approach to the management of patients with undifferentiated chest pain in the ED has emphasized the role of admission for further examination and risk stratification. This long-standing practice pattern was questioned over the past decade as ED diagnoses have become more sensitive. With the development of more sensitive cardiac biomarkers, combined with validated clinical scoring systems, ED physicians have begun to identify a large group of patients who can be rapidly evaluated in the ED and safely discharged. In this cohort of low-to-moderate-risk patients, the traditional emphasis on the need for stimulation cardiac testing in patients presenting to the ED with chest pain has been challenged.

The possible presence of cardiogenic chest pain can be considered as a continuum from full-blown AMI to simple transient angina. Within this spectrum, there is severe cardiac ischemia and minimal myocardial injury in acute coronary syndromes [14]. Three potentially life-threatening causes of chest pain—pulmonary embolism, aortic coarctation, and acute coronary syndrome (ACS)—should be suspected. Of these three causes, ACS is the most common cause of significant chest pain and is identified in approximately 15% of all patients presenting with chest pain [3]. Although history, physical examination, X-rays, and ECG are obtained in almost all patients with chest pain, these components have poor sensitivity and specificity to reliably detect or exclude ACS. Given these limitations, cardiac biomarkers, including creatine kinase MB fraction (CK-MB), myoglobin, and troponin, have been used to assess the presence of myocardial ischemia [15].

ACS describes a spectrum of myocardial ischemic states, including unstable angina, non-ST-segment elevation myocardial infarction (MI), or ST-segment elevation MI. ACS is associated with substantial morbidity and mortality and places a significant economic burden on the healthcare system. The diagnosis of ACS begins with a thorough clinical evaluation of the patient's symptoms, ECG and cardiac troponin levels, and a review of past medical history. Early risk stratification can help clinicians determine whether an early invasive management strategy or an initial conservative strategy is warranted and can help determine appropriate pharmacological therapy. Key components of ACS treatment include coronary revascularization when available; prompt initiation of dual antiplatelet therapy and anticoagulation; and consideration of adjunctive medications, including beta-blockers, renin-angiotensin system inhibitors, and HmG-coenzyme A reductase inhibitor. Clinicians must take an individualized approach when managing patients with a history of ACS after hospital discharge and consider long-term safety and efficacy [14].

10.4 Clinical Assessment

When evaluating patients with acute chest pain, clinicians must address a range of questions related to prognosis and immediate management. Before attempting to decide on a definitive diagnosis, high-priority questions include the following [2, 16]:

1. Clinical stability: Does the patient require immediate treatment for actual or impending circulatory collapse or respiratory insufficiency?
2. Immediate prognosis: If the patient is currently clinically stable, what is his or her risk of developing a life-threatening condition (e.g., ACS, pulmonary embolism, or aortic dissection)?
3. Safety of the bypass protocol: If the risk of life-threatening conditions is low, is it safe to discharge the patient for outpatient treatment, or should he or she receive further testing or observation to guide treatment?

10.5 Assessment and Diagnostic Testing

Most patients with chest pain are initially consulted by their general practitioner (GP), who is faced with the challenge of triage. To accomplish this task, GPs need to know the relevant etiologies and their respective frequencies. In an intuitive probabilistic reasoning process, GPs combine the initial likelihood of a given etiology, namely, pre-test probability, with the findings they derive from the patient's history and clinical examination to attain a final or at least tentative diagnosis, namely, post-test probability [17].

Evaluation of patients with acute chest pain can begin before the patient visits the physician, so validity may depend on the actions of office staff and other nonphysician personnel. The ACC and AHA guidelines emphasize that patients with symptoms of ACS should not be evaluated solely by telephone but should be referred to a facility where a 12-lead ECG can be evaluated and recorded by a physician [4]. These guidelines also recommend that immediate referral to an ED or specialty chest pain department should be strongly considered for patients with suspected ACS who present at rest with chest discomfort for more than 20 min, are hemodynamically unstable, or have recently experienced syncope or near syncope [18]. Traveling as a passenger in a private vehicle is considered an acceptable alternative to an ambulance only if waiting would result in a delay of more than 20–30 min [2].

The National Heart Attack Alert Program guidelines suggest that patients who have the following complaints should be assessed immediately by the triage nurse and referred for further assessment [19]:

1. Chest pain, pressure, tightness, or heaviness; pain radiating to the neck, jaw, shoulders, back, or one or both arms.
2. Indigestion or heartburn; nausea and/or vomiting associated with chest discomfort.
3. Persistent shortness of breath.
4. Weakness, dizziness, light-headedness, loss of consciousness.

For patients with these symptoms, the initial evaluation includes taking a history, performing a physical examination, obtaining an electrocardiogram and chest radiograph, measuring biomarkers of myocardial injury, and a HEART score [2].

10.5.1 Medical History

If the patient requires no immediate intervention as there is no impending or actual circulatory collapse or respiratory insufficiency, the physician's evaluation should begin with a clinical history that documents the features of the patient's pain, including the quality, location, and radiation of the pain, the timing and rhythm of onset (sudden or gradual), the duration of symptoms, activities precipitating or relieving the pain, and any associated symptoms, especially those of the lungs or gastrointestinal tract. ACS is usually described as diffuse substernal chest pressure that begins gradually and radiates to the jaw or arms. It can be aggravated by exertion and mitigated after a rest or use of nitroglycerin. Studies have shown that the response to nitroglycerin may not be a reliable evidence to distinguish between cardiac and noncardiac chest pain [20]. Contrary to the rhythm of chest pain in ACS, chest pain in pulmonary embolism, aortic dissection, and pneumothorax is sudden and severe. In addition, pleuritic or positional pain suggests pulmonary embolism, pericarditis, pneumonia, or musculoskeletal diseases.

Besides the acute onset, the presence of risk factors for atherosclerosis such as advanced age, male, and diabetes amplifies the likelihood that chest pain is provoked by myocardial ischemia. A history of MI not only indicates a high risk of obstructive coronary disease but also suggests an increased likelihood of multivessel disease. Younger patients are at lower risk for ACS, but greater attention should be paid to screening for a history of recent cocaine use.

10.5.2 Physical Examination

The initial examination of patients with acute chest pain should target the identification of potential triggers of myocardial ischemia (e.g., uncontrolled hypertension), significant comorbidities (e.g., chronic obstructive pulmonary disease), and evidence of hemodynamic complications (e.g., congestive heart failure, new mitral regurgitation, hypotension) [4]. Apart from vital signs, examination of the peripheral vessels should contain evaluation of bruising or absence of pulses, which would indicate extracardiac vascular disease.

In patients whose clinical symptoms do not indicate myocardial ischemia, the search for noncoronary causes of chest pain should take potential life-threatening problems such as aortic dissection and pulmonary embolism as a priority and then turn to the possibility of other cardiac diagnoses like pericarditis and noncardiac diagnoses like esophageal discomfort. Differences in blood pressure or pulse rate or a new murmur of aortic regurgitation accompanied by back or midline anterior chest pain suggest aortic regurgitation. In the setting of acute dyspnea and pleuritic chest pain, differences in breath sounds may be a sign of pneumothorax. Tachycardia, tachypnea, and exacerbation of the pulmonary component of the second heart sound (P2) may be the main manifestations of pulmonary embolism on physical examination [21].

10.5.3 Electrocardiography

The ECG serves as a critical source of data and should be attained within 10 min after persistent chest discomfort appears or as soon as possible for patients with a history of chest discomfort but whose discomfort has resolved at the time of evaluation to identify patients who may benefit from immediate reperfusion therapy (mechanical or pharmacological) [18].

The ECG provides significant information for diagnosis and prognosis. An indication of acute ischemia and severe coronary artery disease lies in the new persistent or transient ST-segment abnormalities (≥0.05 mV) in the presence of symptoms at rest and being resolved with symptom resolution. Nonspecific ST-segment and T-wave abnormalities are usually defined as lesser ST-segment deviation or T-wave inversion of 0.2 mV or less; thus, they are less helpful for risk stratification. An entirely normal ECG does not exclude the possibility of ACS; the risk of acute MI is approximately 4% in patients with a history of coronary artery disease and 2% in patients without a history of coronary artery disease [22]. However, patients with a normal or near-normal ECG had a better prognosis than those with a significantly abnormal ECG at the time of presentation. In addition, the negative predictive value of a normal ECG is 80–90%, regardless of whether the patient has chest pain at the time of acquisition [23]. Diffuse ST-segment elevation and PR-segment depression suggest pericarditis. Right-axis deviation, right bundle branch block, T-wave inversion in leads V_1 to V_4, and S-wave in lead I and Q- and T-wave inversion in lead III suggest pulmonary embolism.

The availability of an ECG promotes diagnostic accuracy and lowers the admission rate of patients with abnormal baseline tracings. Continuous ECG tracings enhance the clinician's ability to diagnose acute MI, especially if combined with serial measurements of cardiac biomarkers. Continuous ECG monitoring to detect ST-segment movement is technically feasible, but its contribution to patient management is uncertain. Posterior leads are useful for identifying ischemia in the region supplied by the left coronary artery, which is otherwise relatively silent on the ECG.

10.5.4 Chest Radiography

A chest radiograph is usually taken by all patients presenting with chest pain. Though it is normally not diagnostic in patients with ACS, it may reflect pulmonary edema caused by diastolic or systolic dysfunction due to ischemia. It provides more valuable information for diagnosing or indicating other diseases. For instance, it may present widening of the mediastinum or aortic nodes in aortic dissection. The chest radiograph is normal in the presence of pulmonary embolism but may manifest atelectasis, elevated diaphragm, pleural effusion, or, more rarely, Hampton's hump or Westermarck's sign. The chest radiograph can show pneumonia or pneumothorax.

10.5.5 Biomarkers

Biomarkers of myocardial injury should be measured in patients presenting with chest discomfort that may be consistent with ACS. The preferred biomarker is cardiac troponin (T or I; cTnT or cTnI). And creatine kinase MB isoenzyme (CK-MB) is less sensitive [4].

1. Diagnostic performance

   Studies of the diagnostic performance of cTnI, cTnT, or CK-MB have shown that when any of these test results appear as abnormalities, there is a high probability that the patient has ACS. Nevertheless, it should be acknowledged that defining the diagnostic performance of biomarkers of MI is a challenge in itself since part of the definition of MI includes rising and falling biomarkers of cardiac necrosis. These assays, however, are indispensable in diagnosing MI and using the totality of clinical evidence as a referential standard for diagnosis, considering their excellent sensitivity and specificity.

   (a) Troponins

In cardiac muscle, slow skeletal muscle, and fast skeletal muscle, different genes encode troponin I and T. Therefore, detection of cardiac troponin is more specific for myocardial injury than detection of CK-MB, and cardiac troponin is the diagnostic biomarker of choice. The high specificity of cardiac troponin for myocardium makes false-positive elevations extremely rare such as elevation of cardiac troponin in the absence of myocardial injury. In contrast, in the absence of other clinical data consistent with ACS, elevations of cardiac troponin are usually due to true myocardial injury from causes other than atherosclerotic coronary artery disease. This injury may occur in other forms of myocardial injury such as myocarditis, myocardial contusion or cardioversion or defibrillation, left ventricular strain from congestive heart failure, hypertensive crisis or extreme exercise, right ventricular strain from pulmonary embolism, or acute pulmonary hypertension from other causes [24, 25]. The exact mechanism is unknown, but in patients with a clinical history of ACS, elevated cardiac troponin levels also imply a similarly increased risk of ischemic complications in patients with various renal functions.

The sensitivity of cardiac troponins was higher than 95% and the specificity was 90% when serial sampling to 12 h after the onset of discomfort. When using a single sample at presentation, the performance deteriorates to a large extent, with a sensitivity of 70–75%. However, recently developed sensitive assays have lower detection limit, which is approximately 0.001–0.01 ng/mL, depending on the specific assay and acceptably low-level imprecision, which is now below the 99th percentile of the normal reference population (typically 0.01–0.07 ng/mL). Therefore, the assays can improve the ability to detect myocardial injury. The sensitivity and specificity of the assays for detecting MI using a single sample at the presentation are both approximately 90%, while the negative predictive value is approximately 97–99% [26–28]. In addition, the superior performance of high-sensitivity assays is even more striking in patients presenting within 3 h of chest pain onset, with a sensitivity of 80–85% compared with approximately 55% of older assays. The area under the receiver operating characteristic curve is as high as 0.98 for serial samples using high-sensitivity assays.

Ultrasensitive assays with lower limits of detection such as <0.001 ng/mL or <1 pg/mL are also being developed, allowing almost all individuals to have a quantifiable troponin result, including healthy individuals. Using the assays, among patients with non-ST-segment elevation MI, 72% had circulating troponin levels at baseline above the 99th percentile, and an additional 28% had levels above the limit of detection. In addition, in patients with unstable angina, which is defined as having no elevated troponin levels using a current-generation commercial assay, 44% of patients had circulating troponin levels at baseline above the 99th percentile and an additional 52% had levels above the limit of detection; after 6–8 h, these values were 82% and 18%, respectively [29]. The ultrasensitive assays, likewise, can detect the rise in circulating troponin proportional to the amount of ischemia experienced during exercise stress testing. Consequently, troponin may transform from being a semi-quantitative test (negative in most people and quantitative in some) to semi-quantifiable in all populations. The clinical significance of the very low-level values reported in the ultrasensitive assays should be defined.

(b) Creatine kinase MB isoenzyme

Prior to the application of cardiac troponin assays, CK-MB was the priority biomarker used for the diagnosis of

MI. The greatest limitation of CK-MB as a diagnostic biomarker is its lack of specificity as it can be found in many parts of the human body such as skeletal muscle, tongue, diaphragm, small intestine, uterus, and prostate. Using the CK-MB relative index (ratio of CK-MB to total CK) can overcome its limitation in patients whose pain comes from skeletal muscle. However, the quantity of CK-MB rises in patients with diseases that cause chronic muscle destruction and regeneration, such as muscular dystrophy, high-performance sports like marathon, or rhabdomyolysis [30]. It is common to find increases in CK-MB in ED patients because they are more likely to have histories of alcohol abuse or trauma. On the other hand, one advantage of CK-MB is its short half-life in the circulation, which promotes its application in anticipating the timing of MI and diagnosing reinfarction in patients who have had an MI last week. After all, a normal CK-MB and an elevated troponin level may reflect a mild MI or an MI that occurred a few days earlier.

(c) Other markers

Compared with CK and troponin molecules, serum myoglobin and cardiac-type fatty acid-binding protein (H-FABP) are smaller molecules that diffuse more rapidly in the interstitium after cell death. The abnormality of H-FABP can be detected 30 min after myocardial injury.

Many patients presenting with ACS, including those without evidence of myocardial necrosis, have elevated concentrations of inflammatory biomarkers such as C-reactive protein, serum amyloid A, myeloperoxidase, or interleukin 6 (IL-6). Yet, rare studies have identified exact decision cut points or shown incremental benefits for admission or treatment strategies based on these new markers, resulting in the obstructed clinical utility of these observations.

Ischemia-modified albumin (IMA) has been approved for clinical use by the U.S. Food and Drug Administration. The albumin cobalt-binding assay used to detect IMA is based on the observation that in patients with myocardial ischemia the affinity of the N terminus of human albumin for cobalt is degraded.

D-dimer testing is an effective tool for diagnosing chest pain. It can help exclude pulmonary embolism when 99% of the prediction results provided by the enzyme-linked immunosorbent assay (ELISA) are negative among patients with a low clinical probability. For patients with a high clinical probability of pulmonary embolism, an imaging study should be arranged [31].

B-type natriuretic peptides [BNP and N-terminal pro-BNP (NT-proBNP)] are present under the intensified ventricular wall stress. Natriuretic peptides are always used to identify heart failure. BNP levels may rise when the transient myocardial ischemia occurs, and the magnitude of the elevation in ACS is associated to prognosis. Nevertheless, the elevated natriuretic peptides have no specificity for ACS, restricting its use as a diagnostic indicator.

(d) Prognosis implications of test results

Abnormalities of CK-MB, cTnI, and cTnT reflect the increasing risks of complications. Even if patients do not have elevated CK-MB, cTnI and cTnT are useful for early risk stratification of patients with acute chest pain. The concept of patients with mildly elevated troponin having infarctlet of problematic prognostic implications should be discarded.

2. Test strategies

The 2007 National Academy of Clinical Biochemistry (NACB) practice guidelines recommend the biomarker tests of cardiac injury for patients with ACS symptoms. On the other hand, patients with a low probability of ACS should not take biomarker tests, in case false-positive results cause unnecessary admissions to hospital, examinations, surgeries, and complications [4].

The ACC, AHA, and NACB guidelines recommend cTnI or cTnT as the preferred first-line markers. CK-MB (by mass assay) is an acceptable alternative, but the cardiac troponins have greater specificity and prognostic value than CK-MB. If the initial set of markers is negative in patients visiting hospitals within 6 h after pain presenting, the guidelines recommend that another sample be drawn within a time frame of 8–12 h after the onset of symptoms [4].

10.5.6 HEART Score

The HEART score was developed specifically for unselected patients presenting at the ED with chest pain. Unlike other risk stratification tools, it includes the physician's clinical suspicion and the presence of multiple coronary risk factors in its calculation. In addition, because it is based primarily on simple clinical parameters, it can be easily calculated at the bedside. The score manifests a patient's risk of a major adverse cardiac event (MACE) within 6 weeks after initial presentation. It has been tested and validated in numerous studies conducted in Europe, the United States, and the Asia-Pacific region [32–35]. Generally, a HEART score of 3 or less can help clinicians in diagnosing 35–46% of low-risk patients with very high sensitivity and negative predictive value [36]. Patients with a HEART score of 7 or more are a very high-risk subgroup with more than 50% MACE within 6 weeks, and therefore they should be admitted to the cardiac intensive care unit immediately [32]. Initially, the HEART score was used and validated in combination with cTn assays. Consequently, when using HEART scores based on hs-cTn assay results, clinicians should be cautious since the troponin-related score may vary depending on the assays used. However, in two retrospective cohort studies using the hs-cTn assay, the HEART score identified 31.6–37.2% of low-risk patients with a sensitivity of 93.7–100% and a negative predictive value of 98.3–100%. Such results are very similar to those observed in earlier validation studies [33, 37].

10.5.7 Conclusion

For patients presenting at the ED with chest pain, their diagnosis and management can be greatly improved by following a new clinical diagnostic algorithm based on hs-cTn testing combined with careful evaluation of clinical signs and symptoms, ECG, and other bedside examination techniques. The new diagnostic algorithm allows for more efficient and rapid triage of patients with chest pain. Three-quarters of patients can be ruled out or ruled in for AMI based on hs-cTn measurements on admission or an hour after admission. Up to half of patients are eligible for early discharge if differential diagnoses are ruled out. The new hs-cTn-based diagnostic algorithm, though, does not require the use of a clinical risk stratification score, a HEART score of 3 or less is recommended as an additional criterion for deciding on early discharge because the score predicts a very low risk of MACE in early follow-up. For the rest small percentage of patients whose diagnosis remains uncertain, they have to stay in the ED, CPU, or observation unit till their ECG monitoring, repeat hs-cTn measurements, bedside echocardiography, and additional CCTA or ischemic testing provide clear diagnosis [38, 39].

10.6 Treatments

10.6.1 Acute Coronary Syndrome (ACS)

The management of ACS can be very complicated depending on the patients' conditions. For patients who are diagnosed with ACS, they will firstly be treated with the following initial steps: placing a cardiac monitor, establishing intravascular access (IV), giving 162–325 mg chewable aspirin, clopidogrel, or ticagrelor (unless bypass surgery is imminent), controlling pain, and considering oxygen therapy. It has been shown that nitroglycerin can improve mortality. Thus, using nitroglycerin to lower mean arterial pressure (MAP) by 10% in normotensive patients and by 30% in hypertensive patients. Noticeably, patients with hypotension or inferior ST-segment elevation are contradicted to nitroglycerin. Patients with ST-segment elevation on ECG should receive immediate reperfusion therapy, either pharmacological (thrombolytic) or percutaneous coronary intervention (PCI) in the catheterization laboratory. PCI is the first choice and should be initiated within 90 min at the scene or within 120 min after being transferred to an outside facility. If PCI is not available, thrombolytic agents should be initiated within 30 min. On the other hand, patients with non-ST-segment elevation myocardial infarction (NSTEMI) and unstable angina should be admitted to the hospital for a cardiology consultation and examination. In addition, patients with stable angina may be suitable for examination on an outpatient basis. For elderly patients and those with comorbidities, they should be hospitalized for further observation and cardiac workup [40, 41].

10.6.2 Pneumothorax (PTX)

Pneumothorax should be decompressed with a chest tube [42, 43].

10.6.3 Pericardial Tamponade

Pericardial tamponade can be diagnosed with bedside ultrasonography. A fluid bolus can be adopted as a temporary measure. Needle pericardiotomy or pericardial window is used to relieve pressure in the pericardial pouch [44].

10.6.4 Aortic Dissection

For patients with this condition, they should visit a cardiothoracic surgeon as soon as possible and receive immediate surgery. CT angiography is the most useful test to evaluate dissection. Placing two large-bore IVs to quickly lower the patient's blood pressure to systolic between 100 and 130 mmHg is important. Initiate treatment using beta-blockers therapy, the aim of which is to prevent reflux tachycardia [45–47].

10.6.5 Esophageal Perforation

Esophageal rupture may be indicated by a left pleural effusion on a chest radiograph. A contrast esophagram is the most efficient confirmatory test. It is a medical emergency that requires immediate surgical consultation [46].

10.6.6 Gastrointestinal Reflux Disease (GERD)

Treatment of GERD begins with lifestyle and behavioral adjustments. Recommended measures include weight loss, avoidance of food triggers, and elevation of the head of the bed. Tobacco can also exacerbate GERD-related NCCP symptoms; thus, patients should be persuaded to quit smoking. The American Gastroenterological Association guidelines recommend PPI therapy for GERD-related chest pain and following treatments may depend on patients' response to PPI [48].

Patients can be given viscous lidocaine and Maalox, known as a gastrointestinal cocktail. Yet, it is therapeutic instead of diagnostic. ACS can also present with dyspepsia and may respond to the GI cocktail. Therefore, ACS must be excluded before assuring GERD as the final diagnosis. PPIs or H2 blockers are ideal for long-term treatment of GERD [49].

10.6.7 Pulmonary Embolism (PE)

CT pulmonary angiography (CTPA) is the best confirmatory test for PE. A VQ scan is also a useful diagnostic tool, yet the accuracy of which is compromising when patients have chronic lung disease. Patients whose hemodynamics is unstable should be given thrombolytic agents at the beginning, while patients with stable hemodynamics should be given anticoagulants [50].

10.6.8 Costochondritis

It is a self-healing disease. Additional treatment includes rest, soothing, nonnarcotic analgesics, nonpharmacological pain management (ice or heat), and traction.

10.6.9 Generalized Anxiety Disorder (GAD)

Using certain antidepressants followed by other anxiolytics is effective in treating GAD. NCCP patients whose pain is a psychiatric nature can benefit from reassurance about their prognosis in addition to cognitive therapy, biopsychosocial models, hypnotherapy, and biofeedback [51, 52].

10.6.10 Cognitive Therapy

Addressing the psychological impact of persistent chest pain and psychological comorbidity is an indispensable part of chest pain treatment as patients often suffer decreased quality of life and psychological distress [53]. Cognitive therapy should be individualized to meet the patient's needs, so that patients can better adhere to medical advice, adjust their coping skills, and receive successful treatment. Patients may not fully understand the chest pain they are experiencing and aspire to learn more information. Therefore, interventions aimed at improving knowledge and strategies to address pain and stress may be useful, including a psychiatry department referral. NCCP patients may also benefit from cognitive behavioral therapy [54]. Chambers and colleagues recommend treatment using a biopsychosocial model, which involves supporting patients with explanation and reassurance, connecting them to social resources, administering medication according to clinical indications, teaching relaxation methods, and making referrals to specialists as required [55]. A biopsychosocial approach can lessen the number of chest pain episodes, activity avoidance, psychological distress, and healthcare use and work absence associated with chest pain [56].

References

1. Expert consensus on combined detection of cardiovascular markers in emergency chest pain. Chin J Emerg Med. 2022;31(4):448–58.
2. McClintic BR, Rosenblatt RL. Approach to the patient with chest pain. In: Bisognano J, Beck R, Connell R, editors. Manual of outpatient cardiology. London: Springer; 2012. https://doi.org/10.1007/978-0-85729-944-4_13.
3. Haasenritter J, Biroga T, Keunecke C, Becker A, Donner-Banzhoff N, Dornieden K, Stadje R, Viniol A, Bösner S. Causes of chest pain in primary care—a systematic review and meta-analysis. Croat Med J. 2015;56(5):422–30. https://doi.org/10.3325/cmj.2015.56.422.
4. Anderson JL, Adams CD, Antman EM, et al. ACC/AHA 2007 guidelines for the management of patients with unstable angina/non ST-elevation myocardial infarction: a report of the American College of Cardiology/American Heart Association Task Force on Practice Guidelines (Writing Committee to Revise the 2002 Guidelines for the Management of Patients with Unstable Angina/Non ST-Elevation Myocardial Infarction): developed in collaboration with the American College of Emergency Physicians, the Society for Cardiovascular Angiography and Interventions, and the Society of Thoracic Surgeons: endorsed by the American Association of Cardiovascular and Pulmonary Rehabilitation and the Society for Academic Emergency Medicine. Circulation. 2007;116:e148.
5. Fass R, Achem SR. Noncardiac chest pain: epidemiology, natural course and pathogenesis. J Neurogastroenterol Motil. 2011;17(2):110–23.
6. Weiss AJ, Wier LM, Stocks C, et al. Overview of emergency department visits in the United States. Rockville, MD: Healthcare Cost and Utilization Project: Agency for Healthcare Research and Quality; 2014. p. 1–13.
7. Rushton S, Carman MJ. Chest pain: if it is not the heart, what is it? Nurs Clin North Am. 2018;53(3):421–31. https://doi.org/10.1016/j.cnur.2018.04.009. Epub 2018 Jul 11.
8. Husser D, Bollmann A, Kuhne C, et al. Evaluation of noncardiac chest pain: diagnostic approach, coping strategies and quality of life. Eur J Pain. 2006;10:51–5.
9. Jiang F, Li S, Pan L, et al. Association of anxiety disorders with the risk of smoking behaviors: a meta-analysis of prospective observational studies. Drug Alcohol Depend. 2014;145:69–76.
10. Morrow DA. Chest discomfort. In: Kasper D, Fauci A, Hauser S, editors. Harrison's principles of inter-

nal medicine. 19th ed. New York: McGraw-Hill Education; 2015.
11. Rothberg B, Schneck CD. Anxiety and depression. In: Rakel RE, Rakel DP, editors. Textbook of family medicine. 9th ed. Philadelphia: Elsevier, Saunders; 2016. p. 1090–1107.e3.
12. Plummer F, Manea L, Trepel D, et al. Screening for anxiety disorders with the GAD-7 and GAD-2: a systematic review and diagnostic metaanalysis. Gen Hosp Psychiatry. 2016;39:24–31.
13. Dalrymple KL. Anxiety (generalized anxiety disorder). In: Ferri F, editor. Ferri's clinical advisor 2018. Philadelphia: Elsevier; 2018. p. 110.
14. Smith JN, Negrelli JM, Manek MB, Hawes EM, Viera AJ. Diagnosis and management of acute coronary syndrome: an evidence-based update. J Am Board Fam Med. 2015;28(2):283–93. https://doi.org/10.3122/jabfm.2015.02.140189.
15. DeLaney MC, Neth M, Thomas JJ. Chest pain triage: current trends in the emergency departments in the United States. J Nucl Cardiol. 2017;24(6):2004–11. https://doi.org/10.1007/s12350-016-0578-0. Epub 2016 Sep 8.
16. Ayerbe L, González E, Gallo V, et al. Clinical assessment of patients with chest pain; a systematic review of predictive tools. BMC Cardiovasc Disord. 2016;16:18. https://doi.org/10.1186/s12872-016-0196-4.
17. Doust J. Diagnosis in general practice. Using probabilistic reasoning. BMJ. 2009;339:b3823. https://doi.org/10.1136/bmj.b3823.
18. Antman EM, Anbe DT, Armstrong PW, et al. ACC/AHA guidelines for the management of patients with ST-elevation myocardial infarction: a report of the American College of Cardiology/American Heart Association Task Force on Practice Guidelines (Committee to Revise the 1999 Guidelines for the Management of Patients with Acute Myocardial Infarction). Circulation. 2004;110:e82.
19. National Heart Attack Alert Program Coordinating Committee, 60 Minutes to Treatment Working Group. Emergency department: rapid identification and treatment of patients with acute myocardial infarction. Ann Emerg Med. 1994;23:311.
20. Diercks DB, Boghos E, Guzman H, et al. Changes in the numeric descriptive scale for pain after sublingual nitroglycerin do not predict cardiac etiology of chest pain. Ann Emerg Med. 2005;45:581.
21. Beiser DG, Cifu AS, Paul J. Evaluation and diagnosis of chest pain. JAMA. 2022;328(3):292–3. https://doi.org/10.1001/jama.2022.10362.
22. Lee TH, Goldman L. Evaluation of the patient with acute chest pain. N Engl J Med. 2000;342:1187.
23. Turnipseed SD, Trythall WS, Diercks DB, et al. Frequency of acute coronary syndrome in patients with normal electrocardiogram performed during presence or absence of chest pain. Acad Emerg Med. 2009;16:495.
24. Peacock WF 4th, De Marco T, Fonarow GC, et al. Cardiac troponin and outcome in acute heart failure. N Engl J Med. 2008;358:2117.
25. Becattini C, Vedovati MC, Agnelli G. Prognostic value of troponins in acute pulmonary embolism: a meta-analysis. Circulation. 2007;116:427.
26. Morrow DA. Clinical application of sensitive troponin assays. N Engl J Med. 2009;361:913.
27. Reichlin T, Hochholzer W, Bassetti S, et al. Early diagnosis of myocardial infarction with sensitive cardiac troponin assays. N Engl J Med. 2009;361:858.
28. Keller T, Zeller T, Peetz D, et al. Sensitive troponin I assay in early diagnosis of acute myocardial infarction. N Engl J Med. 2009;61:868.
29. Wilson SR, Sabatine MS, Braunwald E, et al. Detection of myocardial injury in patients with unstable angina using a novel nanoparticle cardiac troponin I assay: observations from the PROTECT-TIMI 30 trial. Am Heart J. 2009;158:386.
30. Leers MP, Schepers R, Baumgarten R. Effects of a long-distance run on cardiac markers in healthy athletes. Clin Chem Lab Med. 2006;44:999.
31. van Belle A, Buller HR, Huisman MV, et al. Effectiveness of managing suspected pulmonary embolism using an algorithm combining clinical probability, D-dimer testing, and computed tomography. JAMA. 2006;295:172.
32. Backus BE, Six AJ, Kelder JC, et al. A prospective validation of the HEART score for chest pain patients at the emergency department. Int J Cardiol. 2013;168:2153–8.
33. Santi L, Farina G, Gramenzi A, et al. The HEART score with high-sensitive troponin T at presentation: ruling out patients with chest pain in the emergency room. Intern Emerg Med. 2017;12:357–64.
34. Carlton EW, Khattab A, Greaves K. Identifying patients suitable for discharge after a single-presentation high-sensitivity troponin result: a comparison of five established risk scores and two high-sensitivity assays. Ann Emerg Med. 2015;66:635–645.e1.
35. de Hoog VC, Lim SH, Bank IE, et al. HEART score performance in Asian and Caucasian patients presenting to the emergency department with suspected acute coronary syndrome. Eur Heart J Acute Cardiovasc Care. 2018;7:591–60.
36. Van Den Berg P, Body R. The HEART score for early rule out of acute coronary syndromes in the emergency department: a systematic review and meta-analysis. Eur Heart J Acute Cardiovasc Care. 2018;7:111–9.
37. Carlton EW, Cullen L, Than M, et al. A novel diagnostic protocol to identify patients suitable for discharge after a single high-sensitivity troponin. Heart. 2015;101:1041–6.
38. Stepinska J, Lettino M, Ahrens I, et al. Diagnosis and risk stratification of chest pain patients in the emergency department: focus on acute coronary syndromes. A position paper of the Acute Cardiovascular Care Association. Eur Heart J Acute Cardiovasc Care. 2020;9(1):76–89. https://doi.org/10.1177/2048872619885346.
39. Kohn MA, Worster A. ED chest pain rules: follow your HEART? Acad Emerg Med. 2019;26(2):261–2.

https://doi.org/10.1111/acem.13647. Epub 2019 Jan 21.

40. de Bliek EC. ST elevation: differential diagnosis and caveats. A comprehensive review to help distinguish ST elevation myocardial infarction from nonischemic etiologies of ST elevation. Turk J Emerg Med. 2018;18(1):1–10.
41. Solhpour A, Chang KW, Arain SA, Balan P, Zhao Y, Loghin C, McCarthy JJ, Vernon Anderson H, Smalling RW. Comparison of 30-day mortality and myocardial scar indices for patients treated with prehospital reduced dose fibrinolytic followed by percutaneous coronary intervention versus percutaneous coronary intervention alone for treatment of ST-elevation myocardial infarction. Catheter Cardiovasc Interv. 2016;88(5):709–15.
42. Habibi B, Achachi L, Hayoun S, Raoufi M, Herrak L, Ftouh ME. [Management of spontaneous pneumothorax: about 138 cases]. Pan Afr Med J. 2017;26:152.
43. Hsu KA, Levsky JM, Haramati LB, Gohari A. Performance of a simple robust empiric timing protocol for CT pulmonary angiography. Clin Imaging. 2018;48:17–21.
44. Shokoohi H, Boniface KS, Zaragoza M, Pourmand A, Earls JP. Point-of-care ultrasound leads to diagnostic shifts in patients with undifferentiated hypotension. Am J Emerg Med. 2017;35(12):1984.e3–7.
45. Zhao DL, Liu XD, Zhao CL, Zhou HT, Wang GK, Liang HW, Zhang JL. Multislice spiral CT angiography for evaluation of acute aortic syndrome. Echocardiography. 2017;34(10):1495–9.
46. Shiber JR, Fontane E, Ra JH, Kerwin AJ. Hydropneumothorax due to esophageal rupture. J Emerg Med. 2017;52(6):856–8.
47. Khoynezhad A, Plestis KA. Managing emergency hypertension in aortic dissection and aortic aneurysm surgery. J Card Surg. 2006;21(Suppl 1):S3–7.
48. Katz PO, Gerson LB, Vela MF. Guidelines for the diagnosis and management of gastroesophageal reflux disease. Am J Gastroenterol. 2013;108:308–28.
49. Alzubaidi M, Gabbard S. GERD: diagnosing and treating the burn. Cleve Clin J Med. 2015;82(10):685–92.
50. Meyer G. Effective diagnosis and treatment of pulmonary embolism: improving patient outcomes. Arch Cardiovasc Dis. 2014;107(6–7):406–14.
51. Rang HP, Ritter JM, Flower RJ, et al. Anxiolytic and hypnotic drugs. In: Rang and Dale's pharmacology. London: Elsevier Churchill Livingstone; 2016. p. 536–45.
52. Kisely SR, Campbell LA, Yelland MJ, et al. Psychological interventions for symptomatic management of non-specific chest pain in patients with normal coronary anatomy. Cochrane Database Syst Rev. 2015;2015:CD004101.
53. Yamasaki T, Fass R. Noncardiac chest pain: diagnosis and management. Curr Opin Gastroenterol. 2017;33:293–300.
54. George N, Abdallah J, Maradey-Romero C, et al. Review article: the current treatment of non-cardiac chest pain. Aliment Pharmacol Ther. 2016;43:213–39.
55. Chambers JB, Marks E, Knisley L, et al. Non-cardiac chest pain: time to extend the rapid access chest pain clinic? Int J Clin Pract. 2013;67:303–6.
56. Chambers JB, Marks EM, Russell V, et al. A multidisciplinary, biopsychosocial treatment for non-cardiac chest pain. Int J Clin Pract. 2015;69:922–7.

11 Pain in Abdominal Viscera

Ming Xia

Pain in the abdominal viscera is more complex than chest pain as most of the human viscera locate in the abdominal region. Evaluating any patient with a complaint of abdominal pain is challenging. Abdominal pain can be benign and self-limited or a harbinger of a serious life-threatening disease. The diagnoses of related diseases require careful consideration and clinical interrogation besides appropriate diagnostic testing to discern whether the entity is indeed the cause of the patient's pain. This chapter centers on irritable bowel syndrome, peptic gastric ulcer, chronic pancreatitis and its acute attacks, biliary dyskinesia, visceral pain due to surgeries, and common pediatric recurrent abdominal pain.

11.1 Abdominal Pain in Irritable Bowel Syndrome

11.1.1 Definition and Classification of Irritable Bowel Syndrome

1. Definition

   Irritable bowel syndrome (IBS) is the most common type of functional gastrointestinal disorder, with abdominal pain, abdominal distension, or abdominal discomfort, accompanied by bowel habits, such as changes in frequency and/or stool characteristics, as the main clinical manifestations. Abdominal pain is associated with defecation and mostly improves after defecation; symptoms tend to be recurrent or chronically prolonged.
2. Classification

   According to Rome IV criteria [1], IBS can be classified into constipation-predominant, diarrhea-predominant, mixed bowel habit-predominant, and unclassified IBS. Postinfectious-IBS (PI-IBS) is IBS that occurs following gastrointestinal infections. Different subtypes of patients are classified to maintain consistency in selection. As a result, we are able to understand pathophysiological mechanisms, diagnose and treat patients more effectively, and recruit patients for clinical trials more effectively.

11.1.2 The Etiology and Pathogenesis of Abdominal Pain in Irritable Bowel Syndrome

It is characteristic of IBS that abdominal pain and changes in bowel movement appear transiently or for a long period of time with some chronic diseases. Among these, abdominal pain is the most common. It usually occurs in the lower or left lower abdomen, intensifies before stools, worsens after cold foods, and is most prevalent in the

M. Xia (✉)
Department of Anesthesiology, Shanghai Ninth People's Hospital, Shanghai Jiao Tong University School of Medicine, Shanghai, China
e-mail: xiaming1980@xzhmu.edu.cn

M. Xia et al. (eds.), *Visceral Pain*, https://doi.org/10.1007/978-981-99-9167-9_11

early hours of the day. It was found by Thompson that people with IBS experience abdominal pain six times more often than people with healthy adult bodies [2]. In addition to being difficult to localize, abdominal pain can migrate around the abdomen and is unpredictable. It is common for patients to experience abdominal pain that is relieved by defecating, to have frequent bowel movements during painful attacks, to have loose stools during painful episodes, and to experience significant abdominal distention. Symptoms of IBS differed according to gender, with women reporting more abdominal pain and constipation and men reporting more diarrhea, according to a meta-analysis. Researchers found that both persons with IBS and those without IBS experienced worse symptoms during menstruation, suggesting that female hormones may contribute to IBS symptoms. The degree of IBS pain varies widely among and within individuals, and the pain episodes are intermittent or persistent, and the degree of pain is difficult to quantify, significantly reducing people's quality of life and resulting in significant medical costs. Currently, research on the pathogenesis of IBS has progressed slowly, and the lack of attention to the mechanisms of abdominal pain has led to the absence of effective methods for treating abdominal pain in IBS. How to reduce the pain of IBS patients is a common concern of clinicians.

1. Etiology of abdominal pain

   The pathogenesis of abdominal pain in IBS is not yet clear, and no single pathogenesis can fully explain all its clinical manifestations. Therefore, most scholars believe that the occurrence of the disease is the result of a combination of pathogenic factors, mainly involving abnormal gastrointestinal dynamics, visceral hypersensitivity, immune abnormalities, psychosomatic factors, infection, gut-brain axis dysregulation, intestinal mucosal barrier dysfunction, and other factors, and there are close links between various possible mechanisms.

   (a) Genetic factors: Some studies have shown that there is a tendency for family clustering in IBS patients, and the prevalence of IBS in identical twins is higher than that in dizygotic twins, suggesting that IBS is associated with genetic abnormalities. Current studies demonstrating the association between IBS and genes have focused on the transcriptional activity of the 5-HT transporter.
   (b) Dietary factors: A random survey of IBS patients' morbidity by some investigators found that 70% of patients reported intestinal symptoms after ingestion [3]. This is because the gastrointestinal tract has the largest mucosal lymphoid tissue in the body and plays an important role in food antigen transmission, recognition, and antibody production. The immune system treats food that enters the body as an abnormal antigen and produces food-specific antibodies, which form immune complexes with food particles and are deposited in the intestinal mucosal tissue, causing a metamorphic reaction in the GI tissues and inducing a series of GI symptoms. Allergenic food antigens enter the lamina propria through the intestinal mucosal barrier, activating immune cells in the lamina propria, increasing antibody and cytokine production, and elevated antibodies and cytokines cause intestinal inflammatory reactions and loss of control of the intestinal neuro-immune-endocrine network, leading to intestinal dysfunction, resulting in symptoms such as abdominal pain, abdominal discomfort, bloating, and diarrhea.
   (c) Inflammatory factors: When an acute infection of the intestine can cause postinfectious IBS in some patients, despite the removal of the pathogen, the intestine still has mild inflammatory changes, as evidenced by an increase in lymphocytes and macrophages in the intraepithelial and lamina propria layers of the mucosa. These immune cells are in close contact with enteric nerve fibers and the release of inflammatory mediators can affect enteric nervous system function and muscle contractility. Inflammatory stimulation

leads to macrophage activation degranulation and release of multiple bioactive substances affecting intestinal motility and sensation, which may be the key to inflammation-induced IBS symptoms.

(d) Spiritual and psychological factors: IBS, as an individual-specific, multicausal, and heterogeneous disease, is closely related to factors such as life stress and mental status of patients. Studies have shown that the proportion of IBS patients with suicidal tendencies is two to four times higher than that of controls.

The pathological essence of functional gastrointestinal symptoms is a power or sensory disorder with impaired innervation regulation. In the central nervous system, there are rich synaptic and loop connections between the higher nuclei of neural activity and the nuclei of gastrointestinal sensorimotor function. Bidirectional pathways exist between the cognitive and affective centers and the neuroendocrine, enteric nervous system, and immune system, with external stimuli and internal information connected to the higher nociceptors via neural links affecting gastrointestinal sensation, dynamics, and secretion, and visceral activity acting in turn on central pain, emotional, and behavioral areas. Therefore, abnormal psychosomatic factors have the potential to lead to simultaneous multisite, multifunctional abnormal changes in the gastrointestinal tract, thus exhibiting different symptomatic features.

2. Pathogenesis of abdominal pain

(a) Abnormal gastrointestinal dynamics: The main clinical symptoms of IBS are abdominal pain or abdominal discomfort, accompanied by changes in bowel habits or stool properties, so the earliest studies on its etiology focused on abnormal gastrointestinal dynamics. Most of the current studies show that gastric emptying is basically normal in IBS patients. Some studies have used gastric electrograms to observe postprandial gastric emptying in patients with IBS and found delayed gastric emptying in patients with IBS. Another study showed that only patients with IBS with dyspeptic symptoms had abnormal gastric motility. The rate of small intestinal content transit can be used directly to assess small intestinal motility. It has been suggested that the rate of small bowel content transit is faster in diarrheal patients and slower in constipated patients, suggesting that small bowel motility plays an important role in the pathogenesis of IBS. The main forms of colonic motility in normal subjects are mixed motility and propulsive motility. Mixed motility is mainly to make full contact between intestinal contents and the intestinal wall, which facilitates the absorption of water and inorganic salts, while propulsive motility is mainly used to transport intestinal contents. At present, there is no characteristic marker and uniform conclusion of complex gastrointestinal dynamics abnormalities in IBS patients, and further clinical research is needed. In addition, the correlation between abnormal gastrointestinal motility and clinical symptoms in IBS is not constant. Therefore, it is one of the future research directions to find effective drugs to improve the symptoms of IBS by starting from the key links affecting gastrointestinal motility.

(b) Visceral hypersensitivity: Visceral hypersensitivity is one of the important pathophysiological mechanisms of IBS and also a biological marker of IBS. It is currently believed that patients with IBS have a state of visceral hypersensitivity (including nociceptive hypersensitivity and nociceptive abnormalities), and the excitability of the spinal cord involved in nociceptive perception is significantly increased. Some studies have reported that pain thresholds for rectal distension are significantly lower in IBS patients compared to normal subjects and patients with functional abdominal pain syndrome, in which the dorsal horn of the spinal cord is a key site for modulating visceral sensitivity. Some studies have found that patients with IBS may have increased visceral neurosensitivity, but not all patients with IBS have abnormal visceral sensations. Current studies on the mechanism of visceral hypersensitivity have mainly focused on animal experiments, which not only differ greatly from humans but also mostly use the colorectal stimulation method for modeling, ignoring that the production of symptoms such as abdominal pain and diarrhea may also be related to the small intestine.

The mechanism of visceral hypersensitivity mainly lies in the altered sensitivity of visceral mechanoreceptors, abnormal sensory nerve afferents, and sensitization of central injurious neurons. Activation of intestinal inflammatory mediator receptors in patients can affect the sensitivity and excitability of intestinal wall mechanoreceptors, spinal nerves, and central injurious neurons, thus affecting the development of visceral hypersensitivity. However, it has also been suggested that the reduced pain threshold and loading sensory threshold in the colon of patients with IBS compared to normal subjects is due to lower reporting criteria for pain rather than due to visceral hypersensitivity, and that this lowering of criteria is generally determined by psychological factors. Therefore, the investigators concluded that visceral hypersensitivity in IBS patients may be determined by psychological rather than physiological factors [4, 5].

(c) Gut-brain axis dysfunction: Gut-brain interaction refers to the process by which gastrointestinal tract information is transmitted to the central nervous system via the enteric nervous system, and the feedback from the latter regulates gastrointestinal activity, which is realized by the gut brain axis composed of neuroendocrine mechanisms involved. The enteric nervous system is located throughout the intestinal wall from the mucosal layer to the plasma layer and is closely linked to the central nervous system. Neurotransmitters such as 5-HT, calcitonin gene-related peptide, substance P, cholecystokinin, enkephalin, nitric oxide, and vasoactive peptide are widely distributed in the enteric nervous system and the central nervous system. They can be involved in regulating gastrointestinal motility, sensation, emotional response, and immunity. Gene microarray screening revealed that nearly 500 genes were abnormally expressed in the gut-brain axis pathway in visceral hypersensitive mice [6]. However, the specific mechanisms of the roles of the above molecules in gut-brain axis dysfunction need to be further investigated. In addition, autonomic dysfunction, an important component of gut-brain interaction, also plays an important role in the pathogenesis of IBS. Increased sympathetic tone and decreased vagal responsiveness are common in IBS patients, but the findings are inconsistent.

(d) Abnormal immune regulation: A large number of studies have shown that not only postinfection IBS but also IBS patients without clear evidence of infection have mild immune abnormalities in the intestine and peripheral blood. Microscopic biopsies of their ileal and colonic mucosa show nonspecific inflammatory changes, and the number of immune cells such as intestinal chromophores, macrophages, T cells, and mast cells is significantly increased compared with healthy volunteers. Immunohistochemical staining showed an increased number of intraepithelial lymphocytes and immune cells in the lamina propria. It is now confirmed that the intrinsic immune destruction of the colonic mucosa in IBS patients is manifested by abnormal expression of Toll-like receptors in colonic mucosal specimens, causing a low-grade inflammatory response in the colonic mucosa, while the increased T cells and mast cells are anatomically adjacent to the axonal fibers of the enteric nervous system, and their increased secretion of inflammatory cytokines and neurotransmitters can act on the enteric plexus and smooth muscle cells to cause sensory and motor abnormalities; in addition, this low-grade inflammation can also disrupt intestinal mucosal epithelial barrier function, resulting in increased intestinal mucosal permeability, and increased intestinal permeability can promote inflammation, promote exposed lower luminal antigens, and subsequently interfere with intestinal sensation and motility. In contrast, immune cells tend to fade slowly after intestinal infectious agents are cleared, and low-grade inflammation can persist for up to 5 years in approximately 50% of patients with IBS after infection [7]. Some studies have shown that 7–32% of IBS patients have a history of gastrointestinal infection and that defects in inflammatory regression mechanisms may be the main cause of post-infection IBS production [8, 9]. The persistence of low-grade inflammation may increase visceral sensitivity and may also lead to changes in smooth muscle cell morphology in some patients, as well as an increase in neuropeptide content or in the number of their immune-responsive neurons, and these abnormalities are closely associated with the development of symptoms in patients. The inflammatory cytokines in the peripheral blood of IBS patients with increased frequency of defecation, watery stools, and abdominal pain are significantly higher than those of IBS patients without these symptoms, and neutralizing the inflammatory factors in the blood significantly improves the bowel function and reduces the abdominal symptoms in IBS patients. The plasma levels of IL-1β and TNF-a were significantly higher in IBS patients compared with those with fibromyalgia, suggesting that these two factors may be closely related to the development of abdominal pain symptoms in IBS patients.

Abnormal immune regulation may also be involved in the development of abdominal pain symptoms in IBS patients, and the mechanism may be related to inflammatory cells and secreted cytokines stimulating nerve fibers distributed in the intestine. Electron microscopy revealed a significant number of activated mast cells close to the nerve fiber endings in the colonic mucosa of patients with IBS and correlated significantly with the degree and frequency of abdominal pain or abdominal discomfort in patients. The mediators released by mast cells from the supernatant of the patients' colonic mucosal specimens were significantly higher, and when human submucosal neurons were stimulated with the supernatant, this resulted in an increase in the frequency of neuronal firing. Peripheral blood mononuclear cells from infected IBS patients activated the pelvic and lumbar visceral nerves innervating the mouse colon, resulting in increased mechanical sensitivity of the mouse intestinal mucosa, muscularis, and plasma membrane layers. The administration of the mast cell stabilizer ketotifen or the immunosuppressive drug mesalazine to patients with IBS significantly increased the patients' sensory threshold to rectal distension stimulation and improved their clinical symptoms such as abdominal distension and diarrhea.

(e) IBS abdominal pain-related factors
   - Capsaicin receptor, transient receptor potential vanilloid 1 (TRPV 1): Capsaicin can cause immediate pain avoidance response, as well as persistent nociceptive hyperalgesia. It was found that capsaicin exacerbated tongue pain induced by 49 °C stimulation, that is, enhanced TRPV1 chan-

nels exacerbated nociceptive hypersensitivity to temperature. TRPV1 plays a key (if not indispensable) role in chemical inflammation-induced visceral nociceptive hypersensitivity. Other investigators suggest that the development of visceral nociceptive hypersensitivity may also be related to the activation of low-threshold rectal mechanoreceptors within the normal physiological range. During colorectal stimulation, on the one hand, the relative ischemic state induced by colorectal dilation can lead to local acidification; on the other hand, mediators produced during dilation such as ATP and endogenous cannabinoids can also activate TRPV1, and the TRVP1-dependent conduction pathway induced by chemical mechanisms is very important for the production of nociceptive allergy, and its triggering factors include inflorescence stimulation, mechanical stimulation, and thermal stimulation.

- 5-HT: As an important gut-brain neurotransmitter, it is involved in the regulation of abdominal pain at all levels. Intestinal chromophobe cells, as the most important endocrine cells in the intestine, can synthesize and store 5-HT and also synthesize other gastrointestinal hormones. Increased intestinal pressure, vagus nerve stimulation, allergic reactions, duodenal acidification, etc. can induce intestinal chromophores to release 5-HT, which can bind to 5-HT receptors in exogenous primary afferent nerve endings in the lamina propria of the mucosa, leading to hypersensitivity of visceral afferent nerves and the enteric nervous system, as well as activation of various neuroactive substances, resulting in disturbance of gut-brain axis signals and abnormal chemical signals to the afferent center, causing visceral hypersensitivity and various IBS symptoms.
- Brain-derived neurotrophic factor (BDNF): A member of neurotrophic substances plays an important regulatory role in the morphological plasticity of the nervous system. The appropriate amount of endogenous BDNF can maintain the normal function of sensory nerves and their neural pathways, but its abnormal elevation can lead to a variety of pain-related abnormal sensations. Some studies have confirmed that the nerve fiber density in the colonic mucosa of IBS patients is significantly increased, and there are obvious structural abnormalities in the nervous system, mainly manifested by neuronal hyperplasia and synaptic hyperplasia, which may be related to the increased secretion of neurotrophic factors in the epithelial and lamina propria tissues of the colonic mucosa. Therefore, it is currently believed that the increase in intestinal mucosal nerve fiber density in IBS patients may be related to the increased expression of BDNF in colonic mucosal epithelial cells.
- Substance P and its receptor: Substance P is one of the first discovered neuropeptides, consisting of 11 amino acids, widely distributed in the central and peripheral nervous system and peripheral tissues in mammals, with the highest content in the gastrointestinal tract and central nervous system, and is a major pro-inflammatory sensory neuropeptide. Its receptor, a member of the guanine nucleotide-binding protein-coupled receptor superfamily, contains seven transmembrane regions and interacts with cellular effector systems via G proteins. It was found that the expression of substance P and its receptor R-positive was significantly increased in the intestinal mucosa of IBS patients, and the expressed substance P, in addition to transmitting sensory information to the central ner-

vous system, has peripheral physiological regulatory effects such as dilating blood vessels, causing histamine release from mast cells and plasma extravasation and affecting macrophages and leukocytes. Substance P has the effect of stimulating the secretion of water and electrolytes from the small intestine and colonic mucosa, which can lead to plasma extravasation and neutrophil infiltration. The current study suggests that substance P activates receptors that cause colonic sensory sensitization, and when the two are combined, they lead to neutrophil aggregation and trigger the chain-linked release of various inflammatory mediator molecules. It can be inferred that the changes in substance P receptor may influence the severity of IBS, and the two together affect the occurrence of IBS, and both play an important role in the pathogenesis of IBS, and the increased expression of substance P receptor in the intestinal mucosa is closely related to the effect of substance P.

- PAR2: The protease-activated receptor family (PAR) is a member of the G protein-coupled receptor family, which is unevenly distributed in mammalian tissues and cells and has both pro- and anti-inflammatory effects. The number of mast cells in the mucosal tissue of the proximal jejunum, terminal ileum, and ascending colon of IBS patients is significantly higher than that of the normal population, and mast cells can release a variety of bioactive transmitters such as PAR2, 5-HT, trypsin-like enzymes, etc. The current study concluded that the infiltration of mast cells and the release of bioactive transmitters are related to the production of abdominal pain sensation in IBS patients, in which PAR2 plays a special role in the information conversion of neurons, and the culture supernatant of biopsied tissues can stimulate the release of calcium signals from PAR2-positive spinal dorsal root nerves, causing continuous excitation of nerve cells, and the instillation of these supernatants into the colons of mice can lead to somatic sensory allergy and visceral sensory allergy, and these effects were blocked by PAR2 antagonists, suggesting that trypsin-like proteins are important in causing visceral sensory sensitization mediated by PAR2. Both cellular and animal model approaches have shown that PAR2 activation causes sustained visceral hypersensitivity or hyperexcitability of enteric neurons, suggesting that PAR2 activation plays an important role in visceral hypersensitivity. Experiments have confirmed the widespread presence of PAR2-positive neurons in the colon. The increased sensitivity of the intestine to mechanical and thermal stimuli after administration of PAR2 agonists also suggests that PAR2 activation plays an important role in the development of visceral hypersensitivity in IBS. The dorsal horn of the spinal cord, as an intermediate station in the gut-brain axis, is a key site in the regulation of visceral sensitization. PAR2-positive injury-sensing neurons terminate in the dorsal horn of the spinal cord and release substance P after PAR2 activation, leading to nociceptive hypersensitivity to heat and mechanical stimuli, and substance P is involved in pain messaging in such a way that PAR2 activation causes hyperexcitation of injury neurons and release of excitatory neurotransmitters, leading to increased visceral sensitivity.

In summary, increased expression and activation of mast cells increases the release of trypsin-like enzymes, which act as potent activators of PAR2 to activate PAR2, the latter positive for increased excitability of injury sensory neurons, leading to increased sensitivity of the gut as well, which in turn releases excitatory neurotransmitter substance P. Its reverse regulation of mast cells increases visceral hypersensitivity in IBS.

11.1.3 Diagnosis and Treatment of Abdominal Pain and Irritable Bowel Syndrome

1. Diagnosis

   IBS is a common functional gastrointestinal disease, and a comprehensive and accurate diagnosis of IBS is a prerequisite for improving the efficacy of treatment. It is internationally recognized that the Rome III criteria [10] proposed in 2006 are symptomatic diagnostic criteria, and the exclusion of organic diseases is still a prerequisite for the diagnosis of IBS. IBS patients often have overlapping symptoms, combined with psychosomatic disorders, and the quality of life is generally reduced, so it is advocated to diagnose the severity of IBS from multiple dimensions to better guide the treatment.

   The 2006 Rome III diagnostic criteria proposed that:

   (a) Recurrent episodes of abdominal pain or abdominal discomfort, at least 3 days per month in the last 3 months, with two or more of the following: (1) improvement after defecation, (2) change in the number of bowel movements during the episode, and (3) change in the nature of bowel movements during the episode.
   (b) Current symptoms have lasted for at least 3 months, and there has been one attack at least 6 months prior to diagnosis.
   (c) Frequency of pain or abdominal discomfort at least 2 days per week as a candidate condition at the time of study or clinical validation.

      In 2016, the Rome Criteria Committee proposed the Rome IV criteria [1], which deleted "abdominal discomfort" from the IBS diagnostic criteria and emphasized "abdominal pain" as a necessary condition for the diagnosis of IBS, while the rest of the diagnostic criteria were the same as the Rome III criteria.

2. Treatment

   (a) Health education

      Most patients have serious misconceptions about IBS, and health education is mainly in the form of doctor's advice, supplemented by other kinds of publicity materials, which is diversified and individualized. It has been proved that effective publicity and education can help reduce self-conscious symptoms, reduce the number of visits, and lower the medical costs of IBS patients.

   (b) Dietary treatment

      Diet has a great influence on symptoms, and certain foods can often trigger the appearance of symptoms, and avoiding certain specific foods can reduce the occurrence of symptoms. The possible pathogenesis is related to gas production in the digestive tract, colonic fermentation, abnormal dynamics after meals, and intolerance to specific foods. For patients with bloating, diarrhea, and increased anal venting, a low-fiber or exclusionary diet therapy can be chosen, while for patients with constipation, a high-fiber diet can be used. The efficacy of different fiber preparations for symptom improvement in BS varies. By monitoring 14 SIgG in the serum of IBS patients and healthy controls, it was found that intervention therapy of eliminating allergic foods in IBS patients with elevated SIgG could completely relieve symptoms in 31.4% of patients, and avoiding large meals and reducing the intake of lactose, fat, sorbitol, xylitol, gas-producing foods, and wheat products could relieve symptoms in some IBS patients [11].

   (c) Antispasmodics

      Anticholinergic drugs such as atropine, bromopamine tylenol, scopolamine, etc. can effectively improve abdominal pain and other symptoms, but attention should be paid to adverse reactions.

Currently, the more commonly used are selective intestinal smooth muscle calcium channel blockers such as pinaverium bromide, oxybutynin, etc., or ion channel modulators such as trimethoprim maleate, all of which have a good safety profile. Such drugs can relax the smooth muscle of the gastrointestinal tract and reduce the colonic response to feeding and stress. A systematic evaluation of 22 studies of 12 different antispasmodics versus placebo-controlled treatment of IBS found that the relative risk value of unimproved symptoms after antispasmodic treatment was 0.68, and the number needed to treat was 5 [12]. Subgroup analysis found that only five antispasmodics, cimetropium bromide, scopolamine, pivelbromine, octreotide, and dicycloverine, were significantly more effective than placebo, while trimebutine, mebeverine, alverine, and pirenzepine were significantly more effective than placebo, Alverine, pirenzepine, piventine bromide, pacivirine, and rosiverine were comparable in efficacy to placebo, and there was no statistical difference in the incidence of adverse reactions between antispasmodics and placebo. Results from a randomized controlled trial (RCT) of IBS treated with peppermint oil have shown that after 4 weeks of treatment, 75% of patients in the treatment group had more than a 50% reduction in total symptom score from the baseline period, while only 38% of patients in the placebo group met this criterion [13]. Overall scores at 4 weeks post-treatment were significantly lower in the peppermint oil treatment group compared to the baseline period, while no significant change was seen in the placebo group.

(d) 5-HT-related drugs

- 5-HT_3 antagonists: They modulate the enteric nervous system, reduce gastrointestinal secretion and peristalsis, and decrease the afferent of nociceptive signals. Such drugs include alosetron, ondansetron, granisetron, and cilansetron, among which only alosetron is approved by the US FDA for clinical treatment of IBS. However, due to the complications of severe ischemic enterocolitis, the drug was withdrawn from the market in 2000 and was reinstated in 2002 after a decision was made to restrict the sale and application of this drug, but the indication was limited to female patients with IBS who had predominantly severe diarrhea and were not responding to conventional therapy. Several randomized controlled trial studies have shown that alosetron is superior to placebo in relieving abdominal pain, abdominal discomfort, anxiety, and overall symptoms of IBS and that alosetron has similar efficacy to that of cilansetron. In addition, cilansetron has similar adverse effects as alosetron, and its main complications are constipation and ischemic enterocolitis, of which the incidence of ischemic enterocolitis is about 1.1/1000 per year [14], so it failed to be approved for marketing by FDA.
- 5-HT_4 agonists: Mainly include cisapride, tegaserod, and lenzapride, which can promote gastrointestinal motility and regulate visceral sensation. In a randomized controlled trial study, tegaserod resulted in more than 15% improvement in overall symptoms in patients with mixed IBS, constipated IBS compared to placebo [15]. The results of another study noted that tegaserod improved overall symptoms of IBS, but not abdominal pain or abdominal discomfort. The study included 29 studies, including 11,614 in the tegaserod-treated group and 7031 in the placebo group. The incidence of cardiovascular events in the tegaserod group was 0.11%, significantly higher than 0.01% in the placebo group [16]. Renzapride has

both 5-HT_4 agonist and 5-HT_3 receptor antagonist effects. The clinical phase IIb drug trial study found that 4 mg of Renzapride daily was significantly better than the placebo group in improving the rate of relief of abdominal pain or discomfort, frequency of bowel movements, and stool properties, and that Renzapride was well tolerated in all dose groups, but the efficacy of Renzapride in the phase III clinical trial was not as good.

(e) Chloride channel-activating drugs: Mainly include lubiprostone, which was found to be effective in improving abdominal pain and abdominal discomfort in IBS patients in the study. In a clinical drug study of lubiprostone in patients with constipated IBS, it was found that 1171 cases of constipated IBS treated with 8 μg of lubiprostone twice daily for 12 weeks had a significantly higher overall efficiency in the treatment of abdominal discomfort than the placebo-treated group and effectively improved the quality of life, anxiety symptoms, and somatic symptoms of IBS patients. The main adverse effects of this drug include nausea and diarrhea [17].

(f) Opioids: Opioids or opioid analogues can have antidiarrheal effects by stimulating intestinal opioid receptors and thus inhibiting colonic peristalsis and secretion; in addition, opioid receptor agonists such as acepromazine can increase the pain threshold of the organism in IBS patients and effectively improve patients' abdominal pain symptoms.

(g) Antidepressants: These drugs mainly include tricyclic antidepressants and new selective 5-HT reuptake inhibitors (SSRI). One investigator studied 596 patients in a randomized controlled trial and found that for patients with diarrheal IBS, amitriptyline was significantly better compared to the placebo group in terms of complete relief of abdominal pain or discomfort, overall symptom relief, abdominal pain score, and frequency of defecation and was well tolerated [18]. Several other randomized controlled trials have shown that low doses of tricyclic antidepressants are effective in improving abdominal pain and abdominal discomfort in patients with IBS. However, some studies have also shown that paroxetine did not significantly improve abdominal pain and stool accumulation, constipation, bloating, diarrhea, and tension.

(h) Microecological agents: The normal intestinal flora is mutually restrained and interdependent, forming a mutually beneficial symbiotic ecological balance in terms of quality and quantity. Intestinal flora dysbiosis is common in patients with IBS. Among them, bifidobacteria and other beneficial probiotics are reduced, while enterobacteria with potential pathogenicity overgrow. Some studies have shown that the use of probiotics to improve intestinal flora disorders in IBS patients can alleviate the symptoms of most patients, and the efficacy is significant in some patients.

(i) Psychotherapy: It mainly includes establishing a good doctor-patient relationship, lifestyle adjustment, cognitive-behavioral therapy, motivational psychotherapy, hypnotherapy, relaxation therapy, suggestion therapy, and antipsychotic medication. A recent randomized controlled trial study showed that cognitive behavioral therapy significantly improved patients' abdominal pain, overall symptoms, health-related quality of life, and IBS severity. Cognitive-behavioral therapy, motivational psychotherapy, and hypnotherapy are now considered to provide more comprehensive symptom improvement than general treatment. A meta-analysis has shown that hypnotherapy significantly relieves GI symptoms and improves the quality of life in patients with IBS and also improves extra-GI symptoms. *2007 British Gastroenterological Society IBS guidelines* [19] recommend hypnotherapy for patients with IBS who do not respond well to conventional treatment and who do not have a severe psychiatric illness. However, current therapeutic studies on psychology generally suffer from the inability to be blinded, the small number of cases included in the studies, unreliable methodology, and unclear treatment mechanisms.

In summary, there is a wide range of drugs and regimens for the treatment of IBS, but no single drug or regimen is completely effective in treating all types of IBS, and in addition, the mechanisms underlying the development of abdominal pain in IBS remain unclear. The current findings suggest that multiple factors and mechanisms are involved in the development of abdominal pain in IBS, and therefore, there is a lack of effective and safe drugs for its treatment. The rapid progress in drug development hides certain risks, such as cisapride and tegaserod, which had been withdrawn from the market due to the discovery of serious complications; therefore, various new drugs must be approached with caution. Simply applying these drugs to patients without selection may be counterproductive. Since IBS is a syndrome diagnosed based on symptom criteria, changes in diagnostic criteria inevitably lead to changes in the detection rate of IBS, which indicates that the diagnosis of IBS is somewhat subjective and arbitrary, so the standardization and rigor of IBS diagnosis and treatment is also the main problem we are currently facing. Further studies on animal models related to IBS can better elucidate the etiology and pathogenesis of IBS, identify biomarker-based diagnoses of IBS that may be better than relying solely on symptomatological criteria, use more valid or clinically meaningful physiological or patient-reported indicators to assess the severity and treatment effects of IBS, conduct basic and clinical studies on the effects of psychological factors on IBS, use more effective treatment, focus on assessing the efficacy of IBS drugs or other treatment modalities, develop more effective drugs for IBS, and a series of other studies will be important topics in the future.

11.2 Peptic Gastric Ulcer

11.2.1 Possible Pathogenesis of Peptic Ulcer Pain

The mechanisms causing peptic ulcer lesions and pain are not fully understood. It is known that in normal people there is an equilibrium between ulcerogenic factors and anti-ulcer protective factors in which the latter prevails. Peptic ulcers can occur if ulcerogenic factors increase and/or anti-ulcer protective factors diminish.

Ulcer pain is visceral in nature, and visceral pain arises mainly from: (1) violent contraction or hyperextension of smooth muscle, (2) inflammation, (3) ischemia, (4) sharp expansion of the peritoneum of substantial organs, (5) direct nerve invasion, etc. The possible mechanism of ulcer pain is speculated as follows: according to the main function of small intestine movement for further grinding, stirring, and mixing of chyme, then the relative small intestine walls must have a certain pressure inward when contracting in order to grind, and when the intestinal contents are less, the relative small intestine walls can contact each other, and in the fasting state, small intestine movement makes the duodenal walls in contact with each other squeeze and grind, and ulcer pain occurs.

In addition, various reasons such as eating lead to increased secretion of gastric acid in peptic ulcer patients, excessive gastric acid promotes the decomposition of pepsinogen into pepsin, and excessive gastric acid and pepsin have stimulating and erosive effects on the gastroduodenal mucosa, which may aggravate gastroduodenitis or ulcer and cause clinical symptoms. At the same time, due to increased secretion of gastric acid, the negative feedback effect causes a decrease in gastrin secretion, and gastrin has a strong effect on the movement of the stomach, which can improve the pyloric pump activity, make the pylorus diastolic, and promote gastric emptying, so too much gastric acid instead inhibits gastric peristalsis, leads to gastric emptying disorders, and aggravates the symptoms of ulcer pain.

11.2.2 Peptic Ulcer Abdominal Pain Site and Characteristics

Epigastric pain is the most common clinical manifestation of peptic ulcer; its pain is often located in the middle of the epigastrium, left or right; and the pain of a duodenal ulcer is mostly located between the glabella and umbilicus, which mostly in the upper abdomen, usually the right side, can be radiated to the back, rib margin, and chest. Gastric ulcer brings left lower anterior chest or left upper abdominal pain, the range of which is about several centimeters in diameter size. Ulcer disease pain may present as vague, dull, stabbing, burning pain, or distension. In patients without complications, the pain is mostly not severe and can be tolerated. The intensity of pain is not clearly related to the size of the ulcer or the level of gastric acid. The occurrence of complications often changes the nature and intensity of ulcer pain.

The active phase of the ulcer is usually accompanied by pressure pain in the epigastrium, which is more limited in its area of pressure, unlike the diffuse pressure pain of chronic gastritis. The pressure point of pancreatic or lesser curvature ulcers is mostly located under or slightly to the left of the saber process in the upper abdomen: pyloric ulcers are mostly located in the midline above the umbilicus or slightly to the right; duodenal ulcers are mostly located in the upper right side of the umbilicus. When the ulcer is combined with pyloric obstruction, the abdominal pain may become persistent and distending without rhythm. Alkaline medication is not effective and is often accompanied by vomiting, which relieves the abdominal pain.

The vast majority of patients have the typical clinical symptoms of chronic, periodic, and rhythmic epigastric pain and discomfort. In contrast, a minority of patients may be asymptomatic, with some patients having bleeding and perforation as the first symptoms.

Since the ulcer can heal on its own after occurrence but is often prone to recurrence after healing, it is often characterized by long-term recurrent epigastric pain. The average duration of the disease is 6–7 years, and some can exceed 10 years, or even longer.

Epigastric pain with recurrent periodic episodes is one of the characteristics of ulcers. Duodenal is more pronounced than a gastric ulcer. The so-called periodicity of pain means that the pain lasts for days, weeks, or months, followed by months to years of remission, and then recurrence. Recurrence can occur throughout the year but is more common in the late fall and early winter when temperatures are colder. In some patients, recurrences are more frequent and last longer after years of attacks, and the remission period is shortened accordingly.

Rhythmicity is another characteristic of peptic ulcer. Since the occurrence of pain is related to the exposure of the ulcer surface to gastric acid and the acidity of gastric acid, food is the main cause of gastric acid secretion. Therefore, the pain of ulcers is related to eating. In the day, the period from 3:00 a.m. to breakfast has the lowest gastric acid secretion, so pain rarely occurs during this time. The pain of duodenal ulcer mostly occurs between meals and continues unabated until the next meal is eaten or relieved by taking antacids. Gastric ulcer pain occurs more irregularly and often occurs within 1 h after a meal, gradually relieved after 1–2 h, until the above-mentioned rhythmic pain occurs again after the next meal. In some patients with duodenal ulcer, midnight pain can occur due to high stomach acid at night, especially in those who have eaten before bedtime. The midnight pain that occurs at regular intervals is another characteristic of duodenal ulcers.

11.2.3 Treatment of Peptic Ulcer Pain

The purpose of peptic ulcer treatment is to eliminate pain, heal the ulcer, and prevent recurrence of the ulcer. In addition to general treatment, drug therapy is particularly important, mainly including the inhibition of gastric acid secretion and elimination of bacterial infection, to distinguish the presence of *Helicobacter pylori* infection in cases with a clear diagnosis of peptic ulcer.

Eradication of *H. pylori* treatment in those with positive infection can shorten the treatment time of ulcers. A triple therapy centered on antacids plus two antibiotics, namely, famotidine 20 mg (twice daily, orally) or omeprazole 20 mg (once daily, orally), amoxicillin 500 mg (four times daily, orally) and tinidazole 400 mg (four times daily, orally), is applied for 2 weeks. One of the antacids can be replaced by bismuth potassium citrate 120 mg (four times daily, orally). The course of antacids is 4–6 weeks in duodenal ulcers and can be extended to 8–12 weeks in gastric ulcers, which should be determined according to whether the ulcer is healing. When mucosal protective drugs are applied instead of antacids, the course of treatment of bismuth potassium citrate does not exceed 8–12 weeks, and the later service can be maintained by H_2 receptor antagonists. Foreign proposed bismuth-centered "standard" program includes bismuth potassium citrate, metronidazole (or tinidazole), and amoxicillin (or tetracycline), 2 weeks of *H. pylori* eradication rate of 80–90% [20]. Domestic according to the characteristics of the national light weight, the last two antibiotic doses by half, that is, "low-dose" triple therapy, *H. pylori* eradication rate of 70–80%, the adverse reactions greatly reduced, and this program is inexpensive and can be applied at the grassroots level. Some foreign reports use quadruple therapy, that is, bismuth-centered triple therapy plus a proton pump inhibitor, which can improve the efficacy, but two groups in China reported that the addition of antacids only early relief of ulcer symptoms, and *H. pylori* eradication rate did not significantly improve.

For *H. pylori* negative patients, an H_2 receptor antagonist or a proton pump inhibitor can be used. The course of treatment for duodenal ulcer is 4–6 weeks and for gastric ulcer is 8–12 weeks [21] and can be shortened or prolonged according to the healing of ulcer: those with recurrent attacks should take maintenance doses for a long time, at least 1 year, or longer, and those who take oral antacids add mucosal protective drugs and bismuth potassium citrate 120 mg (four times daily, before meals orally) for 8 weeks as a course of treatment, which is better than those who take antacids commonly. Patients with peptic ulcers should be diagnosed by endoscopy prior to *H. pylori* eradication therapy, and detailed measurement of ulcer size and Sakita-Miwa staging should be performed to observe ulcer healing. The same examination is performed after eradication treatment to evaluate the effectiveness of the treatment. Fiberoptic gastroscopy is usually performed within 3 days prior to drug administration and 4 weeks after discontinuation of eradication therapy. During the examination, one piece of mucosa from each of the lesser and greater curvatures of the gastric sinus and one piece of mucosa from each of the lesser and greater curvatures of the gastric body were taken 3–5 cm from the pyloric valve for histological examination, and two pieces of mucosa from the lesser curvature of the gastric sinus were taken, one for urease test and the other for *H. pylori* culture. The urinary toxin test was positive before treatment, and at least one of the two tests, histology and *H. pylori* culture, was positive for infection. A negative urease test, histology, and *H. pylori* culture at the 4-week discontinuation of the drug is considered eradication of *H. pylori*. Ulcer healing is determined as healing, improvement, or failure. Healed ulcer means that the patient has no conscious symptoms and the ulcer is healed by gastroscopy: improved means that the patient has conscious symptoms and the ulcer is reduced by more than 50% by gastroscopy [21], and ineffective means that the patient may or may not have conscious symptoms and the size of the ulcer does not change by gastroscopy or is less than 50% healed.

In conclusion, although the etiology and pathogenesis of ulcer disease are not yet fully understood, its causative factors have different clinical manifestations in different patients, and giving targeted treatment is an important step to achieve good results. At present, the main means of treatment for ulcer disease is drugs, which can heal almost all ulcers and eliminate all symptoms.

11.3 Chronic Pancreatitis and Pain Due to Its Acute Attacks

11.3.1 Definition, Epidemiology, and Classification of Chronic Pancreatitis

Chronic pancreatitis refers to persistent damage to pancreatic tissues and functions caused by various etiologies, and its pathology is characterized by pancreatic fibrosis, with recurrent abdominal pain and pancreatic exocrine insufficiency as the main symptoms, which can be combined with endocrine insufficiency, pancreatic parenchymal calcification, pancreatic duct stones, and pancreatic pseudocyst formation.

There are significant geographical differences in the incidence of chronic pancreatitis worldwide. The average annual incidence in Western countries is 10–15 new cases per 100,000 people, but in Sweden, there is an annual increase of 3–8 cases [22]. In the Asia-Pacific region, there is an average of 10 cases per 100,000 people; in southern India and some other regions, there are more than 100 cases per 100,000 people, mainly tropical pancreatitis [23]. There are no definite data on the incidence of chronic pancreatitis in China, as well as epidemiological information based on population censuses, and the published data were obtained from hospitals, and it was estimated that the incidence of chronic pancreatitis increased year by year from 1996 to 2003, with 3.08, 3.91, 5.28, 7.61, 10.43, 11.92, 12.84, and 13.52 cases, especially in the developed eastern regions of China, where the incidence of chronic pancreatitis is increasing at a significantly higher rate than in other regions [24]. This reminds us to pay more attention to and study chronic pancreatitis.

Chronic pancreatitis can be subdivided into different types according to the etiology. Alcoholic chronic pancreatitis is also the most common form of chronic pancreatitis in western industrialized countries. Tropical pancreatitis, which is endemic in India and Indonesia, has a gender-neutral infection rate and is thought to be caused by dietary factors, but the exact pathogenesis of this clinical disease remains unknown. Other types of chronic pancreatitis include hereditary pancreatitis due to genetic mutations (e.g., gallbladder fibrosis gene), chronic pancreatitis due to metabolic disorders such as hypercalcemia or hyperlipoproteinemia, chronic pancreatitis due to pancreatic compartment or duodenal wall cysts, and primary chronic pancreatitis of unknown origin. Multiple etiologies of chronic pancreatitis may cause a superposition of pain types and patterns, with abdominal pain, especially epigastric pain, being the most common type of pain.

11.3.2 Chronic Pancreatitis and Pain

Abdominal pain is the main clinical symptom of chronic pancreatitis, which usually presents as recurrent intermittent episodes of pain in the upper abdomen. As the disease progresses, the frequency of pain episodes gradually increases, and the asymptomatic period progressively shortens and eventually progresses to persistent pain. The site of pancreatitis pain is usually in the upper abdomen, sometimes radiating to the back and left shoulder. Typical symptoms of pancreatitis appear after eating, but the pain itself is often not directly related to eating. The degree of pancreatitis pain varies widely among and within individuals and is difficult to quantify. As the frequency of pain episodes progresses from intermittent to persistent, the degree of pain progresses from mild pain to requiring frequent hospitalization, and patients gradually lose their ability to work. A domestic multicenter survey of 2000 patients with chronic pancreatitis showed that abdominal pain was the first symptom in 72.65% of cases. This is similar to the characteristics of patients in Western countries, and it not only is the main reason for patients to visit the clinic but also seriously affects their quality of life. Therefore, pain relief occupies a considerable place in the treatment of chronic pancreatitis.

Unfortunately, our understanding of the biology of chronic pancreatitis has been slow to advance, especially with regard to the pathogenesis of the basic symptoms of pancreatitis such as pain. Physicians who have treated such patients have noted that pain is not only the most important symptom of chronic pancreatitis but also the most difficult to treat, and it is generally accepted that there is little understanding of chronic pancreatitis pain and that treatment is controversial. As a result, the lack of knowledge about pain in pancreatitis has severely hampered the improvement of patient care, resulting in a variety of empirical treatments often based on purely anatomical aspects that are highly invasive and have limited effectiveness. Despite the variety of treatment approaches, there is no consensus, and none of them are currently satisfactory. How to reduce the pain of patients with chronic pancreatitis is a common concern for clinicians, and this chapter will focus on the mechanisms of the occurrence of pain in chronic pancreatitis and treatment countermeasures.

11.3.3 Mechanisms of the Occurrence of Pain in Chronic Pancreatitis

The traditional theory is that pancreatic tissue hypertension or pancreatic ischemia caused by pancreatic duct obstruction and pancreatic fibrosis is the main cause of chronic pancreatitis pain. With the in-depth investigation of the causes of chronic pancreatitis pain, it has been found that the number of local nerve fibers in the pancreas increases and the diameter increases significantly in chronic pancreatitis, and the nerve bundle membrane is damaged, on the basis of which immune cells, various inflammatory mediators, neurotrophic factors, and neuropeptides infiltrated in the pancreas can sensitize the damaged nerves in the pancreas and cause a series of changes in the sensory transmission pathways, thus inducing the development of nociceptive hypersensitivity in chronic pancreatitis. The development of nociceptive hypersensitivity in chronic pancreatitis. Therefore, the current view is that neurogenic inflammation and neurogenic pain are one of the key factors in the formation and maintenance of pain in chronic pancreatitis.

1. Intraductal pancreatic hypertension

   In our country, chronic biliary system disease is the main cause of chronic pancreatitis pain. The activation of pancreatic enzymes in the pancreas caused by small amounts of bile backflowing into the pancreatic duct several times and long-term repeated chronic irritation are the causes of chronic biliary pancreatitis pain. Especially in the case of combined biliary system stones, the stenosis or obstruction at the junction of the pancreaticobiliary duct caused by stones or infection, the outflow of pancreatic juice is obstructed, which in turn leads to an increase in the internal pressure of the pancreatic duct, resulting in the rupture of the pancreatic alveoli and small ducts, damage to the pancreatic tissue and pancreatic duct system, distortion, and deformation of the pancreatic duct, which increases the number and degree of episodes of chronic pancreatitis pain. Clinically, it is often manifested as intermittent pain in the upper abdomen or around the umbilicus, and in severe cases, it can be persistent and progressively aggravated in the form of cluster-like pain, which can spread to the bilateral quarter rib area and back, chest, scapula, and other places.

   It is believed that obstruction of the lower pancreatic duct forming pancreatic duct dilatation and intraductal hypertension is the main cause of pancreatitis pain, which is the theoretical basis for surgical and endoscopic pancreatic duct drainage and other treatment methods. Studies have shown that intrapancreatic duct stones, intrapancreatic duct stenosis due to chronic inflammation, and dysfunction of the jugular sphincter can lead to a significant increase in intrapancreatic duct pressure, which in turn causes pain. Currently, surgery and endoscopy are the main methods to measure intrapancreatic ductal pressure, and ERCP technique can also provide accurate measurement of intrapancreatic ductal pressure. Studies have shown that intrapancreatic ductal pressure is generally 8–20 mmHg in normal subjects and 8–10 mmHg higher than normal in patients with chronic pancreatitis [25]; however, this view is highly controversial. Although pancreatic duct obstruction is an important factor in causing pain and there is evidence of significant short-term pain relief after endoscopic and surgical pancreatic duct drainage, the failure of the procedure also suggests that pancreatic duct dilatation is not the only etiology of pain. A subset of cases showed a similar probability of pancreatic duct dilatation in patients with and without painful symptoms, while other cases showed patients with severe painful symptoms with or without pancreatic duct stricture and dilatation. Increased intrapancreatic ductal pressure can be measured by surgical and endoscopic methods in patients with chronic pancreatitis, but common bile duct obstruction does not correlate with the degree of pancreatic pain, and endoscopic drainage of common bile duct obstruction does not improve the pain of chronic pancreatitis. In addition, although sphincter of Oddi dysfunction can lead to increased intrapancreatic ductal pressure in chronic pancreatitis and acute recurrent pancreatitis, the magnitude of intrapancreatic ductal pressure and the degree of pain in chronic pancreatitis are also not correlated. At present, the theory that pancreatic duct stones cause pancreatic duct hypertension and pancreatic duct stenosis and obstruction cause pancreatic fibrosis leading to painful pancreatitis is still commonly accepted clinically, although it has not been supported by experimental data.

2. Intrapancreatic parenchymal hypertension

   Pancreatic parenchymal hypertension is another pathological mechanism leading to pain in chronic pancreatitis. This is better explained by the theory of compartmentalization syndrome. The pancreatic parenchyma is completely surrounded by the relatively less stretchable pancreatic tegument. When inflammation irritates the pancreatic parenchyma, the parenchyma can become congested and swollen, and because the tegument restricts its expansion, it leads to a significant increase in tissue pressure within the pancreatic parenchyma, capillary, and venous collapse and reduced perfusion of pancreatic tissue, which in turn leads to anaerobic metabolism and acidosis, causing persistent pain in the pancreas. If the intrapancreatic parenchymal pressure can be reduced by 10 mmHg by surgical means, the patient's pain symptoms can usually be effectively relieved [26]. One-year follow-up showed that the intrapancreatic parenchymal pressure tended to be close to the preoperative level in patients who developed pain again after surgery, indicating that increased intrapancreatic parenchymal pressure is significantly associated with pain in chronic pancreatitis.

3. Oxidative stress response

   The theory that an imbalance in the production and scavenging of reactive oxygen species causes damage to pancreatic alveolar cells is increasingly recognized. In the analysis of studies of patients with alcoholic chronic pancreatitis, serum levels of antioxidants were found to be significantly reduced. Excessive release of oxygen-free radicals caused by alcohol, smoking, and chemical toxins can cause inflammatory responses and tissue damage leading to painful chronic pancreatitis. Alcohol consumption can be a direct cause of pancreatic pain as an independent factor, and this condition is more common abroad. In vitro experiments have shown that patients with alcoholic chronic pancreatitis can have increased production of reactive oxygen species due to the activation of neutrophils, causing cell and tissue damage. Other reports suggest that micronutrient deficiencies in the body can exacerbate oxidative stress. A study investigating the diet of patients with chronic pancreatitis found that their reduced micronutrient intake, which exacerbates oxidative stress, may be related to the development of their pain.

4. Peripheral injury receptor mechanisms

   Possible stimuli of pain receptors in the pancreas: Ductal hypertension triggered by constriction or stones, increased parenchymal pressure due to fibrosis, toxic substances such as ethanol. However, there is no evidence to date that these factors are directly related to pancreatic pain, and even in the absence of these factors, patients with chronic pancreatitis often still have severe pain. It has been shown that substances released by damaged alveolar cells such as protons, bradykinin, hydrogen sulfide, serotonin, and calcium will activate injury receptor nerves through their respective receptors. However, it must be mentioned that the direct activation of these molecules by the injury receptors has not been demonstrated in animal models of chronic pancreatitis or in patients with chronic pancreatitis. Therefore, the activation of damage receptor nerves by these molecules is still a theoretical hypothesis. On the other hand, only two injury receptors have been identified in the pancreas and have been shown to be directly activated by these substances, PAR2 and TRPV1. One study showed that in vivo pancreatic protease activates sensory dorsal root ganglion neurons by binding to PAR2 after entering the pancreatic duct in rats by enhanced immunoreactivity assay of c-fos protein. It is worth stating that the above study used a behavioral assay model rather than a chronic pancreatitis model. In another important study, the investigators induced chronic pancreatitis in rats with trinitrobenzene sulfonic acid, and the experimental group had significantly greater depolarization resting potentials and reduced type A potassium current density in pancreatic-specific dorsal root ganglion neurons compared to the control group. The increased TRPV1 expression and enhanced capsaicin response in pancreatic-specific dorsal root ganglion neurons in the chronic pancreatitis model further validated the direct activation of injury-sensing fibers. In addition, some of the inflammatory mediators mentioned above can also indirectly activate TRPV1 by decreasing its stimulation threshold.

5. Mechanisms of peripheral neuropathic alterations

   The motivation to investigate the peripheral injury perception mechanisms mentioned above stems in part from parallel studies of acute pancreatitis, and the currently accepted concept of neuropathology in chronic pancreatitis and other pancreatic diseases is rooted in the initial identification of neural alterations in histopathological specimens. Keith et al. first reported the presence of chronic pancreatitis with significant infiltration of inflammatory cells, especially eosinophils, into the nerves within the pancreas [27]. They found a significant correlation between pain and the percentage of eosinophil infiltration around these nerves. In a subsequent study, Bockman et al. found increased nerve density and hypertrophy in chronic pancreatitis. More importantly, when they performed ultrastructural analysis of the nerves within the pancreas in chronic pancreatitis, they observed some evidence of nerve injury, such as broken nerve bundle membranes, edematous nerve contents, and inflammatory cell infiltration into the interior of the nerves.

   (a) Pancreatic nerve plasticity: Intrapancreatic nerve injury appears to require many alterations in peripheral nerve plasticity, best evidenced by significant hypertrophy and sprouting of intrapancreatic nerves. The finding of overexpression of GA-43, a marker molecule of neuroplasticity in chronic pancreatitis, also validates this phenomenon. This plasticity was further elucidated when comparing the autonomic innervation of the normal pancreas with that of chronic pancreatitis. When comparing sympathetic and parasympathetic innervation of the pancreas in normal and chronic pancreatitis patients, it was found that sympathetic innervation of the pancreas in chronic pancreatitis was significantly reduced. There was no apparent difference in parasympathetic innervation between the two, but both sympathetic and parasympathetic innervation were significantly reduced in patients with chronic pancreatitis with severe neuropathic abdominal pain and/or severe pancreatic neuritis. When analyzing peripheral nerves, it is important to consider not only the neuronal composition but also the status of the glial cells in these nerves. The aim of the above study was to study not only the autonomic innervation of the pancreas in chronic pancreatitis but also to analyze the role of

Schwann cells in these nerves. Studies have shown that glial cells play a key role in neuropathic pain, especially for inflammatory diseases. To understand their activation status, some investigators quantified the expression of the glial transcription factor Sox10 and neuroepithelial stem cell marker neural stem cell protein in chronic pancreatitis. In principle with neuropathy, the activation status of glial in chronic pancreatitis was also significantly different: Sox10 expression within nerves was extremely reduced, while Nestin immunoreactivity was significantly increased. These findings are of great importance as they help to initially elucidate the role of neuroglia in pancreatic neuropathy.

Upon nerve injury, Schwann cells begin to proliferate and dedifferentiate through the release of neurotrophic substances, axonal growth and myelin regeneration, and pain receptor sensitization. Because Sox10 persists in mature Schwann cells, reduced neural Sox10 expression in chronic pancreatitis is likely a marker of reduced numbers of mature Schwann cells, which may result from the reactive dedifferentiation described above. This elucidation is consistent with the observed Nestin upregulation, as high expression of glial Nestin and subsequent onset of neural sprouting has been demonstrated following muscle denervation at the neuromuscular junction. Therefore, as in multiple other neuropathies, alterations in Sox10 and Nestin in pancreatic neuropathies can indirectly indicate neuroglial activation.

Overall, the neuropathic changes in chronic pancreatitis consist of three main axes: changes in autonomic innervation, glial activation, and associated neuropathic pain, and it can be said that pancreatic neuropathy is characterized by "neural remodeling." This pancreatic nerve alteration may be one of the reasons for the poor efficacy of pancreatic denervation techniques in the treatment of chronic pancreatitis pain. Especially after observing a significant reduction of sympathetic nerves accompanying sensory nerves in the visceral nerves, we should think about the distribution and number of sensory/injury sensory nerves in the visceral and ventral plexus in patients with chronic pancreatitis. As mentioned earlier, pain in chronic pancreatitis may be transmitted via, for example, vagal or somatosensory afferent nerves that reach the dorsal root ganglia rather than afferent nerves that accompany the visceral nerves. The most effective method of pain relief for patients with chronic pancreatitis has been demonstrated in numerous controlled trials to be surgical resection of the head of the pancreas. Therefore, interventions targeting the root cause of pancreatic neuropathy, that is, intrapancreatic interventions, are more effective than surgical or chemical removal of nerve fibers, which may then not be inherently a transmission pathway for pain.

(b) Neuroinflammatory role: The degree of pancreatic neuropathy, the interdependence between nerve remodeling, and pancreatic neuritis should draw our attention to the role of neuroinflammation in the generation of peripheral visceral neuropathy. The actors that produce pancreatic neuritis remain undiscovered. Among dozens of known markers of inflammation, studies have shown that only L-8, derived mainly from inflammatory cells infiltrating hypertrophic nerves, is overexpressed in chronic pancreatitis tissue compared to normal pancreas. There are several factors that attract inflammatory cells to the nerve, thereby mediating nerve injury and neuropathic pain. A typical representative of such molecule is the chemokine CX3, which is likely to induce the aforementioned neuropathic alterations in chronic pancreatitis in three ways: firstly, CX3 is a chemoattractant for immune cells; secondly, it can also induce neuropathic pain through neuroglial activation; and finally, it has a role in promoting tissue fibrosis. In chronic pancreatitis, researchers not only detected overexpression of chemokine CX3 and its receptor CX3CR1 at the protein level but also found increased mean immunoreactivity to chemokine CX3 and CX3CR1 in patients suffering from severe neuropathic pain and pancreatic neuritis. Furthermore, these alterations appeared to be more pronounced in patients with chronic neuropathic pain. Therefore, researchers identified molecular analogs that target neuronal molecules to induce neural affinity for the production of inflammatory cells. It has been suggested that blockade of CX3CR1 may play an important role in improving neuroinflammation in the pancreas and neurogenic nociception in the abdomen. Further studies targeting other cytokine and chemokine receptors are pending. Throughout the study of pancreatic neuropathy, recent findings suggest that neuropathic pain in chronic pancreatitis is the result of a combination of numerous cells and molecules, including immune cells, damaged nerves, nerve regeneration, glial cell activation, chemokines, cytokines, and some other substances that have not yet been identified.

6. Mechanisms of central neuropathic alterations and neuroplasticity
   (a) Sensitization: The evidence of peripheral nerve damage in chronic pancreatitis has laid the foundation for "pancreatic neuropathy" to become a new subclass of peripheral visceral neuropathy. Encouragingly, many recent studies have shown similar alterations in the neuropathic pain symptoms of chronic pancreatitis at the central nervous system level. As mentioned earlier, in peripheral nerve injury, the nerves are susceptible to noxious stimuli from the surrounding environment and secrete factors that further sensitize injury receptors. Continued sensitization of peripheral injury receptors leads to sensitization of spinal neurons, which can transmit peripheral signals to the brain. This overall sensitization is the hallmark of neuropathic pain symptoms. This sensitization leads to the main symptoms of neuropathic pain, namely, abnormal pain and nociceptive hyperalgesia.
   (b) Referred pain: In a prospective study, patients with chronic pancreatitis were stimulated in multiple modalities and multiple organs and observed whether there was an increase in the area of involvement pain and the sensory response of the patient's visceral and body surface organs. They also proposed that patients with chronic pancreatitis have an aggregation of afferent signals from body surface organs and visceral organs and that injurious stimulation of these organs would produce signs of central hyperexcitability. As in the hypothetical case, they found a significant difference in pain response between patients with chronic pancreatitis and controls after single and repeated electrical stimulation. This difference reflects an important feature of neurogenic pain symptoms in chronic pancreatitis, namely, the role of temporal summation. Moreover, the investigators also confirmed a greater increase in the area of involved pain in patients with chronic pancreatitis, thus demonstrating two main features of neurogenic pain in chronic pancreatitis. There is still controversy regarding their findings on nociception. They found reduced sensitivity to mechanical stimuli at the skin, duodenum, and esophagus in patients with chronic pancreatitis. The authors of the article concluded that chronic organic diseases of the gastrointestinal tract such as Crohn's disease, esophagitis, and gastric ulcers also all exhibit diminished nociception to mechanical stimuli. In contrast, Buscher et al. demonstrated that patients with chronic pancreatitis exhibit

significant generalized profound nociceptive hyperalgesia, even under opioid therapy [28]. Because of the complex pathophysiological processes involved in central pain, it is difficult to provide a precise explanation for these conflicting findings. Likewise, it is difficult to explain why Dimcevski et al. reported hyperalgesia in the periphery of patients with chronic pancreatitis, while the center is hyperexcitable and has increased areas of involvement in pain.

(c) Downstream inhibitory system: It is certain that the central nervous system, which ultimately controls nociceptive perception, especially higher centers such as the brainstem, plays a major role in the regulation of neuropathic pain in patients with chronic pancreatitis. This so-called "downward inhibitory control" is activated in the presence of a continuous pain stimulus, which leads to an inhibition of the responsiveness of dorsal horn spinal neuron activity. Although it is possible that patients with chronic pancreatitis may have downward inhibition, some recent findings are inconsistent with this. The presence of downstream "vulnerability" in chronic pancreatitis was confirmed in a study by Vera-Portocarrero et al. [29], and they disrupted the brain stem cells responsible for downstream regulation by a single local injection of dermorphin-saponin in a rat model of chronic pancreatitis and then observed that the abdominal hypersensitivity associated with chronic pancreatitis continued to be maintained without being blocked. In another recent study, this phenomenon of downward easing rather than inhibition was confirmed in patients with chronic pancreatitis. Electrical or thermal stimulation given in the rectosigmoid region resulted in significant distal nociceptive hyperalgesia in patients with chronic pancreatitis compared to controls. Thus, organic gastrointestinal diseases all exhibit hyperalgesia due to the inhibitory control of diffuse toxic substances, but this hypothesis cannot be verified in patients with chronic pancreatitis who have significant generalized hyperalgesia.

(d) EEG alterations: In studies focusing on pain processing in the brain, evidence that chronic pancreatitis is characterized by neuropathic pain can also be found. In one of the earliest studies in this area, investigators performed endoscopic electrical stimulation of the esophagus, stomach, and duodenum in patients with chronic pancreatitis while recording event-associated brain potentials (ERBP) by electroencephalography. Strikingly, the latency of early ERBP characterizing exogenous brain pain processing was significantly lower in patients with chronic pancreatitis compared to controls. Subsequent analysis revealed that these ERBP localized to typical visceral sensory areas in the cerebral cortex, namely, the insula on both sides, the anterior cingulate gyrus, and the second somatosensory area on both sides. Interestingly, the islet dipoles on both sides of the chronic pancreatitis group were positioned more medially, while the cingulate gyrus was positioned more posteriorly, suggesting an important message: there is a reorganization of the cerebral cortex in patients with chronic pancreatitis. In a further study, the investigators confirmed increased 0-wave activity in EEG, which is typical of neuropathic pain, thus providing further evidence for the neuropathic nature of pain symptoms in chronic pancreatitis. Fregni et al. demonstrated increased glutamate levels and found hyperactivity in the right top somatosensory cortical area by magnetic resonance spectroscopy [30]. In essence, there will be reliable evidence of central nervous system remodeling and activity modulation in chronic pancreatitis as a hallmark of neuropathic pain syndrome.

7. Summary and discussion

The elucidation of the mechanisms underlying the development of pain in chronic pancreatitis is a great challenge. The development of pancreatic surgical techniques in the second half of the twentieth century, the emergence of clinical scientists, and the intense interest of basic research scientists and pain specialists have allowed the accumulation of a wealth of information related to the pathogenesis of the disease. The mechanism of pain in chronic pancreatitis can be analyzed in three main aspects: peripheral injury perception, peripheral/pancreatic neuropathy and neuroplasticity, and central neuropathy and neuroplasticity. Chronic pancreatitis appears to be associated with persistent sensitization of pancreatic peripheral pain receptors mediated by neurotransmitters and neurotrophic factors following nerve injury. This peripheral pancreatic neuropathy leads to altered neuroplasticity in the pancreas through "neural remodeling," which is associated with altered autonomic innervation of the human pancreas. It further leads to over-activation of sensory secondary neurons in the spinal cord and presents a state of hyperexcitability. Finally, the brain stem and supraspinal regions of the brain exacerbate this caudal overactivation by downstream facilitation and reorganization to process more peripheral inputs. In chronic pancreatitis neuropathic pain syndrome, the neuropathic pain mechanism is clearly dominant and relies mainly on continuous injurious stimulation from peripheral pain receptors compared to the primary neuropathic pain syndrome. The effectiveness of surgical excision of this "neurological neuropathy" at the origin and the resulting gap in the injury receptors, which would otherwise continue to transmit painful stimuli to the central nervous system. This is an important feature of this syndrome. Therefore, based on the interconnection of injury sensation and neuropathy in chronic pancreatitis, clinicians can consider chronic pancreatitis pain as a "mixed" type of pain that is "predominantly neuropathic." The ideal treatment for chronic pancreatitis pain can only be obtained by carefully considering this particular hybrid mechanism.

11.3.4 Treatment of Chronic Pancreatitis Pain

Chronic pancreatitis pain varies greatly between patients and between stages in the same patient, and factors contributing to this variation include etiology, the natural history of pancreatitis, and the presence or absence of associated complications; in addition, psychosocial factors such as secondary gain and addiction-prone personalities significantly add to the complexity of treatment in these patients. Most of the published literature is for the treatment of pain in patients with alcoholic pancreatitis, as this is the most common form of this disease. Even in such patients, however, pain does not present as a uniform symptom, and its pattern may have implications for treatment and prognosis. The treatment of pain in chronic pancreatitis is a challenge. Despite new imaging and pancreatic assessment tools, the clinical treatment of chronic pancreatitis pain is still highly arbitrary and often ends in failure. If the complexity of chronic pancreatitis pain and its pathological mechanisms are not properly understood, pain management is quite difficult. The American Gastroenterological Association guidelines state that it is very important to determine the presence of treatable complications of chronic pancreatitis such as pseudocysts, bile duct strictures, and duodenal obstruction [31]. Other causes of abdominal pain, such as peptic ulcer, biliary tract disease, and gastrointestinal motility disorders, also need to be ruled out. Chronic heavy alcohol consumption accelerates the progression of endocrine and exocrine pancreatic insufficiency. The altered pancreatic function caused by alcoholic pancreatitis progresses even after the cessation of alcohol intake, although its progression is of course slowed down. In patients with severe alcoholic pancreatitis, cessation of alcohol intake does not change the characteristics of their pancreatic pain, but those who continue to abuse will have a threefold higher mortality rate than those who abstain from alcohol or reduce alcohol intake and, more importantly, a threefold higher incidence of physical defects in the former.

The complexity of the mechanism of abdominal pain in chronic pancreatitis makes clinical management very difficult. It is currently believed that the treatment of abdominal pain in chronic pancreatitis should be multidisciplinary, using a combination of drugs and addressing psychological issues. The treatment of chronic pancreatitis includes various methods, and pseudocysts and pancreatic duct obstruction can be treated by endoscopy or extracorporeal shock wave lithotripsy, and surgical procedures such as local lesion removal, nerve release, and nerve block can be performed. However, for most patients, drug treatment is still the mainstay. Treatment of chronic pancreatitis pain is difficult and often requires the use of strong opioids. The cornerstone of neuropathic pain treatment, on the other hand, is multifunctional drugs acting on different central targets, such as tricyclic antidepressants, gabapentin or pregabalin, tramadol, and eventually opioids of choice. Studies have shown that drugs effective in the treatment of neuropathic pain may also be effective in chronic pancreatitis, as demonstrated by Drewes et al. [32]. Therefore, in the future, the combination of drugs should be considered more often for the pharmacological treatment of chronic pancreatitis pain.

Therefore, medical treatment for pain should be considered first, and measures such as nerve block and destruction resection, endoscopic lithotripsy, drainage, and stent placement should be considered when the results are poor, and only after that, surgical treatment such as decompression, drainage, and pancreatic resection should be considered. Surgery is an effective treatment for patients with chronic pancreatitis who have failed medical and endoscopic treatment, of which 15–20% of patients must undergo surgery, such as pseudocyst infection, rupture, and bleeding [33].

11.3.4.1 Medical Treatment

1. Diet

   Patients with chronic pancreatitis should receive professional dietary guidance. The degree of endocrine and exocrine insufficiency, like micronutrient deficiency, requires professional dietary determination. The conventional recommendation is a low-fat diet with a small total amount of food eaten at each meal to avoid overstimulation of the pancreas. However, a complete evaluation of this idea has not been reported. In addition, reducing alcohol intake is the main treatment for alcoholic pancreatitis. Although most studies have concluded that abstinence from alcohol does not relieve patients' pain, the mortality rate of patients with alcoholic pancreatitis can be reduced to one-third of the original rate after abstinence [34].

2. Drug treatment

   For patients with chronic pancreatitis, pain management inevitably requires the use of analgesics. Analgesic treatment is generally divided into three stages: the first stage can use non-narcotic analgesics, such as nonsteroidal anti-inflammatory drugs, acetaminophen, but non-opioid analgesics to relieve pain is not ideal; the second stage can be used in different strength of action of narcotics, such as the preferred powerful but small adverse effects of analgesics such as tramadol. Tramadol is characterized by small adverse effects (especially gastrointestinal adverse effects) and can be used as the first-line analgesic for chronic pancreatitis. The third stage is usually the application of opioid analgesics considered in the late stage of pancreatic cancer with severe pain. However, even in this stage, we should try to choose a slow-release dosage form to reduce the number of doses to reduce the possibility of drug addiction, and the dose should be adjusted for individual conditions, with the minimum effective dose, avoiding the use of short-acting opioids such as pethidine. In addition, cholecystokinin receptor antagonists, pancreatic enzyme inhibitors, protease inhibitors, and leukotriene receptor antagonists have certain efficacy.

At present, it is still very difficult to treat chronic pancreatitis pain using internal medicine, analgesics are still the main drugs relied on clinically, and the use of pancreatic enzyme preparations, antioxidants, oral protease inhibitors, and octreotide is still more controversial in clinical practice.

11.3.4.2 Endoscopic Treatment

For recurrent acute attacks of intractable pain despite appropriate life conditioning and endoscopic treatment, especially those with markedly increased intrapancreatic pressure, early surgical decompression is mostly advocated to stop or reverse the course of the disease, improve the progressive loss of endocrine and exocrine functions, and relieve pain. With endoscopic decompression therapy alone, about 23% of patients with chronic pancreatitis can have long-term complete or basic pain relief [35].

Endoscopic treatment can relieve the pain of chronic pancreatitis by releasing the obstruction of the pancreatic duct and reducing the pressure in the pancreatic duct and has become a popular means of treating chronic pancreatitis today with its advantages of easy operation, less trauma, less pain, and higher safety. Especially for patients with failed medical treatment and high surgical risk, endoscopic treatment can show its advantageous role.

The mechanism of endoscopic pain relief in chronic pancreatitis lies in the ability of endoscopy to target the treatment of pancreatic duct stones and pancreatic duct dilatation. This has been demonstrated in several studies. A recent study of a large sample of more than 1000 patients included pancreatic duct stenosis, stones, and stones in combination with stenosis [36]. The results of endoscopic treatment showed that the overall effectiveness of endoscopic decompression in chronic pancreatitis was 86%, demonstrating the importance of endoscopic treatment in the management of chronic pancreatitis. While the complication rate of endoscopic treatment is about 25%, the vast majority of them are mild, and the ideal target of endoscopic treatment should be patients with pancreatic duct stenosis with upstream dilatation. In conclusion, endoscopic treatment of chronic pancreatitis pain has a good prospect for development, but at the same time, there are many uncertainties. It is believed that with the accumulation and summary of cases and the continuous improvement of related technology, it will become a major means of treatment of chronic pancreatitis pain.

11.3.4.3 Surgical Treatment

Although chronic pancreatitis is a benign disease, it is potentially malignant and usually requires surgical intervention, and the efficacy is closely related to the choice of surgical method and the control of postoperative complications. When intractable pain is difficult to control with medications, or when chronic pancreatitis is combined with pseudocysts, pancreatic fistula, biliary obstruction, and digestive tract obstruction, surgical treatment becomes the key to disease control. The purpose of surgical treatment is not only to relieve pain and relieve compression symptoms but also to improve endocrine function and obtain pathological results. Surgery is an effective treatment for patients with chronic pancreatitis who have failed medical and endoscopic treatment, and it is necessary in 15–20% of patients [37]. Surgery should minimize the impact on the endocrine and exocrine functions of the pancreas and provide effective pain relief. Patients with pancreatic ducts larger than 7 mm in diameter are considered typical indications for drainage, while the so-called "small pancreatic ducts" smaller than 3 mm in diameter should be considered for pancreatic resection. The surgical procedures can be broadly classified as denervation, pancreatic duct decompression, and pancreatectomy.

11.3.4.4 Comparative Control Study of Surgical and Endoscopic Treatment

The current debate between surgical and endoscopic approaches is mainly a factional one. However, the first prospective randomized controlled study of surgical versus endoscopic treatment of patients with obstructive chronic pancreatitis was recently published. The surgical approach was determined based on patient anatomy and included resection and drainage. Endoscopic treatment included sphincterotomy, stenting, and (or lithotripsy) extracorporeal shock wave lithotripsy. Of the 140 appropriate patients, approximately 50% agreed to randomize to one treatment [38]. However, similar results were obtained whether the analysis included all 140 patients or only those randomly selected. The initial success rate was around 50% for both groups when all patients were included in the analysis, but at the 5-year follow-up period, about 35% of patients in the surgical group were considered completely pain-free, compared with only about 15% in the endoscopic group. All patients had varying degrees of weight gain after treatment. Therefore, the author deduced that for patients with painful obstructive chronic pancreatitis, surgery is superior to endoscopic treatment in the treatment of long-term pain relief.

11.4 Biliary Dyskinesia

11.4.1 Overview

Biliary dyskinesia is a functional disorder characterized by persistent or recurrent pain in the right upper abdomen and/or right upper quadrant, unrelated to biliary stones, and without structural or metabolic abnormalities that could explain the symptoms. Functional biliary pain syndrome can seriously affect the daily life and mental status of patients. There are few studies on the disease, but foreign epidemiological studies have reported its prevalence to be 6–8% in men and more common in women, with a prevalence of 12–25% [39].

Biliary dyskinesia is a complex clinical dilemma commonly seen in two types of patients: those with gallbladders that do not have stones but exhibit typical symptoms of gallbladder stones and biliary colic and and those who are post-cholecystectomy but still have intermittent recurrences similar to biliary pain. In the former group of patients, we generally focus on the examination of the gallbladder and consider whether there is an indication for performing cholecystectomy, while in the second group of patients, we pay more attention to the gallbladder Oddi sphincter to determine whether there is an indication for performing endoscopic sphincterotomy (ES). However, the pathological mechanisms of the above two conditions are not clear, so the corresponding diagnosis and treatment remain controversial.

In recent years, with the continuous research on the dynamics and functional diseases of the GI tract, a new level of understanding of functional diseases of the biliary system has been reached. It is now believed that functional biliary disorders are an independent group of dysmotic disorders with their own unique pathophysiological basis but lacking specific symptoms and signs and easily confused with other gastrointestinal dysfunctions. The Rome III Committee redefined functional biliary pain in an attempt to address this clinical dilemma. Some non-biliary abnormalities can also be excluded based on their clinical features, such as angina pectoris usually caused by exercise, and its duration does not exceed 1 h, and its pain does not have an interval of months to years; pantothenia usually resolves with antacids or acid suppressants; renal stones have abnormalities on routine urinalysis; combined symptoms of the abdomen or chest wall are usually worse with exercise, coughing, or deep breathing. The abdominal discomfort of IBS is often accompanied by a change in bowel habits and may be relieved after defecation.

11.4.2 Possible Mechanisms of Biliary Dyskinesia

Biliary pain is caused by abnormal gallbladder contraction during structural or functional outflow tract obstruction resulting in increased intra-biliary pressure. Possible mechanisms of functional biliary pain include diminished gallbladder motility, partial obstruction of the structural or functional gallbladder outflow tract, dysregulation of gallbladder contraction and sphincter of Oddi relaxation, and visceral hypersensitivity reactions.

1. Gallbladder motility malfunction
    (a) Gallbladder hypokinesis

        Primary gallbladder hypokinesia may be caused by a decrease in CCK receptors, downregulation of CCK receptors, or impaired excitation-contraction coupling mechanism. Secondary causes of hypokinesia include celiac disease, CCK deficiency, long-term parenteral nutrition, long-term starvation, diabetes mellitus, growth inhibitors, birth control pills, VIP tumor, growth inhibitor tumor, etc.

(b) Gallbladder motility dysfunction

- Functional gallbladder motility dysfunction, due to uncoordinated contraction of the gallbladder in response to endogenous or exogenous CCK stimulation, resulting in functional spasm causing obstruction of the gallbladder outflow tract. In a group of patients with non-stone biliary colic, rainfarin induced similar biliary colic symptoms with reduced gallbladder emptying, while nitroglycerin relieved the symptoms induced by rainfarin and restored normal gallbladder emptying. This test confirmed the existence of the above mechanism.
- Organic gallbladder motility dysfunction and stenosis cause obstruction of the gallbladder outflow tract, and the gallbladder strengthens contraction to overcome the obstruction, causing biliary colic. Etiologies include chronic cholecystitis and fibrosis. Long-term recurrent functional spasm can also cause subclinical infection and fibrosis, leading to stricture.

2. Sphincter of Oddi dysfunction (SOD)

SOD refers to the abnormal movement of this sphincter that causes obstruction of bile and pancreatic juice drainage, resulting in increased bile and pancreatic duct internal pressure, with clinical manifestations of biliary stasis, biliary-derived abdominal pain, pancreatic-derived abdominal pain, or recurrent pancreatitis.

SOD consists of two parts:

(a) SO dysfunction, which refers to SO primary motility abnormalities leading to elevated tone and to a lesser extent reduced tone.

(b) SO stenosis, structural changes due to inflammation, and its subsequent fibrosis.

Since it is difficult to study the human sphincter of Oddi at the histological level and there are no clear criteria for mild histological alterations of the sphincter of Oddi and also autopsy findings often reveal histological alterations of the sphincter of Oddi, it is difficult to distinguish functional disorders from histological or minor organic alterations.

3. Visceral hypersensitivity

Projections of visceral pain receptors to the thalamus and cerebral cortex may lead to visceral nociceptive hypersensitivity (mild painful stimuli causing severe pain) and may further lead to abnormal pain (a state in which harmless stimuli produce pain). As with other gastrointestinal dysfunctions, increased sensitivity of the biliary system or its adjacent structures may be associated with pain in patients with gallbladder dysfunction. For example, Desautels et al. showed that in post-cholecystectomy patients with persistent abdominal pain and no type I or type II sphincter of Oddi dysfunction, distension of the duodenum with a constant pressure device reproduced symptoms of duodenum-specific visceral pain hypersensitivity in most patients [40].

In addition, abnormal gallbladder emptying in patients with biliary dyskinesia may also be associated with a history of gallbladder crystallization and chronic cholecystitis. Velanovic et al. prospectively studied 36 patients who underwent cholecystectomy for suspected functional biliary pain and compared them with patients who underwent cholecystectomy with symptoms of cholelithiasis [41]. It was found that, in patients without gallstones, 90% had bile crystals in the gallbladder and 62% were identified as having intramural crystals. In contrast, 81% of patients with gallstones were found to have crystals within the gallbladder wall. The investigators hypothesized that functional gallbladder pain may be a partial response to a series of gallbladder pathological processes of bile saturation and impaired gallbladder motility leading to crystal growth, which leads to gallstone formation and chronic inflammation. These findings are supported by another study by Brugge et al. whose findings showed an association between cholesterol crystals and post-cholecystectomy prognosis in patients with suspected functional gallbladder pain. In addition, in the Velanovich study on functional gallbladder pain, 94% of patients without gallstones and 100% of patients with gallstones had a history of chronic cholecystitis. However, no abnormal gallbladder lesions were found in patients with suspected functional biliary pain who underwent cholecystectomy with postoperative symptom relief, a situation consistent with the lack of histopathology seen in chronic cholecystitis. Indeed, results vary widely between reports in the literature, and it is unclear whether histologic alterations of the gallbladder are the cause or result of diminished gallbladder contraction, although it has been shown that patients with normal histology are less likely to have complete resolution of symptoms.

We still know very little about the pathogenesis of functional gallbladder pain. The reason that warrants further investigation is not the persistence of symptoms after cholecystectomy, but the possibility that pre-cholecystectomy symptoms may be associated with other concomitant gastrointestinal motility disorders. In patients with suspected functional cholecystic pain, various motility disorder-like symptoms commonly occur, and studies have found that patients with abnormal gallbladder emptying often have concomitant gastric muscle bradykinesia and constipation occurring, suggesting that functional gallbladder dysfunction may reflect whole bowel motility disorders.

11.4.3 Diagnosis, Examination, and Treatment of Biliary Dyskinesia

11.4.3.1 Diagnosis and Examination of Biliary Dyskinesia

1. Exclude stones and other possible diseases

   To correctly diagnose functional (non-lithotripsy) biliary pain, it is necessary to first exclude stones and other diseases that may cause biliary pain. Routine laboratory tests include biochemical indices of the liver and pancreas, gastroscopy and colonoscopy, and ultrasound endoscopy, which can detect gallbladder and bile duct stones smaller than 3 mm and is superior to transabdominal ultrasound. In addition, analysis of bile in the duodenum after stimulation by gallbladder contraction allows determination of cholesterol microcrystals or bilirubin salt particles in it. Only if all these tests are negative, the diagnosis of functional biliary pain can be made.

2. Altered gallbladder motor function

   Altered gallbladder motor function has become the basis for the diagnosis of functional biliary pain in most or most cases with in situ gallbladder. The following items should be performed for suspected gallbladder dysfunction.

   (a) Laboratory tests

      Liver function and pancreatic enzyme indices must be normal.

   (b) Abdominal ultrasound

      It can clearly show all sections of the gallbladder and calculate the gallbladder volume. It can initially exclude cholecystitis, gallstone disease, and also can be performed lipid meal or shrink cholecystokinin 8 peptide (CCK-8) stimulation test to understand the gallbladder emptying function. Under normal conditions, SGEF can reach more than 70%, and if it is less than 40%, it is abnormal [42]. However, functional or organic gallbladder hypokinesis can cause emptying disorders, which cannot be identified by simple CCK evoked test, and not only lacks sensitivity and specificity, its results are also unreliable and have little significance in the diagnosis of patients with functional biliary pain. The abdominal ultrasound method is simple and safe, but the detection results are affected by the operator's technical level, the calculation of gallbladder volume is less accurate, and bile reflux cannot be detected; in addition, the repeatability of ultrasound is poor.

   (c) Biliary imaging techniques

- For cholangiography, fat-rich food is eaten at lunch the day before to stimulate the gallbladder to contract and empty, and fat-free food is eaten at dinner, after which no more food is eaten. The contrast agent is administered orally at 10 pm, commonly iodofantrine 3 g, 0.5 g/time, with 5 min interval each time. The best time to take the film is 10 h after oral administration. The film is taken on an empty stomach first, except for organic lesions of the gallbladder, followed by a fatty meal (commonly fried eggs). The gallbladder generally shrinks by one-half in 60 min after the fatty meal. If the gallbladder shrinks by less than one-half in 120 min, the gallbladder is considered to have reduced contractile function. This method is simple and inexpensive, but it is less used now because of its exposure to radiation, lack of accuracy in calculating gallbladder volume, and susceptibility to liver, kidney, and gastrointestinal function.
- Scintigraphy: ^{99m}Tc DIDA is commonly used to determine SGEF, which is currently the most accurate method to detect gallbladder emptying. The excretion fraction can be used to indicate the effect of gallbladder emptying after CCK stimulation. An in vitro model simulating in vivo gallbladder volume has an ejection fraction correlation coefficient of 0.98 for volumetric measurements compared to radiological methods of measurement. Therefore, cholescintigraphy (CCK-CS) is able to measure irregular gallbladder emptying effects by detecting changes in ^{99m}Tc DIDA to observe gallbladder volume changes. Although introduced into clinical practice more than 20 years ago, the dose and rate of CCK administration used to measure the gallbladder excretion fraction (GEF) by this technique have not been standardized in most studies. Because GEF varies with the dose and rate of administration, both the dose and rate of CCK administration are important, but many studies use the same definition of GEF for different doses and rates of CCK administration resulting in different GEFs. Moreover, the standard values for the definition of low GEF obtained with long-term administration of CCK vary widely. Clinically useful standardized values are difficult to obtain in some studies, and it is difficult to compare them with published studies.
- In addition, abnormal GEF does not always mean gallbladder disease, and low GEF is associated with many other factors that should be examined and treated for other etiologies. Tabet et al. found that patients with gallbladder dysmotility had a higher probability of developing complications similar to those seen in IBS compared to patients with cholelithiasis. This may explain why symptoms persist after cholecystectomy in patients with gallbladder motility disorders and supports the hypothesis that gallbladder motility disorders may be a manifestation of systemic gastrointestinal motility abnormalities. Many other conditions such as diabetes, pregnancy, spontaneous slow-transit constipation, obesity, cirrhosis, reduced gastric emptying, and the use of different medications can lead to reduced GEF values. Ignoring these factors at this point of low GEP may lead to unnecessary cholecystectomy if used for standard assessment of surgery.

(d) Pain provocation test: It has been largely abandoned because of its low sensitivity and specificity.

3. Sphincter of Oddi dysfunction (SOD)

   Endoscopic sphincter of Oddi manometry (SOM) is currently the most valuable method for diagnosing SOD, and a basal pressure of more than 40 mmHg is sufficient to diagnose SOD. SOM can also predict the patient's response to treatment with transendoscopic sphincter of Oddi dissection (EST). However, it is prone to complicate postoperative pancreatitis and therefore should be screened first with a noninvasive test.

In recent years, due to the recognition of SOD as the etiology of some acute recurrent pancreatitis and the finding that some patients with SOD have normal bile duct manometry and abnormal pancreatic duct or both sides, simultaneous pancreaticobiliary duct manometry is advocated. And 35–65% of patients with abnormal basal manometry were reported by Raddawi et al. to be confined to one side, and abnormal internal Oddi sphincter pressure was mostly confined to the pancreatic duct in patients with pancreatitis [43]. Aymerich et al. retrospectively analyzed 73 cases of simultaneous pancreaticobiliary duct manometry and found that 19% had normal basal pressure on both sides, 40% had abnormal basal pressure on both sides, and 41% had abnormal pressure on only one side [44]. Among 59 cases with elevated pressure, 19 cases had normal bile duct pressure and abnormal pancreatic duct pressure, and 10 cases had normal pancreatic duct pressure but abnormal bile duct pressure. The sensitivity of diagnosing SOD by measuring only bile duct pressure was 68%, while the sensitivity of diagnosing SOD by measuring only pancreatic duct pressure was 83%. If only bile duct pressure was measured, 26% of SOD would have been missed. Given the high incidence of pancreatitis after manometry, Wehrmann et al. used a microelectronic sensing system for SOM that correlated well with capillary water perfusion SOM with less postoperative pancreatitis [45].

However, there is still controversy as to whether SOD plays a role in the development of biliary pain with a normal gallbladder. Existing studies usually assume that SOD is present prior to cholecystectomy and is thought to be the underlying cause of symptoms in some patients. We then have to consider the following two questions: whether SOD is associated with low GEF and whether sphincterotomy, rather than laparoscopic cholecystectomy, should be the first-line treatment for patients with stone-free biliary pain.

Despite evidence of SOD in patients with normal gallbladder with biliary pain, there is no causal association between GEF values and sphincter of Oddi basal pressure values. The available literature still lacks sufficient evidence to infer whether biliary sphincterotomy is effective in patients with biliary pain with low GEF. Ruffolo et al. studied the relationship between SOD and low GEF in 81 patients without stone biliary type abdominal pain and normal liver enzymes: in patients with normal and abnormal GEF, Oddi sphincter pressure was elevated in 57% and 56% of patients, respectively, while Oddi sphincter pressure normal and elevated patients had no statistically significant difference in GEF values [46]. Kalloo and Pasricha also explored the relationship between GEF and Oddi sphincter pressure in 30 patients with biliary type abdominal pain without a stone gallbladder and found that 7 patients with elevated Oddi sphincter pressure had mean GEF values similar to those of 23 patients with normal Oddi sphincter pressure [47]. In addition, Soto et al. found that elevated basal sphincter of Oddi pressure was prevalent in patients without stone gallbladder symptoms with biliary pain, but GEF and sphincter of Oddi pressure were poorly correlated [48]. Choudhary et al. described 35 patients with normal gallbladder and elevated basal sphincter of Oddi pressure, 43% of whom had persistent pain relief after ES alone, while the remaining 20 patients had ineffective or recurrent ES [49]. Of the remaining 20 patients who were ineffective or had a recurrence after an initial effective treatment with ES, 11 underwent cholecystectomy and 8 of them felt a significant reduction in pain. The results were good or excellent in 66% of patients who underwent combined ES and cholecystectomy. Therefore, the available literature does not provide sufficient evidence that GEF values in patients with biliary pain in the presence or absence of a stone gallbladder accurately predict the outcome of cholecystectomy or biliary sphincterotomy.

11.4.3.2 Treatment of Functional (Non-stone) Biliary Pain

In the absence of reliable and noninvasive treatments, some investigators have suggested that nonsurgical treatment options need to be considered judiciously, including careful assessment of the patient's psychological situation and the use of medications that have a modulating effect on chronic visceral pain, such as tricyclic antidepressants (TCA).

1. Gallbladder dysfunction

   The following alternative measures are currently available clinically.

   (a) Pharmacological treatment: (1) Cisapride, to change the gallbladder motor function and promote gallbladder contraction. (2) Ursodeoxycholic acid, which can reduce biliary abdominal pain although it weakens gallbladder motility. (3) Nonsteroidal anti-inflammatory drugs, which can reduce the visceral pain threshold or inflammatory response.

   (b) Surgical treatment: More and more data show that cholecystectomy, especially laparoscopic cholecystectomy, is currently the most effective treatment for gallbladder motility dysfunction. However, it is difficult to grasp the indications for surgery and the timing of surgery. Some investigators suggest that if no obvious cause of gallbladder emptying dysfunction is found, the gallbladder can be removed. If the gallbladder empties normally, bile can be obtained by duodenal drainage or endoscopy, and cholesterol microstones or bile pigment crystals can be analyzed microscopically. ERCP, magnetic resonance cholangiopancreatography (MRCP), and endoscopic ultrasound (EUS) can also be examined to detect stones and if no stones or other abnormalities are found by ERCP. Endoscopic Oddi sphincter manometry can be considered to decide the next step of treatment.

2. Sphincter of Oddi dysfunction (SOD)

   The principle of treatment is to reduce the resistance to bile and pancreatic juice drainage caused by the sphincter of Oddi.

   (a) Smooth muscle relaxants can be tried, such as anticholinergic drugs, nitroglycerin, and calcium channel blocking drugs. The drugs can only temporarily relieve the symptoms, and the symptoms may recur after stopping the drugs.

   (b) Endoscopic sphincterotomy: It is the standard treatment for SOD. After EST, the sphincter of Oddi function is lost, the pressure is reduced, and the bile drainage is smooth, so it can achieve positive results. For those with abnormal SOD manometry, the symptoms improve significantly after endoscopic duodenal papillary sphincterotomy. A meta-analysis suggested that EST for SOD was effective only for those with elevated SO pressure (>40 mmHg), while for those with normal pressure, there was no difference in the efficacy of EST compared to control. However, some studies have concluded that there is no significant difference in the efficacy of EST for biliary SOD with or without elevated pressure.

11.4.4 Diagnosis, Examination, and Treatment of Biliary Dyskinesia After Cholecystectomy

11.4.4.1 Diagnosis and Examination of Biliary Dyskinesia After Cholecystectomy

It is well known that laparoscopic cholecystectomy is superior to traditional open surgery, so the number of laparoscopic surgery continues to rise, and biliary-type pain after cholecystectomy also rises. However, the treatment of pain in such patients is still controversial until recently.

Such patients are classified into three types according to SOD:

Type I biliary-derived abdominal pain: elevated glutathione, glutathione, and bilirubin concentrations measured on at least two occasions, each time exceeding two times the upper limit of normal, and ERCP showing dilatation of the common bile duct (≥12 mm); ERCP showing prolonged bile duct emptying time (>45 min). Oddi sphincterotomy was recommended.

Type II biliary-derived abdominal pain: only one or two of the above presentations. ERCP is recommended to measure the sphincter of Oddi pressure, and most patients can benefit from sphincterotomy if it is >40 mmHg. A small percentage of patients with type II but normal pressure also has pain relief after sphincterotomy.

Type III biliary-derived abdominal pain: the efficacy of sphincterotomy cannot be predicted even by ERCP manometry in these patients, and only a small percentage of patients feel effective, with different pathophysiology and treatment.

11.4.4.2 Causes of Functional Biliary Pain After Cholecystectomy

The possible etiology of functional biliary pain after cholecystectomy lies in the duodenum, or in the combination of biliary tract problems. One study found that patients with three types of SOD exhibited duodenal-specific visceral pain sensitivity. The prevalence of IBS irritable bowel syndrome is higher in patients with types II and III than the population prevalence, making it difficult to relieve symptoms if only the sphincter of Oddi is targeted.

The symptoms of duodenal pain sensitization are similar to those of biliary type pain, and biliary pain sensitization may or may not be associated with sphincter dysfunction. Studies on the neurobiological basis of this overlap phenomenon are lacking and may include sphincter-gut nerve connections, or sensory convergence of afferent nerve fibers in the dorsal horn of the spinal cord. Bidirectional neural connections have been found to exist between the duodenum and the sphincter, so that duodenal pain sensitivity occurs before or after cholecystectomy due to biliary pain hypersensitivity, and normal stimulation can result in both sites exhibiting hypersensitivity.

Attention to the psychobehavioral characteristics of the patient is also required before and after cholecystectomy, and failure to take this aspect into account is likely to lead to poor long-term outcomes.

11.4.4.3 Clinical Treatment of Functional Biliary Pain After Cholecystectomy

The first treatment of choice for these patients is pharmacological pain desensitization, while attention needs to be paid to the assessment of the presence of psychological dysfunction or irritable bowel syndrome. Continuous administration of low-dose tricyclic antidepressants (10–75 mg/day) is indicated for patients with frequent pain episodes or combined BS. Side effects include sedation, constipation, dry mouth, and vertigo, with a high incidence of amitriptyline and promethazine and a relatively low incidence of nortriptyline and desmethyl promethazine. Patients with gastrointestinal disorders are more sensitive to side effects and sometimes need to be switched to another TCA. Intensive monitoring is needed during medication administration, with a maximum of one dose increase every 3–4 weeks.

Since many patients exhibit mood disorders or psychosocial stress, antidepressants have the potential to further improve efficacy with a full dose of selective 5-hydroxytryptamine reuptake inhibitors or other antidepressants.

11.5 Visceral Pain Due to Surgery (Abdominal Adhesions)

11.5.1 Overview

Abdominal adhesions are abnormal adhesions between the mural peritoneum and the visceral peritoneum after abdominal surgery and are a common complication after abdominal or pelvic surgery. Studies have reported that the incidence of abdominal adhesions after laparotomy ranges from 67% to 93% and up to 97% after open gynecological surgery [50, 51]. On the one hand, adhesion formation is its biological protective mechanism against external stimuli and can limit the presence of abdominal inflammation, which is its beneficial side: however, abdominal adhesions also bring many hazards to patients, such as persistent chronic pain or discomfort due to attachment and pulling and dysfunction caused by pushing or compression of organs, resulting in complications such as adhesive bowel obstruction and female infertility. Therefore, the prevention and treatment of abdominal adhesions is important for the recovery of patients after laparotomy.

Abdominal adhesions are mainly divided into congenital adhesions and acquired adhesions, the latter of which usually have an inflammatory or surgical origin. Inflammatory adhesions mainly originate from inflammatory reactions in the abdominal cavity, such as bacterial and/or chemical peritonitis, appendicitis, chronic pelvic inflammatory disease, inflammatory bowel disease, foreign body reactions, and long-term peritoneal dialysis; postsurgical adhesions are mainly caused by tissue damage caused by surgical operations, such as incisions, cautery, and sutures. Surgeries that tend to lead to adhesion formation include colorectal surgery, obstetrical and gynecological surgery, and emergency appendectomy. The incidence of postoperative abdominal adhesions also increases with the age of the patient, the number of surgeries, and the complexity of the surgical procedure and can lead to complications such as small bowel obstruction, female infertility, and chronic abdominopelvic pain in severe cases.

There are many causes of abdominal adhesive pain. Tension; stretching and contraction of the abdominal and pelvic organs, which stimulate peritoneal nociceptive receptors; and adhesions that limit the mobility and expansiveness of the organs are the main causes of adhesion-related pain. In addition, adhesions themselves can create painful stimuli that are directly involved in the pain mechanism. Studies have shown that post-pelvic surgical adhesions can produce direct nociceptive stimuli; this is corroborated by the recent finding that human abdominal and pelvic adhesions contain nerve fibers. In fact, the adherent tissue is formed by vascularized collagen bundles containing adipose tissue and a certain amount of nerve fibers (myelinated and unmyelinated). However, the function of these nerve structures is not clear and may be involved in local blood flow regulation, neurogenic inflammatory response, and wound healing process.

11.5.2 Pathophysiology of Adhesive Pain

11.5.2.1 Pathogenesis of Abdominal Adhesions

The peritoneum is the largest plasma membrane in the human body, which covers the surface of the abdominal organs and has a supporting and fixing effect on the organs. Under normal physiological conditions, the peritoneum secretes small amounts of plasma to moisten the surface of organs and reduce the role of interorgan friction. Mechanical injury, tissue ischemia, implantation of exogenous substances, inflammation of the abdominal cavity, abdominal radiation, and intraperitoneal injection of chemical drugs can trigger abdominal adhesions. Abdominal adhesions are the result of the combined action of multiple factors, and in recent years, more in-depth studies have been conducted on the formation mechanism of abdominal adhesions, which are now described from three aspects: mesothelial cells, inflammatory cells, and fibrinolytic state.

1. The role of mesothelial cells

   The peritoneal surface consists of a single layer of mesothelial cells, whose repair mechanism is different from that of the skin. The area of peritoneal defect can be repaired by the growth of mesothelial cells in the normal peritoneum at the margin, whose integrity and normal function are closely related to the formation of adhesions. The peritoneum is very sensitive to injury, and mesothelial cells can simultaneously proliferate and differentiate to form sheath cells that participate in peritoneal repair, regardless of the size of the injury. When the peritoneum is traumatized, the damaged mesothelial cell layer detaches from the basement membrane and undergoes ballooning, producing lamellar naked areas that result in adhesions. In addition to integrity, functional alterations of the mesothelial cells are also of great importance. The peritoneal hyperosmotic state can inhibit peritoneal mesothelial cell wandering, resulting in the absence of the mesothelial cell layer, as in patients on long-term peritoneal dialysis.

2. Role of inflammatory cells

   The cells mainly involved in the inflammatory response are macrophages, mast cells, and T lymphocytes.

   (a) Role of macrophages

      Inflammation or injury of the peritoneum triggers the coagulation state, promotes the release of multiple chemical mediators, and activates leukocytes and mesothelial cells, and when macrophages are activated, they also release multiple inflammatory mediators (such as cyclooxygenase and its metabolites, fibrinogen activator, PAL, IL-1, L-6, TNF, etc.) and recruit new mesothelial cells.

   (b) Role of mast cells

      There is a large amount of mast cell secretion in the serum of patients with abdominal adhesions, which is manifested by the secretion of large amounts of fibrous exudate and significant proliferation of fibroblasts. In addition, some researchers found that mast cells were present in a large number in the adherent tissues and abdominal fluid after modeling of abdominal adhesions in mice, and as the adherent tissues became dense, the number of mast cells gradually decreased, and inflammatory cells increased significantly. In vitro experiments revealed that co-culture of mast cell pulverized material into fibroblasts of normal intestinal tissue and adhesion tissue, respectively, both promoted significant proliferation of fibroblasts. Thus, it is believed that mast cells have a role in promoting fiber formation in the early stage of adhesion formation.

   (c) Role of T lymphocytes

      Chung et al. showed for the first time that the immune mechanism of peritoneal adhesion formation is under the regulation of T cells. T lymphocytes have an immunomodulatory role, and T cell-derived cytokines and chemokines play an important role in adhesion formation. T lymphocyte-derived IL-17, neutrophil chemokine CXC, macrophage chemokine inflammatory protein-2/CXC18, and CXCL1 are all associated with adhesion formation, and these factors can enter the peritoneal cavity and colonize the peritoneal mucosa.

3. Role of the fibrinolytic system

   The fibrinolytic system plays a key role in the formation of adhesions. Under physiological conditions, the fibrinolytic system can degrade and remove fibrin deposits in the peritoneal cavity in a timely manner. However, inflammation caused by laparotomy and trauma leads to the secretion of exudate containing large amounts of fibrinogen in the peritoneal cavity. The exudate activates the coagulation cascade in the peritoneal cavity, and the dynamic balance between coagulation and fibrinolysis is disrupted, promoting the conversion of fibrinogen into fibrin, leading to the formation of adhesions in the peritoneal cavity. Researchers have found in multiple animal models that increased adhesion products can occur when fibrinolytic activity is reduced. This explains why peritoneal-specific fibrinolytic activity is often a target for adhesion prevention.

   In addition, inadequate local blood supply and reduced tissue oxygenation often occur after surgery, which can also inhibit fibrinolytic activity, promote continued fibrous tissue proliferation, and ultimately lead to peritoneal adhesions. Suturing, compression, traction, and contact with foreign bodies (operator's gloves, etc.) of the peritoneum can all contribute to local ischemia. In addition, factors such as intraperitoneal hemorrhage can inhibit fibrinolytic activity and promote adhesion formation.

11.5.2.2 Factors in the Development of Adhesive Pain

1. Visceral factors

   Sixteen million patients in the United States complain of abdominal pain each year, and two million of them have severe persistent abdominal pain despite pharmacologic interventions, minimally invasive treatments, and surgical interventions.

   Visceral receptors and their afferent nerves transmit information from the viscera to the central nervous system; the information transmission process itself is rarely perceived, and what humans perceive is often visceral discomfort and pain. When changes in sensation from the viscera occur, they often suggest some functional changes, such as small bowel lesions, interstitial cystitis, and ureteral colic, which usually manifest as visceral nociceptive hypersensitivity. Nociceptive hypersensitivity includes both peripheral and central nervous system components, and theoretically, either peripheral or central can initiate and maintain this process alone.

   Visceral injurious receptors are located in the plasma membrane, mucosa, and muscular layer of the cavernous organs and are conducted via unmyelinated C-fibers and small diameter Aδ fibers. Several studies have reported that visceral nociceptive receptors respond only to strong mechanical stimuli and chemical reactions (e.g., inflammatory products); the same number of nociceptive receptors are present in the cavernous organs and can be activated in response to inflammation in the corresponding organ.

2. Abdominal wall factors

   Chronic abdominal wall pain (CAWP), which is characterized by continuous or intermittent pain for more than 1 month, with a limited and fixed location and abdominal wall muscle pressure point less than 2.5 cm in diameter, is often overlooked or misdiagnosed, but in fact, 10–30% of patients with chronic abdominal pain have pain mainly originating from the abdominal wall, and they often undergo repeated clinical examinations and expensive minimally invasive investigations [52], which not only waste medical resources but also delay diagnosis and treatment.

   Abdominal wall pain mainly originates from entrapment pain of the thoracic and abdominal viscera, injury to the T_{7-12} nerve roots, and nerve injury due to peritoneal and abdominal wall injury. Surgical medical peripheral nerve injury is often the most common cause of chronic abdominal wall pain. The surgical incision itself can directly damage the cutaneous nerves, and suture or crust inlay can also indirectly damage the cutaneous nerves. Abdominal cutaneous nerve entrapment syndrome (ACNES) most often occurs at the outer edge of the rectus abdominis muscle and can be due to either surgical trauma or an anatomical abnormality in the cutaneous nerve. Peripheral nerve entrapment signs tend to occur in locations with altered nerve fiber alignment, such as the bone-fiber canal or inelastic muscle fiber edges and tendon arches, because these sites are most susceptible to mechanical stimulation.

   The most common cause of abdominal wall pain is nerve entrapment at the lateral edge of the rectus abdominis muscle. Within the rectus abdominis sheath, the nerve and blood vessels are surrounded by fat and connective tissue, forming a unit relatively independent of the surrounding tissue, along with the accompanying arteries and veins. When the rectus abdominis muscle is viewed from posterior to anterior, the free inferior border of the posterior layer is seen as an arched line convex to the top, called the arcuate line (semicircular line). The posterior aspect of the rectus abdominis below this line is directly adjacent to the transverse abdominal fascia.

11.5.2.3 Differential Diagnosis of Abdominal Wall Pain

When a patient is suspected of having abdominal wall pain, intra-abdominal lesions should first be excluded. Detailed history, meticulous physical examination, and endoscopic screening, combined with diagnostic imaging and laboratory tests, help to exclude other possible causes of abdominal pain, such as abdominal malignancy, semilunar hernia (presenting similar to T_{10} nerve entrapment), pain caused by other neurological disorders, and iliac inguinal or inferior iliac abdominal nerve entrapment (due to surgery in the inguinal region).

Guaiac chemical or immunoassay fecal occult blood tests (FOBT) are useful in detecting the presence of intra-abdominal organ lesions or intra-abdominal tumors, but it is difficult to assess the sensitivity, specificity, and positive predictive value of FOBT in screening. Therefore, patients with symptoms of chronic abdominal pain but negative intraosseous pathology and negative FOBT should be considered for ACNES.

Notably, in patients with lower abdominal pain, ACNES is difficult to differentiate from iliogastroinguinal nerve, inferior iliac abdominal nerve, and genitourinary nerve branch entrapment. Another difficult distinction from nerve entrapment is myofascial pain of the abdominal wall, as these patients also present with a positive Carnett's test. However, patients with myofascial pain often complain of multiple myofascial pressure points throughout the body. In addition, the diagnosis of ACNES must exclude tumor invasion of nerves, herpes zoster, traumatic radiculitis, rectus abdominis sheath hematoma, hernia, and rib pain.

11.5.3 Treatment of Visceral Pain with Abdominal Adhesions

11.5.3.1 Diagnostic Treatment

1. Carnett's test

   It is a relatively simple method to identify whether abdominal pain originates from the abdominal wall. The test is positive when the patient feels pain on palpation of the abdominal discomfort area when the upper body is elevated or when the straight leg is picked up so that the abdominal wall is tense.

   Gallegos and Hobsley concluded that the Carnett's test is particularly useful for diagnosing abdominal wall pain [53]. When the Carnett's test is positive and the area of pain is adjacent to the surgical scar and the patient feels the pain disappear immediately after the injection of local anesthetic, abdominal wall pain is confirmed; otherwise, the presence of other causes of pain needs to be considered.

2. Differential epidural block

   Local anesthetics act differently on different nerve fibers, so a discriminatory plexus block can help determine the cause of pain. Placebo or local anesthetics given after epidural placement can identify the presence of psychological factors, sympathetic, hurt feelings, or central causes. However, the diagnostic efficacy of this approach for pain etiology needs to be further demonstrated. Reviewing the previous literature, only two studies suggest that differential nerve blocks can predict treatment outcome, but the level of evidence is low, and both studies included a small number of cases.

   The rationale for differential nerve blocks is that nerve fibers differ in their sensitivity to local anesthetics, and the underlying reason is that there are different nerve fibers, with differences in their anatomy and function, such as diameter size and myelin content. The limitation of this approach is that the interaction between local anesthetics and nerve fibers is dynamic and unpredictable and may be influenced by multiple factors. Because of the overlap in diameter size of different types of nerve fibers, it is difficult to accurately distinguish a particular nerve fiber with this method. In addition, discriminatory nerve blocks are time-consuming to perform, and there is a risk of nerve block complications.

3. Rectus abdominis sheath block and transverse abdominis plane block (TAP)

   The target nerve area is different between the two. A rectus abdominis sheath block is usually performed at 45° to the skin at the inferior border of the rib cage, and a local anesthetic is injected between the posterior rectus abdominis sheath and the transversus abdominis fascia to provide a sensory block to the midline of the abdomen. In contrast, TAP is generally performed laterally in the abdomen, with local anesthetic injected between the internal oblique abdominal muscle and the transversus abdominis muscle, and a bilateral block can provide analgesia in the subungual region.

Recent studies have shown that in CAWP, pediatric abdominal wall pain is recommended to be treated with a rectus abdominis sheath block and a transversus abdominis plane block. When the painful point of abdominal wall pain is difficult to locate accurately (as in pediatric patients), rectus abdominis sheath block for diagnosis and treatment is a better option. Due to the anatomical peculiarities of the cutaneous nerve branches, the rectus abdominis sheath block may be ineffective in one-third of patients.

The anterior branches of the T_7 to L_1 nerves cross the gap between the internal oblique and transversus abdominis muscles, the transversus abdominis plane, and a TAP block can achieve the effect of blocking these nerve afferents. In 2009, Soliman and Narouze proposed TAP as an alternative to differential epidural blocks for differentiating visceral pain from abdominal wall pain [54]. Compared to differential epidural blocks, TAP has fewer side effects, especially when performed by experienced physicians under ultrasound guidance: the disadvantage is that TAP is often difficult to differentiate somatosensory pain when used for the differential diagnosis of abdominal pain.

4. Paravertebral nerve block

   It is also useful for the differential diagnosis of abdominal pain. The spinal nerve in the corresponding area has no fascial sheath and is therefore very sensitive to local anesthetics. Local anesthetic is injected into the paravertebral space of the vertebral body, and the drug spreads mainly along the long axis of the paravertebral body, blocking the somatic and sympathetic nerves, including the posterior branch of the thoracic nerve. This interspace is adjacent to the pleura and axons, and there is a risk of pneumothorax or spread of local anesthetics into the epidural and intrathecal areas with improper injection. Contraindications include coagulation disorders, anticoagulation therapy, paravertebral tumors, or abscesses.

   Richardson et al. summarized 12 studies that included a total of 538 patients and found that paravertebral blocks provided better intraoperative and postoperative analgesia for thoracic, abdominal, and gynecologic procedures [55]. Naja et al. also reported that paravertebral blocks could provide better results for refractory myofascial pain syndromes in the thoracic segment [56].

11.5.3.2 Treatment of Pain Due to Visceral Factors

1. Spinal cord stimulation (SCS)

   Because the traditional view is that chronic visceral pain is a kind of somatic pain and spinal cord stimulation is effective for neuropathic pain, it was not considered suitable for chronic visceral pain in the past. Recently, there has been interest in the neuropathological changes of chronic visceral pain, with nociceptive sensitization of peripheral visceral injury receptors and WDR neurons in the spinal cord.

   Pharmacotherapy, sympathetic blockade, and radiofrequency ablation are common treatments for visceral pain but provide only temporary pain relief. Animal studies have shown that spinal cord electrical stimulation can inhibit the visceral-motor reflex and significantly improve the treatment of visceral pain, which can be considered as a long-term treatment option.

   In 2006, Tiede et al. first reported the successful treatment of intractable abdominal pain with SCS in patients with multiple surgical procedures resulting in abdominal adhesions [57]. Kapural reported that patients with chronic abdominal pain treated with SCS were mostly patients with chronic pancreatitis, postoperative abdominal adhesions, and gastroparesis [58]. Placement of electrodes in the posterior epidural space at the midline spinal cord at the $T_{5,6}$ gap level treated most abdominal pain, or at the $T_{11,12}$ level for lower abdominal pain. Sympathetic blockade is also not significantly effective in patients who do not respond well to SCS testing. Conversely, patients with a good response to sympathetic block also have a satisfactory SCS test.

2. Sympathetic nerve block

   Percutaneous block of sympathetic nerve is often used in patients who do not respond well to pharmacological treatment and helps to develop the next treatment plan, such as sympathetic nerve thermocoagulation or chemical disruption, SCS.

   Indications for thoracic sympathetic ganglion dissection: CRPS I and II, thoracic neuropathic pain, chest wall, thoracic visceral, epigastric visceral pain, herpes zoster, postherpetic neuralgia, phantom pain after mastectomy, arterial occlusion ischemia, drug-resistant Raynaud's disease, Burger's disease, upper extremity injury, etc. Complications of thoracic sympathetic nerve block include nerve root injury, spinal cord injury, and pneumothorax.

   Abdominal nerve blocks and visceral nerve blocks are generally used for pain associated with malignant or nonmalignant tumors in the upper abdomen. Preganglionic fibers from T_{5-9} converge to form the large visceral nerve (at the level of $T_{9,10}$), which travels across the diaphragm and terminates in the celiac plexus; preganglionic fibers from $T_{10,11}$ unite to form the small visceral nerve, while preganglionic fibers from T_{12} form the smallest visceral nerve. Therefore, the area of action of the celiac nerve block and visceral nerve block includes the lower third of the esophagus to the transverse colon, liver, bile duct, adrenal glands, and mesentery.

   Indications: Tumors in the abdominal viscera to the splenic region, benign abdominal pain that has failed to respond to drug therapy. Adverse effects include hypotension and diarrhea. Complications include nerve injury, paralysis, pneumothorax, intestinal injury, and bleeding. A review that included analysis of 31 studies suggested that 85–90% of patients had satisfactory pain relief after treatment with nerve plexus block (NCPB) in the abdominal cavity [59]. The findings of another meta-analysis also confirmed the effectiveness and safety of NCPB [60].

   The lumbar sympathetic chain is located in the anterolateral aspect of the lumbar vertebral body. Lumbar sympathetic chain blocks are commonly used for CRPS I and II, peripheral neuropathic pain, and ischemia-related pain. A common side effect of lumbar sympathetic chain block is hypotension due to peripheral vasodilation: complications include bleeding, nerve root injury, genitofemoral nerve injury, paresthesia, and renal puncture injury.

   The inferior epigastric plexus is located in the retroperitoneum, slightly to the left of the midline, from the inferior border of the L_3 vertebrae to the superior border of the S_3 sacral vertebrae, adjacent to the bifurcation of the common iliac vessels. The branches of the plexus descend into the pelvis and enter the inferior abdominal plexus, which receives S_{2-4} parasympathetic fibers and forms the pelvic, mid-rectal, prostatic, and uterovaginal plexuses. The inferior epigastric plexus block is indicated for cancerous or noncancerous pain from the descending colon to the rectum and the pelvic genitourinary system. Complications include intravascular injections, intervertebral discitis, nerve injury, urinary tract injury, bladder, and bowel retention.

   The ganglion impar is the terminal ganglion of the sympathetic chain and has a variable anatomic location, mostly on the caudal side of the sacrococcygeal junction. The ganglion impar block can be used in patients with vulvodynia, chronic perineal pain, and sacrococcygeal pain.

   The effectiveness of sympathetic nerve blocks is still lacking in the literature, and the available reports are of poor quality, with only ventral plexus/visceral nerve blocks reaching evidence level 1B, and well-designed RCT studies with large sample sizes are still needed in the future.

3. Destructive nerve blocks

   Destructive nerve blocks continue to play an important role in the management of patients with cancer pain. There is no definite conclusion as to which is more effective, pharmacologic, or technical disruption. While the afferent nerve fibers of the abdominal and pelvic organs converge at the sympathetic ganglion, nerve disruption techniques interfere with the function of the sympathetic nervous system mainly at the ganglion level.

Several different puncture techniques are used to inject nerve-disrupting drugs, with interpleural blocks, ventral plexus blocks, superior inferior abdominal plexus nerve blocks, and ganglion impar blocks being the most commonly used.

With interpleural blocks, local anesthetics are injected between the mural and visceral pleura to cause unilateral multisegmental torso block of the chest while blocking the sympathetic chain and visceral nerves to relieve acute and chronic pain in the surgical or nonsurgical chest and upper abdomen. Interpleural blocks are effective in the treatment of visceral pain from the esophagus, liver and gallbladder, stomach, and pancreas, while complications include pneumothorax, phrenic nerve palsy, and dyspnea. To achieve a disfiguring effect, phenol concentration was initially reported to be 6% and later increased to 10%. Local anesthetics (bupivacaine or ropivacaine) can also be used for continuous or intermittent injections in patients with intractable severe pain.

The celiac plexus receives parasympathetic fibers from the vagus nerve and autonomic fibers from the liver, pancreas, gallbladder, stomach, spleen, kidney, intestines, and adrenal glands. Abdominal plexus block is effective in relieving chronic pancreatitis pain or epigastric cancer pain. Complications include hypotension, diarrhea, sensory dullness, back pain in the interscapular region, reactive pleurisy, eructation, hematuria, retroperitoneal hematoma, paraplegia, temporary motor paralysis, and abdominal aortic puncture injury. Destruction is done using alcohol or phenol with an alcohol concentration of 50–100%. It causes severe pain prior to nerve fiber destruction and therefore requires advance injection of local anesthetics.

Inferior epigastric plexus block can be used for chronic pelvic pain. Destructive block is effective for lower abdominal or pelvic cancer pain, but sometimes, the side effects are intolerable.

4. Radiofrequency treatment (RF)

   It is also an effective way to treat chronic pain, with the advantages of being minimally invasive and available for outpatient treatment. Due to the target selectivity of RF, there are fewer side effects, and the area of RF destruction is located at the tip of the needle (5–6 mm in cross-sectional diameter), adding accuracy and safety to electrical stimulation and impedance monitoring.

   Radiofrequency can be used for pain due to chronic pancreatitis, pancreatic cancer, liver tumors, or abdominal surgery where drug therapy is ineffective by destroying visceral nerves due to its advantages of referable experience, greater selectivity, and fewer complications. Therefore, RF therapy can be considered for patients with abdominal pain syndrome when nonsurgical and symptomatic treatments are not effective.

   Visceral nerve RF has the advantage of being highly selective and having few complications. The success rate of this technique depends on accurate diagnosis, clear nerve structure, technical proficiency, and reasonable patient expectations. The use of RF as part of a multimodal treatment can avoid or reduce the use of invasive or expensive treatment modalities.

   Pulsed radiofrequency (PRF), which does not require nerve destruction to achieve analgesia, is increasingly used in clinical practice. Because it does not require nerve destruction, PRF avoids the side effects associated with conventional RF for visceral pain, and the effectiveness can be easily monitored. Pulsed radiofrequency may be considered as a second strategy in the WHO ladder of therapies as a first-line treatment for chronic pain.

11.5.3.3 Treatment of Abdominal Wall Pain

Nonsurgical treatment is the first-line option for CAWP. If the pain itself does not affect the patient's quality of life, a diagnostic local nerve block is beneficial to clarify the etiology. In patients with moderate to severe pain, the combination of long-acting glucocorticoids is beneficial to improve the efficacy of long-term analgesia. One study reported that the combined application of local anesthetics and glucocorticoids in pediatric patients with rectus abdominis sheath block significantly improved analgesia. Nonsurgical treatments such as abdominal muscle stretching, local medication, and nerve stimulation can be used for mild to severe pain. However, nonoperative treatment is effective in less than 40% of patients. In addition, botulinum toxin injections or local phenol injections at myofascial trigger points may also help to improve symptoms. Patients with peripheral nerve entrapment (ACNES, iliac inguinal nerve entrapment, inferior iliac abdominal nerve entrapment) should be considered for indications to perform nerve release.

In addition, for recalcitrant cases, the following treatment options may be considered in addition to those described above. Peripheral and central nerve modulation (spinal cord electrical stimulation, peripheral nerve electrical stimulation, peripheral regional stimulation) is effective for neuropathic pain caused by peripheral nerve entrapment or nerve root lesions: pulsed radiofrequency is effective for thoracic nerve root pain; when other methods are not effective for analgesia, continuous intrathecal drug infusion for analgesia is optional.

11.5.3.4 Other Treatment Methods

Unlike the somatic structure, the viscera receive dual innervation, with the sensory branch of the vagus nerve, whose cell is located in the brain stem, and the primary afferent nerve of the spinal cord, whose cell is located in the dorsal root ganglion of the corresponding spinal cord segment. Under normal conditions, the body does not perceive sensations from the viscera and is only aware of discomfort or pain when it occurs.

Intrathecal drug delivery (IDD) system has gradually become an effective alternative treatment option for patients with chronic abdominal pain. The mechanism of action of IDD is to interfere with the transmission of pain signals to the brain, and it has a wide range of indications. The mechanism of action of opioids has been studied more thoroughly. Opioids inhibit nociceptive signaling in C-fibers by binding to pre- and postsynaptic μ-type opioid receptors in the posterior horn of the spinal cord; local anesthetics block the transmission of pain signals by blocking voltage-gated sodium channels in the nerve cell membrane and inhibiting action potential conduction; ziconotide works by blocking N-type calcium channels; other adjuvant drugs can directly inhibit nerve conduction and C-fiber transmission.

There are several different combinations of drugs used in clinical practice, such as opioids and local anesthetics, opioids, and colistin, opioids combined with local anesthetics and chlorambucil, and opioids combined with local anesthetics and colistin. According to the literature, the effectiveness of combination of drugs is positive, but the relevant studies are mainly case reports and retrospective analyses, and there is a lack of prospective studies with a long time course. Reference data on drug interactions, dose ranges, and long-term safety of many drugs are limited; information on whether drug-drug interactions within intrathecal catheters and infusion devices can have adverse effects on humans is also imperfect. The dosing regimens currently used in clinical practice still require further studies to clarify the optimal regimen.

Although there is a theoretical basis to support the use of IDDs for the treatment of chronic abdominal pain, their practical application is very limited. To our knowledge, there are still no reports on the use of DD for adhesion-related abdominal pain. However, Guttman et al. reported that DD can achieve satisfactory results in patients with refractory chronic abdominal pain due to median arcuate ligament syndrome (MAL). In this study, all other treatment options including oral opioids, sympathetic blockade, SCS, and surgery failed to provide adequate pain relief, but by administering morphine through an IDD system implanted at the T_{11} level, the patient experienced complete pain relief and regained a normal quality of life after 10 days. Although we cannot draw conclusions based on a single case report, the results of this study suggest that IDD may be one of the appropriate options for the treatment of visceral pain when all other conventional therapies fail to improve it.

11.5.4 Prevention Strategies for Abdominal Adhesions

The incidence of medically induced abdominal adhesions is as high as 95% after abdominal and pelvic surgery, and the complications associated with adhesions not only cause pain to patients but also increase the medical burden, so it is important to prevent postoperative adhesions. Some procedures are at higher risk of adhesions, such as ileal flap surgery and emergency appendectomy. Unlike skin crusting, adherent tissue is a dynamic structure of excessive cellular proliferation and vascularization. Inhibition of cell proliferation, differentiation, migration, angiogenesis, regulation of death, and anti-host response are potential therapeutic targets.

The prevention strategies for postoperative abdominal adhesions include the following.

11.5.4.1 Barrier Prevention and Control

Peritoneal surface injury is a key cause of adhesion formation. Therefore, prevention and control of peritoneal adhesions involve preventing peritoneal injury and isolating the broken part of the peritoneum prone to adhesion formation with a barrier material to allow sufficient time for mesothelial cells to repair, while tissue adhesions begin to form in the immediate postoperative period. Barrier materials should be selected to avoid inflammatory and immunogenic properties, remain active at the site of injury, and be self-degrading. The most critical time to prevent adhesions is also within 7 days postoperatively.

1. Mechanical barrier

   The plasma membrane injury site is isolated by bioabsorbable membrane, mainly oxidized regenerated cellulose membrane (Intercced), hyaluronic acid plus carboxymethyl cellulose (Seprafil), poly-caprolactone barrier membrane, etc. Oxidized regenerated cellulose (ORC) forms a barrier on the surface of tissue damage, transforms into a gel state within 8 h, effectively reduces the degree of adhesions, can be shaped with organ contour, and requires complete hemostasis before clinical application. Seprafil is an artificial hyaluronic acid anti-adhesion barrier, which has been shown to inhibit inflammatory cell activation and aggregation and reduce the aggregation of fibroblasts and blood fibrinogen. The study showed that Seprafil has the ability to inhibit the activation and aggregation of inflammatory cells and reduce the aggregation of fibroblasts and blood fibrinogen. Poly-ethylene-lactone barrier film is a fatty cluster polyester material, and some researchers fixed poly-ethylene-lactone barrier film on the peritoneal wound of rats to prevent postoperative abdominal adhesions with remarkable effect. Polylactide films are L-lactide and D,L-lactide polymers, which can significantly reduce the formation of postoperative peritoneal adhesions, have good histocompatibility, and can degrade into hemagglutination, epithelial formation, and fibrinolysis in vivo.
2. Drug barrier

   Chitosan is made of polyglucosaminoglycan to promote epithelial cell growth, hemostasis, lubricating effect, and biological barrier to prevent adhesion formation. Some studies have shown that it inhibits exogenous healing of tendons, promotes wound healing, prevents abdominal adhesions, has good histocompatibility, and can be degraded in vivo [61]. It has also been studied that the application of gibberellins to prevent and treat abdominal adhesions in patients with no clinical signs and symptoms of intestinal adhesions in patients followed up for 6 months after surgery [62]. Dextran is an anti-adhesive agent that covers the damaged part of the peritoneum to hinder the attachment of blood clots and fibrinous adhesion formation; it was also reported that the use of metronidazole and dextran in a 1:2 preparation for abdominal lavage in abdominal infection surgery did not reveal intestinal obstruction, abdominal pain, and abdominal distension after surgery, which effectively prevented the occurrence of intestinal adhesions after abdominal infection surgery without significant adverse effects [63].

11.5.4.2 Drug Prevention and Control

The mechanism of drug prevention and control of abdominal adhesions is to inhibit inflammatory reaction and fibroblast growth, promote the decomposition and absorption of fibrin, remove fibrin exudate, and prevent the deposition of fibrin and the formation of adhesion zone, so as to inhibit abdominal adhesions.

1. Promote fibrinolytic drugs

   Recombinant streptokinase (r-sk) can activate fibrinogen, promote fibrinolysis, and eliminate local inflammation, thus achieving the purpose of preventing and controlling abdominal adhesions. Some researchers believe that the application of r-sk can promote the recovery of gastrointestinal function after abdominal surgery and early enteral nutrition, prevent postoperative abdominal adhesions, and reduce postoperative abdominal symptoms.
2. Drugs to prevent fiber deposition

   Octreotide inhibits the release of gastrointestinal hormones, reduces the secretion of digestive juices, and decreases the permeability of intestinal mucosa, so it can significantly inhibit the loss of digestive juices. It has been reported that the application of octreotide can effectively prevent the occurrence of postoperative abdominal adhesions.
3. Drugs to reduce inflammatory response

   COX-2 inhibitors can significantly reduce the density of microvessels in neoadhesive tissues and have a longer-lasting anti-adhesive capacity than nonselective cyclooxygenase inhibitors. Short-term oral administration of COX-2 to experimental animals has been reported to be effective in preventing postoperative abdominal adhesions.

11.5.5 Summary

Given that the occurrence of peritoneal adhesions is closely related to surgery and gentle and careful surgical operation and strict adherence to surgical principles remain the most effective measures to prevent peritoneal adhesions, minimizing mechanical irritation from surgery, proper protection of the intestinal canal, and removal of peritoneal fluid and blood accumulation are all important. If the peritoneal defect is too large, there is no need for reluctant suturing, otherwise the suture tension will be too high and will easily cause tissue ischemia. The absence of sutures for peritoneal defects does not affect their strength against tension.

The formation of postoperative peritoneal adhesions is a complex process involving multiple biochemical and biophysical factors. Although some progress has been made in the formation mechanism and treatment, it is far from satisfactory, and there is no ideal method to effectively prevent and treat abdominal adhesions. The ideal therapeutic approach is to prevent and treat the occurrence of abdominal adhesions by promoting mesothelial cell repair, improving the immune defense function of T cells, reducing tissue inflammatory response and exudation, and promoting the phagocytosis of abdominal macrophages in a multi-targeted and multi-linked manner. Both barrier effects and pharmacological treatments have some clinical application, and whether these tools are definitely effective still needs to be confirmed by further large samples of high-quality clinical studies. With the development of molecular biology, the elaboration of the mechanism of abdominal adhesions from a molecular biology perspective will facilitate the regulation of the fibrin formation and lysis process at the cellular and molecular levels, thus exploring new clinical treatment pathways.

11.6 Common Pediatric Recurrent Abdominal Pain

11.6.1 Overview

Pediatric recurrent abdominal pain (RAP) is a common chronic abdominal pain disease in children caused by a variety of organic and functional causes, which has a wide range of causes and features such as recurrent attacks, long-term persistence, and less than ideal efficacy of conventional treatment, thus becoming a difficult point of clinical diagnosis and treatment and seriously affecting the physical and mental health of children and their family life.

RAP was first proposed by Apley et al. It refers to a kind of recurrent abdominal pain occurring in children aged 3 years or above, which occurs every month for at least 3 months, and can affect the normal activities of the child when the attack is severe but behaves normally in the interval between attacks [64]. According to incomplete statistics in China, RAP accounts for more than 50% of children with abdominal pain, and the literature in Europe and the United States reports that RAP can appear before school age but less frequently occurs before the age of 5 and after the age of 16 and frequently occurs in school age (10–12 years old), with an incidence of 10–19.2% in this age group, with more girls than boys in a ratio of 5:3, and the incidence reported in Japan is 3–4% [65].

With the development of diagnostic techniques, especially the popularization and improvement of gastrointestinal endoscopy in pediatrics, the level of diagnosis and treatment of RAP has been significantly improved. According to the etiology causing abdominal pain, RAP is divided into two categories: organic and functional. In preschool and school age, only 10% of cases have organic disease, while functional RAP accounts for more than 90% of cases. Therefore, in the following sections, we will introduce the etiology, diagnosis, and treatment related to organic and functional RAP, respectively.

11.6.2 Etiology, Diagnosis, and Treatment of Organic RAP

11.6.2.1 Etiology

The etiology of organic RAP includes abdominal factors and systemic factors.

1. Common abdominal diseases
   (a) Gastric and duodenal diseases: Acute and chronic gastritis, gastric or duodenal ulcers, gastric torsion, etc. Inflammatory reactions and ulcers are more common in children. In addition, there are also rare diseases such as duodenal stasis, congenital stenosis, and repetitive malformation. In recent years, studies related to *H. pylori* (Hp) infection and RAP have been reported in different countries with varying conclusions of whether there is an association between childhood Hp infection and RAP [66, 67].
   (b) Intestinal diseases: Various infectious enteritis, inflammatory reactive bowel disease (including ulcerative colitis, Crohn's disease), intestinal obstruction (intestinal malrotation, inguinal hernia, intussusception), and appendicitis.
   (c) Hepatic, biliary, and pancreatic diseases: Hepatitis, biliary tract infection, inflammatory reaction of the pancreas, biliary ascariasis, common bile duct cyst, cricothyroid pancreas, etc.
   (d) Spleen diseases: Splenic cysts, splenic torsion, etc.
   (e) Genitourinary system diseases: Urinary tract infection, hydronephrosis, urinary tract obstruction, urinary calculi, etc.
   (f) Other: Mesenteric lymph node hyperplasia, inflammatory reaction, lactose intolerance, gastrointestinal metaplasia, etc.
2. Systemic or extra-abdominal diseases

   Pneumonia, chondromalacia (cribriform disease), pericarditis, diabetes mellitus, ketoacidosis, uremia, allergic purpura, urticaria, porphyria, etc.

11.6.2.2 Diagnosis and Differential Diagnosis

The following symptoms are often indicative of organic disease in RAP: pain site restriction, weight loss, anorexia, altered urinary habits, oliguria, dysuria, vomiting, hematologic abnormalities, urinary routine and culture abnormalities, significant family history, fever, and painful awakening of the child from sleep.

1. Medical history

   Abdominal pain is the first symptom complained by the child (or parents).

   (a) Duration of abdominal pain attack: The duration of the disease is more than 3 months (or only 1–2 months), and the number of episodes is frequent (>3) during the course of the disease.
   (b) Characteristics of abdominal pain episodes: Functional abdominal pain episodes are more common in the morning, often with sudden abdominal pain on an empty stomach or during meals, each lasting less than 1 h, and most children can relieve themselves without treatment: if each abdominal pain lasts 2–3 h or longer, organic should be considered.
   (c) Abdominal pain site: The pain site of organic pain is mostly deviated from the abdominal midline: if the pain site is around the umbilicus or the upper part of the umbilicus near the abdominal midline, it is mostly functional RAP.
   (d) Nature of abdominal pain: Children with organic pain have obvious pain at night; functional pain is mostly vague or dull, sometimes with spasmodic nature, and when the abdominal pain is intermittent, the patient won't be bothered and rarely wakes up with pain at night.
   (e) Age of first attack: Some researchers believe that organic disease should be considered in children with attacks younger than 3 years old, which can only serve as a reference, because in recent years, children with chronic constipation have a younger age of onset, which often causes functional abdominal pain.
   (f) Concomitant symptoms: Organic is caused by a variety of organic diseases and can be accompanied by fever, frequent bilious vomiting, vomiting blood, painful urination, blood in the stool, anemia, and other manifestations of the original disease, which is noteworthy: while functional abdominal pain is usually accompanied only by lack of appetite, paranoia, constipation, occasional headache, dizziness, etc.

2. Physical examination

   After taking a medical history, the attending physician has a preliminary judgment on the diagnosis of abdominal pain in the child, and physical examination is a more important step.

   (a) The child's developmental and nutritional condition. Functional RAP won't affect development and nutrition; therefore, if the child's height and weight are basically normal, it is generally not considered organic.
   (b) The child's neurological and mental condition. Pay attention to the presence of symptoms of autonomic dysfunction: Functional children are sometimes neurotic, manifesting as tachycardia, mildly elevated blood pressure, sweaty palms, cold extremities, large pupils, and pale face, indicating autonomic instability. This indicates unstable autonomic function.

3. Auxiliary examination

   Some experts believe that if a detailed history and careful physical examination can identify a functional disease, laboratory tests are not necessary: however, more literature reports that routine blood, urine, and fecal tests, erythrocyte sedimentation rate, liver function, urine culture, fecal eggs, and fecal occult blood are necessary screening tests, and if they are normal, 95% of them can exclude organic pathology [68].

   Routine blood, urine, and fecal examinations are performed as routine tests to determine the presence of anemia, urinary tract infections, and intestinal parasites. At present, because the prevalence of intestinal parasitism has been decreasing year by year, fecal microscopy for parasitic eggs is often overlooked. Those with high suspicion should be tested by egg collection method. The fecal occult blood test should not be ignored as it can sometimes be positive in children with peptic ulcers. Through physical examination and routine blood and urine and fecal examinations, preliminary judgments can be made on certain organic causes (such as collagen diseases, neurological diseases, diabetes mellitus, pancreatitis and urinary tract infections, etc.), and if abdominal pain is a concomitant symptom of the primary disease, it should be treated as such.

4. Special Auxiliary Examination

   Special auxiliary examinations are mostly used to identify gastritis, peptic ulcer, inflammatory bowel disease, cholelithiasis, chronic pancreatitis, and systemic diseases with RAP as the first symptom.

   (a) Fiber endoscopy: Gastroscopy should be preferred for children with a lack of appetite, nausea, vomiting, emaciation, and epigastric pain. Its clinical diagnostic value and positive rate have been described previously. Fibrous colonoscopy and some cases of inflammatory bowel disease (nonspecific ulcerative colitis, Crohn's disease) only show abdominal pain and need to be confirmed by endoscopy.
   (b) Barium examination: Including gastrointestinal barium meal and barium enema examination, the positive detection rate is 35–85%, and there are many factors affecting it, but it is still a meaningful examination method for those who do not have endoscopic examination conditions.
   (c) Abdominal ultrasound: It has important diagnostic value for suspected gallstone disease, liver or pancreatic disease, intra-abdominal masses, ascites, and abscesses.
   (d) CT and MRI: These examinations can be done for those with high clinical suspicion of intracranial or intra-abdominal tumors and no positive findings in other examinations.
   (e) Laparoscopy: Pediatric patients with high clinical suspicion of organic lesions and no positive findings on imaging may choose to undergo laparoscopy.

Problems to be noted in diagnosis: RAP has a high incidence in children, and its etiology involves systemic diseases, so in the diagnosis, first of all, attention should be paid not to miss organic diseases; however, the majority of RAP has no organic diseases, so excessive and unnecessary tests should also be avoided. In summary, the diagnosis should be based on the characteristics of the onset of RAP, first distinguish between functional and organic diseases, and then select the necessary auxiliary tests to make the correct diagnosis.

11.6.2.3 Treatment of Organic RAP

Organic RAP should be treated actively after the etiology is clarified, and the corresponding medical or surgical treatment should be performed according to the different etiologies. In children younger than 2 years old, RAP often has organic diseases, such as chronic constipation, parasitic infection, carbohydrate intolerance, genitourinary diseases, recurrent pancreatitis, upper gastrointestinal inflammation and peptic ulcer, inflammatory bowel disease, eosinophilic gastroenteritis, hepatobiliary diseases, irritable bowel syndrome, abdominal migraine, hemolytic anemia, and lead poisoning. Gastrointestinal and genitourinary system diseases are the most common, accounting for about one-third of the cases. Therefore, a clear diagnosis should be followed by active treatment of the cause.

11.6.3 Etiology, Diagnosis, and Treatment of Functional RAP

The typical functional RAP lacks the manifestation of corresponding organic lesions, and the abdominal pain is often spasmodic or colicky in nature. The child may have one to two episodes per day, per week, or per month, or one episode per few months. Each attack does not exceed 1–3 h and may resolve on its own. The attacks are more common in the morning and often worsen suddenly on an empty stomach or during meals but rarely at night when the pain interferes with sleep. The pain is mainly visceral around the umbilicus but can also be in other parts of the abdomen. The attacks may be accompanied by functional and autonomic symptoms such as vomiting, pallor, sweating, flushing, palpitations, headache, lack of appetite, diarrhea, constipation, and recurrent vomiting. In addition, children often have a family history of functional disorders. These children are often depressed, nervous, and reluctant to share the care they receive with others.

11.6.3.1 Etiology and Diagnosis

The etiology of functional RAP is still unclear and is currently thought to be related to the following factors:

1. Functional gastrointestinal disease

   The Rome criteria are the most comprehensive and updated criteria for the classification of functional gastrointestinal disorders (FGID). The Rome IV Committee renamed the term "abdominal pain-related FGID" as FAPD. Functional abdominal pain (FAP) often refers to any FGID associated with abdominal pain, such as irritable bowel syndrome (IBS) and FD, and classifies pediatric FAPD into the following four types: irritable bowel syndrome (IBS), functional dyspepsia (FD), abdominal migraine, and nonspecific FAP that does not fit all three diagnoses (FAP-NOS). Studies have shown that the same child may suffer from more than one type of FAPD. Clinically, FAP will continue to be used; however, in studies, the diagnosis of FAP-NOS may be more difficult but is expected to improve the specificity of the diagnosis of different diseases.

   (a) FD: A survey in the United States showed that 1.4% of children had epigastric pain or discomfort at least once a week, but only 0.2% met the diagnostic criteria for FD in the Rome III criteria [69]. A community-based study in the northeastern United States showed that 5–10% of healthy adolescents had symptoms of dyspepsia [70].

      Diagnostic criteria: One or more of the following conditions were met for at least 2 months prior to diagnosis and were symptomatic for at least 4 days per month: (1) postprandial fullness, (2) early satiety, (3) epigastric pain or burning sensation unrelated to defecation, and (4) symptoms that could not be fully explained by other diseases after appropriate evaluation.

      FD includes the following subtypes: (1) postprandial discomfort syndrome, postprandial fullness, and discomfort or early satiety that interferes with normal eating. Criteria supporting the diagnosis: epigastric distention, postprandial nausea, or excessive hiccups. (2) Epigastric pain syndrome: It must include all of the following conditions: (a) severe epigastric pain or burning sensation that interferes with daily life, (b) pain that is not all over the abdomen and is confined to other parts of the abdomen or the thoracic rib region, and (c) failure to relieve after defecation or exhaustion. Criteria supporting the diagnosis: (a) Pain may be burning-like but not retrosternal, and (b) pain is usually induced or relieved by eating but may also occur on an empty stomach.

      Pathophysiologic features: The pathogenesis of FD includes abnormalities in gastric motor function and visceral sensory sensitization caused by central or peripheral sensitization, hypo-inflammation, and genetic susceptibility. Gastric adaptive diastolic dysfunction caused by decreased gastric diastolic capacity after feeding has been demonstrated. Gastric electrograms and gastric emptying were studied, and 50% of children with FD had abnormal gastric electrograms, and 47% had delayed gastric emptying. And 24% of children with FD were attributed to complications of acute bacterial gastroenteritis. Children with allergic disease and FD had increased numbers of eosinophils and mast cells in the lamina propria of the gastric mucosa and rapid degranulation of mast cells after milk administration. Studies have shown that children with FD have lower sensory thresholds when performing proximal gastric balloon dilation than healthy volunteers using the constant pressure test.

Clinical evaluation: The role of gastroscopy in the diagnosis of FD in children is unclear. One study showed that both symptom duration <1 year and vomiting were risk factors for mucosal inflammation. In a prospective study, 290 children (4–18 years of age) with RAP assessed by Rome III criteria and alarm symptoms underwent gastroscopy, and the investigators evaluated the need for gastroscopy in children with different types of dyspeptic symptoms, children with a family history of peptic ulcer or *H. pylori* infection, children over 10 years of age with symptoms lasting longer than 6 months, or with symptoms that are so severe that they interfere with daily life, including sleep.

Alarm signs of RAP: Focus on possible alarm signs during both medical history review and physical examination. Further testing is recommended if the child has one of the following signs: inflammatory bowel disease, family history of celiac disease or peptic ulcer, persistent upper or lower right abdominal pain, dysphagia, painful swallowing, persistent vomiting, gastrointestinal bleeding, nocturnal diarrhea, arthritis, perirectal disease, uncontrolled weight loss, growth retardation, delayed puberty, and unexplained fever.

(b) IBS: School-based studies in Colombia and Sri Lanka found the prevalence of IBS to be 4.9% and 5.4%, respectively [71]. A study published in 2020 estimated the prevalence of functional gastrointestinal disorders in the United States, Canada, and the United Kingdom using online population-based surveys using the Rome III and Rome IV criteria [72]. According to the Rome IV criteria, the prevalence of irritable bowel syndrome was very similar in the three countries, ranging from 4.4% to 4.8% [73].

Diagnostic criteria: All of the following conditions must be met at least 2 months prior to diagnosis. (1) Abdominal pain on at least 4 days per month and at least one of the following: (a) associated with defecation, (b) episodes accompanied by changes in defecation frequency, and (c) episodes accompanied by changes in stool properties. (2) In children with constipation, the pain does not resolve as the constipation improves (if the pain resolves then the constipation is functional and not IBS). (3) After appropriate evaluation, symptoms cannot be fully explained by other diseases. IBS in children can be typed by subtypes similar to those in adults, reflecting the main defecation patterns, such as constipation, diarrhea, mixed constipation and diarrhea alternating, and undefined IBS.

Pathophysiological features: IBS is considered a gut-brain axis dysfunction. In affected individuals, symptoms (e.g., diarrhea and constipation, severity of pain, psychological distress) reflect the location and extent of the gut-brain axis affected. Children with IBS may exhibit rectal hypersensitivity rather than gastric nociceptive hypersensitivity, which is the opposite of children with FAP-NOS. Visceral sensory hypersensitivity may be associated with psychological distress (anxiety, depression, impulsivity, anger) in the child. It has been suggested that IBS after acute infectious gastroenteritis (post-infectious IBS) may be associated with an increase in mucosal pro-inflammatory cytokines. Alterations in intestinal flora have also been confirmed, but it is unclear whether these changes are a cause of IBS and its symptoms or a consequence of IBS. Self-reported stress, anxiety, depression, and emotional problems may be increased in children with IBS. Adverse early life events (e.g., surgery) place children at greater risk for developing FAPD, including IBS, in childhood.

Clinical evaluation: A detailed history and physical examination can differentiate functional constipation from IBS. Diarrheal IBS should be differentiated from infections, celiac disease, carbohydrate malabsorption, and less commonly inflammatory bowel disease. Children with celiac disease rarely present with constipation, and children with constipated IBS should be evaluated. The more alarming symptoms of abdominal pain, the higher the likelihood of organic disease. Fecal calprotectin assays are used as a noninvasive screening method for intestinal mucosal inflammation and appear to be superior to conventional tests, such as C-reactive protein.

(c) Abdominal migraine: According to the Rome IV diagnostic criteria, the prevalence of abdominal migraine ranges from 1% to 23%. Since the Rome II criteria were replaced by the Rome III criteria, the diagnosis of abdominal migraine in children has increased greatly. The Rome III diagnostic criteria are more inclusive and less specific than the Rome II criteria. The Rome III criteria have a high positive predictive value (100%) but a low negative predictive value (7.7%), which may lead to other FAPDs being misdiagnosed as abdominal migraine.

Diagnostic criteria: Two attacks of abdominal pain at least 6 months prior to diagnosis and all of the following conditions are met: (1) Sudden onset acute periumbilical, midline or diffuse severe abdominal pain lasting 1 h or more (the most severe and painful symptom); (2) attacks occurring weeks to months apart; (3) pain that is intolerable and interferes with normal activities; (4) a specific pattern of onset and symptoms; (5) the pain that may be accompanied by two or more of the following symptoms: anorexia, nausea, vomiting, headache, photophobia, and pallor; and (6) symptoms that cannot be fully explained by other diseases after appropriate evaluation.

The prevalence obtained based on the Rome II criteria better represents the actual prevalence of abdominal migraine. To harmonize with the diagnostic criteria for cerebral vascular spasm (CVS), the committee decided to use the same frequency and number of attacks, that is, at least two attacks in 6 months. The main changes to the criteria were: "midline pain, periumbilical or diffuse abdominal pain" instead of "periumbilical pain"; "weeks to months between attacks" instead of "interstitial health status," as the latter may not take into account the underlying gastrointestinal symptoms, thus confusing the guardians. To improve the specificity of the diagnosis, "the child has a specific pattern of onset and symptoms" was added. The diagnosis also does not exclude the presence of other FAPD symptoms during the interictal period. The committee emphasized that the main symptom of abdominal migraine is abdominal pain.

Pathophysiologic features: Abdominal migraine, CVS, and migraine may share the same pathophysiologic mechanisms, and their onset is episodic, self-limited, and specific, and they all have asymptomatic intervals. Similar triggers (e.g., stress, fatigue, and travel), associated symptoms (e.g., anorexia, nausea, vomiting), and remission factors (e.g., rest and sleep) have been reported in children with both abdominal migraine and typical migraine. Both abdominal migraine and CVS can turn into migraine by adulthood. Increased excitatory amino acid activity is found in patients with classic migraine, which could explain the efficacy of drugs that increase γ-aminobutyric acid.

Clinical evaluation: The presence of nonspecific prodromal symptoms similar to those of children with migraine, such as changes in behavior or mood, photophobia, and vasodilatory symptoms, as well as relief of symptoms with migraine treatment, is present in abdominal migraine. Diseases associated with severe episodes of abdominal pain, such as intermittent small bowel or urinary tract obstruction, recurrent pancreatitis, biliary tract disease, familial Mediterranean fever, metabolic disorders such as porphyria, and psychiatric disorders need to be excluded.

(d) FAP-NOS: FAP-NOS replaces FAP and functional abdominal pain syndrome (FAPS) in the Rome IV diagnostic criteria classification. Weekly abdominal pain has been reported in 35–38% of elementary school children. Of these children, only about one-third met the diagnosis of FAPD. The prevalence of FAP-NOS in school-aged children was 2.7% in Colombia and 4.4% in Sri Lanka, according to conditions corresponding to the Rome III criteria. The prevalence of parent-reported FAP-NOS in children was 1.2% in the US community and 2% in German schools.

Diagnostic criteria: Symptoms for at least 2 months prior to diagnosis met all of the following criteria and at least four episodes of abdominal pain per month, (1) episodic or persistent abdominal pain not exclusively associated with a physiological event (e.g., eating, menstrual period); (2) did not meet diagnostic criteria for IBS, FD, or abdominal migraine; and (3) after appropriate evaluation, the abdominal pain could not be explained by other disorders.

The number of abdominal pains required for diagnosis was changed from one per week to four per month to match the other diagnostic criteria for FAPD. This allows for a clear diagnosis for children who do not meet the diagnostic criteria for FAPD but are at risk of being chronically underdiagnosed. The condition "not exclusively associated with physiological events (e.g., eating, menstruation)" was added to the diagnostic criteria. This is because children with FAPD may have increased symptoms during physiological events (e.g., eating, menstruation) and pain at other times. The committee eliminated the FAPS classification in view of the fact that other FAPDs (e.g., IBS) may accompany the child's dysfunction.

Pathophysiologic features: Studies that treat FAP-NOS independently of IBS have shown that children with FAP-NOS usually do not have rectal hypersensitivity compared with children with IBS. Children with FAP-NOS have been reported to have weaker sinus contraction and slower fluid emptying compared to healthy controls. There is evidence that psychological distress is associated with RAP in children and adolescents. RAP has also been associated with stressful events such as parental divorce, hospitalization, intimidation, and early abuse. The way children and their families cope with pain can affect the consequences of FAPD.

Clinical evaluation: Children with FAP-NOS often have nonspecific extra-gastrointestinal somatic symptoms, but laboratory and imaging tests are not always required [69]. Limited diagnostic testing is usually performed to reassure guardians. Special attention should be paid to children with autonomic symptoms, especially postural tachycardia syndrome. If there are signs of abdominal pain alarm, additional tests are recommended.

2. Family environment and psychosocial factors

   It has been reported that children with IBS families see abdominal pain more often: psychosocial factors can affect the gastrointestinal tract and predispose to symptoms of gastrointestinal dysfunction. Children with RAP often have specific psychological manifestations, such as nervousness, depression, desire for love and care, and pursuit of perfection, and can be influenced by environmental factors such as parental divorce and family discord [74].

3. Autonomic dysfunction

   It has been reported that the pupil response to autonomic stimulation in children with RAP is different from that in normal subjects when the hand cold water test is performed [75, 76]. Also, it is reported that the bronchial smooth muscle response is enhanced in children with RAP in the acetylcholine inhalation test [77].

4. Visceral sensory hypersensitivity

   It is concluded that children with RAP have lower pain thresholds and increased sensitivity to painful stimuli than normal children [78].

5. Gastrointestinal motility dysfunction

   Children with RAP have a stronger gastrointestinal kinetic response to stressors. It is hypothesized that the increased activity of endogenous opioids (B-endorphins) in the body during stress excites the smooth muscle of the gastrointestinal tract and prolongs gastric emptying; the propulsive peristalsis of the small and large intestine is weakened; the anal sphincter tone is increased, and defecation is obstructed; the sphincter of Oddi is contracted, and the pressure in the gallbladder and bile duct is increased. All of the above conditions can cause abdominal pain.

   In conclusion, the occurrence of functional RAP is the result of a combination of factors such as functional gastrointestinal disease and sensory, emotional, and cognitive effects. Different visceral sensitivities can lead to different perceptions of pain, and psychosocial stress can influence the intensity and nature of pain. The pain response can be influenced by the stress state, personality type, and the family's concern for the child's illness. The same abdominal pain can cause one child to stop school and go home, while another child can maintain normal activities.

11.6.3.2 Treatment of Functional RAP

There is no clear and effective evidence-based treatment strategy, and multimodal noninvasive treatment options are currently more recommended, with some patients also potentially benefiting from interventional or surgical treatment. The goals of treatment are to reduce stress; relieve child and parental tension; increase physical activity, social interaction, and school attendance; and reduce the impact of pain on the patient's daily activities.

1. Treatment of functional gastrointestinal disease
   (a) FD: Foods that cause aggravation of symptoms (such as caffeinated, spicy, and fatty foods) and nonsteroidal anti-inflammatory drugs should be avoided. Psychological factors that can aggravate the symptoms should be eased. For children with pain as the main symptom, histamine receptor antagonists and PPIs can be used to suppress acid. Omeprazole is more effective than ranitidine, famotidine, and cimetidine if FD cure is defined as complete remission of symptoms after 4 weeks of treatment. Although convincing data are lacking, low-dose tricyclic antidepressants such as amitriptyline and promethazine are commonly used in difficult cases. Nausea, bloating, and early satiety are more difficult to treat, and prokinetic agents such as cisapride and domperidone may also be applied. A retrospective, open study showed that cisapride is safe and effective in the treatment of FD. Gastric electrical stimulation may be a promising option for children with refractory FD.
   (b) IBS: There are data to support the use of probiotics. A small sample of children in a prospective, double-blind trial reported the efficacy achieved with peppermint oil in reducing pain levels. A recent double-blind crossover trial in children with IBS (including all subtypes) demonstrated the efficacy of a fermentation short-chain carbohydrate restricted (FODMAP) diet,

that is, reduced intake of fermented oligosaccharides, disaccharides, monosaccharides, and polyols. Similar to the treatment of FAP-NOS, behavioral therapies can be used in the treatment of IBS in children.

(c) Abdominal migraine: Treatment options are determined by the frequency, severity, and impact of abdominal migraine attacks on the daily life of the child and family. A double-blind, placebo-controlled crossover trial in 14 children demonstrated the prophylactic effect of oral phenothiazine, a drug with anti-5-HT and antihistamine effects. Prophylactic drugs such as amitriptyline, propranolol, and cycloheximide have been shown to have good efficacy.

(d) FAP-NOS: Most therapeutic evaluations of FAPD are unclassified, limiting the applicability of the results. Although adult studies have confirmed the efficacy of antispasmodics, the application of the antispasmodic mebeverine in children has not been significantly better than placebo. A small sample of amitriptyline trials confirmed its efficacy, while a large sample of multicenter studies found no efficacy. A recent study of citalopram in a large sample found that citalopram was effective in the treatment of children with FAP compared with the placebo group. However, clinicians, children, and guardians should be aware of the black box warning issued by the US Food and Drug Administration regarding the application of citalopram, namely, the increased risk of suicidal ideation in adolescents. Hypnotherapy and cognitive behavioral therapy provide immediate and long-term benefits to these children.

2. Psychotherapy

   It is an important part of the treatment of functional abdominal pain in children. The treatment of functional RAP should focus on psychotherapy. The doctor should explain the condition to the child and his parents, patiently explain the pathogenesis of functional RAP, make them eliminate their worries, realize that RAP is a common disease and that school can be continued in general episodes, help children who have dropped out of school due to abdominal pain to return to school, and increase their confidence in treatment.

3. Cognitive-behavioral therapy

   Abdominal pain often coexists with anxiety and depression, and cognitive-behavioral, a non-pharmacological treatment, has entered the first line of treatment. Specific programs: teaching the child to cope with pain, teaching family members how to care for the child, and encouraging the family to confront the child's complaints about abdominal pain, without reinforcing or ignoring them, may be beneficial to the child's pain control.

4. Dietary treatment

   Establishing good dietary habits in children, eating on time, encouraging more fiber-rich foods, and less gas-producing foods such as white potatoes and beans, etc. are beneficial for children with functional RAP. It has also been suggested that probiotics are beneficial for children with IBS. Discontinuation of dairy or use of low-lactose dairy products is advisable in lactose-intolerant individuals; however, some studies have found that there is no direct link between functional abdominal pain and lactose intolerance and that not consuming lactose does not improve the symptoms of functional abdominal pain. It is also important to note that foods that trigger abdominal pain should be avoided.

5. Drug therapy

   To reduce the symptoms, antispasmodics, gastrointestinal stimulants, drugs regulating autonomic function, and tricyclic antidepressants can be applied appropriately according to the condition. However, the clinical effect of tricyclic antidepressants is uncertain, and some studies have concluded that taking the drugs did not improve the pain. There are some randomized controlled studies of selective 5-hydroxytryptamine reuptake inhibitors, but large samples of randomized controlled trials are needed. Diagnostic laparoscopy is considered in rare cases, such as children with recurrent chronic abdominal pain who have failed other treatments.

6. Establish a follow-up system

   Successful management relies on close follow-up in which a true understanding of the child is achieved, both to relieve the fear of the family and the child and to detect or exclude organic disease over time.

11.6.3.3 Prognosis of Functional RAP

About one-third of children with functional RAP have complete resolution of symptoms, one-third have persistent symptoms, and one-third may have other symptoms such as headache. Apley et al. found that the prognosis for children with a family history of functional RAP was poor in those with an initial age of <6 years and a medical history of more than 6 months prior to presentation [79]. In addition, it has been suggested that surgical history, education level, and socioeconomic status also affect the prognosis of functional RAP.

11.6.4 Perioperative Abdominal Pain in Children

The etiology of pediatric abdominal pain is complex. In addition to the pediatric chronic pain described above, perioperative pain is also a common cause of pediatric abdominal pain. The degree of perioperative abdominal pain varies and is related to the type and site of surgery, surgical technique, and the child's health psychological status, with more challenging pain associated with open abdominal surgery and urologic surgery and relatively mild postoperative pain associated with minimally invasive lumpectomy. Techniques such as opioid analgesics, epidural analgesia, regional nerve blocks, and patient/nurse-controlled analgesia have been reported, but the protocols of clinical trials are poor, and more optimal clinical studies need to be designed.

The following treatment options for perioperative abdominal pain in children are available.

1. Systemic drug administration

   The location and size of the incision in open surgery and its effect on muscle tissue are closely related to postoperative abdominal pain. Opioid infusion was effective in relieving postoperative pain in children over 5 years of age and did not show a significant difference in postoperative abdominal pain, either with a single dose or with a single compound background dose. The efficiency of parental/nurse-controlled analgesia in children was similar to that of adult PCA, but the incidence of respiratory depression was higher at 1.7%. NSAIDs supplemented with opioid analgesia significantly reduced pain levels and decreased postoperative opioid use.
2. Nerve block analgesia

   Regional sacral/epidural block can be performed by single injection of local anesthetics, continuous epidural infusion, patient-controlled epidural analgesia in addition to ultrasound-guided nerve blocks such as transversus abdominis plane block, ilioinguinal and inferior ilioinguinal nerve block, and rectus abdominis sheath block. In conclusion, block of spinal nerves innervating the painful area can provide effective analgesia. Epidural analgesia reduces postoperative complications, improves pulmonary ventilation, and shortens the length of hospital stay, and it can be used at any age, including in neonates. Local anesthetics or combined with epidural infusion of opioids, including morphine, hydromorphone, and fentanyl, are effective for analgesia after abdominal surgery. The side effects include nausea, vomiting, and pruritus and are related to the drug dose and hydrophilicity of the drug. Analgesia can also be achieved with epidural administration of colistin, but there are adverse effects of sedation and hypotension.

   Children over 5 years of age have sufficient cognitive ability to use self-administration correctly, and patient-administered epidural analgesia has been used successfully in pediatric patients. Close attention to the background dose is required to avoid overdose of local anesthetics.
3. Abdominal wall nerve block

   Abdominal wall nerve block can reduce pain caused by tissue or muscle incision, but does not affect visceral pain. It can be used in patients for whom epidural analgesia is contraindicated due to anatomical or coagulation problems and is also more suitable for patients undergoing day surgery.

4. Rectus abdominis sheath block

   This technique is indicated for procedures with a median abdominal incision, such as epigastric hernia repair, umbilical hernia repair, and lumpectomy. Ultrasound-guided injection of analgesic into the posterior aspect of the rectus abdominis sheath blocks the endings of the T_{9-11} intercostal nerves, thereby improving anesthesia and providing effective postoperative analgesia.

5. Transversus abdominis plane block

   The abdominal wall is explored with ultrasound in the mid-axillary line, and the nerves in the T_{9-12} and L_1 segments are blocked with a single injection of drug between the transversus abdominis and the internal oblique abdominal muscles. Ultrasound guidance makes this technique safe and easy, and slightly different in children than in adults. Suresh reported on performing TAP blocks for infants and recommended identifying the rectus abdominis sheath and rectus abdominis next to the navel, followed by sliding laterally to identify the latissimus dorsi, where the transversus abdominis muscle begins, with better diffusion and a more complete block after drug injection.

The overall pain profile of laparoscopic surgery is better than that of open surgery, with a shorter duration of postoperative pain but a similar incidence on the first postoperative day. The use of multimodal analgesia, including local anesthetic infiltration, intravenous or oral opioids, nonsteroidal anti-inflammatory drugs, and acetaminophen, is recommended. Epidural analgesia is generally not required for these procedures.

11.6.5 Summary

Abdominal pain is one of the most common symptoms in the pediatric period. It is not only an important sign of pediatric gastrointestinal diseases but also a manifestation of many diseases outside the abdomen; it can be organic or functional. The causes of abdominal pain are many and involve almost all diseases of all disciplines.

In clinical practice, it is often misdiagnosed and undertreated because its etiology is not completely clear, and in serious cases, it can affect the physical and mental health and growth of children. In the diagnostic procedure of abdominal pain, it is necessary to first exclude, as far as possible, organic diseases causing abdominal pain in children based on medical history, physical examination, and necessary laboratory tests and to be alert to unexplained signs such as weight loss, linear decrease in growth rate, vomiting, chronic severe diarrhea, gastrointestinal bleeding, persistent right upper or right lower abdominal pain, unexplained fever, and family history of inflammatory bowel disease.

Recurrent abdominal pain in children also requires consideration of functional factors such as psychosocial factors. The diagnosis and treatment of functional chronic abdominal pain remains controversial, and psychotherapy, cognitive-behavioral therapy, and dietary therapy have the potential to improve pain and promote recovery; continuous research and exploration are needed for rapid diagnosis and improved treatment.

References

1. Rome IV criteria [Internet]. 2023 [cited 2023 Jun 12]. https://theromefoundation.org/rome-iv/rome-iv-criteria/.
2. Thompson WG. Irritable bowel syndrome in general practice: prevalence, characteristics, and referral. Gut. 2000;46(1):78–82. https://doi.org/10.1136/gut.46.1.78.
3. Saha L. Irritable bowel syndrome: pathogenesis, diagnosis, treatment, and evidence-based medicine. World J Gastroenterol. 2014;20(22):6759. https://doi.org/10.3748/wjg.v20.i22.6759.
4. Farzaei MH, Bahramsoltani R, Abdollahi M, Rahimi R. The role of visceral hypersensitivity in irritable bowel syndrome: pharmacological targets and novel treatments. J Neurogastroenterol

Motil. 2016;22(4):558–74. https://doi.org/10.5056/jnm16001.

5. Spetalen S, Sandvik L, Blomhoff S, Jacobsen MB. Rectal visceral sensitivity in women with irritable bowel syndrome without psychiatric comorbidity compared with healthy volunteers. Gastroenterol Res Pract. 2009;2009:1–8. https://doi.org/10.1155/2009/130684.
6. Singh R, Zogg H, Ro S. Role of microRNAs in disorders of gut–brain interactions: clinical insights and therapeutic alternatives. J Pers Med. 2021;11(10):1021. https://doi.org/10.3390/jpm11101021.
7. Barbara G, Cremon C, Carini G, Bellacosa L, Zecchi L, Giorgio RD, et al. The immune system in irritable bowel syndrome. J Neurogastroenterol Motil. 2011;17(4):349–59. https://doi.org/10.5056/jnm.2011.17.4.349.
8. Berumen A, Edwinson AL, Grover M. Post-infection irritable bowel syndrome. Gastroenterol Clin N Am. 2021;50(2):445–61. https://doi.org/10.1016/j.gtc.2021.02.007.
9. Longstreth GF, Thompson WG, Chey WD, Houghton LA, Mearin F, Spiller RC. Functional bowel disorders. Gastroenterology. 2006;130(5):1480–91. https://doi.org/10.1053/j.gastro.2005.11.061.
10. Shih DQ, Kwan LY. All Roads Lead to Rome: Update on Rome III Criteria and New Treatment Options. Gastroenterol Rep. Winter. 2007;1(2):56–65. PMID: 21544252; PMCID: PMC3085189
11. Tada Y, Ishii K, Kimura J, Hanada K, Kawaguchi I. Patient preference for biologic treatments of psoriasis in Japan. J Dermatol. 2019;46(6):466–77. https://doi.org/10.1111/1346-8138.14870.
12. Ford AC, Talley NJ, Spiegel BM, Foxx-Orenstein AE, Schiller L, Quigley EM, et al. Effect of fibre, antispasmodics, and peppermint oil in the treatment of irritable bowel syndrome: systematic review and meta-analysis. BMJ. 2008;337:a2313. https://doi.org/10.1136/bmj.a2313.
13. Merola JF, Landewé R, McInnes IB, Mease PJ, Ritchlin CT, Tanaka Y, et al. Bimekizumab in patients with active psoriatic arthritis and previous inadequate response or intolerance to tumour necrosis factor-α inhibitors: a randomised, double-blind, placebo-controlled, phase 3 trial (be complete). Lancet. 2023;401(10370):38–48. https://doi.org/10.1016/s0140-6736(22)02303-0.
14. Lucak S. Irritable bowel syndrome and ischemic colitis: evidence supporting the increased use of Alosetron. Ther Adv Gastroenterol. 2012;5(4):215–8. https://doi.org/10.1177/1756283x12450934.
15. Shah ED, Lacy BE, Chey WD, Chang L, Brenner DM. Tegaserod for irritable bowel syndrome with constipation in women younger than 65 years without cardiovascular disease: pooled analyses of 4 controlled trials. Am J Gastroenterol. 2021;116(8):1601–11. https://doi.org/10.14309/ajg.0000000000001313.
16. Madia VN, Messore A, Saccoliti F, Tudino V, De Leo A, De Vita D, et al. Tegaserod for the treatment of irritable bowel syndrome. Antiinflamm Antiallergy Agents Med Chem. 2020;19(4):342–69. https://doi.org/10.2174/1871523018666190911121306.
17. Wilson N, Schey R. Lubiprostone in constipation: clinical evidence and place in therapy. Ther Adv Chronic Dis. 2015;6(2):40–50. https://doi.org/10.1177/2040622314567678.
18. Sinagra E, Morreale GC, Mohammadian G, Fusco G, Guarnotta V, Tomasello G, et al. New therapeutic perspectives in irritable bowel syndrome: targeting low-grade inflammation, immuno-neuroendocrine axis, motility, secretion and beyond. World J Gastroenterol. 2017;23(36):6593–627. https://doi.org/10.3748/wjg.v23.i36.6593.
19. British Society of Gastroenterology Guidelines on the management of irritable bowel syndrome [Internet]. 2022 [cited 2023 Jun 12]. https://www.bsg.org.uk/clinical-resource/british-society-of-gastroenterology-guidelines-on-the-management-of-irritable-bowel-syndrome/.
20. Gebeyehu E, Nigatu D, Engidawork E. Helicobacter pylori eradication rate of standard triple therapy and factors affecting eradication rate at Bahir Dar city administration, Northwest Ethiopia: a prospective follow up study. PLoS One. 2019;14(6):e0217645. https://doi.org/10.1371/journal.pone.0217645.
21. Kim HU. Diagnostic and treatment approaches for refractory peptic ulcers. Clin Endosc. 2015;48(4):285. https://doi.org/10.5946/ce.2015.48.4.285.
22. Yarmol-Matusiak EA, Cipriano LE, Stranges S. A comparison of COVID-19 epidemiological indicators in Sweden, Norway, Denmark, and Finland. Scand J Public Health. 2021;49(1):69–78. https://doi.org/10.1177/1403494820980264.
23. Li C, Jiang M, Pan C, Li J, Xu L. The global, regional, and national burden of acute pancreatitis in 204 countries and territories, 1990–2019. BMC Gastroenterol. 2021;21(1):332. https://doi.org/10.1186/s12876-021-01906-2.
24. Wang LW, Li ZS, Li SD, Jin ZD, Zou DW, Chen F. Prevalence and clinical features of chronic pancreatitis in China. Pancreas. 2009;38(3):248–54. https://doi.org/10.1097/mpa.0b013e31818f6ac1.
25. Hobbs PM, Johnson WG, Graham DY. Management of pain in chronic pancreatitis with emphasis on exogenous pancreatic enzymes. World J Gastrointest Pharmacol Ther. 2016;7(3):370. https://doi.org/10.4292/wjgpt.v7.i3.370.
26. Ashraf H, Colombo JP, Marcucci V, Rhoton J, Olowoyo O. A clinical overview of acute and chronic pancreatitis: the medical and surgical management. Cureus. 2021;13:e19764. https://doi.org/10.7759/cureus.19764.
27. Keith RG, Keshavjee SH, Kerenyi NR. Neuropathology of chronic pancreatitis in humans. Can J Surg. 1985;28(3):207–11. PMID: 3995416.
28. Buscher HCJL, Wilder-Smith OHG, Goor H. Chronic pancreatitis patients show hyperalgesia of central origin: a pilot study. Eur J Pain. 2006;10(4):363. https://doi.org/10.1016/j.ejpain.2005.06.006.

29. Vera-Portocarrero LP, Lu Y, Westlund KN. Nociception in persistent pancreatitis in rats. Anesthesiology. 2003;98(2):474–84. https://doi.org/10.1097/00000542-200302000-00029.
30. Fregni F, Pascual-Leone A, Freedman SD. Pain in chronic pancreatitis: a salutogenic mechanism or a maladaptive brain response? Pancreatology. 2007;7(5–6):411–22. https://doi.org/10.1159/000108958.
31. Endoscopy for recurrent acute and chronic pancreatitis [Internet]. [cited 2023 Jun 13]. https://gastro.org/clinical-guidance/endoscopy-for-recurrent-acute-and-chronic-pancreatitis/.
32. Drewes AM, Bouwense SAW, Campbell CM, Ceyhan GO, Delhaye M, Demir IE, et al. Guidelines for the understanding and management of pain in chronic pancreatitis. Pancreatology. 2017;17(5):720–31. https://doi.org/10.1016/j.pan.2017.07.006.
33. Aghdassi AA, Mayerle J, Kraft M, Sielenkämper AW, Heidecke C-D, Lerch MM. Pancreatic pseudocysts—when and how to treat? HPB. 2006;8(6):432–41. https://doi.org/10.1080/13651820600748012.
34. Nikkola J, Raty S, Laukkarinen J, Seppanen H, Lappalainen-Lehto R, Jarvinen S, et al. Abstinence after first acute alcohol-associated pancreatitis protects against recurrent pancreatitis and minimizes the risk of pancreatic dysfunction. Alcohol Alcohol. 2013;48(4):483–6. https://doi.org/10.1093/alcalc/agt019.
35. Sugumar K, Deshpande A. Outcomes of pain management in chronic pancreatitis: experience from a tertiary care hospital in India. Turk J Surg. 2020;36(4):359–67. https://doi.org/10.47717/turkjsurg.2020.4924.
36. Rösch T, Daniel S, Scholz M, Huibregtse K, Smits M, Schneider T, et al. Endoscopic treatment of chronic pancreatitis: a multicenter study of 1000 patients with long-term follow-up. Endoscopy. 2002;34(10):765–71. https://doi.org/10.1055/s-2002-34256.
37. Bouwense SAW, Kempeneers MA, van Santvoort HC, Boermeester MA, van Goor H, Besselink MG. Surgery in chronic pancreatitis: indication, timing and procedures. Visc Med. 2019;35(2):110–8. https://doi.org/10.1159/000499612.
38. Yadav D, Lowenfels AB. The epidemiology of pancreatitis and pancreatic cancer. Gastroenterology. 2013;144(6):1252–61. https://doi.org/10.1053/j.gastro.2013.01.068.
39. Bielefeldt K. The rising tide of cholecystectomy for biliary dyskinesia. Aliment Pharmacol Ther. 2012;37(1):98–106. https://doi.org/10.1111/apt.12105.
40. Desautels SG, Slivka A, Hutson WR, Chun A, Mitrani C, DiLorenzo C, et al. Postcholecystectomy pain syndrome: pathophysiology of abdominal pain in sphincter of Oddi Type III. Gastroenterology. 1999;116(4):900–5. https://doi.org/10.1016/s0016-5085(99)70073-9.
41. Kharbutli B, Velanovich V. Management of preoperatively suspected choledocholithiasis: a decision analysis. J Gastrointest Surg. 2008;12(11):1973–80. https://doi.org/10.1007/s11605-008-0624-6.
42. Eikenboom J, Van Marion V, Putter H, Goodeve A, Rodeghiero F, Castaman G, et al. Linkage analysis in families diagnosed with type 1 von Willebrand disease in the European study, molecular and clinical markers for the diagnosis and management of type 1 VWD. J Thromb Haemost. 2006;4(4):774–82. https://doi.org/10.1111/j.1538-7836.2006.01823.x.
43. Raddawi HM, Geenen JE, Hogan WJ, Dodds WJ, Venu RP, Kenneth Johnson G. Pressure measurements from biliary and pancreatic segments of sphincter of Oddi. Dig Dis Sci. 1991;36(1):71–4. https://doi.org/10.1007/bf01300090.
44. Aymerich RR, Prakash C, Aliperti G. Sphincter of Oddi manometry: is it necessary to measure both biliary and pancreatic sphincter pressures? Gastrointest Endosc. 2000;52(2):183–6. https://doi.org/10.1067/mge.2000.105985.
45. Wehrmann T, Stergiou N, Schmitt T, Dietrich CF, Seifert H. Reduced risk for pancreatitis after endoscopic microtransducer manometry of the sphincter of Oddi: a randomized comparison with the perfusion manometry technique. Endoscopy. 2003;35(6):472–7. https://doi.org/10.1055/s-2003-39677.
46. Ruffolo TA, Sherman S, Lehman GA, Hawes RH. Gallbladder ejection fraction and its relationship to sphincter of Oddi dysfunction. Dig Dis Sci. 1994;39(2):289–92. https://doi.org/10.1007/bf02090199.
47. Kalloo AN, Pasricha PJ. Therapy of sphincter of Oddi dysfunction. Gastrointest Endosc Clin N Am. 1996;6(1):117–25. https://doi.org/10.1016/s1052-5157(18)30381-7.
48. Soto JA, Alvarez O, Lopera JE, Múnera F, Restrepo JC, Correa G. Biliary obstruction: findings at MR cholangiography and cross-sectional MR imaging. Radiographics. 2000;20(2):353–66. https://doi.org/10.1148/radiographics.20.2.g00mc06353.
49. Choudhary N, Guleria M, Puri R, Sud R. Tubercular lymph nodal mass mimicking pancreatic malignancy with extrahepatic biliary obstruction in a young woman. Endoscopy. 2015;47(Suppl 1 UCTN):E53–4. https://doi.org/10.1055/s-0034-1377769.
50. Ghobrial S, Ott J, Parry JP. An overview of postoperative intraabdominal adhesions and their role on female infertility: a narrative review. J Clin Med. 2023;12(6):2263. https://doi.org/10.3390/jcm12062263.
51. Okabayashi K, Ashrafian H, Zacharakis E, Hasegawa H, Kitagawa Y, Athanasiou T, et al. Adhesions after abdominal surgery: a systematic review of the incidence, distribution and severity. Surg Today. 2013;44(3):405–20. https://doi.org/10.1007/s00595-013-0591-8.
52. Srinivasan R, Greenbaum DS. Chronic abdominal wall pain: a frequently overlooked problem. Practical approach to diagnosis and management. Am J Gastroenterol. 2002;97(4):824–30. https://doi.org/10.1111/j.1572-0241.2002.05662.x.

53. Gallegos NC, Hobsley M. Abdominal wall pain: an alternative diagnosis. Br J Surg. 1990;77(10):1167–70. https://doi.org/10.1002/bjs.1800771026.
54. Soliman LM, Narouze S. Ultrasound-guided transversus abdominus plan block for the management of abdominal pain: an alternative to differential epidural block. Tech Reg Anesth Pain Manag. 2009;13(3):117–20. https://doi.org/10.1053/j.trap.2009.06.004.
55. Richardson J, Lönnqvist PA, Naja Z. Bilateral thoracic paravertebral block: potential and practice. Br J Anaesth. 2011;106(2):164–71. https://doi.org/10.1093/bja/aeq378.
56. Naja ZM, Raf M, El Rajab M, Daoud N, Ziade FM, Al Tannir MA, et al. A comparison of nerve stimulator guided paravertebral block and ilio-inguinal nerve block for analgesia after inguinal herniorrhaphy in children. Anaesthesia. 2006;61(11):1064–8. https://doi.org/10.1111/j.1365-2044.2006.04833.x.
57. Tiede JM, Ghazi SM, Lamer TJ, Obray JB. The use of spinal cord stimulation in refractory abdominal visceral pain: case reports and literature review. Pain Pract. 2006;6(3):197–202. https://doi.org/10.1111/j.1533-2500.2006.00085.x.
58. Kapural L. Spinal cord stimulation for intractable chronic pain. Curr Pain Headache Rep. 2014;18(4):406. https://doi.org/10.1007/s11916-014-0406-7.
59. Arcidiacono PG, Calori G, Carrara S, McNicol ED, Testoni PA. Celiac plexus block for pancreatic cancer pain in adults. Cochrane Database Syst Rev. 2011;2011(7):CD007519. https://doi.org/10.1002/14651858.cd007519.pub2.
60. Kwon HJ, Jang K, Leem JG, Shin JW, Kim DH, Choi SS. Factors associated with successful response to neurolytic celiac plexus block in patients with upper abdominal cancer-related pain: a retrospective study. Korean J Pain. 2021;34(4):479–86. https://doi.org/10.3344/kjp.2021.34.4.479. PMID: 34593666; PMCID: PMC8494952.
61. De Wilde RL, Devassy R, Broek RPGT, Miller CE, Adlan A, Aquino P, Becker S, Darmawan F, Gergolet M, Habana MAE, Khoo CK, Koninckx PR, Korell M, Krentel H, Musigavong O, Pistofidis G, Puntambekar S, Rachman IA, Sendag F, Wallwiener M, Torres-de la Roche LA. The future of adhesion prophylaxis trials in abdominal surgery: an expert global consensus. J Clin Med. 2022;11(6):1476. https://doi.org/10.3390/jcm11061476. PMID: 35329802; PMCID: PMC8950418.
62. Ahmad G, Kim K, Thompson M, Agarwal P, O'Flynn H, Hindocha A, Watson A. Barrier agents for adhesion prevention after gynaecological surgery. Cochrane Database Syst Rev. 2020;3:CD000475. https://doi.org/10.1002/14651858.CD000475.pub4.
63. Kim W, Yang Y, Kim D, Jeong S, Yoo JW, Yoon JH, Jung Y. Conjugation of metronidazole with dextran: a potential pharmaceutical strategy to control colonic distribution of the anti-amebic drug susceptible to metabolism by colonic microbes. Drug Des Devel Ther. 2017;11:419–29. https://doi.org/10.2147/DDDT.S129922. PMID: 28243064; PMCID: PMC5317261.
64. Abbott RA, Martin AE, Newlove-Delgado TV, Bethel A, Whear RS, Thompson Coon J, Logan S. Recurrent abdominal pain in children: summary evidence from 3 systematic reviews of treatment effectiveness. J Pediatr Gastroenterol Nutr. 2018;67(1):23–33. https://doi.org/10.1097/MPG.0000000000001922. PMID: 29470291.
65. Zhijie L. Visceral pain—basic and clinical. Beijing: Science Publishing House; 2018.
66. Shahinyan T, Amaryan G, Tadevosyan A, Braegger C. Clinical, endoscopic, and histological characteristics of Helicobacter pylori positive and negative Armenian children with recurrent abdominal pain and/or dyspepsia. Georgian Med News. 2022;324:71–8. PMID: 35417865.
67. Günel E, Findik D, Cağlayan O, Cağlayan F, Topgaç Z. Helicobacter pylori and hypergastrinemia in children with recurrent abdominal pain. Pediatr Surg Int. 1998;14(1–2):40–2. https://doi.org/10.1007/s003830050431. PMID: 9880693.
68. Kaur K, Zubair M, Adamski JJ. Fecal occult blood test. Treasure Island, FL: StatPearls Publishing; 2023. PMID: 30725823.
69. Hyams JS, Di Lorenzo C, Saps M, Shulman RJ, Staiano A, van Tilburg M. Childhood functional gastrointestinal disorders: child/adolescent. Gastroenterology. 2016;150:1456. https://doi.org/10.1053/j.gastro.2016.02.015. Epub ahead of print. PMID: 27144632.
70. Yeh AM, Golianu B. Integrative treatment of reflux and functional dyspepsia in children. Children (Basel). 2014;1(2):119–33. https://doi.org/10.3390/children1020119. PMID: 27417471; PMCID: PMC4928719.
71. Gomez Alvarez DF, et al. Prevalence of irritable bowel syndrome and associated factors according to the Rome III diagnostic criteria in a general population in Colombia [Spanish]. Gastroenterol Hepatol. 2009;32:395–400.
72. Palsson OS, Whitehead W, Tornblom H, Sperber AD, Simren M. Prevalence of Rome IV functional bowel disorders among adults in the United States, Canada, and the United Kingdom. Gastroenterology. 2020;158:1262–1273.e3.
73. Black CJ, Ford AC. Global burden of irritable bowel syndrome: trends, predictions and risk factors. Nat Rev Gastroenterol Hepatol. 2020;17:473–86. https://doi.org/10.1038/s41575-020-0286-8.
74. Moayedi A, Moayedi F. Psychological aspects of recurrent abdominal pain syndrome in children. J Med Life. 2015;8(Spec Iss 4):56–9. PMID: 28316707; PMCID: PMC5319255.
75. Apley J, Haslam DR, Tulloh CG. Pupillary reaction in children with recurrent abdominal pain. Arch Dis Child. 1971;46(247):337–40. https://doi.org/10.1136/adc.46.247.337. PMID: 5090666; PMCID: PMC1647716.

76. Wildemeersch D, Peeters N, Saldien V, Vercauteren M, Hans G. Pain assessment by pupil dilation reflex in response to noxious stimulation in anaesthetized adults. Acta Anaesthesiol Scand. 2018;62:1050–6. https://doi.org/10.1111/aas.13129.
77. Kumari MV, Amarasiri L, Rajindrajith S, Devanarayana NM. Gastric motility and pulmonary function in children with functional abdominal pain disorders and asthma: a pathophysiological study. PLoS One. 2022;17(1):e0262086. https://doi.org/10.1371/journal.pone.0262086. PMID: 34982797; PMCID: PMC8726504.
78. Tsao JC, Evans S, Seidman LC, Zeltzer LK. Experimental pain responses in children with chronic pain and in healthy children: how do they differ? Pain Res Manag. 2012;17(2):103–9. https://doi.org/10.1155/2012/592108. PMID: 22518373; PMCID: PMC3393051.
79. Apley J, Hale B. Children with recurrent abdominal pain: how do they grow up? Br Med J. 1973;3(5870):7–9. https://doi.org/10.1136/bmj.3.5870.7. PMID: 4717440; PMCID: PMC1587952.

Chronic Abdominal Pain Due to Obstetric and Gynecological Factors

12

Hong Jiang

12.1 Introduction

Chronic pelvic pain (CPP) is a common disorder in clinical practice. Patients who suffer from it often have their daily life being disturbed by the pain for a long time before they visit doctors as CPP is defined as cyclical or noncyclical pain lasting for over 6 months. Patients with CPP may present with dysmenorrhea, dyspareunia, dyspareunia, and dyspareunia. Up to 24% of women worldwide suffer from CPP [1]. Clinically, many patients often fail to detect clear pathological changes through various diagnostic tests, and painful symptoms are the primary presentation at the clinic. Causes of CPP include gastrointestinal, urological, gynecological, oncological, musculoskeletal, and psychosocial factors [2]. When evaluating and treating patients, subspecialists are often inadequate in multidisciplinary training and knowledge of the various causes required. As a result, patients may have seen multiple physicians, undergone multiple tests and examinations, and may have undergone surgical procedures before seeking treatments, yet without significant improvement in associated symptoms. With further research on CPP suggesting that CPP may be just a chronic symptom without any pathological changes and that pain is closely related to sexual function, defecation, and urination due to its location and is often accompanied by emotional and psychological changes in the patient, more medical practitioners have now become interested in the diagnosis and treatment of patients with CPP. This chapter attempts to provide a multidisciplinary overview of CPP with an evaluation focus, including its etiology, epidemiology, diagnosis, and treatment of common CPP syndromes.

12.2 Definition of CPP

CPP is a multifactorial group of conditions relating to pain in the pelvis, anterior abdominal wall, or abdomen below the umbilical, lumbosacral back, and buttocks lasting for more than 6 months, or presenting cyclically for over 3 months. Such pain is associated with negative cognition, behavior, sexual activities, and emotions, accompanied by lower urinary tract symptoms and bowel, pelvic floor, and gynecological or sexual dysfunction. The main clinical manifestations of CPP include chronic lower abdominal pain (anatomical pelvic area), dysmenorrhea, and dyspareunia. Although dysmenorrhea and dyspareunia are diagnostic evidence of CPP, they should ideally be viewed separately because of their unique etiology, diagnosis, and treatment.

In a narrower sense, CPP refers to pain caused by lesions in the pelvic organs, also known as lower abdominal pain, and the etiological

H. Jiang (✉)
Department of Anesthesiology, Shanghai Ninth People's Hospital, Shanghai Jiao Tong University School of Medicine, Shanghai, China

M. Xia et al. (eds.), *Visceral Pain*, https://doi.org/10.1007/978-981-99-9167-9_12

diagnosis is also limited to diseases of the uterus and organs other than the uterus in obstetrics and gynecology, such as endometriosis, pelvic inflammatory disease (PID), pelvic adhesions and pelvic congestion syndrome, adenomyosis, and uterine leiomyoma. In a broader sense, all lesions that ignite lower abdominal pain in patients should be included in the etiological diagnosis, including some somatic diseases of obstetrics and gynecology, such as irritable bowel syndrome (IBS), hernia, pelvic floor myalgia (anal raphe spasm), interstitial cystitis and neuropathic diseases, such as dual personality, depression, abdominal epilepsy, and abdominal migraine. In conclusion, the diagnosis of CPP may depend on the clinician's professions, so the diversity of diagnosis requires more diagnostic thinking, extraction of complete medical history data, and a complete systematic review of diseases, especially symptoms related to the gastrointestinal, urological, orthopedic, and reproductive tracts conditions that must not be ignored. The CPP:ACOG (American College of Obstetricians and Gynecologists) Practice Bulletin listed a number of diseases that are thought to cause CPP. There is ample evidence proving how CPP was caused by several common disorders such as endometriosis, interstitial cystitis, and IBS.

12.3 Prevalence of CPP

Several studies have reported the prevalence of CPP in women, while the majority of them used sampling frames, such as hospital patients, which do not allow for an accurate estimation of CPP prevalence in the general population [3, 4]. The relatively few population-based studies have reported prevalence rates ranging from 6.4% in Mexico [5] to 25.4% in New Zealand [6]. These studies were carried out by randomly selecting women from a representative sampling frame, with sample sizes ranging from 1160 [6] to 5263 [7]. It should be noted that differences in study designs, case definitions, and survey methods may have profoundly impacted the variations in reported prevalence among different areas.

In 1994, the earliest population-based survey was conducted in the United States, the result of which showed that the prevalence of CPP was 14.7% [7]. Other studies conducted in the United Kingdom, New Zealand, and Australia reported prevalence rates of 24%, 25.4%, and 21.5%, respectively [2–6, 8]. From the statistics, it could be found that the prevalence in the latter three studies was higher than that reported by the first US study, the reason of which probably lay in the exclusion of women with mid-cycle pain in the first study. While, in the studies in the United Kingdom and New Zealand, if the same exclusion criterion was adopted, namely, excluding women with mid-cycle pain, the prevalence would be reduced to 16.9% and 16.5%, respectively. Data from Mexico obtained in 2005, based on face-to-face interviews with relatively older (25–54 years) women, reported a 12-month prevalence of 6.4% [5], which was the lowest prevalence identified, although a similar definition of CPP to previous studies was used.

All of the abovementioned studies included subjects of women of reproductive age. Women of older ages, who are regarded as less susceptible to CPP, were excluded from prevalence studies. In 1994, a cross-sectional analysis of a UK primary care database reported a higher prevalence of CPP in women aged between 61–73 years compared with women in younger age groups (monthly prevalence of approximately 27/1000 vs. 21/1000) [9]. Such a trend was also verified by recent population studies [10–12], one of which found the highest prevalence in women aged 18–25 years (17%) compared with 13% in women aged 75 years and older [12].

12.4 Pelvic Anatomy and Pathogenesis of CPP

12.4.1 Pelvic Anatomy

12.4.1.1 Innervation of Female Genital Organs

The nerves of the womb, fallopian tubes, and ovaries consist of sympathetic, parasympathetic, and spinal nerves. The pelvic nerves are mainly composed of sympathetic nerves from the anterior sacral plexus, parasympathetic nerves from the 2nd–fourth sacral nerves (containing a small amount of sympathetic nerves), and a small portion of parasympathetic nerves from the pudendal nerves of the spinal nerves. Branches of the pelvic plexus innervate the fallopian tubes, bladder, rectum, and womb. The nerves in the ovaries are of multiple origin, including the ovarian plexus, which consists of nerve fibers from the renal plexus, fibers from the inferior abdominal plexus and pelvic plexus, and sympathetic nerve fibers extending from the uterine body. The ovaries are extremely insensitive to nerve stimulation and are mainly regulated by incretion. The pelvic plexus extends to the paracervical plexus on both sides of the cervix, which enters the uterus in parallel with branches of the uterine artery at the isthmus and spreads to the myometrium of the uterus and cervix. The nerves stretching to the myometrium continue to branch in parallel with the sagittal artery through the myometrium to the endometrium and are distributed around the helicine artery. A few other nerves lateral to the body of the uterus ascend in parallel with the upper branches of the uterine arteries to the fundus and divide into smaller nerve fibers that innervate the ovaries and proximal oviducts.

12.4.1.2 Function of Nerves in Female Genital Organs

Sensory Nerve

The sensory nerve fibers of the sympathetic nerve mainly transmit nociception of the uterine corpus to the central nerve via $T_{11, 12}$. While the sensory nerve fibers of the parasympathetic nerve mainly transmit nociception of the upper part of the cervix and vagina to the center via $S_{2\text{–}4}$. Nociception in the urethra and the middle and lower part of the vagina is transferred via the pudendal nerves and then to the center via $S_{2\sim4}$. The sensory plexus around the isthmus uteri and the internal cervical orifice are extremely sensitive, consisting of both sympathetic and parasympathetic nerves that transmit the pain to the central nerves.

Motor Nerve

The motor nerve fibers of the pelvic nerve are transmitted through $T_{7, 8}$. The sympathetic nerves constrict the blood vessels in the pelvic organs and inhibit the secretion of the glands of the gastrointestinal tract; the parasympathetic nerves, on the other hand, relax the blood vessels of the pelvic organs and stimulate the secretion of the glands of the gastrointestinal tract.

12.4.2 Pathogenesis of CPP

The pathogenesis of CPP may be related to physical and inflammatory stimulations. For most CPP patients, pelvic inflammations and tissue fibrosis cause pelvic adhesions, which leads to pain due to pulling or twisting of tissues and organs after the movement of pelvic organs when the patients change their positions. Pelvic adhesions are complications and sequelae of many pelvic diseases. Inflammatory cell aggregated at the initial stage of the disease, and then tissues fiberize and scars form, resulting in the extensive adhesions between pelvic tissues and organs. Pulling of the adnexa, change of uterine position, etc., can bring problems such as obstruction of ovulation, severe dysmenorrhea, and painful intercourse dyspareunia. In addition, space-occupying lesions in the pelvic area may block the arterial and venous systems and cause obstruction to the lymphatic system as the tumor gradually expands, resulting in local edema and exudation, and referred pain in swelling interfascial space of the organs. Moreover, mechanical factors such as pelvic organ prolapse, abnormal position of the intrauterine device, and ligament or soft tissue injury after delivery may cause CPP.

CPP is commonly associated with the local inflammatory response of the body, release of inflammatory factors, and stimulation of peripheral nerve endings. Common inflammatory factors include interleukin (IL), tumor necrosis factor, transforming growth factor β, etc.

1. IL can be produced by a variety of cells and is not only involved in regulating the immune

response, but also widely involved in regulating the physiological and pathological processes of the body. About 18% of patients with PID are not treated promptly or properly after the acute attack of the disease, often causing chronic pain in the pelvis. Inhibiting the inflammatory response can significantly mitigate the pain. An animal study found that the rats in the pelvic inflammatory model group had necrotic detachment of mucosal epithelial cells, glandular deformation, structural disorder, fibroblast proliferation, massive inflammatory cell infiltration and inflammatory exudation, and increased levels of L-1B, IL-8, and TNF-α in serum and uterine tissues [13].

2. Tumor necrosis factor-α (TNF-α) is a kind of pro-inflammatory and immunomodulatory factor that is mainly secreted by Th1 cells. The periodic bleeding of ectopic endometrium in patients with endometriosis stimulates the body to present an immune response, resulting in an increase in the number of macrophages in their peritoneal fluid and lymphocytes in peripheral blood, which secrete large amounts of TNF-α and cytokines such as IL-6 and IL-8. And the content of TNF-α is positively correlated with the severity of endometriosis. In patients with PID, the endometrium is infiltrated by a large number of inflammatory cells, leading to a significant increase in the TNF-α content in the tissues. When the inflammation of uterine tissues is mitigated, the TNF-α level also comes down. When inflammation occurs, mast cells, monocytes, and lymphocytes are activated, and degranulation begins. During the process, the inflammatory mediator TNF-α is released and the NF-κB signaling pathway is activated to enhance the genetic transcription of TNF-α and promote the expression of TNF-α, while TNF-α reactivates the NF-κB signaling pathway through a positive feedback mechanism. They promote each other, and at the same time induce the production and release of other pro-inflammatory cytokines, forming a cascade response that leads to further amplification of the initial inflammatory signal to cause chronic pain.

3. Transforming growth factor-β (TGF-β) is involved in the inflammatory response with a bidirectional nature, with both anti-inflammatory and pro-inflammatory effects, and its levels can reflect the degree of inflammation in pelvic disease. TGF-β can inhibit the translation/transcription of DNAX-activated protein 12 on the surface of NK cells by inducing the expression of miRNA-183, which destabilizes the receptor on the surface of NK cells and its downstream signaling, resulting in ectopic endometriotic cells being more likely to migrate and invade to distant sites. Secondly, TGF-β can activate the Wnt/β-catenin signaling pathway to participate in the fibrosis process of endometriosis. In addition, TGF-β can increase the expression of miRNA-183 by elevating lactic acid content in endometriosis patients, creating a favorable environment for local lesion vascularization and promoting nerve growth and sensitization of local lesions, thus leading to recurrent pelvic pain.

Berkley et al. summarized the pathogenesis of CPP associated with menstruation in combined interstitial cystitis and IBS in their experimental studies on rats. (1) Female genital organs are innervated by highly sensitive afferent nerves originating from the lower abdomen (fundus, horn of the uterus) and pelvis (vagina, cervix). (2) Sensory nerve impulses in the uterus and vagina are influenced by the function of the pelvic reproductive organs. (3) Neurons throughout the central nervous system (CNS) respond to stimuli originating from both the reproductive and visceral skin systems, and this response can be influenced by the functional state of the reproductive organs and by peripheral pathophysiological disorders. (4) Afferent nerves from different parts of the body pass through the dorsal nucleus and the nucleus tractus solitarii of the spinal cord when extensive neural connections occur and converge into the CNS to complete normal physiological processes. (5) The convergence of nerve impulses in the CNS is also manifested by the extensive mutual nerve projections within the nervous system and the influence of mutual nerve impulses between visceral nerve fibers, thus completing the normal physiological responses of the body. (6) Some reciprocal systems have a wide range of effects, such as cystitis, which affects uterine contractions and the effects of drugs acting on the uterus; colitis, which produces an inflammatory response in the normal uterus and bladder; endometriosis, which produces vaginal hyperalgesia and lowers the bladder volume threshold; and ureteral stones, which exacerbate the painful symptoms of endometriosis.

12.4.2.1 Common CPP-Related Syndromes

CPP can be associated with the gynecological, gastrointestinal, urinary, musculoskeletal, oncology, and psychosocial systems [14]. In this chapter, the focus will be on the obstetric and gynecological considerations.

Endometriosis

Endometriosis is the appearance of ectopic tissue with the structure and function of endometrial tissue outside the uterine cavity and is one of the most common causes of CPP. Although endometriosis is a benign proliferative process that develops, it exhibits several characteristics of cancer, including invasion of surrounding healthy tissue, causing severe pain, and a tendency to recur. Approximately 10% of women of childbearing age have endometriosis, and this number is currently on the rise as laparoscopy continues to spread. Endometriosis is a chronic disease that causes CPP and infertility [15]. Several theories have been proposed to explain endometriosis, including retrograde menstruation, pelvic chemosis, embryonic shock, and lymphatic vascular spread [16]. The exact mechanism of endometriosis is not fully understood, but the most popular explanation is the "menstrual reflux theory," which mainly refers to the reflux of menstrual blood and fallopian tubes into the pelvic cavity, where endometrial cells in the growth phase are planted in the pelvic organs outside the uterus, growing and reproducing and eventually forming endometrial tissue. Genetic defects and immune deficiencies in the individual are important factors that lead to "retrograde implantation of menstrual blood." Depending on the cause of discomfort, the pathophysiology may vary. For example, endometriosis causes cyclic discomfort due to recurrent bleeding from endometrial implants. In patients with pelvic congestion syndrome, the pelvic veins are congested and dilated, resulting in inadequate venous flushing, which causes pain. About one-third of patients are asymptomatic. Symptoms often coexist. Some of the typical combinations of symptoms include CPP (cyclic and non-cyclic), dysmenorrhea, dyspareunia, pain during defecation and urination, fatigue and depression, sub/infertility, and bleeding disorders [17, 18].

Adenomyosis

A common condition in gynecology clinics is adenomyosis, often referred to as endometriosis. Older women aged around 40 years are more likely to develop this disease. The disease often coexists with endometrial cancer, benign uterine fibroids, and pelvic endometriosis. Some women are asymptomatic, while others may present with pelvic discomfort, back pain, menstrual irregularities, difficulty urinating, and progressively worse dysmenorrhea. Although adenomyomas rarely cause symptoms of uterine hypertrophy and bulkiness, they can cause a similar painful sensation by inflaming the myometrium [19]. Most gynecologists prefer MRI to ultrasound in the diagnosis of this condition because MRI shows hypoechoic or anechoic areas in the uterine wall [20]. Histological diagnosis is the ultimate method to diagnose adenomyosis [8].

Hydrosalpinx

A tubal effusion is described as a collection of fluid in the lumen of the fallopian tubes, which causes them to swell. Most patients with tubal effusion do not experience any symptoms. As a result, patients may not realize they have a health problem until they are unable to conceive. People with signs of tubal effusion may experience abnormal vaginal discharge, and pelvic and abdominal pain, and these symptoms may worsen during the menstrual cycle. Tubal effusion is bilateral in most cases. In general, the walls of the fallopian tubes are translucent and very thin. Some researchers believe that tubal effusions are mobile and can be twisted. Tubal effusion can be caused by sexually transmitted infections (STIs), endometriosis, previous tubal surgery, and tubal infections. Gynecologists can confirm tubal effusion by hysterosalpingogram (HSG) or laparoscopy [21].

Pelvic Inflammatory Disease (PID)

PID is an infection of the upper genital tract that is commonly seen in young women and in sexually active people. *Neisseria gonorrhoeae* and *Chlamydia trachomatis* are the prevalent causative organisms. If left untreated, PID may lead to intra-abdominal infection, infertility, ectopic pregnancy, and CPP [10]. Risk factors for PID include age younger than 25 years, multiple sexual partners, unprotected sex, sex with a symptomatic partner, first sexual intercourse at a younger age (under 15 years), or any previous history of STIs or PID [11]. The sudden onset of lower abdominal or pelvic pain in sexually active women is the typical feature of PID. Signs and symptoms are mild, including mild bilateral lower abdominal pain that worsens during intercourse, difficulty with intercourse, abnormal uterine bleeding, dysmenorrhea, increased frequency of urination, irregular menstruation, difficulty urinating, or abnormal vaginal discharge [12].

Pelvic Congestion

Pelvic stasis syndrome is a clinical syndrome with CPP as a progressive symptom based on the pathology of ovarian varicose veins with pelvic plexus stasis, similar to scrotal varicocele in men, and very common in women aged 20–30 years. In general, symptoms are usually worse before menstruation and during the day. In addition, patients may describe intense dyspareunia or post-coital pain. Imaging studies, including duplex venography, MRI, and laparoscopy, show vasodilatation. In addition to capillary endothelial hypertrophy and hyperplasia, pathological findings include fibrosis of the intima and mesentery [22]. Ovarian suppression and embolization therapy have the potential to alleviate clinical symptoms, with studies showing success rates of embolization therapy ranging from 24% to 100% [23].

Dysmenorrhea

Dysmenorrhea is a periodic lower abdominal pain that occurs during and/or around the menstrual period, often before and during the menstrual period, and occasionally within a few days after the menstrual period. The lower abdominal pain is crampy and distending and may radiate to the lumbosacral region, inner thighs, and around the anus. It may be accompanied by pallor, nausea, vomiting, body or lower abdominal coldness, increased frequency of defecation, and collapse in severe pain.

It can be a manifestation of a disease of the reproductive tract, but it is also a diagnosis in itself. When dysmenorrhea is not a symptom of another disease, it is called primary dysmenorrhea, and when it is a symptom of a pelvic disease, it is called secondary dysmenorrhea. The degree of dysmenorrhea depends on subjective sensations and there are no objective criteria, leading to the varying incidence. Usually, dysmenorrhea occurs 2 years after menarche, but the age and duration of secondary dysmenorrhea due to different diseases vary, so the occurrence of dysmenorrhea also varies.

Primary dysmenorrhea is very common in adolescents and is associated with spasmodic hypercontraction of the uterus. Secondary dysmenorrhea is caused by clear underlying pelvic pathological changes, and common disorders include endometriosis, pelvic inflammatory disease, ovarian cysts, adenomyosis, and fibroids. Endometriosis is the most common cause of secondary dysmenorrhea and is commonly seen in young women. Studies have shown that laparoscopy in adolescent women with dysmenorrhea treated unsatisfactorily with nonsteroidal anti-inflammatory drugs (NSAIDs) and oral contraceptives reveals varying degrees of endometriosis in about 70% of patients. In multipara women, the possibility of adenomyosis should be considered if dysmenorrhea is accompanied by menorrhagia and a uniformly enlarged uterus. Submucosal fibroids or endometrial polyps may cause cervical stenosis, which in turn may cause pain during menstruation. In patients with a history of cervical surgery, including cerclage of cervix, cervical cryotherapy, and cervical conization, dysmenorrhea occurring after surgery may be caused by secondary cervical stenosis. When sudden onset or worsening of dysmenorrhea occurs in patients with no history of dysmenorrhea or mild dysmenorrhea, pelvic inflammatory disease or pregnancy should first be considered to be ruled out.

The possible mechanisms for dysmenorrhea are related to various factors such as abnormal contractions of the uterus leading to uterine ischemia and hypoxia, cyclic changes in sex hormones, and stimulation of the isthmus uteri plexus. The primary dysmenorrhea is associated with increased uterine tension and excessive spasmodic contractions due to increased uterine muscle activity. The basal tension in the uterine cavity during normal menstruation is <10 mmHg (1.33 kPa); the pressure during contractions does not exceed 120 mmHg (16 kPa); and the uterine contractions are coordinated with a frequency of 3–4 contractions per 10 min. In dysmenorrhea, the basal tension in the uterine cavity increases and the pressure exceeds 120–150 mmHg (16–20 kPa) during contractions, leading to the increased, uncoordinated, or unrhythmic contraction. Due to the enhanced abnormal contractions of the uterus, the uterine blood flow decreases, causing uterine ischemia and hypoxia, which then leads to dysmenorrhea. The causes of excessive uterine contractions have been found to be prostaglandins, leukotrienes, vasopressin, oxytocin, etc.

Vulvodynia or Vestibulodynia

Vulvodynia, often accompanied by difficulty with intercourse, is also known as vulvar vestibulodynia and is characterized by burning pain with itching, but patients usually have no signs of dermatological diseases or vulvar infection. The pain may be spontaneous or induced by palpation or friction of the perineum area. There are five subtypes of vulvar pain, classified as skin diseases of the vulva (such as chronic dermatitis and eczema), periodic vulvovaginitis (*Candida* infection), papillomatous hyperplasia of the perineum (possibly associated with human papillomavirus infection), hyperalgesia or vulvar pain (diffuse sensory hypersensitivity), and vulvovaginitis syndrome (manifested by difficulty with intercourse and tenderness to touch).

Although the mechanism of vulvodynia is unknown, possible factors involved include neuropathic pain, where the human vaginal wall nerve supply comes primarily from the uterovaginal plexus and the vagina receives abundant nerve fibers containing substance P, a neuropeptide in nociceptive afferent fibers. Low levels of estradiol may cause an increase in the number of vaginal pain fibers and an increase in avoidance response behavior to vaginal dilation, which may be associated with delayed sensory vulvodynia. Estrogen has been used to treat vulvodynia. Delayed sensory vulvodynia occurs primarily in postmenopausal women because estrogen levels decline after menopause.

12.5 Diagnostic Ideas for CPP in Women

12.5.1 Medical History

More than 80% of patients with CPP experience pain for more than 1 year, and about 1/3 of patients have a history of pain of more than 5 years [24]. Medical history and physical examination are powerful diagnostic tools for CPP that provide clues to the diagnosis.

What must be emphasized in the management of CPP is the completeness of the history taking as each question may be suggestive for the diagnosis of the disease. For example, age is an important factor. Most of the female patients with CPP is in their reproductive ages. The suspicion of malignancy tumors should be raised for CPP female patients beyond childbearing years. CPP may also be a result of trauma to the pelvic and low back muscles during pregnancy and childbirth such as relaxation of the pelvic floor muscles and ligaments. Relaxation of the pelvic floor muscles is often accompanied by prolapse of organs such as bladder prolapse, uterine prolapse, and intestinal prolapse, all of which may induce CPP. A history of previous pelvic and abdominal surgery is associated with CPP. For instance, undetected cholorrhagia and gall stones during cholecystectomy, together with cervical canal stenosis caused by previous surgery, will lead to endometriosis.

Locating the patient's pain is essential for an accurate diagnosis as most pain is induced by gynecological organ lesions that are difficult to identify the exact site where pain is felt. Since the neck of the uterus, the body of the uterus, adnexa, bladder, distal ureteral, lower part of the ileum, rectum, and sigmoid colon are innervated by the same neurotome, it is difficult for patients to distinguish whether the pain in the abdominal and pelvic cavity is of gynecological, urological, or intestinal origin. About 60% of CPP is unilateral, while the rest are bilateral or widespread. Generally, unilateral pain tends to happen in the adnexa or sigmoid colon; pain in the midline of the abdomen or below the umbilicus may be secondary to the uterus, the fundus uteri ligaments, the posterior Douglascul-de-sac, the cervix, but may also be due to mild distension of the left colon or the right colon.

Clarifying the nature of the pain helps in the diagnosis. For example, neuropathic pain is usually described as burning or stabbing pain accompanied by electric shock-like feelings; muscle pain may be sore in nature or accompanied by sharp and knife-like pain after a change in position: visceral pain is of paroxysmal sharp and radiating characteristics; and pain of endometriosis is usually spasmodic or colic.

Learning the time of the pain occurrence is helpful for diagnosis. When the episodes of the pain match with the cycle of menstruation, it is mostly associated with gynecological diseases. Endometriosis, adenomyosis, and pelvic congestion syndrome are common gynecological conditions associated with CPP. Although gynecological pain often worsens before and during menstruation, it is not unique as other CPP diseases also share such features, such as irritable colon syndrome and other gastrointestinal, urinary, or musculoskeletal pain.

Identifying the specific triggers is conducive to diagnosis. A history of trauma or surgery suggests that the musculoskeletal pain is induced by musculoskeletal reasons rather than gynecological diseases. Pain felt after pregnancy or delivery suggests perinatal pelvic pain syndrome. Dysmenorrhea that begins at or shortly after menarche and worsens progressively and persists suggests endometriosis. If the pain begins after somatic or sexual assault, it may be influenced by musculoskeletal or psychological changes. All factors aggravating or relieving the patient's pain should be consulted. In addition, the intestinal functions, bladder functions, and especially sexual intercourse are crucial. Patients with CPP are more likely to have dysmenorrhea and dyspareunia, with more than 80% of them experiencing dysmenorrhea (compared to about 50% in the general population) and at least 40% having dyspareunia (compared to 10–15% of the general population).

Ask patients if they have sexually transmitted diseases or PID. It is estimated that 18–27% of patients with acute PID developing into CPP, the exact mechanism of which remains unknown, but not all PIDs and genital injuries will progress to CPP. The epidemiological studies of CPP have shown that PID occurs most often in women before the age of 25, which is about 10 years younger than the average age of women with CPP. Treatments of PID do not affect the probability of developing into CPP subsequently, and the probability of developing into CPP with outpatient or inpatient treatment is 34% and 30%, respectively. Physical factors and sexual promiscuity are significantly associated with various types of CPP. About 40–50% of patients with CPP have a history of sexual promiscuity. Those with a history of sexual promiscuity and high Symptom Checklist scores are more likely to have nonphysical CPP, suggesting that the link between sexual promiscuity and CPP may be psychological or neurological. In patients with CPP, it is important to know whether they have a sexual promiscuous history or similar behavior.

Using hormonal contraceptives may conceal some of the conditions that cause gynecological pain, such as endometriosis and adenomyosis. Asking patients about their contraceptives taking history can reveal whether pain episodes or exacerbations are associated with discontinuation of hormonal contraceptives. If they are taking those medications, their treatment should exclude them.

A thorough inquiry into previous treatments for CPP and their effectiveness is a critical part of the process. The inquiry should cover the type, dosage, and effectiveness of the analgesics used, and any previous surgeries, including not only those for pain, but also postoperative surgical pain that may be a risk factor or trigger for CPP. Carefully learning the patient's previous treatments and their outcomes not only prevents the physicians from repeating invasive and costly diagnostic tests and treatment measures, but also prompts them to develop a treatment strategy for recurrent pain. For example, an RCT performed by Peters et al. clearly demonstrated that a second-time laparoscopy for women who have done it before or had a laparotomy with negative results was less helpful compared with that for women who underwent comprehensive treatments without a laparoscopy [25]. In addition, a good response to gonadotropin-releasing hormone agonists including a pregnancy and 2–3 years of pain relief suggests that gonadotropin-releasing hormone agonists are a good treatment option for the recurrent CPP. Similarly, if the response to the surgical treatment of endometriosis is ideal, another surgery may be considered when the disease recurs.

12.5.2 Physical Examination

Physical examination is also a powerful diagnostic tool, as is history taking. The main purpose is to determine, as much as possible, the anatomic site of tenderness and the pain site stated. The patients should be asked if this pressed pain is identical to the pain complained of.

The physical examination of CPP should be systematic and orderly, and all relevant examinations should not be ignored. Some scholars have divided the examination of CPP into standing, sitting, supine, and Trendelenburg positions, so that the examination can cover any system causing CPP. In this chapter, the obstetrical and gynecological examinations for CPP are described in detail taking the Trendelenburg position as an example.

After the patient is placed in the Trendelenburg position, the area of the external genitalia is observed first for inflammation, discharge, abscess, excoriation, perineal fistulas, perineal ulcers, pigment changes, warts, dystrophic changes (thinning, pallor, loss of vaginal folds, protrusion of the urethral mucosa), and trauma. Confirm whether there are anal fistulas and fissures as these are sometimes the primary objective evidence of inflammatory bowel disease. Inspection also includes the view obtained from the vaginoscopy, including prolapse of the uterus, cystocele, and rectocele. While the position of the cervix should also be noted as the lateral displacement of the cervix indicates the possible presence of endometriosis in the sacrum.

Palpation is the primary means of physical examination for CPP of obstetric and gynecological origin, with the goal of performing basic sensory tests to determine whether it is sharp, dull, or light tenderness. The painful areas of vulvar vestibulitis are mainly in the vestibule and also include the labia, vulva, hymen, and vestibular glands. When using a swab to palpate the patient with vulvar vestibulitis, the tenderness can be precisely felt in the vestibular glands outside the hymen. The pain-sensitive areas of the cervix, on the other hand, are mainly located in the areas of 1, 3, 6, and 9 o'clock.

Palpation of the lower abdomen using a single finger through the vagina is more sensitive than traditional two-handed abdominal palpation. Among patients with vaginismus, 75% can be diagnosed through single-finger palpation. The levator ani muscle can be easily palpated through bimanual examination and can be identified by asking the patient to lift the pelvis forcefully. The anus will be lifted together with pelvis. In normal patients, touching the levator ani muscle causes only a sensation of pressure, but in patients with pelvic floor pain syndrome it can cause constant pain. Cervical pressing pain is most often indicative of cervicitis, repeated cervical trauma (often due to sexual intercourse), or pelvic infection. Vaginal vault pressing pain may indicate pelvic infection and endometriosis. Uterine pressing pain can be evaluated by palpating the uterus with one finger and squeezing it toward the sacrum. It can present in adenomyosis, pelvic congestion syndrome, pelvic infection, or premenstrual syndrome. Immobilization of the uterus, especially in a retroflexed position, may be due to endometriosis or uterine adhesions. Palpation of the adnexal region includes checking the thickness, mobility, and volume of the adnexa. Patients with asymmetrical, enlarged ovaries, especially if fixed to the broad ligament or pelvic wall, may have endometriosis. Bilateral or unilateral ovarian tenderness may be associated with pelvic congestion syndrome. Finally, carefully examine whether there is pressing pain in the rectovaginal septum, and if present, it is a typical sign of endometriosis.

In addition, the timing of the gynecological physical examination is also of interest. For example, many patients with endometriosis have significant tenderness only during their menstrual period. Therefore, it is very helpful to perform this examination on the +first or second day of menstruation, which will improve the detection rate of endometrial papules in the rectovaginal septum. At the end of the physical examination, the physician must discuss and describe any positive or negative findings and infer the reasonableness of the hypothetical diagnosis.

12.5.3 Laboratory Tests and Imaging

In patients with CPP, it is reasonable to perform some exclusionary tests to look for an etiology when physical examination does not reveal significant positive signs.

12.5.3.1 Laboratory Tests

First of all, screening for sexually transmitted diseases is necessary. Tests related to gonorrhea, chlamydia, viruses, hepatitis, AIDS, etc., can be included as part of the patient's primary health examination. For patients with dyspareunia, tests for sexually transmitted diseases, especially urine, cervical secretion culture, and chlamydia PCR tests, are necessary. Patients with urinary tract symptoms with frequent lower abdominal pain may have interstitial cystitis; thus, they should accept urine analysis, urine culture, and thinprep cytology test (TCT). For patients with vulvar vestibulitis, urinary oxalate crystallization index test is indispensable for the oxalate crystals are the primary stimulus. In patients suspected to have residual ovary syndrome, their estradiol and follicle-stimulating hormone remain at a high level. For female patients with depression, thyroid-stimulating hormone, thyroid hormone, T3, T4 and, if necessary, thyroid antibodies to exclude thyroid diseases. The level of CA125 is substantially higher in patients with lower abdominal pain than in patients with endometriosis; thus, it can be regarded as an important diagnostic and follow-up indicator for endometriosis, though its sensitivity and specificity are low.

12.5.3.2 Ultrasound

Gynecological ultrasound is a useful tool for diagnosing gynecological disorders. It can diagnose whether a pelvic mass originates from the uterus and adnexa or from the gastrointestinal tract and bladder. In the case of adnexal masses, the location, size, quality, and composition of the cyst wall can be determined. If endometriosis is suspected, ultrasound has a greater diagnostic value than laparoscopy as it can follow up patients with endometriosis after surgery and determine the recurrence of the disease. If a lesion of the uterus itself is suspected, such as a fibroid, ultrasound can confirm the diagnosis and the number, location, calcification, and growth rate of the myoma. In addition, ultrasound can distinguish leiomyoma from adenomyosis, diagnose endometrial polyps, and detect intrauterine devices. At the same time, ultrasound is effective in the differential diagnosis of uterine polyps and thickened endometrium. Transvaginal ultrasound has a 50–85% true-positive rate for the diagnosis of abdominal masses in ovarian remnant syndrome.

It can diagnose obstructive cervical stenosis and inspect fluid and tissue fragments in the uterine cavity.

12.5.3.3 Pelvic Venography

Pelvic venography is the only reliable method to diagnose pelvic congestion syndrome. According to the diameter of the uterine plexus, the degree of congestion and the time of disappearance of the contrast are recorded and scored, with the score of 3–4 being normal and 5–9 being abnormal. The sensitivity of this method for diagnosis is 91% and the accuracy rate is 89%. Some scholars consider this invasive examination as a way to diagnose varicose pelvic veins, the standard of which is the ovarian veins being over 10 mm in diameter, ovarian venous plexus congestion, congested veins crossing the midline, and varicose vulvar or thigh veins.

12.5.3.4 Laparoscopy

Laparoscopy is widely used by gynecologists to evaluate pelvic pain. In a meta-analysis of 105 patients who underwent laparoscopy for CPP, clear pathological changes were found in 95.24% of cases, including endometriosis in 56 cases (53.33%), chronic PID in 27 cases (25.23%), mucinosis in 10 cases (9.52%), and pelvic congestion syndrome in 7 cases (6.67%) [26]. However, in clinical practice, many gynecologists prefer laparoscopy as the final or definitive diagnosis of CPP when in fact laparoscopy in CPP is mainly used to diagnose endometriosis and pelvic adhesion diseases. A negative result of laparoscopy means that the patient does not have pain associated with endometriosis or pelvic adhesion diseases, while it does not indicate that the patient has no organic pathology.

12.6 Treatments for CPP

There is only limited evidence-based literature reporting the treatments of CPP. For nonspecific CPP, the treatment normally targets symptomatic pain relief [27]. The treatments of chronic pelvic disorders should focus on both the underlying pathology and the psychological factors of pain, including comorbid mood disorders. For CPP with a known source of pain, the underlying disease process should be treated primarily. In cases where the sources of the pain remain unknown, patients should be advised to undergo further evaluation to identify the underlying disease process.

For CPP with unknown sources, the first choice of treatment is using over-the-counter analgesics such as acetaminophen and NSAIDs which are usually well tolerated. If sufficient pain relief is achieved, no further pain management is required. Yet, if pain relief is not adequate and the patient has cyclic pelvic pain, hormone alternative therapy (oral contraceptives, depot medroxyprogesterone, or intrauterine device) is recommended. If hormonal therapy is ineffective, or if the patient's pain is not cyclic, or if it is suspected that their pelvic pain is neurological, it is important to assess the patient for an underlying mood disorder. If a mood disorder is presumed, antidepressant therapy (selective 5-hydroxytryptamine reuptake inhibitor) may be useful. If there is no underlying mood disorder in patients with CPP secondary to suspected neuropathic pain, various treatment options may be adopted. For example, depending on patients' preference and their various comorbidities, treatment options ranging from tricyclic antidepressants (TCAs), pregabalin, gabapentin, or 5-hydroxytryptamine-norepinephrine reuptake inhibitors (SNRIs) such as venlafaxine or duloxetine have been shown to be effective. If these treatment options do not achieve the ideal effect, referral to a pain medicine specialist and consideration of trying opioid analgesics is recommended. In cases of CPP secondary to suspected neuropathy, gabapentin has been shown to be more effective than amitriptyline alone either as a single agent or in combination with amitriptyline [28–31].

Complementary nonpharmacological treatments should also be provided if necessary. Pelvic floor physical therapy may be helpful in relieving CPP and also in diagnosing the musculoskeletal origin of CPP [32]. Cognitive-behavioral therapy is also an integral part of treatment that reduces pain, stress, and improves function [33]. Mindfulness can be taught as an integral part of physical therapy and cognitive-behavioral therapy [34]. In severe cases, peripheral nerve blocks and sacral neuromodulation may also be required. For CPP secondary to the uterus, hysterectomy may be considered, but this is often a last resort. Oral contraceptives are not helpful to patients without cyclic pelvic pain [35]. Cyclobenzaprine is an effective analgesic for patients with CPP and can also improve sleep [36]. If sacral nerve injury is suspected, local corticosteroid injections can be both diagnostic to identify peripheral nerve involvement in CPP and therapeutic to provide pain relief. Some clinicians administrated pharmacological treatment along with various interventional procedures.

If local steroid injections are successful, radiofrequency ablation, peripheral nerve blocks, or neuromodulation with a spinal cord stimulator may be a viable treatment option. Botulinum toxin injections in patients with CPP have been shown to reduce pain during sexual activity and decrease pelvic pressure and persistent noncyclical pelvic pain [37]. Cutaneous treatment option can be considered for relieving short-term pain, such as trigger point injections of local anesthetics like lidocaine. These injections are usually used to relieve hypertonicity and pain secondary to the pelvic floor or abdominal wall muscles. If trigger point injections are effective, they could be both therapeutic and diagnostic of myofascial pain syndrome. Combining cognitive-behavioral therapy that educates patients about their CPP, including the psychological aspects of their pain, is beneficial as well [38].

12.6.1 Treatments for Endometriosis

Treatment of endometriosis-related pelvic pain is complex and should be planned with a patient-centered approach that takes into account a variety of factors. The patient's age, fertility requirements, duration of infertility, and attitude toward surgery or hormonal therapy are major concerns. In addition, the patient's initiative and emotional state can also influence the choice of treatment. Current treatment options for endometriosis-related pain include hormone suppression therapy, analgesic drug combinations, palliative conservative surgery, and radical surgery. Treatment guidelines based on studies of pharmacological and surgical treatment of endometriosis-related pelvic pain are available [39].

1. NSAIDs: Relieving pain associated with endometriosis (Level of Evidence: A, 1b).
2. Hormonal therapy: Suppressing ovarian function to reduce estrogen levels for 6 months can relieve painful symptoms associated with endometriosis. The main therapeutic agents include danazol, combined oral contraceptives (COC), medroxyprogesterone acetate (MPA), and gonadotropin-releasing hormone (GnRH) agonist, with the difference being the adverse effects of the drugs (Level of Evidence: A, 1a).
3. GnRH agonists (GnRHa): In terms of pain relief, GnRHa therapy for 3 months is as effective as for 6 months; a combined GnRHa and add-back therapy for more than 2 years significantly reduces bone mineral density loss while alleviating pain (Level of Evidence A, 1b).
4. Endometrial ablation together with laparoscopic uterine nerve ablation: The less severe the endometriosis, the less significant the treatment effect; however, there is no evidence that 1 laparoscopic uterine nerve ablation is necessary because it has no therapeutic effect on primary dysmenorrhea associated with endometriosis (Level of Evidence: A, 1b).
5. Hysterectomy together with bilateral tubectomy and ovariectomy: In patients with severe endometriosis, it is feasible to consider resection of all diseased tissues, and if the entire uterus is to be removed, then resection of bilateral oviducts and ovaries must also be considered (Level of Evidence: A, 1b).
6. Postoperative treatment: Postoperative GnRH agonist therapy for 6 months significantly reduces the recurrence of endometriosis at 12 and 24 months postoperatively compared with

placebo therapy, while postoperative oral contraceptives have no such effect (Level of Evidence: A, 1b).

7. Hormone replacement therapy: This therapy is recommended for young women who have undergone bilateral ovariectomy, but no exact strategy is decided (Level of Evidence: D, 4).

To relieve the CPP associated with endometriosis, presacral neurectomy is recommended. Data from clinical trials show that presacral neurectomy relieves pain through surgical treatment of endometriosis. However, presacral neurectomy may result in incurable constipation and urgent urination in up to 5% of patients. Surgical complications vary depending on the severity of the disease, but damage to the pelvic organs is a potential risk for women with endometriosis, and untreated endometriosis can cause ureteral and bowel obstruction, as well as urethral and venereal invasion, but is rarely life-threatening. In endometriosis with CPP, there is no guarantee that medication or surgical treatment will be effective in relieving the pain of endometriosis. In contrast, although treatment of endometriosis in women with pelvic pain is based on randomized, double-blind, placebo-controlled clinical trials, only 40–70% of CPP associated with endometriosis achieve the desired outcome after 6 months or more of treatment [40]. In addition, the recurrence rate of CPP after pharmacological and surgical treatment is high. Women with endometriosis need differential diagnoses for all sources of chronic abdominal and pelvic pain (including nongynecological) to ensure the treatments they received are appropriate.

12.6.2 Treatment for Dysmenorrhea

The treatments of dysmenorrhea mainly include nonpharmacological treatment, pharmacological treatment, surgical interventions, and complementary therapies. Nonpharmacological treatment methods mainly include physical exercise (mainly yoga), transcutaneous thermal stimulation, acupuncture, traditional Chinese medical massage, and local thermotherapy. Pharmacological treatments mainly include NSAIDs and sex hormone therapy. Surgical treatments include hysterectomy, presacral neurectomy, and utero-sacral neurectomy in laparoscopy. Supplementary and alternative drugs include vitamin B_1, vitamin E, combination of fish oil and vitamin B_{12}, magnesium, and combination of vitamin B_6 and fish oil.

12.7 Summary

CPP is a common female disease. Patients often present to the clinic with pain that has seriously affected their daily lives, with a long course and complex symptoms, involving multiple sites in the lower abdomen, pelvis, and perineum, and possibly related to multiple systems such as urinary, digestive, and reproductive, and patients are often accompanied by emotional and psychological changes. A clear diagnosis of CPP pain requires detailed patient history and meticulous physical examination. Imaging is helpful in diagnosing most CPP patients with organic lesions. Ultrasound diagnosis, nerve block therapy, trigger point therapy, and pelvic rehabilitation therapy for CPP are more and more widely used in clinical practice.

References

1. Latthe P, Latthe M, Say L, Gülmezoglu M, Khan KS. WHO systematic review of prevalence of chronic pelvic pain: a neglected reproductive health morbidity. BMC Public Health. 2006;6:177.
2. Evidence-based management of chronic pelvic pain. Reiter RC. Clin Obstet Gynecol. 1998;41:422–35.
3. Marszalek M, Wehrberger C, Temml C, Ponholzer A, Berger I, Madersbacher S. Chronic pelvic pain and lower urinary tract symptoms in both sexes: analysis of 2749 participants of an urban health screening project. Eur Urol. 2009;55(2):499–507.
4. Muhammad YY, Nossier SA, El-Dawaiaty AA. Prevalence and characteristics of chronic pelvic pain among women in Alexandria. Egypt J Egypt Public Health Assoc. 2011;86(1–2):33–8.
5. Garcia-Perez H, Harlow SD, Erdmann CA, Denman C. Pelvic pain and associated characteristics among

women in northern Mexico. Int Perspect Sex Reprod Health. 2010;36(2):90–8.
6. Grace VM, Zondervan KR. Chronic pelvic pain in New Zealand: prevalence, pain severity, diagnoses and use of the health services. Aust Nz J Public Health. 2004;28(4):369–75.
7. Mathias SD, Kuppermann M, Liberman RF, Lipschutz RC, Steege JF. Chronic pelvic pain: prevalence, healthrelated quality of life, and economic correlates. Obstet Gynecol. 1996;87(3):321–7.
8. Abbott JA. Adenomyosis and abnormal uterine bleeding (AUB-A)-pathogenesis, diagnosis, and management. Best Pract Res Clin Obstet Gynaecol. 2017;40:68–81.
9. Drossman DA. The functional gastrointestinal disorders and the Rome II process. Gut. 1999;45(Suppl 2):II1–5.
10. Curry A, Williams T, Penny ML. Pelvic inflammatory disease: diagnosis, management, and prevention. Am Fam Physician. 2019;100:357–64. https://www.aafp.org/pubs/afp/issues/2019/0915/p357.html.
11. Simms I, Stephenson JM, Mallinson H, et al. Risk factors associated with pelvic inflammatory disease. Sex Transm Infect. 2006;82:452–7.
12. Workowski KA. Centers for Disease Control and Prevention sexually transmitted diseases treatment guidelines. Clin Infect Dis. 2015;61(Suppl 8):S759–62.
13. Zheng Y, Jin Y, Zhu HB, Xu ST, Xia YX, Huang Y. The anti-inflammatory and anti-nociceptive activities of Patrinia villosa and its mechanism on the proinflammatory cytokines of rats with pelvic inflammation. Afr J Tradit Complement Altern Med. 2012;9(3):295–302. https://doi.org/10.4314/ajtcam.v9i3.
14. Juganavar A, Joshi KS. Chronic pelvic pain: a comprehensive review. Cureus. 2022;14(10):e30691. https://doi.org/10.7759/cureus.30691.
15. Nisenblat V, Bossuyt PM, Shaikh R, et al. Blood biomarkers for the non-invasive diagnosis of endometriosis. Cochrane Database Syst Rev. 2016;2016(5):CD012179.
16. Arafah M, Rashid S, Akhtar M. Endometriosis: a comprehensive review. Adv Anat Pathol. 2021;28:30–43.
17. Saunders PT, Horne AW. Endometriosis: etiology, pathobiology, and therapeutic prospects. Cell. 2021;184:2807–24.
18. Mechsner S. Endometriosis: an often unrecognized pain disorder (article in German). Schmerz. 2016;30:477–90.
19. Senapati S, Atashroo D, Carey E, Dassel M, Tu MF. Surgical interventions for chronic pelvic pain. Curr Opin Obstet Gynecol. 2016;28:290–6.
20. Dueholm M, Lundorf E, Hansen ES, Sørensen JS, Ledertoug S, Olesen F. Magnetic resonance imaging and transvaginal ultrasonography for the diagnosis of adenomyosis. Fertil Steril. 2001;76:588–94.
21. Baradwan S, Baradwan A, Baradwan A, Al-Jaroudi D. Hydrosalpinx with acute abdominal pain during the third trimester of pregnancy: a case report. Case Rep Womens Health. 2018;20:e00077.
22. Liddle AD, Davies AH. Pelvic congestion syndrome: chronic pelvic pain caused by ovarian and internal iliac varices. Phlebology. 2007;22:100–4.
23. Tu FF, Hahn D, Steege JF. Pelvic congestion syndrome-associated pelvic pain: a systematic review of diagnosis and management. Obstet Gynecol Surv. 2010;65:332–40.
24. Yongjun Z, Tingjie Z, Xiaoqiu Y, Zhiying F, Feng Q, Guangke X, Jinfeng L, Fachuan N, Xiaohong J, Yanqing L. A survey of chronic pain in China. Libyan J Med. 2020;15(1):1730550. https://doi.org/10.1080/19932820.2020.1730550.
25. Peters AA, van Dorst E, et al. A randomized clinical trial to compare two different approaches in women with chronic pelvic pain. Obstet Gynecol. 1991;77:740–4.
26. Li Hui LY, Jie Z. Laparoscopic diagnosis and therapy for chronic pelvic pain. China J Endosc. 2004:04.
27. Cheong YC, Smotra G, Williams AC. Non-surgical interventions for the management of chronic pelvic pain. Cochrane Database Syst Rev. 2014;3:CD008797.
28. Cottrell AM, Schneider MP, Goonewardene S, Yuan Y, Baranowski AP, Engeler DS, Borovicka J, Dinis-Oliveira P, Elneil S, Hughes J, Messelink BJ, de C Williams AC. Benefits and harms of electrical neuromodulation for chronic pelvic pain: a systematic review. Eur Urol Focus. 2020;6(3):559–71.
29. Sator-Katzenschlager SM, Scharbert G, Kress HG, Frickey N, Ellend A, Gleiss A, Kozek-Langenecker SA. Chronic pelvic pain treated with gabapentin and amitriptyline: a randomized controlled pilot study. Wien Klin Wochenschr. 2005;117(21–22):761–8.
30. Allen C, Hopewell S, Prentice A, Gregory D. Nonsteroidal anti-inflammatory drugs for pain in women with endometriosis. Cochrane Database Syst Rev. 2009;2:CD004753.
31. Lewis SC, Bhattacharya S, Wu O, Vincent K, Jack SA, Critchley HO, Porter MA, Cranley D, Wilson JA, Horne AW. Gabapentin for the Management of Chronic Pelvic Pain in women (GaPP1): a pilot randomised controlled trial. PLoS One. 2016;11(4):e0153037.
32. Haugstad GK, Kirste U, Leganger S, Haakonsen E, Haugstad TS. Somatocognitive therapy in the management of chronic gynaecological pain. A review of the historical background and results of a current approach. Scand. J Pain. 2018;2(3):124–9.
33. Haugstad GK, Haugstad TS, Kirste UM, Leganger S, Wojniusz S, Klemmetsen I, Malt UF. Continuing improvement of chronic pelvic pain in women after short-term Mensendieck somatocognitive therapy: results of a 1-year follow-up study. Am J Obstet Gynecol. 2008;199(6):615.e1–8.
34. Louw A, Zimney K, O'Hotto C, Hilton S. The clinical application of teaching people about pain. Physiother Theory Pract. 2016;32(5):385–95.
35. Harada T, Momoeda M, Taketani Y, Hoshiai H, Terakawa N. Low-dose oral contraceptive pill for dys-

menorrhea associated with endometriosis: a placebo-controlled, double-blind, randomized trial. Fertil Steril. 2008;90(5):1583–8.

36. Moldofsky H, Harris HW, Archambault WT, Kwong T, Lederman S. Effects of bedtime very low dose cyclobenzaprine on symptoms and sleep physiology in patients with fibromyalgia syndrome: a double-blind randomized placebo-controlled study. J Rheumatol. 2011;38(12):2653–63.
37. Abbott JA, Jarvis SK, Lyons SD, Thomson A, Vancaille TG. Botulinum toxin type a for chronic pain and pelvic floor spasm in women: a randomized controlled trial. Obstet Gynecol. 2006;108(4):915–23.
38. Montenegro ML, Braz CA, Rosa-e-Silva JC, Candido-dos-Reis FJ, Nogueira AA, Poli-Neto OB. Anaesthetic injection versus ischemic compression for the pain relief of abdominal wall trigger points in women with chronic pelvic pain. BMC Anesthesiol. 2015;15:175.
39. Royal college of Obstetricians and Gynaecologists, 2015. The initial management of chonic pelvic pain, May 2012. https://www.rcog.org.uk/media/muab2gj2/gtg_41.pdf.
40. Howard FM. An evidence-based medicine approach to the treatment of endometriosis-associated chronic pelvic pain: placebo-controlled studies. J Am Assoc Gynecol Laparosc. 2000;7(4):477–88. https://doi.org/10.1016/s1074-3804(05)60360-x.

13 Visceral Pain and Pelvic Pain Related to Urogenital System

Bifa Fan

13.1 Introduction

Chronic urogenital or pelvic pain is frequently encountered by clinical practitioners in the clinical practice, especially urologists, gynecologists, and gastroenterologists. In most cases, patients have been suffering from pain for a long time and often do not visit the clinicians until the pain becomes severe enough to interfere with their daily life. The complaint of pain is in the lower abdomen, pelvis, and perineum, suggesting possible acute or chronic injury to the lower abdominal and pelvic organs. However, many healthcare providers often question the presence of chronic pelvic pain (CPP) and urogenital pain, especially when no clear pathological changes can be detected by examinations [1]. Therefore, it is important to realize that a patient's pain is not only a sign of pelvic and urogenital pathology, but also an indication that the patient is suffering as chronic pain is itself a condition that needs to be managed. Moreover, such pain is particularly important because its location is closely related to sexual function, defecation, and urinary function. In addition, emotional and psychological changes closely related to pain are often considered to be the cause of pain [1]. Whereas, from the perspective of pain management, healthcare professionals should update the concept that patients' emotional and psychological changes and pain can be causal and mutually reinforcing. This chapter discusses the mechanisms and classification of CPP and the management of CPP in men, while for CPP in women, please refer to Chap. 11.

B. Fan (✉)
Department of Pain Medicine, China-Japan Friendship Hospital, Beijing, China

13.2 Definition of Chronic Pelvic Pain

CPP is the chronic or persistent pain felt in the structures associated with the male or female pelvis. The etiology of CPP is not fully understood and may be related to cognitive, behavioral, sexual and emotional, and lower urinary tract, bowel, pelvic floor, or gynecological dysfunction. Clinicians should confine pain to a designated pelvic region in light of medical history and physical examinations whenever possible. It is generally accepted that nociceptive pain that lasts or is recurrent for over 6 months could be regarded as chronic pain. Yet, when central sensitization is confirmed, then the pain can be directly determined as chronic pain regardless of the duration of pain.

Generally, CPP can be divided into two categories, namely, pain with clear pathological causes, which is also known as specific disease-associated pelvic pain, and pain without precise pathological causes, which is also known as CPP syndrome. For many years, the treatment of CPP has been focused on the peripheral organ diseases,

M. Xia et al. (eds.), *Visceral Pain*, https://doi.org/10.1007/978-981-99-9167-9_13

such as inflammatory or infectious diseases. However, animal and clinical studies have shown that many of the mechanisms of CPP syndrome are rooted in the central nervous system (CNS). Although external stimuli such as infection may initiate the onset of pelvic pain, pain may eventually become spontaneous that exists even without external stimuli because of the involvement of the CNS in nociceptive modulation. In addition to pain, abnormal CNS modulation can lead to other sensory, functional, behavioral, and psychological abnormalities [2].

CPP poses a major challenge to medical practitioners due to its complex etiology and treatment. Medical professionals need to understand all organ systems within and outside the pelvis and their relationship to other systems and systemic conditions, including the musculoskeletal, neurological, urological, gynecological, and psychological systems, to promote multidisciplinary diagnosis and treatment [1].

13.3 Mechanisms of CPP

13.3.1 Central Sensitization

There are essentially three processes involved in central sensitization at the spinal cord level. The activity of existing proteins is the earliest, and changes in the genetic transcription of proteins and even structural changes in neuronal connections may also play a role, the latter probably occurring within a few days. The early chemicals involved include neurotransmitters such as glutamate, substance P, calcitonin gene-related peptide (CGRP), prostaglandin E_2 (PGE_2), and brain-derived neurotrophic factor (BDNF) [3].

Repeated noxious stimulus afferents result in elevated glutamate levels, which release magnesium ions embedded in *N*-methyl-D-aspartate (NMDA), which further allows calcium ions to enter neurons and enhances depolarization. Glutamate also binds aminomethyl phosphonic acid (AMPA), which may be an additional pathway to increase intracellular calcium. Other modulators of concentrated release include substance P, which acts on neurokinin receptors, PGE_2, which binds endogenous prostaglandin receptors, and BDNF, which acts on tyrosine kinase B receptors, all of which also increase intracellular calcium ions. Calcium ions decrease neurological excitation and increase signaling to higher centers. The first important feature of increased calcium ions is internal translational processing, which usually involves the addition of phosphate groups to amino acids via kinases. Phosphorylation can significantly alter the properties of the protein, usually decreasing the channel opening threshold and keeping the channel opening period. As a result, noxious stimulus signals are amplified in these neurons [3].

13.3.2 Mechanisms of Spinal Cord and Visceral Hyperalgesia

Central sensitization leads to a decrease in the body's perceptual threshold to injurious stimuli, increasing reaction time and the number of dorsal horn neurons in the spinal cord. This increases signaling to the central nervous system and amplifies the signal perceived by the organism from peripheral stimuli. For example, among skin stimuli, soft touch does not usually induce pain; however, with central sensitization, soft touch may induce pain (touch-induced pain). Visceral nociceptive sensitization may manifest as a visceral stimulus that is usually felt as a subthreshold and is not perceived as such. For example, in central sensitization, subthreshold stimuli may produce a sensation of holding and distension that requires urination or defecation to be relieved. Thus, many of the clinical symptoms of bladder painful syndrome (BPS), also known as interstitial cystitis (IC), and irritable bowel syndrome (IBS) can be explained by central sensitization. The muscle pain of fibromyalgia has a similar explanation [4].

13.3.3 Advanced Central Modulation of Nociceptive Pathways in Spinal Cord

The International Association for the Study of Pain (IASP) defines pain as "an unpleasant sensory and emotional experience associated with actual or potential tissue damage." This definition reflects the complexity of pain, which involves not only the activation of nociceptive pathways, but also the emotional response of the individual. The brain may influence the regulation of pain pathways at the spinal cord level. Current research generally suggests that both the downstream pain inhibition and vulnerability pathways originating in the brain are diminished. The periaqueductal gray (PAG) plays an important role in spinal cord modulation by receiving thought- and emotion-related signal transmissions. Several neurotransmitters and neuromodulators are involved in reducing pain inhibition pathways, while opioids, 5-hydroxytryptamine, and norepinephrine can enhance pain inhibition [5].

13.3.4 Emotional, Cognitive, Behavioral, and Sexual Response Mechanisms

13.3.4.1 Neuromodulation and Psychology

The mental processes of emotion, thought, and behavior involve complex networks, and the interaction of these processes with pain processing is even more complex. As mentioned above, many links and mental processes are associated with prostaglandins, which is also a mechanism that affects pain transmission at the spinal cord level. At the spinal cord level, the level of visceral nociception is dependent on the intensity encoding system. The main afferents for both normal sensation and nociception in the viscera appear to arrive within the same small nerve fibers of the spinal cord, and the difference between normal and noxious information depends on the number of afferent signals conducted to the dorsal horn (A-fibers and C-fibers transmit nociception and A-fibers also transmit soft touch). Accordingly, it is believed that mental adjustments can alter intensity encoding, and thus pain perception more readily than dual nerve fibers encoding [6]. Various psychological processes influence superior pain neuromodulation, inhibiting or facilitating the nociception signal to reach the level of being felt, as well as the evaluation and interpretation of the signal. It also modulates the response to the nociception, thereby altering the pain experience. In addition, the downstream pathway represents cognitive, emotional, and behavioral states at the spinal and peripheral levels. Functional magnetic resonance imaging (fMRI) has shown that the psychological modulation of visceral pain may involve multiple pathways [7]. For example, shifting the focus of attention may relieve pain by inhibiting the active brain regions aroused by pain.

Stress is an internal or external force that may threaten the physical or psychological homeostasis of an organism. Stress-induced adaptive responses involve the endocrine system, the autonomic nervous system, and the immune system, which may also have feedback loops. Long-term stress can substantially alter the nervous system, a process that may also be associated with chronic pelvic pain syndrome. In addition, major adverse events, including rape, sexual abuse, sexual trauma, and sexual threats, such as during detention or torture, may produce long-lasting changes and effects in the nervous system and the patient's emotion, cognition, and sexual response.

13.3.4.2 Autonomic Nervous System

Little is known about the role of the autonomic nervous system in chronic pelvic pain, but there is evidence that injured afferent fibers may be sensitized to sympathetic stimulation at the site of injury and in the dorsal horn [8]. In visceral pain, alterations in CNS efferent information may produce significant organ dysfunction. These functional abnormalities may have a significant impact on quality of life and must be managed appropriately.

13.3.5 Other Mechanisms

13.3.5.1 Endocrine System

The endocrine system is involved in the visceral function. Major life events, especially early life events, may alter the release of hypothalamic–pituitary–adrenal axis and related chemicals, increase the expression of corticotrophin-releasing hormone (CRH) genes, and increase pain susceptibility. CRH upregulation may involve several pain states, such as rectal hypersensitivity to distension. A number of stress-related disorders have been proposed, such as IBS and BPS, and there is evidence that sex hormones also modulate nociception and pain perception [9].

13.3.5.2 Genetics and Chronic Pelvic Pain

Family history of chronic pelvic pain syndrome is an important risk factor. A number of genetic variants have been identified that can explain pain in some cases, many of which are associated with subtle changes in neurotransmitters and their receptors. However, the situation is further complicated by the involvement of growth, environmental, and social factors.

13.4 Classification of Chronic Pelvic Pain

Proper classification of chronic pelvic pain is important to distinguish the similarities and differences between different types of CPP, thereby facilitating research and treatments. As the classification becomes clearer, clinicians can adopt more specific and research evidence-based treatment approaches. At the same time, basic research can only be better translated and applied in the clinical practice if the phenotypes being studied are clearly defined. In addition, the diagnosis or name of a group of symptoms can provide patients with a sense of being understood and hope for curing rather than being blind and confused about the disease conditions. Thus, accurate classification helps alleviate patient concerns and promotes patients' participation in treatment and self-management [2].

13.4.1 Guidelines for the Classification of Chronic Pelvic Pain Syndrome

1. Pain syndromes are defined by a process of exclusion, especially without evidence of infection or inflammation. Therefore, ultimately the pain physician's examination should aim to obtain a differential diagnosis but it should be noted that repeated and unnecessary examinations are not conducive to the management of chronic pain as a clear pathological cause is often not found in chronic pain syndromes [10].
2. Subdivided phenotypes should be used only when supported by sufficient evidence. For example, in nonspecific, poorly limited pelvic pain without an obvious pathological cause, only the name chronic pelvic pain syndrome should be used. If the pain is limited to an organ, a more specific term such as rectal pain syndrome may be used. If the pain is confined to multiple organs, then the syndrome is still a regional pain syndrome; thus, chronic pelvic pain syndrome should be considered for use [10].

In addition to defining the patient by a specific organ phenotype, other factors need to be considered as well, including psychological (e.g., cognitive or emotional), sexual, behavioral, and functional factors. Psychological and behavioral factors are associated with the quality of life and prognosis [10, 11].

13.4.2 Classification of Common Chronic Pelvic Pain [11]

Chronic pelvic pain refers to pain originating from nonmalignant tumors of the pelvic organs, chronic continuous or recurrent pain caused by injurious stimuli for >6 months, or if the pain can be proven to be caused by acute onset of central nervous system sensitization regardless of the duration of the disease; pain accompanied by cognitive, behavioral, sexual, and emotional changes.

Pelvic pain syndrome is a persistent or recurrent, noninfectious pelvic pain associated with lower urinary tract, sexuality, defecation, and gynecological dysfunction.

Bladder pain syndrome is suprapubic pain associated with bladder filling, accompanied by increased daytime and nocturnal urinary frequency without evidence that the symptom is caused by urinary tract infection or other pathological changes.

Urethral pain syndrome is recurrent urethral pain, usually during urination, accompanied by frequent urination and increased nocturia without evidence of infection or other pathological changes.

Penile pain syndrome is pain in the penis that does not originate in the urethra, without evidence of infection or other pathological changes.

Prostate pain syndrome is persistent or recurrent prostate pain with symptoms of urethral and/or sexual dysfunction, without evidence of infection or other pathological changes. According to the classification system released by the National Institutes of Health (NIH), prostate pain syndrome can be subdivided into type A (inflammatory) and type B (noninflammatory syndrome) [2].

Scrotal pain syndrome is recurrent scrotal pain with symptoms of urethral or sexual dysfunction without evidence of infection or other pathological changes.

Testicular pain syndrome is persistent or recurrent pain that occurs on physical examination of the testicles, accompanied by symptoms of urethral or sexual dysfunction. It is not epidididymo-orchitis and without other obvious pathological changes. It refers specifically to testicular pain in contrast to scrotal pain.

Post-vasectomy pain syndrome is a painful scrotal syndrome that occurs after vasectomy.

Epididymal pain syndrome is persistent or recurrent pain that occurs on physical examination of the epididymis, accompanied by symptoms of urethral or sexual dysfunction It is not epidididymo-orchitis and without other obvious pathological changes. It refers specifically to epididymal pain in contrast to scrotal pain.

Endometriosis-associated pain syndrome is chronic or recurrent pelvic pain, where endometriosis is present but does not fully explain all symptoms.

Vaginal pain syndrome is persistent or recurrent vaginal pain with urethral or sexual dysfunction, with no evidence of vaginal infection or other pathological changes.

Vulvar pain syndrome is persistent or recurrent vulvar pain with or without symptoms of micturition cycle or urethral or sexual dysfunction and without evidence of vulvar infection or other pathological changes.

Generalized vulvar pain syndrome is burning sensation in the vulva and pain that cannot be localized on pressure testing. The pain extends to the vulvar vestibule, but is not limited to it. In the absence of irritation, pain may be present at any time.

Localized vulvar pain syndrome is pain that is persistent and closely localized to one or more parts of the vulva to which pressure is mapped. Clinically, the pain usually occurs after irritation.

Vestibular pain syndrome is the pain confined to one or more parts of the vulva where pressure is mapped.

Clitoral pain syndrome is the pain confined to the area of the clitoral band where pressure is mapped.

Pudendal pain syndrome is a kind of neuropathic pain that is located in the area innervated by pudendal nerves, accompanied by dysfunction of related innervated organs, such as rectum, lower urethra, and sexual dysfunction; there are no obvious pathological changes in the related area.

Perineal pain syndrome is persistent or recurrent perineal pain accompanied by altered micturition cycles or symptoms of urethral or sexual dysfunction, without definite infection or other obvious pathological changes.

Pelvic floor muscle pain syndrome is persistent or recurrent pain located at trigger points related to the pelvic floor, accompanied by altered micturition cycles or symptoms associated with urethral, bowel, or sexual dysfunction, without definite infection or other significant pathological changes.

13.5 Urogenital/Pelvic Pain in Men

Urogenital/pelvic pain in men is a prominent clinical problem among patients encountered by urologists. These patients are often unable to speak out their pain, and the pain is often poorly expressed or downplayed as there is a lack of clinical sign. Consequently, such pain is difficult to diagnose and treat. Generally, the diagnosis of urogenital/pelvic pain in men can be divided into two categories, namely, descriptive and pathological diagnoses. The descriptive diagnosis is considered to be independent lesions of peripheral sites, which is mainly a description of symptoms rather than pathologies. Commonly seen diseases diagnosed with this method include bladder pain syndrome, IC, urethral pain syndrome, urethritis/urethralgia, prostate pain syndrome, chronic aseptic prostatitis, scrotal pain syndrome, testicular pain, post-vasectomy "granulomatous" pain, and epididymal pain. On the other hand, pathological diagnosis often refers to a clear pathological cause, such as infective cystitis, infective prostatitis, infective urethritis, infective testicular epididymitis, and urethral calculi, treatments of which are etiological treatment. However, all treatments seem to provide relief for a certain period of time, but all are difficult to completely relieve the pain. For example, scrotal pain persists after orchiectomy on the affected side in patients with testicular pain, after epididymitis with epididymectomy, and after sarcoid resection after vasectomy. Therefore, a comprehensive assessment of the treatment approaches to male pelvic pain is necessary. This section focuses on the use of neuropathological principles to assess the role of the nervous system in the etiology and maintenance of pain, and evaluate the conditions and surrounding environmental factors of persistent pain syndromes [12].

13.5.1 Mechanism of Urogenital/Pelvic Pain in Men

13.5.1.1 Innervation and Pelvic Floor Structure of Pelvis

The pelvic organs are primarily innervated by parasympathetic nerves from $S_{3,\,4}$ and sympathetic nerves from T_{12}–L_2, and the testes are also considered to be innervated by the sacral nerves. Sympathetic nerves play an important role in the male reproductive system. Stimulation of the hypogastric nerves is known to cause contraction of the epididymis, vas deferens, seminal vesicles prostate, and bladder neck. Moreover, because of the importance of sympathetic nerves in sensory and neurogenic inflammation, they may also play an important role in the maintenance of urogenital pain in men. The sites with a rich sympathetic innervation (bladder neck, prostate, vas deferens, and epididymis) are all tissues that are prone to present hypersensitivity reactions in men. These findings provide positive implications for explaining the role of the central nervous system in the persistent pain of the male genital system and for differentiating between referred pain and organ-specific pain [12].

The pelvic floor consists of two functional layers: the deep layer of levator muscles (innervated by $S_{3,4}$ nerves) and the superficial layer (innervated by the S_2 nerve and pudendal nerves). These two layers of muscles can be clearly observed when the pelvic floor muscles contract due to the stimulation of different sacral nerves. Specifically, the relaxation or contraction of the levator muscles produces a marked deepening or flattening of the gluteal lines as the pelvic organs are pulled toward the pubic side. A bellows-like movement can also be seen in the perineum. The second functional layer of the pelvis is composed of all the muscles below the levator muscle layer, including the transverse muscles, the puborectalis, the bulbocavernosus, the urethral sphincter, and the superficial anal sphincter, which are innervated by the pudendal nerves, mainly originating from the S_2 nerve. Stimulation of the pudendal nerves produces anterior–posterior compression, like the movement of a pincer. The bellows-like movement and the pincer-like movement are very different from a functional point of view. Normally the two movements are mixed, whereas the bellows-like movement is more pronounced and easily recognizable in many pelvic pain syndromes where the two movements are separated from each other or relatively uncoordinated and are inharmonious with bladder movements

13.5.1.2 Key Role of the Central Nervous System in Persistent Pain

Just as tendonitis and myalgia are the result of inappropriate muscle activities, repetitive non-functional movements of the pelvic muscles can predispose them to neuroinflammatory chain reactions that include the central nervous system. These chain reactions include alterations in structure and transmission function within the CNS, increased dendritic switching on motor neurons, and enhanced responses of afferent neurons to a range of peripheral sensations. The maintenance of these related phenomena is achieved through the upregulation of the production of labile peptides within the spinal dorsal root ganglia and spinal dorsal horn (e.g., glutamatergic facilitation). Inappropriate convergence of information tends to produce a mixed-line phenomenon, splitting C-sensory fibers into two parts, which can produce the wind up in the laminae of the dorsal horn of the spinal cord, in the brainstem, and at other relevant central neural levels. Motor neurons finally receive enhanced afferent information from multiple sources. Further disruption of sensory processes, accompanied by excitatory neurotransmitter release and abnormal sympathetic reflex activity, ultimately leads to the formation of peripheral sensitized tissues, irritable urination, uncoordinated urination movements, and neurogenic inflammation within the sensitized tissues [3].

Sensitization of the receptive areas, wind-up phenomena, and regional generalization are typical responses of the central nervous system to nociceptive afferent information. Symptoms such as abnormal urethral sensation, referred pain, increased urinary frequency, and urgency are consistent with these alterations in the central nervous system. Similarly, as in the case of nociceptive hyperalgesia of the sphincter (localized pain), tenderness of the pelvic floor, motor tonicity, and ineffective uncoordinated movements, interrupting any of the normal pathways that ensure central coordination of pelvic floor muscle movements (e.g., absence of gate regulation) only enhances the lesions [8].

13.5.2 Clinical Manifestations

13.5.2.1 Abnormal Urinary Function

The symptoms of abnormal urinary function mainly include urgent and frequent urination, dribbling, urinary incontinence, and chronic urinary retention, and the causes include primary and secondary factors. The primary factors are mainly hypuria and frequent urination caused by prostate lesions. In addition, inflammatory lesions of the pelvic organs are also common primary causes of urinary dysfunction. Common secondary causes are sexual dysfunctions, such as impotence accompanied by testicular pain. Abnormalities in central neuromodulatory conduction are also a common secondary factor causing voiding dysfunction, such as urgent urination caused by excessive perception of bladder expansion, or frequent and urgent urination caused by stimulation of painful symptoms in the lower urinary tract [13, 14].

Most patients with pelvic pain with voiding dysfunction regard the pain and dyspareunia as a localized lesion and assume that the symptoms will be resolved by reasonable and necessary local surgical treatment. However, the fact is that the results of local surgical interventions are often unsatisfactory. A reasonable explanation of such results is that the mechanisms behind the pain and dyspareunia are not only due to local lesions, but that central nervous system facilitation may be involved and play an important role.

The mechanisms of CNS facilitation in patients with persistent pelvic pain have been described in detail earlier in this chapter, and it is important to emphasize here that, similar to persistent pelvic pain, CNS activation or facilitation imposes a significant impact on urinary function and the sensory nervous system.

13.5.2.2 Abnormality of Urodynamics

The vicious cycle of pain and functional abnormalities is often the multifactor result accumulated over years, but often only a single contributing factor is recognized. The massive transmission of information from inappropriate or somatic nociceptive stimuli can be very harmful to the sensitive central regulation of the voiding circuit and, over time, can affect the overall central regulation of the pelvic organs. Continuous or repeated harmful behaviors can gradually damage the normal gating role of the central nervous system, such as incorrect urinary postures and habits learned in childhood, frequent urinary holding, long-term body postural imbalances kept till adulthood, instruments during surgical examinations and procedures, and straining and psychological confusions. All these constitute the stressors of nociception, which eventually stimulate the neural component chain reactions that are normally parts of the traumatic tissue repair reactions, often accompanied by hypersensitivity of the lower urinary tract.

13.5.2.3 Hypersensitivity of Genitourinary System

Symptoms include localized tenderness and referred discomfort, primarily in the lower abdomen, pubic area, and medial femur, and to a lesser extent in the ribs, the feet, mandible, shoulders, and hands. Many diagnoses are unrelated to the patient's initial symptoms, and without proper evaluation, it will be difficult to discover the true causes of the symptoms [15].

13.5.3 Treatment

Chronic pelvic pain has been clearly implicated in multiple mechanisms as previously described, and therefore treatment requires a holistic plan that includes bio-psychological and social factors and active patient involvement. Three aspects can be considered: (1) treatment of pelvic floor dysfunction and reduction of psychological stress; (2) medication to reduce pain, anxiety, and muscle tension; and (3) surgical removal of definite lesions. All these aspects are important. Surgery is important but should not be the preferred treatment method. In fact, there are few indications for surgery for male urogenital pain, and it should only be planned when there is a theoretical hope of benefit. Testicular ligation, epididymectomy, prostatectomy, and nerve ligation must be carefully considered and decided if only for pain relief [16, 17].

There are a number of medications available, but the most commonly used are p-acetaminophen, nonsteroidal anti-inflammatory drugs (NSAIDs), opioid analgesics (e.g., oxycodone), tricyclic antidepressants (e.g., amitriptyline), anxiolytics (e.g., alprazolam), anticonvulsants (e.g., pregabalin), and alpha-adrenergic receptor antagonists (e.g., alfuzosin), as well as different combinations thereof. For using any of these drugs, the aim is to relieve pain and improve function. Regular titration and optimization of the drug dose should be considered, and if there is no benefit then the drug should be withdrawn. Alternatively, bupivacaine, ropivacaine, or lidocaine mixed with glucocorticoids may be considered and injected at specific sites once a week for 2–3 weeks. Concomitantly, local injections of botulinum toxin may be administered, but this approach requires experimental studies and is not yet definitive. Additional treatments include nerve blocks, transcutaneous electrical nerve stimulation (TENS), and neuromodulation [18–20].

13.6 Common Male Pelvic Pain Syndromes

13.6.1 Primary Prostate Pain Syndrome

Primary prostate pain syndrome (PPPS) is a condition of persistent or recurrent pain in the prostate region that occurs at least three times within 6 months, with pain on palpation of the prostate, without definite infection or other significant local pathological changes. It is usually associated with negative cognitive, behavioral, or emotional consequences and may be accompanied by clinical manifestations of lower urinary tract dysfunction or sexual dysfunction. According to the classification developed by the National Institute of Diabetes, Digestive and Kidney Diseases (NIDDK), prostatitis can be classified into five types: acute bacterial prostatitis (ABP), chronic bacterial prostatitis (CBP), PPPS, and asymptomatic inflammatory prostatitis [21]. PPPS is a noninflammatory pelvic pain syndrome with significant urinary symptoms and pelvic floor muscle tension pain, but a normal prostate on rectal examination and a culture of sterile specimens from prostate-specific specimens (i.e., semen, prostatic secretions, and urine collected after prostate massage) are associated with significant or nonsignificant white blood cell counts.

Epidemiologically, there is very limited information on the true prevalence of PPPS in the population. Because symptoms are so similar to other conditions (e.g., benign prostatic hyperplasia syndrome and painful bladder syndrome), a case definition based solely on symptoms may not reflect the true prevalence of PPPS.

13.6.1.1 Pathogenesis

No single etiological explanation has been found, and most believe that this condition may occur in susceptible populations exposed to one or more triggering factors. Several potential triggering factors have been proposed, including infectious, genetic, anatomical, neuromuscular, endocrine, immune (including autoimmune), or psychological mechanisms [2]. These factors may lead to a peripheral autoimmune inflammatory state and/or neurogenic injury that produces acute and chronic pain [22]. Sensitization of the peripheral and central nervous systems may explain why significant tissue damage is not usually found in PPPS. There is increasing evidence that altered plasticity of the peripheral and central nervous systems, that is, neuropathological changes, is an important etiology of PPPS. There are several theories as to the possible mechanisms by which PPPS arises.

Theories of Spastic Pain in Pelvic Floor Muscle Groups

In urodynamic studies of patients with painful chronic prostatitis, decreased maximum and mean urinary flow rates were found with abnormally high maximum urethral closure pressures. Partial incomplete relaxation of the urethra to the external urethral sphincter in the bladder neck and prostate, and varying degrees of bladder and/or urethral muscle dysfunction, which have no difference between patients with and without evidence of chronic prostatitis, suggest that pathological changes in the prostate itself are not necessarily the direct cause of pain, and that some patients can be treated with prostate and/or pelvic floor massage. Therefore, many scholars believe that the pain of chronic prostatitis may be essentially a spastic pain in the pelvic floor muscles [23]. The pain is a reflexive, spasmodic pain of the pelvic floor perineal muscles caused by the stimulation of the prostate through the spinal reflex, pelvic floor muscle spasm, and/or bladder neck dysfunction; this increases the pressure in the urethra of the prostate during urination, leading to urine reflux in the prostate, thus causing "chemical prostatitis" that induce a vicious cycle of pelvic floor muscle dysfunction and prostatitis. PPPS patients have obvious mental and psychological disorders, such as anxiety and depression, and somatic tension. As a result, systemic autonomic dysfunction occurs, leading to or aggravating posterior urethral neuromuscular dysfunction. Continuous physical and psychological stimulations can cause elevated muscle tone and muscle spasm, and reduced muscle blood supply. Tense muscle activity in turn leads to the accumulation of metabolites such as potassium, lactate, histamine, and kinins. Ischemia and increased metabolites in turn lead to intensified pain, creating a vicious cycle of pain and pelvic floor muscle dysfunction. Therefore, spasm of the pelvic floor muscle groups may be both a cause and a consequence of PPPS [24].

Theory of Neurogenic Inflammation

Recently, it has been suggested that neurogenic inflammation plays an important role in the development of prostate pain. Studies have shown that stimulation of sensory nerve fibers in the proximal spinal cord can lead to both cis-conduction of impulses to spinal sensory neurons and simultaneous reverse conduction to the periphery, and when the reverse impulse reaches activated primary injury receptors, the nerve endings release neuropeptides (e.g., substance P, kinin) that induce neurogenic inflammation and local hyperalgesia [25]. The presence of neurogenic inflammation was confirmed by electrical stimulation of the prostate, which revealed that the vasodilatation and plasma exudation in the perineum of the painful patients were more pronounced than in the control group. The distribution of neurogenic plasma exudation on the body surface was found to be similar to the clinical site of prostate pain, mainly located in the L_5–S_1 dermatomes, using capsaicin to stimulate the bladder and prostate; thus, prostate pain is closely related to neurogenic inflammation was proved.

Cytokines Theory

Cytokines are associated with the production of pain in prostate inflammation [26]. Nerve growth factor (NGF) increases the sensitivity of the body to injurious stimuli by participating in the regulation of gene and protein expression. During tissue inflammation, NGF released by fibroblasts and Schwann cells stimulates the release of histamine from mast cells, which acts directly on peripheral sensory nerve endings and increases their excitability. NGF upregulates the expression of substance P expression, and increased release of substance P at peripheral and central endings accelerates the production of hyperalgesia. Tissue injury and inflammation can activate immune cells to release large amounts of cytokines such as IL-1, IL-6, and TNF, which upregulate the release of substance P by stimulating the synthesis of NGF. Studies have reported that in patients with prostate pain, the level of NGF in semen is significantly elevated and positively correlated with the level of pain. Thus, feedback regulation can be formed between cytokines and neuropeptides, and participate in the formation and maintenance of chronic pain. Oxygen-free radicals, histamine, and prostaglandins may also play a role in the mechanism of pain development, while specific mechanisms remain unknown [22].

Mechanism of Referred Pain

Studies have shown that visceral and somatic primary sensory afferent information from the pelvic region converges directly or indirectly in the L_5–S_1 joint nucleus neurons, and that the neurons receiving nociceptive afferents from the prostate and perineum overlap or cross over significantly in the spinal cord, which constitutes the anatomical basis for referred pain in prostatitis [27, 28]. In prostatitis, referred pain in the perineum can develop through the visceral–somatic–visceral reflex. An important feature of prostatitis is that the pain cannot be treated effectively with persistent medical treatment, which is associated with a long and slow accumulation of central neuronal excitability. Repeated stimulation of C-fibers by inflammation increases afferent excitement and thus raises activity in the posterior horn of the spinal cord. Moreover, this accumulation of stimulation causes a decrease in the excitability threshold of neurons in the posterior horn of the spinal cord and a significant increase in the number of spontaneous active cells. The decrease in the threshold of nociception and the altered excitability of neurons in the posterior horn of the spinal cord may be important causes of hyperalgesia and spontaneous pain. This could explain the persistence of pain in many patients despite the absence of inflammatory manifestations in the prostatic fluid after treatment. Thus, in patients with prostate pain, both the visceral–somatic and visceral–visceral reflexes of the spinal cord can cause referred pain in the pubic area and other areas of the perineum.

In conclusion, considering the complex etiology, the pathogenesis of prostatitis is still not well understood. The association between different pathogens and prostatitis, the immune status of prostatitis patients, the existence of susceptibility genes in prostatitis patients, and the association between prostatitis and neuroinflammation all need to be studied further.

13.6.1.2 Clinical Manifestation

Prostate pain is prevalent in young and middle-aged men who have nonspecific symptoms of prostatitis, but usually have no history of urinary tract infection [29]. Pain is the main clinical manifestation of PPPS. And it is also the main reason why patients visit the hospital and the most important factor affecting their quality of life. The main symptoms include recurrent episodes of pain in the perineum, penis, scrotum, and retropubic area unrelated to urination. The pain is not located in the prostate, resembling referred pain; patients have manifestations of prostatitis from mild, moderate to severe, and few have clear pathogens of infection [29]. The majority of patients with prostate pain have varying degrees of emotional impairment and abnormal psychosocial experiences, suggesting that psychosocial factors play an important role in the pathogenesis of prostate pain. Several studies have demonstrated that patients with prostate pain have more concern and anxiety about physical discomfort and pain than normal people, and have overly stressful behavioral patterns [9].

13.6.1.3 Diagnosis

PPPS lacks objective signs; thus, the diagnostic process is actually a differential diagnosis, that is, a systematic and comprehensive examination of patients with symptoms of prostatitis, to rule out bacterial prostatitis and nonbacterial prostatitis that may cause confusion with PPPS, as well as some other less common diseases such as IC, carcinoma in situ of the bladder, and osteomyelitis pubis.

13.6.1.4 Differential Diagnosis

The symptoms of ABP are typical and may not be easily confused with PPPS.

The symptoms of PPPS, CBP, and chronic nonbacterial prostatitis (CNBP) are very similar, with patients complaining of irritating symptoms such as difficult and painful urination, frequent daytime urination, and increased enuresis nocturna, the severity of which can vary over time. In the case of CBP and CNBP, the leukocytes on microscopic examination of prostatic fluid are ≧ 10/HP, while in patients with PPPS, the leukocytes in prostate fluid are <10/HP, prostatic fluid and urine sediment are free of bacteria, and the urine culture is negative. CBP patients, on the other hand, may have abnormally high white blood cells on routine microscopy, bacteria on urine sediment microscopy, and bacterial growth on urine culture due to the possible presence of bacteriuria. The symptomatic relief from the antibiotic therapy or other nonspecific treatments in the medical history is an important reference for the diagnosis and differential diagnosis of PPPS [20]. Most CBP patients treated with antibiotics have their symptoms completely relieved due to the clearance of bacteria from the urine and is not related to bacteriological changes in the prostate infection. However, if the treatment is not complete, the infection can recur within months. Some CNBP and PPPS can be relieved with antibiotic therapy. Unlike CBP, however, these symptoms' relief is transient or similar to that of poorly treated CNBP. CNBP or PPPS often responds better to nonspecific treatment [30].

IC and carcinoma in situ of the bladder can sometimes present symptoms similar to those of PPPS. Through history, physical examination, and prostatic fluid analysis, if IC and carcinoma in situ of the bladder cannot be excluded or suggested, cystoscopy and/or tissue examination and urine exfoliation cytology can be considered to help the differentiation.

In assessing and diagnosing PPPS, the European Urological Association gave the following evidence and recommendations in 2014 [31].

1. Conclusions
   (a) PPPS is associated with negative cognitive, behavioral, sexual, or emotional consequences and may be accompanied by clinical manifestations of lower urinary tract or sexual dysfunction.
   (b) PPPS has no known single etiology.
   (c) Pain in PPPS involves mechanisms of neuroplasticity and neuropathic pain.
   (d) PPPS has a significant impact on quality of life.
   (e) Depression and catastrophic thinking are associated with more pain and poorer adjustment.
   (f) Population-based studies (>2%) have shown a high prevalence of PPPS-like symptoms.
   (g) There are reliable tools to assess symptom severity and phenotypic differences.
2. Recommendations
   (a) Diagnostic procedures for the patient should be adopted. Specific diseases with similar symptoms must be excluded.
   (b) Validated symptom and quality-of-life scoring instruments (e.g., NIH-CPSI)

should be considered for initial assessment and follow-up.

(c) Assessment of negative cognitive, behavioral, sexual, or emotional consequences associated with PPPS, as well as lower urinary tract symptoms and sexual dysfunction, is recommended.

13.6.1.5 Treatment

The pathogenesis of prostate pain has not been fully elucidated, so there is no specific treatment. The general principles of treatment are avoiding triggering factors, reducing patient pain, treating both mind and body, and preventing recurrence of the disease. In most patients, symptomatic treatment is the main concern, and the management and treatment of complications should be considered at the same time.

The recommended treatments are that for patients with PPPS who suffer from the pain for less than a year, α-blockers are effective treating drugs and using antibiotics alone for 6 weeks also works; and using high-dose sulfated polysaccharide to improve quality-of-life scores and symptoms is recommended. Other medications and treatments such as NSAID, phytotherapy, perineal extracorporeal shock wave therapy, acupuncture with electric stimulation, PTNS, and psychological therapy specific to pain are recommended as well, but their adverse effects should be measured and balanced.

13.6.2 Bladder Pain Syndrome/ Interstitial Cystitis

Bladder pain syndrome/interstitial cystitis (BPS/IC) is a chronic inflammatory bladder disease characterized by irritable excretion, pain in the pubic arch or pelvis, and the absence of detectable bacteria in the urine. The prevalence of IC in women with chronic pelvic pain is as high as 38%, and other studies also report a high incidence of IC, indicating that the possibility of IC should be considered seriously when patients have pelvic pain [32]. For patients with bladder pain, BPS is a more accurate descriptive diagnostic term. Thus, IC belongs to a specific type of chronic bladder inflammation, whereas BPS refers to perceived pain in the bladder region and is a more accurate term to be used in this section.

13.6.2.1 Definition and Overview

The history of IC becoming a separate pathological type can be traced back to 1878, when Skene first described an inflammatory condition that "damages part or all of the bladder mucosa and even invades the muscular layer of the bladder" [33]. In 1978, Walsh introduced the concept of "hemorrhagic spots" to describe the cystoscopic findings of bleeding and petechiae in the bladder wall [33]. Caucasian women are the main population group of IC, the diagnosis of which is usually based on clinical symptoms, cystoscopy, and bladder biopsy. The diagnosis of BPS/IC must include signs of bladder irritation with pain in the bladder region, such as daytime or nocturnal dysuria, and exclude other confounding etiologies.

13.6.2.2 Etiology and Pathophysiology

Although more than 100 years have passed since the first diagnosis of BPS/IC, its exact etiology still remains unknown. The known pathogenesis includes infection, inflammation, autoimmune mechanisms, defects in the uroepithelial glucosaminoglycan layer, hypoxia, and central nervous system. Multiple studies have confirmed the involvement of neurogenic inflammation in causing BPS followed by altered neuroplasticity and neuronal sensitization of the peripheral and central nervous system in patients with BPS. Some clinical and histopathological features are similar to autoimmune phenomena [22]. However, autoantibodies, immune deposits, or complement activation are rarely seen.

13.6.2.3 Diagnosis

The diagnosis of IC should be excluded diagnosis, which is based on history, clinical symptoms, tests, and exclusion of other possible causes. While the diagnosis of BPS is based on bladder-related pain, pressure or discomfort with at least one other symptom, such as increased white size and/or nocturnal frequency, and excludes confounding conditions.

Patients who present at the hospitals often have prolonged clinical symptoms and a history of recurrent episodes, and antibiotic treatment is not effective. The nature of the pain is key to the definition of the disease. BPS/IC pain is a bladder-related pain with pressure or discomfort increasing with bladder contents, located on pubis, and sometimes radiating to the groin, vagina, rectum, or sacrum; it is eliminated by emptying bladder but soon reappears and may be aggravated by eating or drinking.

The typical symptoms of IC are suprapubic pain associated with filling of bladder, frequent and urgent urination, and increased enuresis nocturna, but without urge incontinence; and pelvic floor pain, including urethrovaginal irritation or vaginal pain in women and perineal pain in men, which is relieved after urination. Some of these patients will have predominantly painful symptoms with little or no urinary tract symptoms, while others will have bladder-related symptoms without pain [13, 14].

According to the Guidelines for the Treatment of IC, patients who are suspected to have IC should receive tests of urinalysis, urine culture, and urine cytology. The purpose of urinalysis and urine culture is mainly to exclude urinary tract infections. Even if urinary tract infections are present, if there are severe bladder pain symptoms between two infections, IC cannot be excluded. Lower urine pH value may cause BPS. Urine cytology is used primarily for excluding urinary epithelial tumors, especially extensive carcinoma in situ of the bladder, which is the most common reason leading to bladder pain. If urine cytology is not reliable, random biopsy of the bladder mucosa may be an alternative. In addition, the guidelines categorize cystoscopy as an elective test, mainly for random biopsy of the bladder mucosa, especially in the elderly. Cystoscopy can detect IC, and along with hydrodilation under anesthesia, can exclude other local lesions of the bladder and urethra, such as cystitis tuberculosa, eosinophilic cystitis, urethral diverticula, and tumors. Potassium sensitivity test is recommended for those specific patients to diagnose whether the moderate bladder pain is of bladder origin. And patients with a positive test result can be referred to predict the efficacy of mucosal protective drugs. In addition, bladder hydrodilation is also recommended for special patients. Erythema is the traditional criterion for IC diagnosis, but it needs to be combined with clinical symptoms. Random biopsies can be performed at the same time. It showed that 60–70% of patients have postoperative pain relief, which helps build patient confidence, but the efficiency rate at 6 months is the same as placebo. If the symptoms can be relieved to some extent after hydrodilation, it is beneficial to the next step of treatment, and immediately starting medical treatment after hydrodilation achieves better effects. Bladder mucosal biopsy is recommended for those patients with a high suspicion of bladder pathology and can exclude other localized bladder pathologies causing bladder pain and other symptoms similar to IC [11, 13].

In addition, certain features of the inflammation of the interstitial tissue, including the bladder muscle layer, may help in the choice of treatments. Bladder mucosal biopsy is recommended for severe symptoms with poor outcomes or in the elderly. According to the NIDDK diagnostic criteria, filling cytometry is one of the necessary tests to know the patient's bladder volume, that is, IC can be ruled out if the bladder volume is more than 350 mL or more than 150 mL without urgent urination. Evidence suggests the possible presence of a hypo-compliant bladder, such as an intravenous pyelography (IVP), indicating an altered bladder volume pattern or possible impairment of upper urinary tract function due to a bladder lesion.

13.6.2.4 Treatment

Because the pathogenesis is not clearly defined, the majority of patients are treated with strategies for relieving clinical symptoms, including education and self-care, oral medication, intravesical instillation therapy, and neuromodulation.

13.6.3 Scrotal Pain Syndrome

Scrotal pain syndrome (SPS) is persistent or recurrent episodes of pain within the scrotal organ and may be associated with symptoms of urethral or sexual dysfunction without definite infection or other significant local pathological changes. Scrotal pain syndrome is usually associated with negative cognitive, behavioral, sexual, or emotional consequences and symptoms indicating lower urinary tract and sexual dysfunctions. Scrotal pain syndrome is a general concept referring to pain without a definite site, being either in the testes or epididymis. The pain is not felt on the skin of the scrotum, but in its contents [34].

The pathogenesis of chronic scrotal pain is varied and in most cases unknown. Pain in the scrotum can be classified as direct pain confined to the scrotum or referred pain from other parts or systems of the body. Direct pain is located in the testes, epididymis, inguinal nerve, or vas deferens.

13.6.3.1 Diagnosis

Patients suffering from scrotal pain must take physical examinations. Light palpation of all parts of the scrotum can identify lumps and painful spots. The rectal examination can inspect prostate abnormalities and the pelvic floor muscles. Scrotal ultrasound (US) is of limited value in finding the cause of pain in more than 80% of patients whose US does not show clinically significant abnormalities. However, if the results of physical examinations are normal, US can still be performed to ensure that the patient does not have pathologic changes that require surgical treatments. US can be used to diagnose scrotal effusions, seminomas, and varicocele when abnormalities such as cysts are found and may facilitate the treatment decisions.

13.6.3.2 Treatment

The treatment of chronic scrotal pain is based on the principles of treating chronic pain syndromes. Consideration of surgical treatment should be preceded by multidisciplinary pain management strategies, including nonsurgical treatment, which may delay the need for surgeries or even make surgeries unnecessary [18]. For nonsurgical treatments, in addition to medication, myofasciitis treatment by a professional physiotherapist should be considered [19]. Pelvic floor muscles should be tested as excessive contraction is often found, which means adequate relaxation is needed. Pelvic hypermobility should be treated with physical therapy. More specific myofascial trigger points are located in the pelvic floor and are also seen in the lower abdominal muscle tissues. Treatments involve applying pressure to the trigger points and stretching the muscles [24].

13.6.4 Urethral Pain Syndrome

Urethral pain syndrome (UPS) is a chronic or recurrent pain in the urethra without infection or other obvious local pathological changes. UPS is usually associated with negative cognitive behaviors, sexual or emotional consequences and symptoms suggesting lower urinary tract, sexual behavior, bowel, or gynecological dysfunctions. UPS can occur in both men and women.

In terms of pathogenesis, there is no clear pathogenetic mechanism for the UPS. The close relationship between the urethra and the bladder (both covered with uroepithelium) makes them have the same pathological changes. The pathological changes similar to those of BPS are found in the urethra. Therefore, the classification of UPS refers to that of BPS. Apparently, the etiology that causes BPS may also be the cause of urethral pain. It is currently believed that the basic mechanism of BPS is also applicable to UPS since the pain is also induced by epithelial leakage. Another possible mechanism is neurological hypersensitivity following urinary tract infection. The symptoms recorded in patients with UPS can also be classified as so-called pain in other organs or in the myofascial system. Referred pain is important.

There are no specific recommended treatments for UPS, which should be multidisciplinary and multimodal [18]. Laser treatment of the germarium may be a specific treatment approach. Most publications on the treatment of UPS have come from psychologists. In a 2007 treatment review, Kaur and Arunkalaivanan concluded that the best treatment method is "behavioral therapy, including biofeedback, meditation, bladder retraining and hypnosis," which have been successful [35]. Baldoni et al. reported a high incidence of anxiety and depression in patients with UPS and the worsening stress-related symptoms [36, 37]. They described how psychotherapy "in some cases" enables patients to recognize the "emotional meaning" of their urinary problems, leading to physical and psychological improvement. This may mean exposure to emotional conflicts or similar effects, and the psychological disorder is one of the etiologies of urethral pain.

References

1. Hakenberg OW, Wirth MP. Chronic pelvic pain in men. Urol Int. 2002;68(3):138–43. https://doi.org/10.1159/000048438.
2. Sandhu J, Tu HYV. Recent advances in managing chronic prostatitis/chronic pelvic pain syndrome. F1000Res. 2017;6:F1000 Faculty Rev–1747. https://doi.org/10.12688/f1000research.10558.1.
3. Harte SE, Harris RE, Clauw DJ. The neurobiology of central sensitization. J Appl Behav Res. 2018;23:e12137. https://doi.org/10.1111/jabr.12137.
4. Cervero F, Laird JMA. Spinal Mechanisms of Visceral Pain and Hyperalgesia. In: Malcangio M, editor. Synaptic Plasticity in Pain. New York, NY: Springer; 2009. https://doi.org/10.1007/978-1-4419-0226-9_13.
5. Bardoni R. Serotonergic Modulation of Nociceptive Circuits in Spinal Cord Dorsal Horn. Curr Neuropharmacol. 2019;17(12):1133–45. https://doi.org/10.2174/1570159X17666191001123900.
6. Westlund KN. Visceral nociception. Curr Rev. Pain. 2000;4(6):478–87. https://doi.org/10.1007/s11916-000-0072-9.
7. Rotman JA, Kierans AS, Lo G, Gavlin A, Guniganti P. Imaging of chronic male pelvic pain: what the abdominal imager should know. Abdom Radiol (NY). 2020;45(7):1961–72. https://doi.org/10.1007/s00261-019-02353-0.
8. Grundy D. Neuroanatomy of visceral nociception: vagal and splanchnic afferent. Gut. 2002;51 Suppl 1(Suppl 1):i2–5. https://doi.org/10.1136/gut.51.suppl_1.i2.
9. Maniam J, Antoniadis C, Morris MJ. Early-Life Stress, HPA Axis Adaptation, and Mechanisms Contributing to Later Health Outcomes. Front Endocrinol (Lausanne). 2014;5:73. https://doi.org/10.3389/fendo.2014.00073.
10. Cerruto MA. Chronic Pelvic Pain and Chronic Pelvic Pain Syndrome: Classification and Epidemiology. In: Giammò A, Biroli A, editors. Chronic Pelvic Pain and Pelvic Dysfunctions. Urodynamics, Neurourology and Pelvic Floor Dysfunctions. Cham: Springer; 2021. https://doi.org/10.1007/978-3-030-56387-5_4.
11. Chronic Pelvic Pain Guidelines. EAU. (2022). Retrieved from https://uroweb.org/guidelines/chronic-pelvic-pain/summary-of-changes/2022
12. Baranowski AP. Urogenital/pelvic pain in men. Curr Opin Support Palliat Care. 2012;6(2):213–9. https://doi.org/10.1097/SPC.0b013e3283523f19.
13. Kim SJ, Kim KH. Clinical approach to recurrent voiding dysfunction, dysuria, and pelvic pain persisting for at least 3 months. Int Neurourol J. 2022;26(3):179–89. https://doi.org/10.5213/inj.2244200.100.
14. Stabholz Y, Sandhu JS. Management of voiding dysfunction associated with pelvic malignancies. Int J Urol. 2021;28(1):17–24. https://doi.org/10.1111/iju.14405.
15. Polackwich AS, Shoskes DA. Chronic prostatitis/chronic pelvic pain syndrome: a review of evaluation and therapy. Prostate Cancer Prostatic Dis. 2016;19(2):132–8. https://doi.org/10.1038/pcan.2016.8.
16. Moise G, Capodice JL, Winfree CJ. Treatment of chronic pelvic pain in men and women. Expert Rev. Neurother. 2007;7(5):507–20. https://doi.org/10.1586/14737175.7.5.507.
17. Franco JV, Turk T, Jung JH, Xiao YT, Iakhno S, Garrote V, Vietto V. Non-pharmacological interventions for treating chronic prostatitis/chronic pelvic pain syndrome. Cochrane Database Syst Rev. 2018;1(1):CD012551. https://doi.org/10.1002/14651858.CD012551.
18. Magistro G, Wagenlehner FM, Grabe M, et al. Contemporary Management of Chronic Prostatitis/Chronic Pelvic Pain Syndrome. Eur Urol. 2016;69(2):286–97. https://doi.org/10.1016/j.eururo.2015.08.061.
19. Burzynski B, Jurys T, Burzynski K, Cempa K, Paradysz A. Physiotherapeutic assessment and management of chronic pelvic pain syndrome: A case report. Medicine (Baltimore). 2021;100(15):e25525. https://doi.org/10.1097/MD.0000000000025525.
20. Pena VN, Engel N, Gabrielson AT, et al. Diagnostic and Management Strategies for Patients with Chronic Prostatitis and Chronic Pelvic Pain Syndrome. Drugs Aging. 2021;38:845–86. https://doi.org/10.1007/s40266-021-00890-2.
21. https://www.niddk.nih.gov/health-information/urologic-diseases/prostate-problems/prostatitis-inflammation-prostate
22. Chen L, Zhang M, Liang C. Chronic Prostatitis and Pelvic Pain Syndrome: Another Autoimmune Disease? Arch Immunol Ther Exp (Warsz). 2021;69(1):24. https://doi.org/10.1007/s00005-021-00628-3.

23. Murphy AB, Macejko A, Taylor A, Nadler RB. Chronic prostatitis: management strategies. Drugs. 2009;69(1):71–84. https://doi.org/10.2165/00003495-200,969,010-00005.
24. Cohen D, Gonzalez J, Goldstein I. The Role of Pelvic Floor Muscles in Male Sexual Dysfunction and Pelvic Pain. Sex Med Rev. 2016 Jan;4(1):53–62. https://doi.org/10.1016/j.sxmr.2015.10.001.
25. Matsuda M, Huh Y, Ji RR. Roles of inflammation, neurogenic inflammation, and neuroinflammation in pain. J Anesth. 2019;33(1):131–9. https://doi.org/10.1007/s00540-018-2579-4.
26. Jang TL, Schaeffer AJ. The role of cytokines in prostatitis. World J Urol. 2003;21:95–9. https://doi.org/10.1007/s00345-003-0335-2.
27. Udit S, Blake K, Chiu IM. Somatosensory and autonomic neuronal regulation of the immune response. Nat Rev. Neurosci. 2022;23:157–71. https://doi.org/10.1038/s41583-021-00555-4.
28. Sengupta JN. Visceral pain: the neurophysiological mechanism. Handb Exp Pharmacol. 2009;194:31–74. https://doi.org/10.1007/978-3-540-79,090-7_2.
29. Potts JM. Chronic pelvic pain syndrome: a non-prostatocentric perspective. World J Urol. 2003;21(2):54–6. https://doi.org/10.1007/s00345-003-0327-2. Epub 2003 Apr 4
30. Rees J, Abrahams M, Doble A, Cooper A. Diagnosis and treatment of chronic bacterial prostatitis and chronic prostatitis/chronic pelvic pain syndrome: a consensus guideline. BJU Int. 2015;116:509–25. https://doi.org/10.1111/bju.13101.
31. https://uroweb.org/guidelines/chronic-pelvic-pain/chapter/diagnostic-evaluation
32. Clemons JL, Arya LA, Myers DL. Diagnosing interstitial cystitis in women with chronic pelvic pain. Obstet Gynecol. 2002;200:337–41.
33. Meijlink JM. Interstitial cystitis and the painful bladder: a brief history of nomenclature, definitions and criteria. Int J Urol. 2014;21(Suppl 1):4–12. https://doi.org/10.1111/iju.12307.
34. Moubasher A, Waqar M, Raison N, Brunckhorst O, Ahmed K. A Review of the Management of Chronic Scrotal Pain. Cureus. 2020;12(12):e11979. https://doi.org/10.7759/cureus.11979.
35. Kaur H, Arunkalaivanan AS. Urethral pain syndrome and its management. Obstet Gynecol Surv. 2007;62(5):348–51; quiz 353–4. https://doi.org/10.1097/01.ogx.0000261645.12099.2a.
36. Baldoni F, Baldaro B, Ercolani M, Emili E, Trombini G. Urethral syndrome: a study in psychosomatic urology. Psychother Psychosom. 1989;52(1–3):114–8. https://doi.org/10.1159/000288310.
37. Baldoni F, Ercolani M, Baldaro B, Trombini G. Stressful events and psychological symptoms in patients with functional urinary disorders. Percept Mot Skills. 1995;80(2):605–6. http://www.ncbi.nlm.nih.gov/entrez/query.fcgi?cmd=Retrieve&db=PubMed&dopt=Citation&list_uids=7,675,600

14 Visceral Cancer Pain

Ming Xia

Visceral cancer pain is very commonly seen in patients with cancer who are often unable to clearly express the nature of the pain, but the pain is difficult to tolerate. Visceral pain is not caused exclusively by internal organs, or associated with internal injuries, but it is often involved in other areas, as the pain is diffuse and difficult to locate.

Visceral pain can be a concomitant symptom of strong motor and autonomic reflexes. All forms of visceral pain are vaguely localized, and most patients feel a significantly larger area of pain than the original visceral area. Moreover, when the pain is intense, the area of the torso where the pain is felt is larger. This suggests that the representative areas of visceral organs in the central nervous system are not very precise.

In this chapter, visceral cancer pain is introduced from the perspectives of its causes, clinical manifestations, epidemiology, and treatment.

14.1 Causes of Visceral Cancer Pain and its Clinical Manifestations

Most often observed in patients with tumors in their abdominal or pelvic organs, visceral cancer pain accounts for about 28% of cancer pain (the other type, cancer pain of the skeletal system, accounts for about 42%) [1]. Cancer pain can also originate from cavernous or substantial organ damage caused by malignant tumors of the thoracic organs. Cancer pain in the abdominal cavity is mainly caused by primary or metastatic tumors invading the abdominal or pelvic viscera, as well as pain caused by somatosensory nerves in the abdominal cavity. There is a great deal of complexity in its clinical manifestations, causes, and mechanisms.

Symptoms of abdominal tumors or concomitant abdominal diseases can result in pain sensations due to mechanical stimulation, including twisting and pulling of the mesentery, dilation of the hollow viscera, stretching of the plasma membrane, or compression of certain organs. When pressure in hollow organs surpasses a certain threshold, pain can be felt in their lumens. Pain can result, for example, from obstructions or inflammation in the bile duct or pancreatic duct, both of which result in an increase in blood pressure and the release of pain mediators. A biliary obstruction or distension can cause epigastric pain. It may also be exacerbated by medically derived inmates such as morphine, which can cause spasms of the biliary sphincter, causing pain. Patients may also be experiencing empty stomachs and vomiting leaves. Due to morphine's ability to dilate the biliary system, it can also lower the threshold of pain perception. As a result of smooth muscle contractions, mesenteric traction, and intestinal ischemia, patients with

M. Xia (✉)
Department of Anesthesiology, Shanghai Ninth People's Hospital, Shanghai Jiao Tong University School of Medicine, Shanghai, China
e-mail: xiaming1980@xzhmu.edu.cn

M. Xia et al. (eds.), *Visceral Pain*, https://doi.org/10.1007/978-981-99-9167-9_14

abdominal or pelvic tumors can experience abdominal pain. The dislodged cancerous embolus can cause obstruction of the bladder or bowel due to tumor invasion of the rectum or bladder. In addition to neuropathic pain, patients with pelvic tumors may also experience pain in the iliopsoas muscle, the lumbosacral plexus, and the anterior sacrum. In advanced stages of tumors, visceral malignancies often spread to invade the pleura or peritoneum, producing localized pain in more superficial body organs.

The diffuse and milder visceral pain in early stages of cancer arises from the nature of visceral nerve afferents to the spinal cord. Probably, due to higher pain stimulus perception thresholds, viscera are relatively insensitive to nociception and require adequate and specific stimulation, and some visceral organs are insensitive to damage and usually do not show clinical manifestations until late in the tumor. Only when the tumor involves structures innervated by somatic nerves, such as the mural peritoneum, can there be a clearer localization of pain, because the dorsal horn neurons of the spinal cord receive afferent signals from both visceral and somatic nerves. Because of the scattered distribution of visceral afferent nerves in the spinal cord, visceral pain is dull and difficult to localize exactly, so the pain site of cancerous visceral pain is hardly directly related to visceral damage.

Although visceral pain cannot be classified as neuropathic pain under the new definition (the definition of neuropathic pain given by IASP is limited to somatosensory system) [2], when the tumor invades the visceral plexus, especially the thoracoabdominal wall and other somatic nerve regions, the patient's pain can still have distinct neuropathic pain characteristics. Therefore, cancer visceral pain is a mixture of injury-receptive pain and neuropathic pain. In fact, it is difficult to distinguish visceral cancer pain as neuropathic pain or injury-receptive pain. A study by IASP showed that 72% of people with visceral cancer pain were neuropathic in origin.

In addition, when certain visceral and somatic sites share sensory nerve afferents to the same dorsal horn neurons of the spinal cord, the pain of these visceral sites can be localized to the corresponding somatic site, that is, referred pain. Often, visceral cancer pain is misdiagnosed as lesions in other parts of the body due to involvement pain or tumor invasion of the thoracoabdominal wall [3, 4]. Common referred pains include abdominal back pain in the case of pancreatic cancer and right shoulder pain in the case of liver tumors, gallbladder tumors, or liver metastases. Visceral tumors may also have indirect effects, such as abdominal distension caused by a large subdiaphragmatic tumor that can irritate the diaphragm, thus causing right shoulder pain and spacing. These phenomena help explain some of the phenomena that occur when nerve blocks are performed for abdominal cancer pain and the response of cancerous visceral pain to analgesic drugs. Ineffective or partial failure of abdominal or infra-abdominal plexus block may be due to metastasis of the tumor that has exceeded the innervation of the abdominal plexus, such as pain caused by tumor invasion of the mural peritoneum, retroperitoneal lymph node metastasis, or bone metastasis.

Visceral cancer pain can also be caused by tumor treatment, such as visceral pain after tumor surgery, pain caused by chemotherapy drugs, tissue damage caused by radiotherapy, or visceral pain caused by mediator treatment such as embolization [5]. Pelvic tumors or pelvic radiation therapy can produce progressive pelvic and perineal pain, as well as other complications, including ureteral obstruction and obstruction of lymphatic and venous return. Embolization therapy for liver tumors can also cause pain.

The relationship and interactions between cancer pain production and tumor development are very complex, and the etiology and mechanisms of pain production often vary greatly among patients with cancer pain. In recent years, new perspectives on the biology of pain caused by tumor invasion have emerged. Cancer pain is increasingly considered to be the result of interactions between tumor cells and the host immune system and the peripheral central nervous system. In contrast to previous perceptions, the nervous system may be an important participant in the production of cancer pain, for example, squamous cell carcinoma secretes high levels of nerve growth factor (NGF), and the use of anti-NGF antibodies may alleviate cancer pain.

Visceral cancer pain is usually progressively worse. Although pain can strike at any time during the course of the disease, generally the more severe the cancer progresses, the more intense the pain suffered by the patient, and without effective intervention, the pain often remains with the patient until death. In addition, as the disease progresses, the original pain can be chronic and become chronic and persistent, while the newly occurred pain can be acute pain or acute aggravation on the basis of chronic pain [6], such as pathological fracture and severe pain caused by spasm or obstruction of cavity organs: therefore, cancer visceral pain is also characterized by the coexistence of acute pain and chronic pain.

Even if the underlying pain of cancer patients is adequately treated with medication, including the use of strong opioids, patients may still experience acute, sudden, and severe pain (break through pain). Breakthrough pain is a frequent clinical problem for cancer patients, and studies have shown that the incidence of breakthrough pain in cancer patients can be as high as 19–95% [7]. It can occur spontaneously or can be triggered by various factors. It is the worst part of cancer pain treatment and is also the focus and difficulty of cancer pain treatment. The European Association for Palliative Care (EAPC) classify it as one of the core indicators for cancer assessment and guidance [8].

Most patients with cancer pain have pain that is more pronounced at night, the cause of which is unknown. Similar to other cancer pains, visceral cancer pain is characterized by nocturnal resting pain. The impact of nocturnal pain is that the patient's sleep is directly disturbed, and thus, the impact on quality of life is more pronounced.

14.2 Current Treatment of Cancer Pain

Cancer pain is the most important factor affecting the quality of life of patients with malignant tumors, especially those with mid- to late-stage malignant tumors, and pain becomes more frequently progressive with the development of malignant tumors, with one-third of reports stating that 60–80% of patients with advanced cancers have cancer pain. Tumor growth and metastasis can cause pain in any organ.

Previously, pain was treated as a symptom only and was not taken seriously except to guide diagnosis and treatment. Now we recognize that pain can cause pathophysiological changes. Chronic pain causes neurological alterations that increase the intensity of pain and diminish the effectiveness of treatment and is therefore defined as a disease. In other words, some intractable pain is actually medical in origin, the result of pain that is not treated in a timely manner or pain that is difficult to treat. In addition, the lack of pain relief may have multiple psychological, spiritual, and practical effects on patients and their families. In the past 30 years, the concept of pain has been elevated; corresponding pain treatment, especially cancer pain treatment, has received increasing attention; and related pain treatment techniques have been significantly developed and applied in clinical practice.

Even so, the current status of cancer pain treatment is still unsatisfactory. A retrospective study by the European Society of Medical Oncology (ESMO) showed that 43% of cancer pain patients had a negative PMI index, which means that about one in two cancer pain patients had inadequate cancer pain control [9]. A retrospective, case-control study in China [10], which included 475 patients with malignant solid tumors with bone metastases, was divided into a control group (no GPM, 244 cases) and a GPM group (231 cases) according to whether they underwent standardized cancer pain management (GPM), and the results showed that about 60% of cancer pain patients had moderate cancer pain, and only 16.1% of moderate cancer pain patients received strong opioids.

In developing countries, many cancer patients are not diagnosed in time, or have difficulty in affording treatment, or miss the best time for treatment, resulting in more severe disease and pain becoming a major problem for patients and their families. Many factors limit access to effective pain management for cancer pain patients in developing countries, including perceptions of pain, overly strict opioid regulation, and lack of specialized health-care professionals, health-care infrastructure, materials, and funding.

14.3 Perineural Infiltration and Visceral Cancer Pain

It is well known that in addition to cancer cell metastasis found in the vascular system and lymphatic system, cancer cells can also spread and metastasize through the perineural area. Some studies have reported the growth of tumor cells along the nerves surrounding the tumor to confirm the neuroinvasive ability of tumor cells. Earlier views suggested that this pathway of tumor cell migration along the peripheral nerves had the least resistance. However, other studies have successively disproved this idea. For example, studies have confirmed that tumor cells coexist with Schwann cells in the intraneural space and that tumor cells are equally present in the neural fasciculus space [11]. Similarly, recent studies have defined the distribution of tumor cells along the perineurium and simultaneously (or partially) in the perineural space with the nerve sheaths of the outer nerve membrane, nerve fasciculus, and nerve endothelium as perineural infiltration (PNI), with tumor cell infiltration occupying at least 33% of the nerve [12]. Thus, PNI, previously described as the spread of tumor cells along the perineural space, can now also be described as nerve infiltration (NI) based on the presence of tumor cells in the three spaces surrounding the nerve sheath. Therefore, some scholars have used the term "nerve infiltration" instead of "perineural infiltration." The cause of tumor cell infiltration into the nerve is still not fully understood, but it has been hypothesized that once tumor cells infiltrate the outer layer of the nerve sheath, they become part of a favorable environment that promotes tumor growth. Our knowledge of the presence of tumor cells within the nerve sheath at the present stage provides further evidence that the movement of tumor cells is achieved through a highly coordinated signaling system between the tumor cells and the surrounding nerve, with many signaling factors, including neurotrophic factors, inflammatory chemokines, and cell surface ligands and receptors, acting in the course of PNI. In many cases, PNI is accompanied by pain, and the PN-related factors mentioned above are also associated with pain production. In recent years, researchers have devoted great efforts to the study of targeted therapeutic aspects of cancer pain. In this section, we review the molecular mechanisms of PNI and associated cancer pain with a focus on pancreatic cancer.

14.3.1 Perineural Infiltration of Tumors

Since PNI was first reported in head and neck tumors, it has been successively reported in tumors including pancreatic, prostate, colorectal, and other tumors. Although the rate of PNI varies among tumors, PNI-positive cases are often associated with poorer prognosis and lower survival rates.

Pancreatic ductal adenocarcinoma (PDA) has the highest incidence of PNI among all types of tumors, ranging from 80% to 100% [13]. The reason for the high rate of PNI in pancreatic adenocarcinoma is not fully understood, but the highly neurophilic nature of PDA cells and the high proximity of the pancreas to several nerve plexuses could partially explain this phenomenon. The fact that the pancreas receives such abundant innervation from the plexus provides very favorable conditions for tumor cells to fully interact with the nerves. Even so, to some extent, the underlying molecular mechanisms explaining the high incidence of PNI in pancreatic cancer remain unknown. Moreover, although tumor cells have a tendency to disseminate along nerves, nerves likewise preferentially tend in the direction of the tumor due to chemotaxis by tumor-secreted factors.

14.3.2 Molecular Mechanisms of Peripheral Nerve Infiltration

The understanding of the mechanism of PNI has changed as the molecular mechanisms that determine what drives PNI have been studied in depth. The current view is that a coordinated and interacting signaling system between tumor cells and nerves is the fundamental basis for the occurrence of PNI. Studies have shown that high expression of transforming growth factor alpha (TGF-α) in peripancreatic nerves and expression of epidermal growth factor receptor (EGFR) on pancreatic tumor cells increase the affinity between nerve and tumor cells [14, 15]. This early study also paved the way for exploring the role of other nerve-associated growth factors in PNI. Subsequent studies have successively demonstrated the potential role of multiple factors in PNI development, including neurotrophins and their receptors, protease classes, cytokine classes, inflammatory chemokine classes, and cell surface markers, all of which have altered expression on tumor cells and/or nerves.

PNI is a multifactorial process that includes multiple signaling molecules from different signaling pathways. The interrelationship between molecules expressed on tumor cells and peripheral nerves plays an important role in PNI development. These signaling molecules include secreted neurotrophins such as nerve growth factor (NGF), a specific ligand for tyrosine kinase receptor A, and brain-derived neurotrophic factor (BDNF), a TrkB ligand. There is also the low-affinity receptor p75 neurotrophic factor receptor (p75NTR). Other secreted factors include the glial cell-derived neurotrophic factor (GDNF) family. GDNF forms compounds and rearranges with the GDNF receptor α1 (GFRCα1) transfected receptor tyrosine kinase (RET), while GDNF family members artemin and GFR α3-RET form compounds. In addition, inflammatory chemokines and their receptors are associated with other cell surface molecules, such as mucin 1 (MUC1), myelin-associated glycoprotein (MAG), and neural cell adhesion molecule (NCAM). L1 cell adhesion molecule (L1CAM) and CD74 are also associated with PNI. In addition, differential expression of genes and proteins contribute to tumor cell infiltration and PNI. These include mucosa-associated lymphoid tissue lymphoma translocation gene 1 (MALT1) and tumor necrosis factor receptor-associated factor 2 (TRAF2), synaptic nuclear protein γ (SNCG), RHOGGDP dissociation inhibitor β (ARHGDI β), microtubule phase protein RPEB family member 2 (MAPRE2), YPEL1, and kinesin family member 14 (KIF14).

14.3.3 PNI and Pain Production in PDA

Pain production in PDA is one of the prominent symptoms of PNI. Many patients complain of the presence of abdominal or back pain on the side of the tumor. The use of traditional analgesic drugs such as opioids and non-cardiogenic anti-inflammatory drugs has been effective in the treatment of pancreatic cancer pain. Unfortunately, these drugs are not always effective, and their serious adverse effects often affect the quality of life of patients. The application of ganglion blocks can sometimes be effective for cancer pain, but such operations are often associated with some adverse effects. For example, abdominal ganglion blocks to reduce pain associated with pancreatic cancer are technically demanding to perform and are associated with shorter patient survival, in addition to several significant adverse effects and complications. Therapeutic approaches targeting PNI and pain-specific targets have the potential to overcome these drawbacks and achieve better outcomes.

The incidence of pain is also usually higher in the presence of concomitant PI, and certain molecular mechanisms associated with the development of PN are likewise associated with the production of pancreatic cancer pain. These include secreted nerve growth factor (NGF), glial cell-derived nerve growth factor (GDNF), artemin, granulocyte colony-stimulating factor (G-CSF) and granulocyte G macrophage colony-stimulating factor (GM-CSF) and their corresponding receptors tyrosine kinase receptor A (TrkA) and p75 neurotrophic factor receptor (p75NTR), GDNF receptor a1 (GFRa,)-rearranged transfection (RET) complex (GFRa, GRET), GFRo3GRET, G-CSF receptor (G-CSFR), and GM-CSF receptor α (GM-CSFR α).

The causes of pain in pancreatic cancer patients are the result of a combination of multiple factors. For example, infiltration of cancer cells disrupts the nerve sheath, making the nerve synapses vulnerable to injurious stimulation from the ECM, and signaling between pancreatic cancer cells and nerves leads to accelerated growth of pancreatic cancer cells and accelerated growth of nerves [16]. In addition, infiltration of the perineural space may promote the growth of tumor cells, which in turn induces tumor metastasis and leads to pain [16, 17]. Tumor neovascularization, which accompanies new nerve fibers during tumor progression, also contributes to pain production. It is hypothesized that one of the reasons for this is molecular factors including vascular endothelial growth factor (VEGF), ARTN, ILGl, EphrinB2, and prostaglandins that affect the growth of new capillaries and nerve fibers [18].

Although various neurotrophins and their receptors can promote pancreatic cancer growth and nerve infiltration, their functional analysis in pancreatic cancer pain production has been relatively little studied. Among the signaling pathways associated with pain production, the most widely studied is the NGF signaling pathway. It has been theorized that NGF secreted by tumor-associated immune cells and fibroblasts can directly activate and sensitize sensory nerves adjacent to pancreatic tumor periphery by binding to TkA and/or p75NTR expressed on the nerve bundle membrane. This pathway that contributes to pain production is known as the "neurogenic infection" pathway. Recently, using a mouse model of pancreatitis, Malin et al. [19] found that NGF modulates the expression and function of the nonselective cation channel capsaicin receptor (TRPV1), the activation of which stimulates sensory nerves. TRPV1 can be activated by the chemical capsaicin or by thermal and mechanical stimulation, which subsequently triggers pain signals. Following capsaicin stimulation, TRPV1 acts as a sodium and calcium channel, leading to depolarization of neurons and the release of the pain-related transmitters calcitonin gene-related peptide (CGRP) and substance P (SP), which signal pain through the central nervous system. Similarly, the GDNF signaling pathway can increase the expression of TRPV1, which induces a capsaicin-related response and generates pain via TRPV1 in isolated neurons [20]. Increased ARTN expression in pancreatic cancer cells and Schwann cells can also increase TRPV1 expression and increase their capsaicin-related responses. In addition, co-expression of ARTN receptor GFRα and TRPV1 may also enhance the function of TRPV1 with pain signaling. Thus, the role of multiple neurotrophins in PNI and pain production makes it a favorable target for the reduction of PNI and its associated pain treatment. Granulocyte colony-stimulating factor (G-CSF) and granulocyte G macrophage colony-stimulating factor (GM-CSF) were identified in human PDA samples, while increased expression of their receptors G-CSFR and GM-CSFRα was found in peripancreatic nerves. Interestingly, G-CSF and GM-CSF and their receptors were associated with increased expression of CGRP in the nerves, which can lead to neurogenic infections and pain. It is also suggested that G-CSF and GM-CSF generate signals through the signal transducer and activator of transcription (STAT) pathway Janus kinase (JAK) and that inhibition of this pathway can sincerely reduce pain. Further evidence for a role of the G-CSF and GM-CSF pathways in pain is that peripheral nerve sprouting, thermal nociception, and mechanical nociceptive sensitization are reduced following the use of neutralizing antibodies or sRNAs against this pathway were reduced. Thus, PDA-derived hematopoietic signaling molecules could be developed to target new therapeutic tools for cancer pain and pain associated with various diseases

14.3.4 Treatment Strategies for PN and Pain

Considering the clinical consequences associated with PI (metastasis and pain), treatment targeting PNI becomes a potentially attractive treatment approach for patients with cancerous visceral pain. It is conceivable that treatment strategies targeting PNI could not only stop the spread of cancer cells but also reduce pain and thus improve the quality of life of patients. To date, the NGF-TrkA signaling pathway has been most intensively studied, and it is also the most promising therapeutic measure. The most commonly used measure to target this pathway is a neutralizing antibody to inhibit NGF, thereby preventing it from binding to TrkA. A monoclonal antibody against NGF, muM-ab911, in mice greatly reduced bone cancer pain in a mouse model [21]. Tanezumab (also known as RN624), a humanized muM-ab911, is currently in phase II clinical trials. These trials are focused on reducing pain in patients with osteoarthritis, as well as reducing severe pain from bone metastases in patients with prostate cancer, breast cancer, multiple myeloma, or other cancers. In addition, other humanized neutralizing antibodies against NGF are being investigated for the treatment of pain. Similarly, MNACI3, a selective high-affinity antibody targeting the TrkA receptor, prevents NGF from binding to TrkA both in vivo and in vitro [22]. In mice, a model of neuropathic pain and inflammation, MNAC13, and opioid analgesia has synergistic effects. Furthermore, through the d5 ectodomain of NGF-specific binding to TrkA, the recombinant Trk-Ad5 protein can be used to block NGF binding to TrkA, allowing activation of TrkA survival signals and thus cutting off its downstream pain signals. Indeed, in several in vivo models of inflammation, mature recombinant Trk-Ad5 attenuates pain signaling in models of pancreatitis and interstitial cystitis. In addition, NGF isolation caused by Tk-Ad5 reduced neuronal axon prolongation in PC12 cells [23]. The fusion protein marker of the extracellular domain of TrkA and the Fc tail of IGG immunoglobulin constructed another way to collect and isolate NGF, a molecule that captures NGF with picomolar levels of affinity. Although the fusion protein marker successfully attenuated pain and reduced thermal and mechanical NGF, peptide fusion proteins can also reduce nociceptive hypersensitivity in various pain states, such as tactile abnormal pain and thermal nociceptive sensitization in rats. However, the short half-life and potential for immune response limit its clinical use.

Given the role of TrkA in pro-survival signaling, various small molecule inhibitors of TrkA kinase activity have been used as anticancer agents, several of which are in clinical trials. For example, a TRK inhibitor, ARRYG470, largely attenuates bone cancer pain in a mouse sarcoma model and reduces nerve fiber remodeling associated with cancer pain. In addition, PHAG848125, a dual inhibitor of cell cycle protein-dependent kinase (CDK) and TrkA, inhibited tumor growth in a pancreatic implantation tumor model and is currently in phase I and II clinical trials [24]. PHAG848125 has the potential to target PNI and reduce pain production in the treatment of pancreatic cancer patients. These findings suggest that drugs targeting the NGF-TrkA signaling pathway may not only have a direct effect on tumor growth but also inhibit PNI and thereby reduce pain associated with pancreatic cancer. Several TRPV1 antagonists are in clinical use for the treatment of various pain states. A drug called resiniferatoxin (RTX), a capsaicin analogue, has been shown to induce apoptosis in pancreatic cancer cells, potentially controlling the pain produced by pancreatic cancer [25]. In addition, antagonists of TRPV1 can reduce pain in bone cancer pain models. Recently, investigators have found that antagonists of CX3CR1 can alleviate various inflammatory pains. In addition, application of neutralizing antibodies to CX3CR1 can alleviate cancer pain in a rat model of bone cancer pain. Much evidence suggests that PNI is associated with high disease recurrence and low survival rates in cancer patients, and PNI is likewise associated with pain production in cancer patients. Thus, treatment for PNI presents a potentially attractive new approach to treating cancerous visceral pain. However, it is not clear whether such therapies will have a positive effect on improving patient survival. Furthermore, while targeting a single signaling pathway such as the NGF pathway may reduce PNI and pain occurrence, it may be necessary to target multiple signaling pathways associated with PNI to improve the outcome of cancer patients, including improving quality of life and survival. Therefore, a better understanding of the mechanisms involved in the development of PNI and its role in the development of PNI in cancer one by one, especially in pancreatic cancer progression, is essential.

14.4 Pharmacological Treatment of Visceral Cancer Pain

Pharmacological analgesia is the main treatment method for cancer pain, and most cancer pain can be better controlled by using appropriate and sufficient amount of drugs. It is generally believed that more than 80% of patients' cancer pain can be well relieved by pharmacological treatment. The analgesic drugs commonly used in clinical treatment of cancer pain include opioids, NSAIDs, and "adjuvant drugs," among which opioids are the most commonly used and most important drugs in cancer pain treatment, while NSAIDs have an important position in cancer pain treatment, especially in visceral cancer pain and bone metastasis pain [26]. With the deepening of research on neuropathic pain, the importance of these drugs has been increasingly emphasized, especially in the clinical treatment of cancer pain and eruption pain, which are more difficult to control.

14.4.1 Opioids

Opioids, also known as narcotic analgesics, are the most potent class of drugs found to date and can alter the emotional response to pain. Opioids have strong analgesic effects and no organ toxicity, and most of them have no ceiling effect, so they are the most important drugs for long-term treatment of cancer pain. Opioids are addictive when used improperly; however, studies have shown that the potential for addiction is extremely low when opioids are used regularly in clinical pain management.

The analgesic effect of strong opioids increases with increasing dose, so theoretically even unlimited doses are possible, and there is no such thing as a maximum or optimal dose. For individual patients, the optimal dose is determined mainly by the balance between analgesic effects and adverse effects. Therefore, it is important to manage opioid-related adverse effects while obtaining analgesic effects.

14.4.1.1 Routes of Drug Administration

1. Noninvasive administration (oral, transdermal, transrectal, transmucosal administration, etc.): It is the preferred mode of administration for the treatment of cancer pain. For patients whose noninvasive methods of administration are ineffective and for surgical and postsurgical analgesia, continuous or single intravenous administration, continuous or single epidural administration, and continuous subcutaneous administration or temporary intramuscular injection can also be used.

   Oral administration has a slower absorption in the gastrointestinal tract, and the first-pass number should be obvious, so its onset of action is longer than that of intravenous administration, and the dose should be larger. Oral administration is simple, reliable, safe, and easy to titrate the dose, and the duration of analgesic effect can last 12–24 h with opioid-controlled slow-release preparations.

   Transrectal administration: It is an alternative option when patients cannot take drugs orally; the pharmacological characteristics are generally considered to be similar to those of oral administration, but the operation is inconvenient and easily affected by defecation.

   Transdermal administration: Mainly for fentanyl and buprenorphine transdermal patches, with high lipid solubility, small molecular weight, strong analgesic effect, no local irritation and skin metabolism, and high transdermal absorption bioavailability.

Fentanyl transdermal patch is applied to the skin and slowly released through the controlled release film to reach the peak blood concentration in about 12 h, and the analgesic effect can be maintained for up to 72 h, while the analgesic effect of buprenorphine can be up to 7 days. Transdermal administration is mainly used for patients who are not suitable for oral opioids, avoiding hepatic first pass effect and reducing the occurrence of gastrointestinal side effects such as nausea, vomiting, and constipation.

Transmucosal administration: Most opioids with high lipid solubility can be administered through the oral mucosa, nasal mucosa, and conjunctiva; commonly used drugs include buprenorphine, buprenorphine, fentanyl, and sufentanyl. The drug is absorbed through the mucosa and directly into the blood circulation, with a faster onset of action, avoiding the first-pass effect of the liver, significantly reducing the drug binding to the gastrointestinal opioid receptors, and reducing the incidence of nausea, vomiting, and constipation. However, there is a lack of corresponding preparations in China.

2. Injectable administration includes subcutaneous, intramuscular, and intravenous injections, and patient-controlled analgesia (PCA) methods can be adopted. Intravenous injection is the most widely used method, and subcutaneous PCA is simple and can be used at home.

14.4.1.2 Precautions for Clinical Application of Opioids

The efficacy and side effects of opioids for individuals are uncertain and unpredictable, and most patients with cancer pain need long time analgesic treatment, so the use of opioids in clinical practice should be based on full assessment of patients and full understanding of drug characteristics, following the principle of maximum analgesic effect and no intolerable side effects and formulating an overall treatment plan. The use of opioids in clinical practice should be based on a thorough assessment of the patient, a thorough understanding of the characteristics of the drug, and a holistic treatment plan that includes both pharmacological and non-pharmacological therapies.

14.4.2 Nonsteroidal Anti-Inflammatory Drugs

Nonsteroidal anti-inflammatory drugs (NSAIDs), also known as antipyretic and analgesic drugs, are a class of anti-inflammatory drugs with different structures but are not steroids. Compared with the strongest anti-inflammatory effect of adrenocorticotropic hormones (both steroidal structure), NSAIDs are not steroidal in chemical structure. NSAIDs mostly have similar pharmacological effects such as antipyretic, analgesic, anti-inflammatory, and anti-rheumatic.

There are many varieties of NSAIDs, starting from the earliest aspirin, more than 100 kinds and thousands of brands of NSAIDs have been developed over the past 100 years, which is one of the most used drug classes worldwide and widely used in the treatment of osteoarthritis, rheumatoid arthritis, many kinds of fever, and various pains including cancer pain.

In both WHO 1986 three-step cancer pain treatment protocol [27] and the modified three-step analgesic protocol, NSAIDs play an important role: it can be used alone for mild to moderate cancer pain or in combination with opioids and other analgesic drugs to improve the analgesic effect and reduce the dosage of opioids throughout the cancer pain treatment. Therefore, for mild to moderate cancer visceral pain and metastatic bone cancer pain, NSAIDs can be considered first if not contraindicated.

Due to the characteristics of visceral cancer pain and NSAID itself, the systemic conditions of patients should be taken into consideration when using them, especially the safety of gastrointestinal, cardiovascular, and hepatic and renal functions, and the principle of risk-benefit balance should be noted: (1) In addition to the low incidence of gastrointestinal side effects, there have been many studies confirming that high expression of COX-2 is associated with the occurrence and deterioration of colorectal, gastric, pancreatic, and ovarian cancers, and COX-2-specific inhibitors such as celecoxib may have a certain inhibitory effect on the development of related tumors in addition to analgesia; (2) pay attention to the prevention and control of NSAID side effects, and proton pump inhibitors (PPI) can be given simultaneously to those with potential gastrointestinal risks; (3) active upper gastrointestinal ulcer and bleeding should be prohibited, and those with severe hepatic and renal dysfunction should be prohibited; (4) no overdose should be given, and two types of NSAIDs should not be used simultaneously, and when one type of NSAIDs is not effective, other NSAIDs may still have a better effect.

14.4.3 Anticonvulsant Drugs and Antidepressants

Cancer pain is a mixed type of pain containing both nociceptive pain and neuropathic pain (NP), and according to research, NP accounts for about 40% of cancer pain [28]. Neuropathic pain is one of the most complex phenomena in the cancer pain syndrome, but in practice, the definition and classification of neuropathic pain in cancer patients is not clear, especially in cancer visceral pain. Therefore, although the neuropathic pain component has received increasing attention in the clinical practice of cancer pain treatment, including cancer visceral pain treatment, it still lacks systematic and clear description. The author believes that, at present, cancer neuropathic pain can be classified as follows: (1) pain caused by tumor compression, indirect injury or direct invasion of nerves; (2) neuropathic pain caused by nerve damage from tumor treatment such as surgery, chemotherapy, or radiotherapy; and (3) pain with unclear classification but with neuropathic pain characteristics, including pain caused by visceral nerve and sympathetic nerve damage and eruption pain.

Neuropathic pain is one of the important reasons for the poor treatment effect of cancer pain. Opioids are the pillar of treatment for cancer pain, but they are ineffective in treating neuropathic pain; NSAIDs are also not significantly effective in neuropathic pain. In the past 20 years, significant progress has been made in the treatment of neuropathic pain, and a number of new therapeutic drugs have been used for the treatment of neuropathic pain with good results. These drugs are classified as adjuvants and include anticonvulsants, antidepressants, glucocorticoids, N-methyl-D-aspartate antagonists, and cannabinoids. Among them, anticonvulsants (e.g., gabapentin, pregabalin) and antidepressants (tricyclic antidepressants, duloxetine, and venlafaxine) are recommended by several guidelines as first-line agents for the treatment of neuropathic pain.

The dorsal root ganglion plays a central role in the central nervous system, as the downregulation of its action leads to the inhibition of spontaneous peripheral injurious signaling. Gabapentin and pregabalin may reduce excessive calcium inward flow by modulating the overexcited 0–2δ voltage-gated calcium channel subunit, which reduces the release of glutamate, norepinephrine, and substance P. The efficacy of both drugs was established, with therapeutic effects on NP alone or in combination with other drugs such as opioids, while enhancing opioid effects and reducing opioid requirements. Multiple RCTs have shown that gabapentin and pregabalin are effective for cancerous neuropathic pain.

Gabapentin has relatively mild side effects, good tolerability, and a proven safety profile (over ten million doses worldwide without serious adverse effects). The starting dose of gabapentin is 900 mg daily, usually given as 300 mg on the first day, taken in the evening, 300 mg twice/day on the second day, and 300 mg three times/day on the third day, maintaining this dose for 1 week, and if therapeutic effect is not achieved, it can be gradually increased to 3600 mg daily in three divided doses by increasing the amount by 300 mg weekly [29]. Gabapentin has a relatively late onset of action and takes several days to weeks to achieve steady-state plasma levels. The most common side effects of gabapentin are dizziness, drowsiness, peripheral edema, weight gain, weakness, and dry mouth.

Pregabalin has a similar mode of action to gabapentin but has a greater affinity for voltage-gated calcium channels. It has a faster onset of action than gabapentin and a mild antidepressant effect. Small doses of pregabalin combined with opioids have been shown to be effective in improving sleep, quality of life, and ability to perform activities of daily living in patients with cancerous neuropathic pain. It is recommended to start with a small dose such as 25 mg daily and gradually increase the dose to 600 mg daily, but the minimum dose of both domestic imported and domestic formulations is 75 g, so this is usually the starting dose in clinical practice [30]. The most common side effects are similar to those of gabapentin.

TCA has a dual mechanism for neuropathic pain, that is, direct pain inhibition and pain-related depression inhibition. TCA analgesic doses are lower than those required to treat depression. The most common side effects are anticholinergic results, including dry mouth, constipation, blurred vision, cognitive impairment, and upright hypotension. Therefore, clinical use of TCA should be aware of the presence of cardiac disease in patients, especially in the middle-aged and elderly. In addition, the pharmacokinetic variability of TCA is large, and individualized treatment should be taken. Amitriptyline is the representative drug of TCA, and compared with antidepressant treatment, clinical treatment of NP generally starts with a small dose (e.g., 6.25 mg), and the dose is gradually adjusted according to the patient's pain control status and side effects.

The analgesic effect of selective 5-HT reuptake inhibitors is unknown, but the therapeutic effect of selective 5-HT-norepinephrine inhibitors (SNRI) such as venlafaxine and duloxetine on cancerous neuropathic pain has been supported by clinical evidence. Among them, venlafaxine is an effective treatment for cancerous neuropathic pain, but low doses (75 mg/d are ineffective and higher doses (150 mg/d are required [31]. The main side effect of venlafaxine is gastrointestinal disturbance, but it rarely leads to discontinuation of the drug, and the dose should be reduced for severe hepatic and renal insufficiency, and blood pressure needs to be monitored regularly during treatment. Duloxetine is another first-line drug in the SNRI family for the treatment of NP, and it has much lower cardiotoxicity. Duloxetine is effective for NP at doses of 60–120 mg daily but ineffective at lower doses. Duloxetine has a slow onset of action, and its dose should be titrated for no less than 2 weeks [32].

14.5 Minimally Invasive Treatment of Visceral Cancer Pain

Generally speaking, minimally invasive treatment for cancer pain is the choice when drug treatment is ineffective or when intolerable side effects occur. However, with the update of cancer pain treatment technology and the development of clinical practice, this concept is gradually changing.

Usually, when the tumor patient's disease has progressed to a more serious level and has lost its effect after a longer period of treatment with high-dose opioids and other analgesic drugs, the pain may have formed a vicious cycle and evolved into intractable pain, and minimally invasive or invasive treatment may also be difficult to be fully effective or the best time for treatment has been missed. Therefore, the timing of minimally invasive treatment should be decided according to the actual situation of patients.

Due to the special situation of cancer visceral pain, such as more combined visceral symptoms, in fact, some minimally invasive treatments can be performed at the early stage of cancer pain treatment at the right time, such as pancreatic cancer patients with abdominal plexus destruction, which can control pain more effectively without affecting the patient's general status, level of consciousness and psychophysiology, and daily activities; reduce the side effects of drugs including opioids; and improve the quality of life.

At present, the minimally invasive treatment methods for cancer pain mainly include neurointervention (nerve block, modulation, and destruction), intrathecal analgesic device implantation, vertebroplasty, and neurosurgical interventions, the latter of which has more types of procedures, such as peripheral neurectomy, dorsal root ganglionectomy, dorsal root destruction into the medullary area, anterolateral spinal cord column dissection, median spinal cord dissection, medial thalamic destruction, cingulate gyrus destruction, midbrain destruction, and pituitary gland removal. However, the clinical application of these techniques is limited by the need for general anesthesia and the fact that most of the procedures have excessive side effects and are not easily tolerated by patients with mid- to late-stage tumors.

14.5.1 Nerve Block/Destruction

Pharmacological treatment of cancer pain, including WHO's three-step therapy, has been widely accepted by physicians in oncology and pain-related specialties. However, there are still 10–20% of cancer patients whose pain is not effectively dug in after the implementation of the three-step therapy. Interventional pain treatment can be considered for this part of refractory cancer pain patients. Moreover, interventional treatment for cancer pain should not only be regarded as a kind of "hospice care," but the early implementation of interventional treatment to relieve refractory cancer pain can reduce patients' pain and even help prolong their lives.

14.5.1.1 Neurolytic Celiac Plexus Block

This is one of the most commonly used interventional techniques for cancer pain. Blocking the visceral nerves by pharmacological or chemical destruction is very effective in treating cancerous visceral pain in the upper abdomen. Since Kappis first proposed the Neurolytic Celiac Plexus Block (NCPB) in 1919, the visceral plexus block technique has become a common method for the treatment of abdominal cancer pain and is widely used in clinical practice. For pain caused by tumors of upper abdominal organs above the splenic flexure of the colon, including the pancreas, liver and gallbladder, lower esophagus and stomach, or metastatic cancer in the upper abdomen, NCPB can often achieve satisfactory results.

1. Indications: NCPB is suitable for cancerous visceral pain above the splenic flexure of the colon, and pancreatic cancer and bile duct cancer are the most typical indications. NCPB is safe and effective and can reduce the dosage of analgesic drugs, especially opioids, and their side effects, so it should be considered early in the treatment of any upper abdominal cancer pain. A study showed that abdominal plexus block provided great pain relief in 70–80% of patients immediately after surgery, and in 60–75% of the patients, pain relief could last until the end of life [33].
2. Anatomy of the celiac plexus: The celiac plexus is composed of one to five ganglia interconnected by a dense network of nerves, which is characterized by variability and complexity. The visceral nerves include preganglionic sympathetic fibers in the upper abdominal viscera, which are connected synaptically to the visceral ganglia, and superior afferent nerve fibers that conduct stimulus signals from the pancreas, gallbladder, other hepatobiliary structures, the distal stomach, small intestine, and large intestine up to the end of the transverse colon. Direct blockade of the visceral nerve as an alternative to NCPB has been reported clinically and can also achieve better results.
3. NCPB methods: There are several methods of abdominal plexus block, and the relevant literature shows no statistical differences between methods in terms of complication rates and immediate and long-term mortality. The most common technical approach is the posterior puncture method, in which the patient is placed prone, given light sedation, and one or two needles are inserted into the vicinity of the celiac plexus or visceral nerves with the aid of X-ray fluoroscopy or CT. A contrast agent is injected to make sure that the needle tip is in the correct and safe position, and a local anesthetic is injected first. If there

is significant pain relief, a nerve-destroying drug (e.g., 70% ethanol) is injected. Depending on the method of puncture, the posterior puncture method can be divided into single-needle and double-needle methods. The abdominal plexus is localized at the intersection of the abdominal aorta and its abdominal trunk branches, so the puncture needle can be placed on either side of the abdominal aorta near the abdominal trunk, or directly through the abdominal aorta, but this is less commonly used.

NCPB can also be performed in several other ways, such as the anterior approach, in which the patient is placed in the supine position and the puncture needle is passed percutaneously through the abdominal cavity to the intersection of the abdominal aorta and the branches of its abdominal trunk, which carries the risk of damaging abdominal organs such as the intestinal canal, while ultrasound gastroscopic NCPB can clearly locate the abdominal aorta and abdominal trunk, which can be positioned in real time, and the puncture needle can be passed through the stom ach wall to the abdominal plexus, and the distribution of anhydrous ethanol can be observed. The abdominal plexus can also be destroyed under direct vision while performing a dissection.

14.5.1.2 Superior Hypogastric Plexus Block

For pain of tumor origin in the lower abdomen and pelvic viscera, intervention of the inferior abdominal plexus is feasible. The primary indication for a disruptive superior hypogastric plexus block is intractable pelvic visceral pain that has failed to respond to pharmacologic therapy, with good or excellent pain relief achieved in approximately 70% of patients, resulting in a reduction in opioid dosage without significant adverse effects or complications. The clinical course of inferior epigastric plexus destruction is essentially similar to that of NCPB, and both are used to control visceral pain, but the former is less effective than NCPB because pelvic tumors are more likely than pancreatic cancer to invade somatosensory innervated tissues and more likely to cause somatic involvement pain or localized somatic pain. Somatic pain due to pelvic tumors is usually caused by compression of the sciatic nerve but can also invade the myofascia and cause pain. Compression of the piriformis muscle may present with pain in the buttock or rectum and may be accompanied by pain in the posterior thigh, which worsens with sitting or activity. Pelvic tumor may also invade the iliopsoas muscle to cause low back pain. Once the tumor invades the lumbosacral plexus in the presacral area or spreads behind the peritoneum and invades the nerve roots, nerve trunk pain will occur, often radiating to the lower extremities. Motor reflexes cause muscle spasm and corresponding somatic pain. Pain may also be caused by surgery or radiation therapy. Pain caused by pelvic tumors often has multiple factors intermingling with each other, so cases must be carefully selected when performing superior inferior abdominal plexus blocks.

14.5.1.3 Ganglion Impar Block

Perineal visceral pain caused by malignant tumors can be analgesically treated with a ganglion impar block. The ganglion impar is located at the level of the sacrococcygeal union and is the terminus of two sympathetic chains. Indications for the ganglion impar block are vague and difficult to localize pain in the perineum with burning sensation and urinary urgency. The puncture is performed with the patient preferably in a prone position and the needle is inserted 2–3 cm through the midpoint of the sacrococcygeal ligament until the tip of the needle reaches the posterior rectum. However, there are few results of studies on its long-term effects.

Pain of celiac plexus, inferior inferior abdominal plexus, and ganglion impar origin may be considered for neurointervention using physical or chemical methods as early as possible. If the tumor invades both the abdominal wall and the posterior peritoneum, sometimes a spinal nerve block is required in conjunction to achieve optimal results. The main complications of visceral plexus intervention are decreased blood pressure and diarrhea. The visceral plexus intervention should be performed under imaging-guided positioning such as X-ray, CT, and ultrasound, and recently, MR guidance and positioning have been reported for NCPB. X-ray positioning is clear, intuitive, holistic, dynamic, and inexpensive but lacks stereoscopic positioning and cannot indicate whether the organ is punctured or not, nor can it accurately determine the distance of the needle tip or the actual spread of the injection. Positioning can clearly and visually show the relative positions of the vertebrae, blood vessels, and abdominal organs; design the puncture access; and accurately determine the distance of the needle tip, but it has a slightly poorer sense of wholeness and is not dynamic for real-time observation. Ultrasound guidance can show the structures of abdominal aorta, abdominal trunk, and superior mesenteric artery more clearly and can dynamically observe the process of needle tip puncture and injection, as well as the diffusion range of nerve destructive agent, with the characteristics of three-dimensional positioning and economic simplicity, but the overall view is poor, and the position of the probe and operating experience also have some influence.

14.5.2 Intrathecal Analgesia

Intrathecal analgesia can be considered for cancer pain patients whose pain is not effectively relieved even after the use of large amounts of opioid drugs or complex medication, or who experience uncontrollable adverse effects such as nausea, vomiting, and excessive sedation. The purpose of intralesional analgesia is to improve the analgesic effect and reduce the dosage of systemic opioids and adverse effects by applying small doses of opioids and/or local anesthetics intralescularly. In addition, cancer pain with predominantly neuropathic pain (e.g., tumor invasion of the plexus, complex regional pain syndrome, etc.) may respond better to intrathecal treatment than conventional treatment, especially when adjuvants such as local anesthetics and colistin are used.

Intrathecal analgesia requires the placement of a catheter in the epidural or subarachnoid space and administration of the drug via an external or implanted micropump. The choice of an epidural or subarachnoid placement and an external or implanted micropump requires consideration of a variety of factors, including duration of treatment, type and location of pain, tumor progression, opioid dosing, physician experience and medical conditions, and economic factors.

Intrathecal administration is the injection of drugs into the cerebrospinal fluid (CSF), which acts directly on central nervous system targets (nerve and opioid receptors), and has the characteristics of targeted drug delivery, which can achieve more rapid analgesia while requiring a smaller dose of drugs and a lower incidence of systemic side effects. In contrast, analgesic treatment by the epidural route has more influencing factors, such as inadvertent catheter displacement and the appearance of epidural fibrosis that can impede drug diffusion, higher drug-demanding doses, and even higher requirements for drug volume or infusion speed (e.g., for local anesthetics), resulting in a higher rate of poor analgesic treatment outcomes. In terms of complication rates due to expertise, long-term epidural infusions (55%) have proven to be higher than intrathecal injections (5%). Moreover, in terms of management of complications, the epidural analgesic route may be more complex, except for cerebrospinal fluid leakage, such as infection, and intrathecal analgesia can be effectively treated by cerebrospinal fluid replacement. The above factors make intrathecal analgesia more widely used in clinical practice.

14.5.2.1 Intrathecal Analgesic Drug Treatment

1. Opioids: Intrathecal μ opioid receptor agonists directly activate opioid receptors in the dorsal horn and brain stem. The local opioid concentration in the spinal cord and brain opioid receptors is higher during subarachnoid administration, while the systemic absorption is less, thus significantly reducing the opioid demand dose and mitigating the adverse effects of opioids. It is generally accepted that the analgesic strength of oral, intravenous, epidural, and subarachnoid opioids is

1:3:30:300, that is, to achieve the same analgesic effect, the amount of opioid used in the subarachnoid space is equivalent to 1/300 of the oral dose or 1/10 of the epidural dose. However, it should be noted that in clinical practice, the equivalent dose, including the equivalent dose between different opioids and between different routes of administration, is only a rough concept and often varies from patient to patient. Therefore, regardless of the route of opioid application, patients need to be closely followed, and the dose should be adjusted in time to achieve effective analgesia with minimal adverse effects. The choice of opioid class and dose is largely individual-specific, based on drug availability and physicochemical properties (e.g., hydrophilic versus lipophilic), and no comparative outcome studies are available.

Numerous opioids, including morphine, hydromorphone, fentanyl, sufentanil, pethidine, and methadone, have been used successfully intrathecally. However, morphine remains the most commonly used opioid for intrathecal analgesia. Morphine has low lipid solubility, and the onset of action of intrathecal morphine is slow, but it can maintain the analgesic effect for a long time. It is difficult to determine the dosage of opioids when administered for the first time, and the dosage and ratio of opioids, local anesthetics, and other drugs should be adjusted in a timely manner according to the patient's pain condition and side effects thereafter, taking into account the dosage of previous opioids, age and pain mechanism, and other factors.

2. Local anesthetics: Such as bupivacaine, ropivacaine, and lidocaine, which are sodium channel blocking drugs, block the nerve action potential of sensory, and motor nerves. When injected intrathecally, local anesthetics can block sensory nerve afferents and produce a more complete analgesic effect. However, the hyperalgesia, motor blockade, and sympathetic nervous system blockade associated with local anesthetics may be the price for pain control, which may result in discomfort, weakness, and hypotension. In appropriate doses, local anesthetics will be a good adjunct to intrathecal opioids, especially for neuropathic pain. In terminally ill patients who are bedridden, have weakness in the lower extremities, and are less affected, higher concentrations and doses of local anesthetics may even be applied to provide deeper analgesia without cognitive adverse effects, but measures to assist with continence must be prepared in advance.
3. Colistin: A 2-adrenoceptor agonist that acts on the dorsal horn neurons of the spinal cord and acts as an analgesic by modulating the transmission of noxious sensory signals. This modulation works by mimicking the descending norepinephrine receptor pathway and inhibiting neurotransmitter release. Colistin is a very useful complement to opioids and local anesthetics, and studies have shown that colistin combined with morphine provides better analgesia for neuropathic pain than morphine treatment alone. The highest analgesic success rate is achieved with the combination of opioids, local anesthetics, and colistin for intrathecal analgesia. Adverse effects of colistin include excessive sedation and hypotension in a dose-related manner.
4. Other drugs: A number of other drugs have also been reported as useful complements to intrathecal drugs; these include baclofen, ketamine, neostigmine, midazolam, ketorolac, haloperidol, and ziconotide (prialt). Haloperidol is used for refractory nausea and vomiting. Ziconotide is a novel snail peptide, an N-type voltage-sensitive calcium channel blocker. Ziconotide can only be used for intrathecal administration, acting on the dorsal horn to reduce sensory signal transmission by a different mechanism of action than other intrathecal drugs. Although it has been approved by the FDA for intrathecal use in intractable pain, ziconotide has not been universally used, primarily because of its adverse effects, including cognitive dysfunction and psychiatric disorders. Clinical experience suggests that most of these adverse effects are dose-related and can be avoided by slow and careful titration.

14.6 Summary

Visceral cancer pain is one of the most common cancer pains, mostly seen in patients with malignant tumors of abdominal or pelvic organs. Like other cancer pains, visceral cancer pain has various clinical manifestations and many combined symptoms, and it gradually worsens with the disease and is affected by many factors, with acute and chronic pain, injury-receptive pain, and neuropathic pain co-existing, which is a complex all-round pain that seriously reduces patients' quality of life. The goal of analgesic treatment is to maintain the highest possible quality of life for patients, and therefore, pain control should be accompanied by the least possible side effects.

So far, the cancer pain treatment system is a comprehensive treatment system with etiological treatment as the premedication, opioids as the core, pharmacotherapy as the main body, and invasive pain treatment techniques as the characteristics. Among them, opioids are the drugs with the strongest analgesic effect and are the main body of cancer pain treatment, but because of their serious side effects including respiratory depression, dependence, addiction and other persistent side effects such as constipation, prevention, and treatment of opioid adverse reactions are as important as pain treatment itself, and measures to prevent and deal with opioid analgesic adverse reactions should be regarded as an important part of the analgesic treatment plan. NSAIDs, anticonvulsants, antidepressants, and anxiety drugs should also be used in combination to improve analgesic effects and reduce opioid dosage and side effects.

References

1. Davis MP. Drug management of visceral pain: Concepts from basic research. Pain Res Treat. 2012;2012:1–18.
2. Neuropathic pain—international association for the study of pain (IASP). 2022. https://www.iasp-pain.org/advocacy/global-year/neuropathic-pain/.
3. Caraceni A, Portenoy RK. An international survey of cancer pain characteristics and syndromes. Pain. 1999;82(3):263–74.
4. Li M, Zhang L, Xu X-J, Shi Z, Zhao X-M. CT and MRI features of tumors and tumor-like lesions in the abdominal wall. Quant Imaging Med Surg. 2019;9(11):1820–39.
5. Facts about cancer pain: Pain from cancer; cancer treatment. American Cancer Society. 2022. https://www.cancer.org/treatment/treatments-and-side-effects/physical-side-effects/pain/facts-about-cancer-pain.html.
6. Whitten C. Chronic pain is a chronic condition, not just a symptom. Perm J. 2005;9(3):43–51.
7. Margarit C, Antón A, Escobar Y, Casas A, Cruz JJ, López R, et al. Breakthrough cancer pain—still a challenge. J Pain Res. 2012;5:559–66.
8. Mercadante S, Radbruch L, Caraceni A, Cherny N, Kaasa S, Nauck F, et al. Episodic (breakthrough) pain. Cancer. 2002;94(3):832–9.
9. Mitera G, Zeiadin N, Kirou-Mauro A, DeAngelis C, Wong J, Sanjeevan T, et al. Retrospective assessment of cancer pain management in an outpatient palliative radiotherapy clinic using the pain management index. J Pain Symptom Manag. 2010;39(2):259–67.
10. Yang Y, Ma Y, Huang Y, Zhao Y, Xu F, Tian Y, et al. The good pain management (GPM) Ward Program in China and its impact on chinese cancer patients: The SYSUCC experience. Chinese J Cancer. 2014;33(7):323–9.
11. Dwivedi S, Krishnan A. Neural invasion: A scenic trail for the nervous tumor and hidden therapeutic opportunity. Am J Cancer Res. 2020;10(8):2258–70. https://www.ncbi.nlm.nih.gov/pmc/articles/PMC7471340/
12. Fu Y, Zhang X, Ding Z, Zhu N, Song Y, Zhang X, et al. Worst pattern of perineural invasion redefines the spatial localization of nerves in oral squamous cell carcinoma. Front Oncol. 2021;11:766902.
13. Becker AE. Pancreatic ductal adenocarcinoma: Risk factors, screening, and early detection. World J Gastroenterol. 2014;20(32):11182.
14. Fujisawa T, Shimamura T, Goto K, Nakagawa R, Muroyama R, Ino Y, et al. A novel role of interleukin 13 receptor alpha2 in perineural invasion and its association with poor prognosis of patients with pancreatic ductal adenocarcinoma. Cancer. 2020;12(5):1294.
15. Demir IE, Ceyhan GO, Liebl F, D'Haese JG, Maak M, Friess H. Neural invasion in pancreatic cancer: The past, present and future. Cancer. 2010;2(3):1513–27.
16. Sha L, Yanlai S, Dongwei G. Role of the nervous system in cancer metastasis. Oncol Lett. 2013;5(4):1101–11.
17. Wang J, Chen Y, Li X, Zou X. Perineural invasion and associated pain transmission in pancreatic cancer. Cancer. 2021;13(18):4594.
18. Niu G, Chen X. Vascular Endothelial Growth Factor as an anti-angiogenic target for cancer therapy. Curr Drug Targets. 2010;11(8):1000–17. https://www.ncbi.nlm.nih.gov/pmc/articles/PMC3617502/
19. Malin S, Molliver D, Christianson JA, Schwartz ES, Cornuet P, Albers KM, et al. TRPV1 and TRPA1 function and modulation are target tissue dependent. J Neurosci. 2011;31(29):10516–28.

20. Premkumar L, Sikand P. TRPV1: A target for next generation analgesics. Curr Neuropharmacol. 2008;6(2):151–63.
21. Xu L, Nwosu LN, Burston JJ, Millns PJ, Sagar DR, Mapp PI, et al. The anti-NGF antibody mumab 911 both prevents and reverses pain behaviour and subchondral osteoclast numbers in a rat model of osteoarthritis pain. Osteoarthr Cartil. 2016;24(9):1587–95.
22. Covaceuszach S, Cattaneo A, Lamba D. Neutralization of NGF-trka receptor interaction by the novel antagonistic anti-trka monoclonal antibody MNAC13: A structural insight. Proteins. 2004;58(3):717–27.
23. Ito H, Nomoto H, Furukawa S. Growth arrest of PC12 cells by nerve growth factor is dependent on the phosphatidylinositol 3-kinase/Akt pathway via P75 neurotrophin receptor. J Neurosci Res. 2003;72(2):211–7.
24. Kazi A, Chen L, Xiang S, Vangipurapu R, Yang H, Beato F, et al. Global phosphoproteomics reveal CDK suppression as a vulnerability to kras addiction in pancreatic cancer. Clin Cancer Res. 2021;27(14):4012–24.
25. Hartel M, Di Mola FF, Selvaggi F, Mascetta G, Wente MN, Felix K, et al. Vanilloids in pancreatic cancer: Potential for chemotherapy and pain management. Gut. 2006;55(4):519–28. https://gut.bmj.com/content/55/4/519
26. What is cancer pain—ESMO. 2022. https://www.esmo.org/content/download/211169/3738827/file/EN-Cancer-Pain-Management-Guide-for-Patients.pdf.
27. WHO. Cancer pain relief. 2022. https://apps.who.int/iris/bitstream/handle/10665/43944/9241561009_eng.pdf.
28. Caraceni A, Shkodra M. Cancer pain assessment and classification. Cancers. 2019;11(4):510.
29. Yang J-Y, Lee WI, Shin W-K, Kim CH, Baik S-W, Kim K-H. Administration of four different doses of gabapentin reduces awakening from breakthrough pain and adverse effects in outpatients with neuropathic pain during the initial titration. Korean J Anesthesiol. 2013;65(1):48.
30. Cross AL, Viswanath O, Sherman AL. Pregabalin. National Center for Biotechnology Information. U.S. National Library of Medicine; 2022. https://pubmed.ncbi.nlm.nih.gov/29261857/.
31. Gallagher HC, Gallagher RM, Butler M, Buggy DJ, Henman MC. Venlafaxine for neuropathic pain in adults. Cochrane Database Syst Rev. 2015;2015(8):CD011091.
32. Lunn MPT, Hughes RAC, Wiffen PJ. Duloxetine for treating painful neuropathy, chronic pain or fibromyalgia. Cochrane Database Syst Rev. 2014;2014(1):CD007115.
33. Cornman-Homonoff J, Holzwanger D, Lee K, Madoff D, Li D. Celiac plexus block and neurolysis in the management of chronic upper abdominal pain. Semin Interv Radiol. 2017;34(04):376–86.

New Technologies and Prospects in the Treatment of Visceral Pain

15

Ming Xia

This chapter will present advances in the treatment of visceral pain. Various treatments for visceral pain have been described in detail in the previous sections (Chaps. 6, 7, 8, and 9), and this chapter will focus on the major discoveries and advances in clinical applications of treatments for visceral pain in recent years.

New advances in medical and nonmedical treatments have been achieved in managing visceral pain. The use of adjunctive classes of drugs, such as GABA analogs and tricyclic antidepressants, may be considered for inclusion early in treatment to avoid central sensitization (nociceptive hyperalgesia and touch-induced pain) and to enhance the effectiveness of chronic pain treatment. Unconventional analgesic drugs, such as TRPV1 receptor antagonists, are currently effective supplements to conventional pharmacotherapy for pain, but are taking on an increasingly important role in the treatment of visceral pain as research continues. Nonmedical treatment methods such as transcranial direct current stimulation, transcranial magnetic stimulation, transcutaneous electrical nerve stimulation, bilateral thoracoscopic splanchnotomy, psychological intervention therapies, probiotic therapy, and low-FODMAP diet greatly broaden the idea of visceral pain treatment. These developments allow clinicians to respond to traditionally intractable visceral pain through multiple means and methods, which coincides with the concept of multimodal analgesia that is commonly promoted in today's medical community.

15.1 Progress in Medical Treatment of Visceral Pain

The overall long development courses of new drugs, techniques, and therapies restrict the number of literature reporting the updates on the clinical treatment of visceral pain. Nevertheless, it should be noticed that compared with a few years ago, the treatment of visceral pain with new technologies is achieving significant development and progress recently. At the same time, a large number of new drugs or techniques are tested in animals or in early clinical context, which may be gradually put into clinical practice in the next few years. At present, the treatment methods of visceral pain usually adopted are the therapeutic strategies and schemes of somatic pain, such as the "three-step ladder analgesia" developed by the World Health Organization (WHO) for the treatment of cancer pain [1]. However, because of the differences between the visceral innervation and the mechanism of visceral pain and somatic pain, the nature and most effective treatments of visceral pain are also significantly different from those of the somatic pain. Therefore,

M. Xia (✉)
Department of Anesthesiology, Shanghai Ninth People's Hospital, Shanghai Jiao Tong University School of Medicine, Shanghai, China
e-mail: xiaming1980@xzhmu.edu.cn

M. Xia et al. (eds.), *Visceral Pain*, https://doi.org/10.1007/978-981-99-9167-9_15

it is pivotal to propose treatment methods specific to visceral pain.

The previous chapters have comprehensively described various treatment methods of visceral pain, which can be summarized as follows: (1) conventional medical treatment, (2) unconventional medical treatment, and (3) nonmedical treatment. Among them, drugs used in conventional medical treatment are generally similar to those used in the treatment of somatic pain, but according to the characteristics of visceral pain, the choice and use of drugs are slightly different. Specifically, weak analgesics, strong analgesics, adjuvant analgesics, and so on can be used. The weak analgesics include acetaminophen and NSAID, while the strong analgesics mainly refer to opioids, such as morphine and oxycodone, and auxiliary drugs include GABA analogues and tricyclic antidepressants (TCA). Conventional treatment includes TRPV1 receptor antagonists, ketamine, humanized anti-NGF monoclonal antibody, central α_2-adrenoceptor agonists, quetiapine and neurokinin-1 receptor (NK-1R) antagonists, etc. In general, nonmedical treatment is often considered clinically as an effective supplement to conventional treatment for chronic visceral pain. Nonmedical treatments include transcranial direct current stimulation (tDCS), transcranial magnetic stimulation (TMS), peripheral transcutaneous electrical nerve stimulation analgesia, neurodestructive therapy, intestinal probiotic therapy, dietotherapy, and psychotherapy. Since the corresponding chapters have systematically described the medical treatment of visceral pain and some of the nonmedical treatment methods, this chapter will allocate more space for the main findings and clinical application of the treatment of visceral pain in recent years.

15.1.1 Adjuvant Drug Therapy

Generally, patients will achieve better results of visceral pain relief after receiving standard analgesic interventions, but there are still considerable numbers of patients whose pain is not effectively controlled. Therefore, when chronic visceral pain is not satisfactorily treated by ladder analgesia, adjuvant analgesics is a good choice. At the same time, clinicians should be aware that when visceral pain is chronic, there may exist central sensitization (hyperalgesia and mechanical allodynia). Under such circumstance, adjuvant drugs should be considered in the early treatment of pain as well as GABA analogues and TCA [2].

15.1.1.1 GABA Analogues

Clinically used GABA analogues are mainly gabapentin and pregabalin [3]. These drugs have certain therapeutic efficacy in clinical models of visceral hypersensitivity [4]. Meanwhile, pregabalin has been proved to be effective in clinical trials of visceral pain caused by chronic pancreatitis. These compounds may indirectly affect the GABAergic system, acting primarily on the $\alpha_2\delta$ subunit of voltage-gated calcium channels (Ca_v) [5]. In addition, GABA-positive allosteric modulator provides a new therapeutic target for visceral pain management, and the sites of action of these drugs are mainly concentrated in the spinal dorsal horn [6]. Gabapentin and pregabalin have been shown to reduce experimental pain in chronic pancreatitis and irritable bowel syndrome (IBS). In an RCT, adjunctive pregabalin was more effective than placebo in relieving pain and improving health in patients with chronic pancreatitis [7]. Therefore, according to the existing research results, pregabalin may be considered as an intensive adjunctive class of therapeutic agent for treating visceral pain that is difficult to be alleviated with ordinary drugs. In addition, TCA, selective serotonin reuptake inhibitors (SSRI), and serotonin-norepinephrine reuptake inhibitors (SNRI) can also be used for the treatment of chronic visceral pain, especially functional pain diseases. TCA has analgesic and neuromodulation effects and should be administered in low dose slow titration in the first few weeks. A recent study has shown that TCA and SSRI have similar effects on pain treatment in patients with IBS [8]. However, the evidence on the analgesic effect of SNRI in functional visceral pain is insufficient, so it is not recommended [9]. When the above-mentioned adjuvant drugs or other new drugs are applied, it is important to develop highly individualized pain treatment plans for each patient due to the varying characteristics of the drug's action, efficacy, and pharmacokinetics and individual differences among patients.

15.1.1.2 Antispasmodics

In addition to visceral hypersensitivity, abnormal GI motility is also considered to be an important pathophysiological mechanism of GI visceral pain. Studies have found that GI motility is increased in diarrhea-type irritable bowel syndrome (IBS-D), whereas it is decreased in constipation-type irritable bowel syndrome (IBS-C). In addition, the small intestine mobility is enhanced in patients with IBS by dietary intake and the action of stress hormones and corticosteroid-releasing factor (CRF). In some cases, this is associated with abdominal pain manifestations. Antispasmodics can reduce GI tract contraction, so the GI application of this kind of drugs may be beneficial and widespread.

A European systematic review found that among 12 placebo-controlled studies on the use of antispasmodics in IBS. Abdominal pain was improved in four of these studies, intestinal symptoms were significantly improved in six studies, and IBS symptom severity scores was reported to be improved in six studies. Overall results of clinical trials were generally favorable, suggesting that antispasmodics can improve abdominal pain symptoms, including modulating gastrointestinal motility disorders, altered bowel movements, and abdominal pain/discomfort with an excellent safety profile. Yet more evidence of high credibility is expected as most studies included did not use standardized patient selection criteria and all studies included were of low to medium quality since they were done before the Rome IV criteria [10].

Another study suggested that while it was not clear which drugs were effective when used alone, there was evidence of abdominal pain and overall symptom relief in some patients. A recent meta-analysis of IBS treatment showed that in RCTs, antispasmodics were superior to placebo in relieving IBS symptoms, but there was a significant imbalance between studies. Otilonium bromide (OB) was the most convincing among the 12 drugs studied [11].

The target of OB is L-type and T-type calcium channels, as well as troponin T2 and neurokinin 2 (NK2) receptor, which may help to improve its efficacy. The efficacy of OB was demonstrated in four studies, including significant improvement in the severity of abdominal pain and swelling [12–14]. Compared with placebo, OB reduced the numbers of pain episode and the severity of abdominal distension and improved the overall assessment of symptoms, but did not improve bowel symptoms. In an international placebo-controlled trial where 356 patients were randomized to take OB (40 mg three times daily) or placebo for 15 weeks, OB was found to be significantly more effective than placebo in reducing abdominal pain, distension, and overall symptoms over a 10-week follow-up period [12]. In general, antispasmodics have few adverse reactions and may only lead to atropine-like side effects or constipation.

15.1.1.3 Antidepressants

Functional dyspepsia (FD) is a chronic gastroduodenal disease, which is characterized by visceral hypersensitivity, epigastric pain, burning sensation, postprandial fullness, early satiety, and so on [15]. The main causes are psychological and spiritual adverse stress, bad eating habits, environmental temperature changes, and so on [16]. A recent estimation on expanses of disease demonstrated that FD costs US $18 billion per year and costs UK £1 billion per year [17, 18]. *Helicobacter pylori* eradication therapy and proton pump inhibitors (PPIs) are the known treatment methods, but their effects are not ideal [19, 20].

As with most other functional GI disorders, FD patients exhibit higher levels of anxiety, depression, and other psychological conditions than healthy individuals [21]. In addition, increased inflammatory cells (e.g., eosinophils) and changes in mucosal integrity have also been demonstrated in FD patients, and these changes may be associated with psychological stress [22, 23]. In addition to the benefits of improving emotional and pain symptoms, psychotropic drugs, including TCA, SSRI, and 5- hydroxy tryptamine 1A(5-HT_{1A}) receptor agonists such as buspirone, and L-carnitine, have been shown to affect gastric motility, but whether they are effective in treating FD is unclear [24, 25]. Although the guidelines for the management of dyspepsia of American College of Gastroenterology (ACG) have highlighted the lack of evidence to support the use of these agents, they have been proposed as potential treatments for FD [26].

At present, there are few studies about antidepressants in the treatment of visceral pain. The efficacy of antidepressants in the treatment of FD has been observed in 1241 patients, of whom 673 received active treatment and 568 received placebo. Overall, 388 (57.7%) of the 673 patients had no improvement in FD symptoms after treatment, compared with 407 (71.7%) of the 568 patients in the placebo group [27]. Among them, psychoactive drugs were more statistically significant than placebo in the differences between persistent or no improvement of FD symptoms after treatment. The subgroup analysis showed that effective psychotropic drugs appeared to be limited to antipsychotic and TCA. When individuals with comorbid mood disorders were excluded, the effect of psychotropic drugs on FD was no longer significant [27]. In terms of adverse drug reactions, the incidence of adverse drug reactions was significantly higher in patients taking psychotropic drugs than in those taking placebo. When psychotropic drugs were analyzed alone, the total number of adverse events if TCA was found to be large.

Thus, psychotropic drugs may be one of the effective treatments for FD and associated abdominal pain, but their effectiveness appears to be limited to antipsychotics (e.g., sulpiride and levosulpiride) and TCAs (e.g., amitriptyline and imipramine) [27]. It should be noted that tandospirone, a 5-HT_{1A} receptor agonist, also has significant advantages [28]. Yet, more high-quality RCT data are needed to support the study of tandospirone.

15.1.2 Unconventional Treatment

Based on the evolving understanding of pain mechanisms of functional and organic visceral pain disorders, new analgesic drugs will likely be developed soon. The emerging new drugs for treating visceral pain are generally less commonly used for generalized somatic pain, and therefore, they are currently referred to as "unconventional analgesics," but as research continues, these drugs perhaps become increasingly important in the treatment of visceral pain. Consequently, they will be incorporated into the category of conventional drugs in the future, with the criteria for classification dependent more on pharmacological mechanism. Currently, it is believed that unconventional treatment in the clinical practice of chronic visceral pain can be an effective complement to conventional treatment for pain.

15.1.2.1 TRPV1 Receptor Antagonist

As described in the previous section, the TRPV1 receptor, also known as the capsaicin receptor, is a nonselective cationic channel of a homotetramer that is fully expressed in nociceptors [29]. TRPV1 can be activated by capsaicin, acidic environment (low pH) and nociceptive thermal stimulation, and is considered as an integrator of pain stimulation [30]. In recent years, a large number of studies have shown that TRPV1 is a highly effective target for pain therapy. The reasons include: (1) TRPV1 agonists, such as capsaicin, can induce desensitization of TRPV1 channels to alleviate pain behaviors in preclinical species [31], and (2) TRPV1 antagonists reduce inflammatory, arthritis, and cancer pain behaviors in rodents models [32]. Despite inconsistent reports of actual efficacy and ongoing controversies over the feasibility of its clinical application, there were still a large number of clinical trials conducted to evaluate the potential analgesic effects of TRPV1 agonists and antagonists. The analgesic effect of TRPV1 antagonists on visceral pain has been demonstrated in a variety of inflammatory diseases, such as acute colitis and chronic pancreatitis, in which TRPV1 receptor sensitization may contribute to enhanced peripheral sensitization [33]. In IBS patients, the increase of TRPV-1 nerve fibers may contribute to visceral hypersensitivity and pain [34]. Other studies have found that blocking the function of TRPV1 can alleviate visceral hyperalgesia in IBS model animals. Therefore, the TRPV1 receptor is a very meaningful pharmacological target in the treatment of inflammatory and functional visceral pain, but the clinical research on TRPV1 receptor antagonists is relatively lagging behind compared with pharmacological studies and animal experiments.

15.1.2.2 Ketamine

Ketamine is a noncompetitive NMDA receptor antagonist. As a special general anesthetic, it has been used in clinical anesthesia for many years because of its unique advantages [35]. In the past decade, studies have found that subanesthetic doses of ketamine have antidepressant effects, and its analgesic effects and inhibition of hyperalgesia have also received more and more attention [36]. Intravenous ketamine has been shown to significantly reverse pressure hyperalgesia in patients with chronic pancreatitis, but the effect is transient [37]. Moreover, a clinical trial evaluated the possible analgesic effect of orally taking ketamine after intravenous administration of ketamine in patients with chronic pancreatitis [38]. In addition, ketamine has also been shown to prevent and reverse the onset and maintenance of acute esophageal hypersensitivity in healthy volunteers. Thus, the treatment of visceral pain with ketamine is still at a very early stage and needs to be validated in further prospective clinical trials, which may bring exciting progress in the near future.

15.1.2.3 Anti-NGF Monoclonal Antibody

Based on the study of the pathophysiological mechanism of chronic visceral pain, it has been found that antagonists of specific receptors can inhibit the release or inhibition of some pain-related pro-nociceptive mediators and thus may be effective in relieving visceral pain [39]. A large amount of experimental and clinical evidence indicated that nerve growth factor (NGF) plays a key role in the production and maintenance of pain [40]. In many studies on visceral pain animal models, it was observed that the expression of NGF was upregulated in the pain animal group. Therefore, various human anti-NGF monoclonal antibodies as potential analgesic drugs are now gradually entering the clinical trial stage [41]. The role of NGF antagonists was clear in somatic pain disorders, but up to now, their effect on visceral pain still remains unclear. A monoclonal NGF antagonist has been proved to be effective in relieving pain in patients with interstitial cystitis.

15.1.2.4 Linaclotide

With the deepening of basic research, specific or potential targets for visceral pain treatment are gradually being discovered [42]. At the same time, other nonconventional drugs have been used to treat chronic visceral pain in animal experiments or clinical cases. Linaclotide, a guanylate cyclase-C (GC-C) agonist, is currently indicated for the treatment of IBS-C [43]. The activation of GC-C can cause the secretion of chloride and carbonate in the intestinal lumen and finally lead to the increase of fluid secretion in the lumen and the enhancement of intestinal peristalsis [43, 44]. In addition, linaclotide also has a laxative effect [45]. It has been suggested that linaclotide may also exert analgesic effect by inhibiting colonic nociceptors [46, 47]. The results of the Phase III clinical trial of linaclotide have been released, which proved that linaclotide has analgesic effect in patients with IBS-C [48].

15.1.2.5 Other Unconventional Drugs

It was found that central α_2- adrenoceptor agonists, quetiapine, and neurokinin-1 receptor (NK-1R) antagonists have analgesic effects [49–51]. Benzodiazepines such as midazolam or antipsychotics may also provide relief from visceral pain in certain conditions. Other studies have found that P2X3 receptor inhibitor TNP-ATP blocks hypersensitivity to visceral pain induced by neoplastic colonic inflammation. Therefore, P2X receptor may also be an effective potential target in the treatment of visceral pain [52–54]. In conclusion, with the development of modern pharmacology, more unconventional drugs may be used in the treatment of visceral pain in the future.

15.2 Progress in Nonmedical Treatment of Visceral Pain

15.2.1 Transcranial Direct Current Stimulation

Transcranial direct current stimulation (tDCS) is a noninvasive technique that uses electrical current to regulate brain function. It is relatively safe and mature in clinical application [55].

tDCS is a type of transcranial direct current stimulation and is a type of neurostimulation (also known as neuromodulation) in which a very low level of constant current is delivered to a specific target area of the brain, often producing profound effects. It was originally used to help patients with brain injuries such as stroke [56]. However, tests on healthy adults have shown that tDCS can improve cognitive performance on a variety of tasks, depending on the area of the brain stimulated. Scientific research has shown that tDCS has the effect of improving language and mathematical ability, attention span and problem-solving ability, memory, and coordination [57–60]. In addition, tDCS has been shown to have great potential in the treatment of depression, anxiety, post-traumatic stress disorder and chronic pain [61–63].

Given that the brain is the most complex organ in the human body, made up of complex networks of nerve cells, these special cellular controls reflect everything that happens in human bodies. The electrochemical synapses of neurons in the brain are different from chemical synapses and can carry out nerve impulses faster. In general, the direct effect usually lasts for 5–90 min after the stimulation period ends. Some studies have shown that repeated stimulation, such as once a day, can prolong and consolidate the effect. In addition, studies on depression found that the beneficial effects of tDCS stimulation were evident throughout the month after treatment.

The vast majority of studies involving this technique have used currents in the range of 0.5–2.0 mA, and it seems that currents below 0.5 mA do not produce significant results, but currents above 2 mA have not been fully studied in terms of safety and effectiveness. Depending on the application, higher treatment intensities are generally considered to be more likely to have longer effects after stimulation ends. The general consensus is that a treatment session of tDCS should last between 5 and 30 min, with the most common specialist procedures lasting 20 or 30 min.

The key point of this technique is to conduct a low-amplitude electric current through scalp electrodes to specific areas, such as the cortex, which in turn relieves pain. This technique can lead to a polarization-dependent shift of the resting membrane potential of neurons, resulting in changes in the excitability of nerve cells in the stimulation site and its contiguous region. At present, tDCS has been used in many aspects of clinical treatment, including neuropathic pain, chronic visceral pain, and depression caused by enteritis [64–66].

15.2.2 Transcranial Magnetic Stimulation

Transcranial magnetic stimulation (TMS) is a noninvasive treatment technique similar to tDCS (Fig. 20.2). In general, TMS is used to treat neurological and psychiatric disorders, including mood and dyskinesia [67]. TMS can also treat several types of chronic neuropathic pain. The pain relief mechanism of cortical stimulation may be the change of neuronal excitability caused by electric current generated from magnetic field. Currently, depression is a common disease and may occur together with chronic pain or chronic visceral pain. Therefore, pain and depression should be treated simultaneously in order to achieve better results. In addition, patients with chronic pain are often accompanied by insomnia [68, 69]. In recent years, several studies have proposed the hypothesis of applying TMS for pain management, and currently, this technique has been used to treat multiple types of chronic visceral pain, including organic and functional pain syndromes [70].

In patients with chronic pancreatitis pain, TMS can alleviate pain and bring corresponding changes in brain metabolites. Recent studies have shown that TMS can elevate the pain threshold of mechanical and electrical stimulation of the colon in patients with IBS and have a therapeutic effect on clinical pain [71]. There are case reports indicating that in palliative care for patients with cancer whose pain is difficult to control by conventional treatments, TMS, due to its noninvasive nature, can be used as an adjunctive treatment to mitigate pain from various causes and even improve the patient's mood. Repetitive transcranial magnetic stimulation (rTMS) can reduce the severity of adverse reactions by reducing the dose of analgesics, thereby improving the quality of life of patients. A recent review has also evaluated the therapeutic effects of rTMS and found that many studies reported that rTMS can significantly relieve pain, especially during continuous treatment through high-frequency stimulation of motor cortex [72]. In the research, the pain was relieved by 30% in the intervention group compared with the control group [73]. The types of pain included are neuropathic pain, fibromyalgia, and complex regional pain syndrome [74]. However, due to the limitation of research methods, there are controversies about the clinical application of this technique. Consequently, more in-depth researches are needed in studying the methods of its maintenance treatment and evaluating its therapeutic effects accurately. Above all, TMS is currently considered safe for the clinical treatment of chronic visceral pain, but it must be performed in a professional healthcare center by a professional physician.

15.2.3 Transcutaneous Electrical Nerve Stimulation

With the rapid development of electrical nerve stimulation, transcutaneous electrical nerve stimulation (TENS) may become one of the most rapidly expanding field in chronic pain, especially chronic visceral pain. TENS is an electrotherapy method that delivers a specific low-frequency pulse current into the human body through the skin to achieve the purpose of treating pain [75]. Emerged in the 1970s, it has been proved to be effective in analgesia and applied in clinical practice. Whereas in China, it is not widely used.

The difference between TENS and traditional nerve stimulation techniques is that the latter mainly stimulate motor fibers, while the former is designed to stimulate sensory fibers. Therefore, the therapeutic apparatus must possess the following conditions: (1) high frequency, mostly in the range of 2 ~ 160 Hz, belonging to the low frequency range; (2) short pulse, the pulse width is mostly 9 ~ 350 μs, and if the pulse is too long, the pain-transmitting fibers will be activated and the ionization will be increased; (3) appropriate intensity, using a subthreshold intensity that makes the patient comfortable and does not cause muscle contraction. Thus, TENS can selectively stimulate the response of the sensory afferent nerve fibers without triggering the response of the efferent nerve fibers; and (4) variable current patterns, currently commonly used waveforms including symmetric two-way square wave, moderate or high frequency current modulated by one-way square wave, symmetric two-way pulse. Besides, there are several hypotheses of the mechanisms of technique (1) gate control hypothesis. It is considered that TENS is a stimulus that excites the crude fibers and closes the gate of the pain afferent, thereby relieving the pain symptoms; (2) hypothesis of endogenous morphine-like release. Low-frequency pulsed current stimulation may activate the endogenous morphine-like peptide neurons in the brain, leading to the release of endogenous morphine-like peptides; and (3) promotion of local blood circulation. Besides analgesia, electrical stimulation of peripheral nerve can also promote local blood circulation. After treatment, local skin temperature can be raised by 1–2.5 °C.

There are many indications for TENS, including headache, migraine, neuralgia, causalgia, phantom limb pain, arthralgia, abdominal pain, postoperative pain, cancer pain, and so on [76–79]. In conclusion, TENS has effects on acute, chronic, and neuropathic pain, and short-term treatment is more effective than long-term treatment [80, 81]. The technique is contradicted in patients with cardiac pacemakers, stimulation of carotid sinus, pregnant women, local anesthesia, and patients who is allergy to electric. It has been reported that TENS may be an effective treatment for chronic shoulder pain [82]. And it also reduces shoulder-related disability and pain complications, thus improving activities and quality of life. After all, TENS is safe and effective and may be a new treatment for patients with chronic diseases. In addition, the vagus nerve stimulation (VNS) technique is also gradually applied to the treatment of visceral pain. Studies have suggested that direct electrical stimulation of the greater splanchnic nerve or gastric electrical stimulation (GES) can also relieve visceral hyperalgesia and gastric pain [83–85]. However, up to now, most of these therapeutic methods are only in the stage of animal experiments, and more trials are needed to verify the practical application of these techniques.

15.2.4 Neurolysis

Even if many strong opioids are used, the clinical pain symptoms of patients with advanced pancreatic cancer, liver cancer, bladder cancer, and complex refractory visceral pain cannot be effectively mitigated. Conversely, the significant side effects of opioids may seriously affect the patients' quality of life. In order to improve the quality of life of these patients with intractable visceral pain, it is possible to consider the intervention of neurolysis, which mainly refers to celiac plexus neurolysis with ethanol [86]. This method is mainly used to treat pain caused by malignant tumors located in the retroperitoneum or upper abdomen, but there is no consensus on the indication and time of applying neurolysis for the control of benign visceral pain. In terms of convenience, low cost, and good analgesic effect, this technique has a certain clinical practice values. But visceral pain is poorly controlled after the procedure in a few patients. Given that, radiofrequency thermocoagulation (RTFC) of splanchnic nerves can be considered, which is performed on the corresponding splanchnic nerve under the guidance of real-time radiographic imaging with the help of contrast media and the electrophysiological stimulation technique to achieve the purpose of neurolysis. In general, the purpose of this method is similar to the absolute ethanol injection technique, but the former has higher degree of accuracy and safety and can significantly lower the pain scores of postoperative patients, highly reduce the demand for opioid analgesics, and greatly improve their quality of life.

In addition, neurolytic splanchnic nerve block and thoracoscopic splanchnicectomy (TS) performed in surgery also belong to this category of treatment. Certain malignant tumors secondary to chronic pancreatitis or mesentery are often accompanied by severe pain that is difficult to be relieved. For example, in the event of pancreatic cancer that cannot be surgically resected, even medical treatment that includes the application of high-dose opioids, the pain is still not effectively controlled. Besides, high-dose opioids may lead to significant drug side effects, seriously affecting the quality of life of patients with advanced tumors. Under such circumstance, visceral nerve block or neurotomy can reduce the patient's dependence on opioids, improve the quality of life, and even prolong the survival period to a certain extent.

Bilateral thoracoscopic splanchnotomy (BTS) is often misnamed as splanchnicectomy because it involves neurotomy of the splanchnic nerves. But essentially, it is a denervation of sympathetic in charge of visceral pain sensation in upper abdomen. In the early 1993, this technique has been reported, but it was rarely performed and no consensus on the surgical plan [87]. Given the lack of evidence for this procedure so far, the researchers from the United Kingdom have reported their experience on the treatment of chronic pain of pancreatic origin with BTS [88]. The study reviewed data from five patients (two men, average age 51 years) who received BTS in the hospital where the investigators worked over the past decade. It can be found that two patients with pain secondary to pancreatic cancer, three patients with pain from chronic alcoholic pancreatitis, and a patient also had acute necrotizing pain. Three of them received NCPB, the effect was obvious but limited. All patients were dependent on opioid analgesics and not sensitive to other medications. In addition, all patients received BTS, expect for one patient who underwent unilateral (right) thoracoscopic splanchnotomy (UTS) due to thoracic adhesions.

The patient undergoing BTS takes the prone position under the general anesthesia with double-lumen endotracheal intubation. Right side first and after single lung collapse, the patient is tilt to the anterior end of left scapula, and a 5 mm observation hole is made in the sixth intercostal space of midaxillary line. Carbon dioxide is inflated to maintain the intrathoracic atmospheric pressure at 8 mm Hg and depress the diaphragm to have better view of surgical field. A 5 mm incision is made at the eighth intercostal space of the posterior axillary line as the operating hole. The splanchnic nerves are seen behind the parietal pleura.

After the surgery, the lungs are inflated, and the chest is sewed up. Commonly, no chest drainage tube is needed after surgery. Postoperative chest radiographs should be reexamined to ensure that no pneumothorax occurs. Patients are allowed to be discharged on the same day of surgery if their general conditions are good.

The visceral nerves, including the major and minor splanchnic nerves, are easy to be identified and dissected, but not in cases of the least splanchnic nerve. In the opinion of the investigators, transection of the major and minor nerves alone can provide excellent therapeutic effect without increasing the difficulty and risk of surgery. The average follow-up period for these patients was approximately 18 months, and there were no significant adverse reactions after surgery. Four of these patients reported significant improvement in pain control postoperatively. Until patients with pancreatic cancer passed away, the demand of opioid was significantly reduced after surgery. The other two patients with chronic pancreatitis had pain control for approximately 12 months. The pain of patients undergoing UTS was also alleviated rapidly, but the therapeutic efficacy lasted less than 3 months, after which opioids were used to control the pain [88].

This research provided an enlightenment that when drugs and other treatments are ineffective, surgical treatment can be used as one of the ultimate ways of pain management, especially minimally invasive surgery, the effect of which is obvious and lasting, which may bring benefits to patients with advanced tumor who may suffer from intolerable severe pain.

15.2.5 Psychological Intervention

Psychotherapy, as one of the comprehensive intervention measures for chronic visceral pain, had certain clinical effect compared with conventional standard nursing care. The methods of psychotherapy mainly include dynamic psychotherapy, cognitive behavior therapy (CBT), and hypnotherapy. CBT is a kind of psychotherapy that helps patients understand the thoughts and feelings that influence behaviors. CBT is commonly used to treat a variety of disorders, including phobias, addiction disorder, depression, and anxiety. Generally, as a short-term therapy, CBT focuses on helping patients deal with a specific problem. During the treatment, people learn how to recognize and change deficits or troubling thought patterns that have a negative impact on behavior and mood.

Research has found that CBT can significantly improve the treatment efficacy of patients with IBS compared with conventional nursing methods [89]. Among factors that affect the pain of patients with chronic pain syndrome (CPS), psychological factor may be one of the most important causes. Therefore, hypnotherapy has become one of better ways to treat CPS. Hypnotherapy for the treatment of GI pain is a specific type, aiming at enhancing patients' tolerance to pain symptoms of GI diseases, thereby promoting changes in their cognitive function and reducing their responsiveness to visceral pain. Also, it was found that a significant number of female IBS patients has anxiety [90]. For this group of patients, hypnotherapy is superior to standard nursing interventions in alleviating pain. Besides, hypnotherapy can also improve the quality of life of patients [91]. In addition, early research found hypnotherapy can reduce a few patients' sensitivity to experimental colorectal distension (CRD) [92].

In general, the number of studies on psychotherapy is significantly fewer than that of other medical and nonmedical treatments, and there is a lack of forceful evidence of its clinical application. Nevertheless, compared with the side effects of medical treatment, hypnotherapy is still one of the safe, effective, and noninvasive options for treatment of patients with visceral pain.

15.3 Other Progress in Treatment of Visceral Pain

15.3.1 Dietotherapy

Recently, the interactions between diet, gut function, and GI tract symptoms have aroused great interests. Fermentable carbohydrate can increase the volume of water in the small intestine and gas production in the colon, but in patients with visceral hypersensitivity disorders such as IBS, it may cause GI symptoms. At present, limited intake of fermentable oligosaccharide, disaccharide, monosaccharide, and polyol (FODMAP) diet is increasingly applied in clinical practice. Initial studies evaluating the efficacy of low-FODMAP diets were limited by retrospective study designs and lack of comparison groups, but results from recent well-designed clinical trials have been published. At present, at least ten RCTs or randomized paired trials have shown that a low-FODMAP diet will lead to clinical response in 50–80% of patients with IBS, especially in terms of improvement in abdominal distension, bloating, diarrhea, and overall symptoms [93]. Nevertheless, despite such obvious advantages of this approach, studies have also shown that low-phosphorus diet leads to significant changes in the microbiome and metabolome, but its duration and clinical result are not fully understood [94].

15.3.1.1 Role of Diet Management in IBS Treatment

First-line dietary advice for patients with IBS often focuses on modifying dietary fiber intake and limiting potential triggers such as caffeine, alcohol, and fat. Studies found that moderate fiber supplementation in IBS can significantly improve systemic symptoms compared with placebo [95]. In contrast, the effects of caffeine, alcohol, and fat were reported only in cross-sectional studies, and the individual limiting effects of these items were not investigated.

With regard to the exclusion diet, the effect of gluten restriction on IBS is not fully defined. Evidence from recent studies and controlled trials of gluten-free diets suggests that gluten-free diets improve symptoms in IBS patients with genotypes of HLA-DQ2 or HLA-DQ8 [96, 97]. Nevertheless, a short-term, double-blind, placebo-controlled, crossover trial showed that no benefit was observed when controlling the background diet [98]. In addition, recent studies on food allergy of specific food such as such as soy, milk, wheat, and yeast found that food antigens may activate response and alter the permeability of the intestinal mucosa [99, 100].

The range and quality of evidence proving the benefits of intestinal probiotic supplementation remains limited [101, 102]. Nevertheless, in the past decade, the evidence of mechanism and clinical efficacy of low-FODMAP diet has surpassed any other dietary interventions except probiotics, indicating its prospect and great potential.

15.3.1.2 Introduction of Low-FODMAP Diet

As an important part of human diets, carbohydrate consists of a range of molecules with different chemical and physical structures and has different physiological and functional properties. Digestibility of carbohydrate varies due to the lack or reduction of hydrolytic enzymes, and such indigestible carbohydrate include some non-starch polysaccharides (NSP), resistant starch (RS), olive sugars, and some polyols.

1. Oligosaccharides: Oligosaccharides mainly consist of fructooligosaccharide (FOS) and galactooligosaccharide (GOS). FOS is composed of a linear chain of less than ten fructose molecules polymerized and terminated by a glucose molecule, and GOS consists of one fructose + one glucose + one raffinose composed of galactose and one fructose + one glucose + two stachyoseg composed of alactose. FOS is difficult to be digested by amylo-

lytic enzymes as the absorption rate is less than 5%, and the α-galactosidase, which is used to digest GOS, cannot be synthesized in the human body, so GOS cannot be absorbed at all.

2. Disaccharides: Disaccharides mainly refer to lactose. The deficiency or reduction of lactase is prevalent, resulting in lactose malabsorption. A meta-analysis showed that the incidence of lactose malabsorption in patients with IBS ranged from 4% to 78% due to the different populations and diagnostic criteria, but this percentage was not higher than that of the normal population in the same region [103, 104].
3. Monosaccharides: Monosaccharides mainly refer to fructose. Fructose is an isomer of glucose and lacks a specific fructose transporter in the intestinal tract. Instead, it is transported by the glucose transporter. Thus, fructose can be fully absorbed only if it coexists with glucose and at concentrations equal to or lower than glucose. At least one-third of patients with IBS also have fructose malabsorption, and this rate is similar to that of the healthy population, suggesting that IBS symptoms may not be directly related to the problem [105, 106]. Another study showed that even in IBS patients whose fructose absorption was good, a low-fructose diet still relieved symptoms [105].
4. Polyols: Polyols are larger molecules that cannot be absorbed by the body through cellular diffusion in the small intestine, and a small amount can cause a dramatic increase of osmotic pressure in the intestinal lumen.
5. Total FODMAP content in food: The biggest difference between the low FODMAP diet and other previous dietary intervention strategies is that the low FODMAP diet aims to control the total daily intake of FODMAP rather than emphasizes avoiding a specific food. However, the total FODMAP content of food is difficult to be quantified precisely. Different species, regions, climates, harvesting seasons, degree of ripeness, and cooking methods all have impacts. For example, blanching can remove a large amount of soluble FODMAP from foods. Therefore, it is feasible in clinical practice to categorize foods into high FODMAP foods and low FODMAP foods. The former include cereals such as barley, wheat, rye, and their products; fruits such as apples, pears, apricots, dates, cherries, figs, guavas, custard apple, mango, nectarines, peaches, grapefruit, plums, persimmons, and watermelon; vegetables such as cauliflower, mushrooms, cabbage, garlic, onions, chives, broccoli, asparagus, okra, and sweet corn; beans; milk and dairy products such as creme, cheese, ice cream, yogurt, and liquid milk (cow's milk, goat's milk, condensed milk, evaporated milk); non-milk beverages such as soymilk and soya-bean milk; condiments such as garlic sauce, and honey; artificial sweeteners such as isomalt, mannitol, sorbitol, xylitol, high fructose corn syrup (HFCS), And nuts such as pistachio, almonds, and cashews.

15.3.1.3 Mechanisms of Low FODMAP Diet

In the dietary treatment of IBS, the lack of knowledge about the mechanisms by which food components are related to symptoms restricted the recommendation of what to eat. Nonetheless, the effects of the FODMAP diet on GI function are supported and proved by a range of studies on its mechanisms.

Specific mechanisms may include the following:

1. Fluid and gas are increased in the intestinal lumen. As FODMAP is difficult to be absorbed, it may lead to increase in osmotic pressure and expanded volume of water in the intestinal lumen, promote intestinal peristalsis and transit, and cause osmotic diarrhea. Undigested FODMAP is decomposed and fermented by intestinal bacteria, which increases the content of short-chain fatty acids (SCFA) and gas. Different FODMAPs have different effects on different intestinal segments. Pure fructose significantly increases the water volume in the lumen of the small intestine and dilates the small intestine, whereas mixtures of glucose and fructose and

inulin do not expand the water volume in the lumen of the small intestine but increase the volume of gas in the colon. The increased hypertonicity and gas in the intestinal lumen may alter the excitability of colorectal afferent nerves in patients with IBS and induce CRD hypersensitivity.
2. The low FODMAP diet regulates endocrine cells. The abnormality of endocrine cells is often indicated in the GI of patients with IBS, which may be related to their symptoms. Several studies have found that the density of endocrine cells in the stomach and colorectum of patients with IBS was restored to a similar level as that in healthy volunteers after 3–9 months of following the low FODMAP diet, such as Ghrelin cells, G cells, 5-HT cells, D cells, chromogranin A (CGA), etc. [107].
3. The low FODMAP diet influences intestinal microbiomes. The low FODMAP diet reduces the absolute richness of the stool bacterial community and alters the relative richness of various bacteria, such as the decrease of mucus-associated bacteria and the increase of *Ruminococcus* torques. Besides, it can increase the diversity of the microbiome. These changes may contribute to improve the barrier function of GI and enhance the metabolism of bowel wall and anti-inflammation.

15.3.1.4 Effectiveness of Low FODMAP Diet

Short-Term Clinical Outcome

Over the past few years, a multitude of trial results on the efficacy of the low-FODMAP diet in reducing IBS symptoms has been published. Two latest systematic reviews have different conclusions, yet their publication revealed the growing interest in this field [108, 109]. The results of many studies on the low FODMAP diet in patients with IBS were limited to some extent as most of them were retrospective studies, lack of control or comparison groups, and randomization of patient selection [110]. Furthermore, the low FODMAP diet lacks dietary assessment and therefore has poor compliance in practice. A number of better-designed study of RCTs are undertaking.

In sum, the recent evidence indicates that the low-FODMAP diet is beneficial to 50–80% patients with IBS in the short term, and data from trials suggest that the regimen is at least as effective as standard dietary and lifestyle interventions [111, 112]. Different expectations on treatment may contribute to different feelings of patients and documented symptoms. The management results are subjectively assessed and are highly sensitive to patients' behaviors, and the effect of placebo is considerable. Likewise, the determination of the relief of visceral pain is based on the subjective description of patients in most case, and there is lack of objective indicators used to determine or compare changes. Thus, placebo-controlled trials have already provided forceful evidence for its clinical treatment efficacy. Moreover, a meta-analysis of RCTs studies on the low-FODMAP diet showed higher possibility of improvement in abdominal pain, abdominal distension, and all IBS symptoms compared with all other interventions [108]. Consistent with these results, the Eatwell Guide (UK) recommend that previous basic diets and lifestyles (such as the well-known NICE guidance) are not considered as a success yet in respect of the actual efficacy of the low-FODMAP diet [113].

Long-Term Clinical Outcome

At present, most clinical trials of the low-FODMAP diet focused on assessing short-term (typically within 12 weeks) clinical outcomes. In consideration of the chronic symptom of IBS, the durability of dietary efficacy in the long term is more significant, yet related data are limited so far. This is important because the current standard practice is introducing FODMAP therapy systematically after symptoms have been controlled. The study by Staudacher et al. was the first prospective study to follow 18 patients with IBS after completing the three phases of the low FODMAPs diet (restriction, reintroduction, and personalization) and investigated clinical symptoms, nutrient intake, and gut microbiota at baseline and 12 months later. The results showed that two-thirds of the patients experienced symptomatic improvement after long-term exposure to a structured and personalized low-FODMAP diet, suggesting that the therapy is safe and effective in long-term [114].

RCT studies observed the long-term prognosis of patients with IBS by comparing the low-FODMAP diet treatment with hypnotherapy. It was found that some indicators were indeed improved, but most of the long-term prognostic improvements were not statistically significant [115]. Therefore, further high-quality long-term RCTs are still needed to clarify the symptomatic response time in patients who receive low FODMAP dietary recommendations, especially those who have FODMAP reintroduced after individual tolerance. In addition, given the chronic symptoms of the patients, the impact of long-term dietary control on nutritional intake needs to be further evaluated.

15.3.1.5 Potential Risks of Low FODMAP Diet

Microbiota in the Gastrointestinal Tract

Even though the low FODMAP diet has clinical effects on IBS, some potential adverse effects of clinical effects still exist. In particular, the low FODMAP diet leads to a high intake of prebiotic and fructose food, whereby the substrate of colonic fermentation may be drastically reduced. Thus, strict dietary restrictions would alter the composition and function of the microbiota in the gastrointestinal tract. Currently, several studies have demonstrated that the low FODMAP diet has influence on the gut flora in the intestinal tract [116, 117].

The effects of a low FODMAP diet on the GI microbiota may require further investigations. It is unclear whether the low-FODMAP diet has an effect on specific groups of bacteria (e.g., *Bifidobacteria*) or the entire microbiota community and whether it has a negative effect on their downstream metabolic output or on colonic health. It is also uncertain whether the GI mucosa, the concentration, and pH of proximal colonic SCFA are affected. Meanwhile, if the microbiota is altered at a key moment, there may be consequences for gut function, but it is not known whether these changes alter short- or long-term prognosis. To date, most studies are descriptive observations of the microbiome and metabolome in clinical trials of the low-FODMAP diet. It is equally important to study the changes in the human microbiome and its production guided by low FODMAP in vitro study. Tolerance of the low FODMAP diet may decrease the abovementioned changes, and research on the combined treatment of FODMAP restriction with probiotic supplementation is ongoing.

Nutritional Intake

Studies have shown that the nutritional needs of most patients with enteropathy are met, and the nutritional intake does not show any difference compared with the control group. During the clinical treatment, there are always inevitable contradictions between the clinical effectiveness of therapeutic diets, the maintenance of appropriate nutritional intake, and adherence to dietary habits. Treatment decisions should be made based on the measurement of advantages and disadvantages of the abovementioned aspects. It is suggested that the low FODMAP diet leads to lower carbohydrate intake compared with the habitual diet [118]. Nevertheless, carbohydrate intake (150–200 g/d) reflects health status although its effect is small. It was reported a substantial reduction in energy intake of patients following a low FODMAP recommendation, which probably arouses concerns, especially for patients who have formed long-term eating habits [118]. Nonetheless, the same changes were present in patients following standard IBS recommendations, so they may not necessarily be induced solely by the low FODMAP diet, but may result from objective changes in the diet.

Measurement error due to lack of data on the composition of low-lactose foods may also be a factor affecting the results of the study. However, whether the intake of calcium or other micronutrients affects the prognosis of patients with IBS who follows the low-FODMAP diet needs to be confirmed by further studies. In summary, assessment of nutrient intake and dietary diversity after the introduction of the low FODMAP diet is important to determine whether the dietary profile poses any long-term nutritional risk for IBS.

In conclusion, at present, there is sufficient evidence that the low FODMAP diet has certain clinical efficacy in IBS, which may be a milestone of IBS treatment as the disease was difficult to be treated with drugs and diets. The low FODMAP diet not only alleviates the symptoms of IBS but also relieves the visceral hypersensitivity and visceral pain related to IBS. There are evidence showing that the low FODMAP diet profoundly affects the microbiota and its metabolites, but further research is necessary to clarify the duration, nature, and impact of the changes in both short and long terms. At present, most of the data comes from relatively small-scale, short-term, single-center, single-blind, or unblinded controlled trials, and there is a lack of long-term efficacy and safety data. Further large-scale, multicenter, long-term, double-blind clinical studies are needed to determine the ideal duration of maintenance on the low-FODMAP diet and to search for possible stool/serum markers or other indicators for predicting which patients with IBS are best suited to the low-FODMAP diet therapy. Meanwhile, interventions associated with the low-FODMAP diet are used as a significant dual prevention and combination therapies to prevent potentially adverse effects on the microflora. In addition, prediction of response to dietary modifications will help optimize the management of patients with IBS and reduce unnecessary dietary restrictions in patients who may response poorly to this treatment.

15.3.2 Probiotic Therapy

As a group of active microorganisms colonized in the human intestinal system and beneficial to the host, intestinal probiotics can produce precise health effects such as improving the microecological balance. Beneficial bacteria or fungi in the human body include *Clostridium butyricum*, *Lactobacillus*, *bifidobacterium*, Actinomycetes, yeast, and so on. Techniques for regulating intestinal microbial homeostasis through probiotics have shown that intestinal probiotics such as *Bifidobacterium* and *Lactobacillus* can reverse visceral hypersensitivity [119, 120].

In studies of modeling mother-infant separation in the neonatal period in mice, IBS and visceral hypersensitivity found the that the application of VSL#3, a mixture of several probiotics, can prevent the progression of hypersensitivity [121, 122]. Furthermore, in a model of inflammatory visceral hypersensitivity induced by the injection of 4% acetic acid in colonic, prophylactic application of probiotics can reduce visceral sensitization of rats while also decreasing defecation rate and colonic permeability and increasing the expression of tight junction proteins [123–125]. It has also been demonstrated that *Bifidobacterium* spp., especially *Bifidobacterium longum* subspecies *infantis*, is effective in ameliorating stress-induced visceral hypersensitivity in rats and colitis [126]. Overall, there are fewer clinical applications and research reports on the therapeutic effects of probiotics on visceral pain, and their mechanisms and roles need to be further explored and clarified.

On the clinical side, some studies have evaluated the potential effects of gut microbiota on peristalsis, the sympathetic nervous system (SNS), the autonomic nervous system (ANS), the hypothalamic-pituitary-adrenal (HPA) axis, the enteric nervous system (ENS), the mucosal barrier, and neuroimmune signaling. Interactions can occur between gut flora, the stress system, and ANS [127]. Changes associated with the microbiota may be one option for the treatment of visceral pain-related disorders and have therapeutic effects on visceral hypersensitivity and visceral pain [128]. All the observations suggest that therapeutic interventions that modify the gut flora through oral probiotics or other measures may be beneficial for patients with IBS [129].

Early studies have shown that patients with functional gastrointestinal disorders (FGIDs) and flatulence were affected by probiotics such as bifidobacteria or co-probiotics alone [130]. Studies in recent years have reported the advantages of probiotics over placebo treatment in terms of systemic symptoms or abdominal pain scores [131, 132]. However, these data did not provide enough information to clearly assess the impact of probiotics on abdominal pain. The systematic review and meta-analysis of intestinal probiotics in 2015 included 15 trials, only two of which had enough data to assess their impact on abdominal pain. These studies used mixed *Escherichia coli* (DSM 17252) and *Enterococcus* (DSM 16440) or *E. coli* (DSM 17252) as probiotics and compared them with placebo. In patients with abdominal pain caused by IBS, the response rate to probiotics was higher than the placebo [133]. Yet, the RCT of probiotic preparations found that probiotics did not have significant advantages over placebo in controlling the pain of adult patients with IBS, though some clinical trials have found that probiotics can improve the frequency and intensity of abdominal pain in children with IBS [134].

Overall, the role of probiotics in the treatment of abdominal pain depends on the strain types, and the effect on children may be more obvious. Therefore, future research is needed to explore which strains and patient groups will benefit most from the treatment.

15.4 Conclusion

There is a great demand for safe and effective visceral analgesics in clinical practice. Currently, the improvement of FGIDs is the most effective treatment for visceral pain, such as the application of 5-HT receptor antagonists. The actual efficacy of antidepressants for visceral pain remains highly controversial due to research methodology or patient selection. As for drugs acting on ion channels or receptors, the proper efficacy against visceral hypersensitivity can only be achieved if subtypes selected by identifying biomarkers works well on compounds. Besides, it is necessary to develop visceral analgesics for peripheral application on central nervous system without adverse effects by the combined application of basic neurobiology and pharmacology. Advances in nonmedical treatment significantly broaden the range of visceral pain treatment and allow clinicians to deal with traditionally intractable visceral pain through various approaches, which coincide with the concept of "multimodal analgesia (MMA)" that is widely advocated today. MMA refers to the analgesic modality of combining multiple medical and nonmedical methods, which overcomes deficiencies in treatment to achieve the best analgesic effect while minimizing adverse reactions and side effects. Besides, latest findings on models of gene expression in mucosa, miRNA in human biopsy, epigenetic marks, and animal models of visceral hypersensitivity suggested that the future treatment of abdominal or visceral pain may be based on novel mechanisms or clinical study outcomes instead of research and clinical applications related to somatic pain.

References

1. WHO guidelines for the pharmacological and radiotherapeutic management of cancer pain in adults and adolescents. World Health Organization. 2019. https://www.who.int/publications/i/item/9789241550390. Accessed 17 Aug 2023.
2. Urits I, Li N, Berardino K, Artounian KA, Bandi P, Jung JW, Kaye RJ, Manchikanti L, Kaye AM, Simopoulos T, Kaye AD, Torres M, Viswanath O. The use of antineuropathic medications for the treatment of chronic pain. Best Pract Res Clin Anaesthesiol. 2020 Sep;34(3):493–506. https://doi.org/10.1016/j.bpa.2020.08.007.
3. Khan MI, Walsh D, Brito-Dellan N. Opioid and adjuvant analgesics: compared and contrasted. Am J Hosp Palliat Care. 2011;28(5):378–83. https://doi.org/10.1177/1049909111410298.
4. Gurusamy KS, Lusuku C, Davidson BR. Pregabalin for decreasing pancreatic pain in chronic pancreatitis. Cochrane Database Syst Rev. 2016 Feb 2;2(2):CD011522. https://doi.org/10.1002/14651858.CD011522.pub2.
5. Thorpe AJ, Offord J. The alpha2-delta protein: an auxiliary subunit of voltage-dependent calcium channels as a recognized drug target. Curr Opin Investig Drugs. 2010;11(7):761–70.
6. Bayer K, Ahmadi S, Zeilhofer H. Gabapentin may inhibit synaptic transmission in the mouse spinal cord dorsal horn through a preferential block of P/Q-type Ca2+ channels. Neuropharmacology. 2004;46(5):743–9. https://doi.org/10.1016/j.neuropharm.2003.11.010.
7. Olesen SS, Bouwense SA, Wilder-Smith OH, van Goor H, Drewes AM. Pregabalin reduces pain in patients with chronic pancreatitis in a randomized, controlled trial. Gastroenterology. 2011;141(2):536–43. https://doi.org/10.1053/j.gastro.2011.04.003.

8. Bonilla-Jaime H, Sánchez-Salcedo JA, Estevez-Cabrera MM, Molina-Jiménez T, Cortes-Altamirano JL, Alfaro-Rodríguez A. Depression and pain: use of antidepressants. Curr Neuropharmacol. 2022;20(2):384–402. https://doi.org/10.2174/1570159X19666210609161447.
9. Verdu B, Decosterd I, Buclin T, Stiefel F, Berney A. Antidepressants for the treatment of chronic pain. Drugs. 2008;68(18):2611–32. https://doi.org/10.2165/0003495-200868180-00007.
10. Annaházi A, Róka R, Rosztóczy A, Wittmann T. Role of antispasmodics in the treatment of irritable bowel syndrome. World J Gastroenterol. 2014;20(20):6031–43.
11. Ford AC, Talley NJ, Spiegel BM, Foxx-Orenstein AE, Schiller L, Quigley EM, Moayyedi P. Effect of fibre, antispasmodics, and peppermint oil in the treatment of irritable bowel syndrome: systematic review and meta-analysis. BMJ. 2008 Nov;13(337):a2313. https://doi.org/10.1136/bmj.a2313.
12. Clavé P, Acalovschi M, Triantafillidis JK, Uspensky YP, Kalayci C, Shee V, Tack J; OBIS Study Investigators. Randomised clinical trial: otilonium bromide improves frequency of abdominal pain, severity of distention and time to relapse in patients with irritable bowel syndrome. Aliment Pharmacol Ther. 2011;34(4):432–42. https://doi.org/10.1111/j.1365-2036.2011.04730.x.
13. Glende M, Morselli-Labate AM, Battaglia G, Evangelista S. Extended analysis of a double-blind, placebo-controlled, 15-week study with otilonium bromide in irritable bowel syndrome. Eur J Gastroenterol Hepatol. 2002;14(12):1331–8. https://doi.org/10.1097/00042737-200212000-00008.
14. Battaglia G, Morselli-Labate AM, Camarri E, Francavilla A, De Marco F, Mastropaolo G, Naccarato R. Otilonium bromide in irritable bowel syndrome: a double-blind, placebo-controlled, 15-week study. Aliment Pharmacol Ther. 1998;12(10):1003–10. https://doi.org/10.1046/j.1365-2036.1998.00397.x.
15. Talley NJ, Ford AC. Functional dyspepsia. N Engl J Med. 2015;373(19):1853–63. https://doi.org/10.1056/NEJMra1501505.
16. Lee KJ, Kindt S, Tack J. Pathophysiology of functional dyspepsia. Best Pract Res Clin Gastroenterol. 2004;18(4):707–16. https://doi.org/10.1016/j.bpg.2004.04.007.
17. Lacy BE, Weiser KT, Kennedy AT, Crowell MD, Talley NJ. Functional dyspepsia: the economic impact to patients. Aliment Pharmacol Ther. 2013 Jul;38(2):170–7. https://doi.org/10.1111/apt.12355.
18. Moayyedi P, Mason J. Clinical and economic consequences of dyspepsia in the community. Gut. 2002;50:iv10–2.
19. Ford AC, Tsipotis E, Yuan Y, Leontiadis GI, Moayyedi P. Efficacy of *helicobacter pylori* eradication therapy for functional dyspepsia: updated systematic review and meta-analysis. Gut. 2022;12:gutjnl-2021-326583. https://doi.org/10.1136/gutjnl-2021-326583.
20. Pinto-Sanchez MI, Yuan Y, Hassan A, Bercik P, Moayyedi P. Proton pump inhibitors for functional dyspepsia. Cochrane Database Syst Rev. 2017;11(11):CD011194. https://doi.org/10.1002/14651858.CD011194.pub3.
21. Aro P, Talley NJ, Ronkainen J, Storskrubb T, Vieth M, Johansson SE, Bolling-Sternevald E, Agréus L. Anxiety is associated with uninvestigated and functional dyspepsia (Rome III criteria) in a Swedish population-based study. Gastroenterology. 2009;137(1):94–100. https://doi.org/10.1053/j.gastro.2009.03.039.
22. Vanheel H, Vicario M, Vanuytsel T, Van Oudenhove L, Martinez C, Keita ÅV, Pardon N, Santos J, Söderholm JD, Tack J, Farré R. Impaired duodenal mucosal integrity and low-grade inflammation in functional dyspepsia. Gut. 2014;63(2):262–71. https://doi.org/10.1136/gutjnl-2012-303857.
23. Van Oudenhove L, Aziz Q. The role of psychosocial factors and psychiatric disorders in functional dyspepsia. Nat Rev Gastroenterol Hepatol. 2013;10(3):158–67. https://doi.org/10.1038/nrgastro.2013.10.
24. Singh R, Zogg H, Ghoshal UC, Ro S. Current treatment options and therapeutic insights for gastrointestinal Dysmotility and functional gastrointestinal disorders. Front Pharmacol. 2022;13:808195. https://doi.org/10.3389/fphar.2022.808195.
25. Tack J, Janssen P, Masaoka T, Farré R, Van Oudenhove L. Efficacy of buspirone, a fundus-relaxing drug, in patients with functional dyspepsia. Clin Gastroenterol Hepatol. 2012;10(11):1239–45. https://doi.org/10.1016/j.cgh.2012.06.036.
26. Moayyedi P, Lacy BE, Andrews CN, Enns RA, Howden CW, Vakil N. ACG and CAG clinical guideline: management of dyspepsia. Am J Gastroenterol. 2017;112(7):988–1013. https://doi.org/10.1038/ajg.2017.154. Erratum in: Am J Gastroenterol. 2017 Sep;112(9):1484.
27. Ford AC, Luthra P, Tack J, Boeckxstaens GE, Moayyedi P, Talley NJ. Efficacy of psychotropic drugs in functional dyspepsia: systematic review and meta-analysis. Gut. 2017;66(3):411–20. https://doi.org/10.1136/gutjnl-2015-310721.
28. Miwa H, Nagahara A, Tominaga K, Yokoyama T, Sawada Y, Inoue K, Ashida K, Fukuchi T, Hojo M, Yamashita H, Tomita T, Hori K, Oshima T. Efficacy of the 5-HT1A agonist tandospirone citrate in improving symptoms of patients with functional dyspepsia: a randomized controlled trial. Am J Gastroenterol. 2009;104(11):2779–87. https://doi.org/10.1038/ajg.2009.427.
29. Caterina MJ, Schumacher MA, Tominaga M, Rosen TA, Levine JD, Julius D. The capsaicin receptor: a heat-activated ion channel in the pain pathway. Nature. 1997;389(6653):816–24. https://doi.org/10.1038/39807.
30. Frias B, Merighi A. Capsaicin, nociception and pain. Molecules. 2016;21(6):797. https://doi.org/10.3390/molecules21060797.
31. Luongo L, Costa B, D'Agostino B, Guida F, Comelli F, Gatta L, Matteis M, Sullo N, De Petrocellis L,

de Novellis V, Maione S, Di Marzo V. Palvanil, a non-pungent capsaicin analogue, inhibits inflammatory and neuropathic pain with little effects on bronchopulmonary function and body temperature. Pharmacol Res. 2012;66(3):243–50. https://doi.org/10.1016/j.phrs.2012.05.005.

32. Honore P, Chandran P, Hernandez G, Gauvin DM, Mikusa JP, Zhong C, Joshi SK, Ghilardi JR, Sevcik MA, Fryer RM, Segreti JA, Banfor PN, Marsh K, Neelands T, Bayburt E, Daanen JF, Gomtsyan A, Lee CH, Kort ME, Reilly RM, Surowy CS, Kym PR, Mantyh PW, Sullivan JP, Jarvis MF, Faltynek CR. Repeated dosing of ABT-102, a potent and selective TRPV1 antagonist, enhances TRPV1-mediated analgesic activity in rodents, but attenuates antagonist-induced hyperthermia. Pain. 2009;142(1–2):27–35. https://doi.org/10.1016/j.pain.2008.11.004.
33. Kimball ES, Wallace NH, Schneider CR, D'Andrea MR, Hornby PJ. Vanilloid receptor 1 antagonists attenuate disease severity in dextran sulphate sodium-induced colitis in mice. Neurogastroenterol Motil. 2004;16(6):811–8. https://doi.org/10.1111/j.1365-2982.2004.00549.x.
34. Akbar A, Yiangou Y, Facer P, Walters JR, Anand P, Ghosh S. Increased capsaicin receptor TRPV1-expressing sensory fibres in irritable bowel syndrome and their correlation with abdominal pain. Gut. 2008;57(7):923–9. https://doi.org/10.1136/gut.2007.138982.
35. Wang X, Lin C, Lan L, Liu J. Perioperative intravenous S-ketamine for acute postoperative pain in adults: a systematic review and meta-analysis. J Clin Anesth. 2021;68:110071. https://doi.org/10.1016/j.jclinane.2020.110071.
36. Zanos P, Gould TD. Mechanisms of ketamine action as an antidepressant. Mol Psychiatry. 2018;23(4):801–11. https://doi.org/10.1038/mp.2017.255.
37. Bouwense SA, Buscher HC, van Goor H, Wilder-Smith OH. S-ketamine modulates hyperalgesia in patients with chronic pancreatitis pain. Reg Anesth Pain Med. 2011;36(3):303–7. https://doi.org/10.1097/AAP.0b013e3182177022.
38. Juel J, Olesen SS, Olesen AE, Poulsen JL, Dahan A, Wilder-Smith O, Madzak A, Frøkjær JB, Drewes AM. Study protocol for a randomised, double-blinded, placebo-controlled, clinical trial of S-ketamine for pain treatment in patients with chronic pancreatitis (RESET trial). BMJ Open. 2015;5(3):e007087. https://doi.org/10.1136/bmjopen-2014-007087. PMID: 25757947; PMCID: PMC4360788.
39. Owolabi JB, Rizkalla G, Tehim A, Ross GM, Riopelle RJ, Kamboj R, Ossipov M, Bian D, Wegert S, Porreca F, Lee DK. Characterization of antiallodynic actions of ALE-0540, a novel nerve growth factor receptor antagonist, in the rat. J Pharmacol Exp Ther. 1999;289(3):1271–6.
40. Hefti FF, Rosenthal A, Walicke PA, Wyatt S, Vergara G, Shelton DL, Davies AM. Novel class of pain drugs based on antagonism of NGF. Trends Pharmacol Sci. 2006;27(2):85–91. https://doi.org/10.1016/j.tips.2005.12.001.
41. McKelvey L, Shorten GD, O'Keeffe GW. Nerve growth factor-mediated regulation of pain signalling and proposed new intervention strategies in clinical pain management. J Neurochem. 2013;124(3):276–89. https://doi.org/10.1111/jnc.12093.
42. Lu CL. Spinal microglia: a potential target in the treatment of chronic visceral pain. J Chin Med Assoc. 2014;77(1):3–9. https://doi.org/10.1016/j.jcma.2013.08.008.
43. Bryant AP, Busby RW, Bartolini WP, Cordero EA, Hannig G, Kessler MM, Pierce CM, Solinga RM, Tobin JV, Mahajan-Miklos S, Cohen MB, Kurtz CB, Currie MG. Linaclotide is a potent and selective guanylate cyclase C agonist that elicits pharmacological effects locally in the gastrointestinal tract. Life Sci. 2010;86(19–20):760–5. https://doi.org/10.1016/j.lfs.2010.03.015.
44. Busby RW, Bryant AP, Bartolini WP, Cordero EA, Hannig G, Kessler MM, Mahajan-Miklos S, Pierce CM, Solinga RM, Sun LJ, Tobin JV, Kurtz CB, Currie MG. Linaclotide, through activation of guanylate cyclase C, acts locally in the gastrointestinal tract to elicit enhanced intestinal secretion and transit. Eur J Pharmacol. 2010;649(1–3):328–35. https://doi.org/10.1016/j.ejphar.2010.09.019.
45. Andresen V, Camilleri M, Busciglio IA, Grudell A, Burton D, McKinzie S, Foxx-Orenstein A, Kurtz CB, Sharma V, Johnston JM, Currie MG, Zinsmeister AR. Effect of 5 days linaclotide on transit and bowel function in females with constipation-predominant irritable bowel syndrome. Gastroenterology. 2007;133(3):761–8. https://doi.org/10.1053/j.gastro.2007.06.067.
46. Castro J, Harrington AM, Hughes PA, Martin CM, Ge P, Shea CM, Jin H, Jacobson S, Hannig G, Mann E, Cohen MB, MacDougall JE, Lavins BJ, Kurtz CB, Silos-Santiago I, Johnston JM, Currie MG, Blackshaw LA, Brierley SM. Linaclotide inhibits colonic nociceptors and relieves abdominal pain via guanylate cyclase-C and extracellular cyclic guanosine 3′,5′-monophosphate. Gastroenterology. 2013;145(6):1334–46.e1–11. https://doi.org/10.1053/j.gastro.2013.08.017.
47. Johnston JM, Kurtz CB, Macdougall JE, Lavins BJ, Currie MG, Fitch DA, O'Dea C, Baird M, Lembo AJ. Linaclotide improves abdominal pain and bowel habits in a phase IIb study of patients with irritable bowel syndrome with constipation. Gastroenterology. 2010;139(6):1877–1886.e2. https://doi.org/10.1053/j.gastro.2010.08.041.
48. Quigley EM, Tack J, Chey WD, Rao SS, Fortea J, Falques M, Diaz C, Shiff SJ, Currie MG, Johnston JM. Randomised clinical trials: linaclotide phase 3 studies in IBS-C - a prespecified further analysis based on European medicines agency-specified endpoints. Aliment Pharmacol Ther. 2013;37(1):49–61. https://doi.org/10.1111/apt.12123.

49. Nguyen V, Tiemann D, Park E, Salehi A. Alpha-2 Agonists. Anesthesiol Clin. 2017;35(2):233–45. https://doi.org/10.1016/j.anclin.2017.01.009.
50. Abed A, Khoshnoud MJ, Taghian M, Aliasgharzadeh M, Mesdaghinia A. Quetiapine reverses paclitaxel-induced neuropathic pain in mice: role of alpha2-adrenergic receptors. Iran J Basic Med Sci. 2017;20(11):1182–8. https://doi.org/10.22038/IJBMS.2017.9500.
51. Yang Y, Zhou W, Xu X, Ge X, Wang F, Zhang GQ, Miao L, Deng X. Aprepitant inhibits JNK and p38/MAPK to attenuate inflammation and suppresses inflammatory pain. Front Pharmacol. 2022 Jan;11(12):811584. https://doi.org/10.3389/fphar.2021.811584.
52. Honore P, Mikusa J, Bianchi B, McDonald H, Cartmell J, Faltynek C, Jarvis MF. TNP-ATP, a potent P2X3 receptor antagonist, blocks acetic acid-induced abdominal constriction in mice: comparison with reference analgesics. Pain. 2002;96(1–2):99–105. https://doi.org/10.1016/s0304-3959(01)00434-1.
53. Luo HM, Ye JR, Pu FQ, Luo HL, Zhang WJ. Role and therapeutic target of P2X2/3 receptors in visceral pain. Neuropeptides. 2023;101:102355. https://doi.org/10.1016/j.npep.2023.102355.
54. Xu GY, Shenoy M, Winston JH, Mittal S, Pasricha PJ. P2X receptor-mediated visceral hyperalgesia in a rat model of chronic visceral hypersensitivity. Gut. 2008;57(9):1230–7. https://doi.org/10.1136/gut.2007.134221.
55. Woods AJ, Antal A, Bikson M, Boggio PS, Brunoni AR, Celnik P, Cohen LG, Fregni F, Herrmann CS, Kappenman ES, Knotkova H, Liebetanz D, Miniussi C, Miranda PC, Paulus W, Priori A, Reato D, Stagg C, Wenderoth N, Nitsche MA. A technical guide to tDCS, and related non-invasive brain stimulation tools. Clin Neurophysiol. 2016;127(2):1031–48. https://doi.org/10.1016/j.clinph.2015.11.012.
56. Villamar MF, Santos Portilla A, Fregni F, Zafonte R. Noninvasive brain stimulation to modulate neuroplasticity in traumatic brain injury. Neuromodulation. 2012;15(4):326–38. https://doi.org/10.1111/j.1525-1403.2012.00474.x.
57. Camacho-Conde JA, Del Rosario G-BM, Carretero-Rey M, Khan ZU. Therapeutic potential of brain stimulation techniques in the treatment of mental, psychiatric, and cognitive disorders. CNS Neurosci Ther. 2023;29(1):8–23. https://doi.org/10.1111/cns.13971.
58. Fregni F, El-Hagrassy MM, Pacheco-Barrios K, Carvalho S, Leite J, Simis M, Brunelin J, Nakamura-Palacios EM, Marangolo P, Venkatasubramanian G, San-Juan D, Caumo W, Bikson M, Brunoni AR, Neuromodulation Center Working Group. Evidence-based guidelines and secondary meta-analysis for the use of transcranial direct current stimulation in neurological and psychiatric disorders. Int J Neuropsychopharmacol. 2021;24(4):256–313. https://doi.org/10.1093/ijnp/pyaa051.
59. Manji A, Amimoto K, Matsuda T, Wada Y, Inaba A, Ko S. Effects of transcranial direct current stimulation over the supplementary motor area body weight-supported treadmill gait training in hemiparetic patients after stroke. Neurosci Lett. 2018;662:302–5. https://doi.org/10.1016/j.neulet.2017.10.049.
60. Marshall L, Mölle M, Hallschmid M, Born J. Transcranial direct current stimulation during sleep improves declarative memory. J Neurosci. 2004;24(44):9985–92. https://doi.org/10.1523/JNEUROSCI.2725-04.2004. Erratum in: J Neurosci 2005 Jan 12;25(2):1 p following 531.
61. Palm U, Hasan A, Strube W, Padberg F. tDCS for the treatment of depression: a comprehensive review. Eur Arch Psychiatry Clin Neurosci. 2016;266(8):681–94. https://doi.org/10.1007/s00406-016-0674-9.
62. Freire RC, Cabrera-Abreu C, Milev R. Neurostimulation in anxiety disorders, post-traumatic stress disorder, and obsessive-compulsive disorder. Adv Exp Med Biol. 2020;1191:331–46. https://doi.org/10.1007/978-981-32-9705-0_18.
63. Knotkova H, Hamani C, Sivanesan E, Le Beuffe MFE, Moon JY, Cohen SP, Huntoon MA. Neuromodulation for chronic pain. Lancet. 2021;397(10289):2111–24. https://doi.org/10.1016/S0140-6736(21)00794-7.
64. Sinopoulou V, Gordon M, Akobeng AK, Gasparetto M, Sammaan M, Vasiliou J, Dovey TM. Interventions for the management of abdominal pain in Crohn's disease and inflammatory bowel disease. Cochrane Database Syst Rev. 2021;11(11):CD013531. https://doi.org/10.1002/14651858.CD013531.pub2.
65. Santos DS, Lopes BC, Medeiros LF, Assumpção JAF, de Souza A, Salvi AA, da Silva LS, Fregni F, Caumo W, Torres ILS. Transcranial direct current stimulation (tDCS) induces analgesia in rats with neuropathic pain and alcohol abstinence. Neurochem Res. 2020;45(11):2653–63. https://doi.org/10.1007/s11064-020-03116-w.
66. Nitsche MA, Boggio PS, Fregni F, Pascual-Leone A. Treatment of depression with transcranial direct current stimulation (tDCS): a review. Exp Neurol. 2009;219(1):14–9. https://doi.org/10.1016/j.expneurol.2009.03.038.
67. Somaa FA, de Graaf TA, Sack AT. Transcranial magnetic stimulation in the treatment of neurological diseases. Front Neurol. 2022;13:793253. https://doi.org/10.3389/fneur.2022.793253.
68. Sun H, Li Z, Qiu Z, Shen Y, Guo Q, Hu SW, Ding HL, An S, Cao JL. A common neuronal ensemble in nucleus accumbens regulates pain-like behaviour and sleep. Nat Commun. 2023;14(1):4700. https://doi.org/10.1038/s41467-023-40450-3.
69. Choy EH. The role of sleep in pain and fibromyalgia. Nat Rev Rheumatol. 2015;11(9):513–20. https://doi.org/10.1038/nrrheum.2015.56.
70. Li G, Jin B, Fan Z. Clinical application of transcranial magnetic stimulation for functional bowel disease. Front Med (Lausanne). 2023;10:1213067. https://doi.org/10.3389/fmed.2023.1213067.

71. Nizard J, Levesque A, Denis N, de Chauvigny E, Lepeintre A, Raoul S, Labat JJ, Bulteau S, Maillard B, Buffenoir K, Potel G, Lefaucheur JP, Nguyen JP. Interest of repetitive transcranial magnetic stimulation of the motor cortex in the management of refractory cancer pain in palliative care: two case reports. Palliat Med. 2015;29(6):564–8. https://doi.org/10.1177/0269216315574260.
72. Lefaucheur JP. Pain Handb Clin Neurol. 2013;116:423–40. https://doi.org/10.1016/B978-0-444-53497-2.00035-8.
73. Galhardoni R, Correia GS, Araujo H, Yeng LT, Fernandes DT, Kaziyama HH, Marcolin MA, Bouhassira D, Teixeira MJ, de Andrade DC. Repetitive transcranial magnetic stimulation in chronic pain: a review of the literature. Arch Phys Med Rehabil. 2015;96(4 Suppl):S156–72. https://doi.org/10.1016/j.apmr.2014.11.010.
74. Moisset X, Lefaucheur JP. Non pharmacological treatment for neuropathic pain: invasive and non-invasive cortical stimulation. Rev Neurol (Paris). 2019;175(1–2):51–8. https://doi.org/10.1016/j.neurol.2018.09.014.
75. Gibson W, Wand BM, Meads C, Catley MJ, O'Connell NE. Transcutaneous electrical nerve stimulation (TENS) for chronic pain - an overview of Cochrane Reviews. Cochrane Database Syst Rev. 2019;4(4):CD011890. https://doi.org/10.1002/14651858.CD011890.pub3.
76. Sbruzzi G, Silveira SA, Silva DV, Coronel CC, Plentz RD. Transcutaneous electrical nerve stimulation after thoracic surgery: systematic review and meta-analysis of 11 randomized trials. Rev Bras Cir Cardiovasc. 2012;27(1):75–87. https://doi.org/10.5935/1678-9741.20120012.
77. Bjordal JM, Johnson MI, Lopes-Martins RA, Bogen B, Chow R, Ljunggren AE. Short-term efficacy of physical interventions in osteoarthritic knee pain. A systematic review and meta-analysis of randomised placebo-controlled trials. BMC Musculoskelet Disord. 2007;8:51. https://doi.org/10.1186/1471-2474-8-51.
78. Bedwell C, Dowswell T, Neilson JP, Lavender T. The use of transcutaneous electrical nerve stimulation (TENS) for pain relief in labour: a review of the evidence. Midwifery. 2011;27(5):e141–8. https://doi.org/10.1016/j.midw.2009.12.004.
79. Hurlow A, Bennett MI, Robb KA, Johnson MI, Simpson KH, Oxberry SG. Transcutaneous electric nerve stimulation (TENS) for cancer pain in adults. Cochrane Database Syst Rev. 2012;2012(3):CD006276. https://doi.org/10.1002/14651858.CD006276.pub3.
80. Johnson MI, Paley CA, Jones G, Mulvey MR, Wittkopf PG. Efficacy and safety of transcutaneous electrical nerve stimulation (TENS) for acute and chronic pain in adults: a systematic review and meta-analysis of 381 studies (the meta-TENS study). BMJ Open. 2022;12(2):e051073. https://doi.org/10.1136/bmjopen-2021-051073.
81. Walsh DM, Howe TE, Johnson MI, Sluka KA. Transcutaneous electrical nerve stimulation for acute pain. Cochrane Database Syst Rev. 2009;2:CD006142. https://doi.org/10.1002/14651858.CD006142. Update in: Cochrane Database Syst Rev. 2015;6:CD006142
82. Chitneni A, Hasoon J, Urits I, Viswanath O, Berger A, Kaye A. Peripheral nerve stimulation for chronic shoulder pain due to rotator cuff pathology. Orthop Rev (Pavia). 2022;14(3):37494. https://doi.org/10.52965/001c.37494.
83. Guo Y, Gharibani P. Analgesic effects of Vagus nerve stimulation on visceral hypersensitivity: a direct comparison between invasive and noninvasive methods in rats. Neuromodulation. 2023;S1094-7159(23):00153–8. https://doi.org/10.1016/j.neurom.2023.04.001.
84. Sun Y, Tan Y, Song G, Chen JD. Effects and mechanisms of gastric electrical stimulation on visceral pain in a rodent model of gastric hyperalgesia secondary to chemically induced mucosal ulceration. Neurogastroenterol Motil. 2014;26(2):176–86. https://doi.org/10.1111/nmo.12248.
85. Lahr CJ, Griffith J, Subramony C, Halley L, Adams K, Paine ER, Schmieg R, Islam S, Salameh J, Spree D, Kothari T, Kedar A, Nikitina Y, Abell T. Gastric electrical stimulation for abdominal pain in patients with symptoms of gastroparesis. Am Surg. 2013;79(5):457–64.
86. Noble M, Gress FG. Techniques and results of neurolysis for chronic pancreatitis and pancreatic cancer pain. Curr Gastroenterol Rep. 2006;8(2):99–103. https://doi.org/10.1007/s11894-006-0004-x.
87. Worsey J, Ferson PF, Keenan RJ, Julian TB, Landreneau RJ. Thoracoscopic pancreatic denervation for pain control in irresectable pancreatic cancer. Br J Surg. 1993;80(8):1051–2. https://doi.org/10.1002/bjs.1800800842.
88. Bosanquet DC, Wilcox CR, Rasheed A. Bilateral Thoracoscopic Splanchnotomy to alleviate pain in chronic pancreatic disease. Ann Thorac Surg. 2016;101(3):e91–3. https://doi.org/10.1016/j.athoracsur.2015.10.019.
89. Kinsinger SW. Cognitive-behavioral therapy for patients with irritable bowel syndrome: current insights. Psychol Res Behav Manag. 2017;10:231–7. https://doi.org/10.2147/PRBM.S120817.
90. Kim YS, Kim N. Sex-gender differences in irritable bowel syndrome. J Neurogastroenterol Motil. 2018;24(4):544–58. https://doi.org/10.5056/jnm18082.
91. Montgomery GH, DuHamel KN, Redd WH. A meta-analysis of hypnotically induced analgesia: how effective is hypnosis? Int J Clin Exp Hypn. 2000;48(2):138–53. https://doi.org/10.1080/00207140008410045.
92. Peters SL, Muir JG, Gibson PR. Review article: gut-directed hypnotherapy in the management of irritable bowel syndrome and inflammatory bowel disease. Aliment Pharmacol Ther. 2015;41(11):1104–15. https://doi.org/10.1111/apt.13202.
93. van Lanen AS, de Bree A, Greyling A. Efficacy of a low-FODMAP diet in adult irritable bowel syn-

drome: a systematic review and meta-analysis. Eur J Nutr. 2021;60(6):3505–22. https://doi.org/10.1007/s00394-020-02473-0.

94. Zhang JY, Niu C, Zhang Q, Wang MJ, Ni L, Liu JF, Rong XY, Zhao C, Chen J. Full-scale clinical data and reshaped intestinal microbiome on a short-term low-phosphorus diet among healthy adults. J Ren Nutr. 2021;31(5):448–58. https://doi.org/10.1053/j.jrn.2020.11.004. Epub 2021 Feb 25
95. Nagarajan N, Morden A, Bischof D, King EA, Kosztowski M, Wick EC, Stein EM. The role of fiber supplementation in the treatment of irritable bowel syndrome: a systematic review and meta-analysis. Eur J Gastroenterol Hepatol. 2015;27(9):1002–10. https://doi.org/10.1097/MEG.0000000000000425.
96. Aziz I, Trott N, Briggs R, North JR, Hadjivassiliou M, Sanders DS. Efficacy of a gluten-free diet in subjects with irritable bowel syndrome-diarrhea unaware of their HLA-DQ2/8 genotype. Clin Gastroenterol Hepatol. 2016;14(5):696–703.e1. https://doi.org/10.1016/j.cgh.2015.12.031.
97. Vazquez-Roque MI, Camilleri M, Smyrk T, Murray JA, Marietta E, O'Neill J, Carlson P, Lamsam J, Janzow D, Eckert D, Burton D, Zinsmeister AR. A controlled trial of gluten-free diet in patients with irritable bowel syndrome-diarrhea: effects on bowel frequency and intestinal function. Gastroenterology. 2013;144(5):903–911.e3. https://doi.org/10.1053/j.gastro.2013.01.049.
98. Mohseni F, Agah S, Ebrahimi-Daryani N, Taher M, Nattagh-Eshtivani E, Karimi S, Rastgoo S, Bourbour F, Hekmatdoost A. The effect of low FODMAP diet with and without gluten on irritable bowel syndrome: a double blind, placebo controlled randomized clinical trial. Clin Nutr ESPEN. 2022;47:45–50. https://doi.org/10.1016/j.clnesp.2021.12.019.
99. Aguilera-Lizarraga J, Florens MV, Viola MF, Jain P, Decraecker L, Appeltans I, Cuende-Estevez M, Fabre N, Van Beek K, Perna E, Balemans D, Stakenborg N, Theofanous S, Bosmans G, Mondelaers SU, Matteoli G, Ibiza Martínez S, et al. Local immune response to food antigens drives meal-induced abdominal pain. Nature. 2021;590(7844):151–6. https://doi.org/10.1038/s41586-020-03118-2.
100. Perrier C, Corthésy B. Gut permeability and food allergies. Clin Exp Allergy. 2011;41(1):20–8. https://doi.org/10.1111/j.1365-2222.2010.03639.x.
101. Dale HF, Rasmussen SH, Asiller ÖÖ, Lied GA. Probiotics in irritable bowel syndrome: An up-to-date systematic review. Nutrients. 2019;11(9):2048. https://doi.org/10.3390/nu11092048.
102. Fatahi S, Hosseini A, Sohouli MH, Sayyari A, Khatami K, Farsani ZF, Amiri H, Dara N, de Souza IGO, Santos HO. Effects of probiotic supplementation on abdominal pain severity in pediatric patients with irritable bowel syndrome: a systematic review and meta-analysis of randomized clinical trials. World J Pediatr. 2022;18(5):320–32. https://doi.org/10.1007/s12519-022-00516-6.
103. Rana SV, Malik A. Breath tests and irritable bowel syndrome. World J Gastroenterol. 2014;20(24):7587–601. https://doi.org/10.3748/wjg.v20.i24.7587.
104. Ghoshal UC, Shukla R, Ghoshal U. Small intestinal bacterial overgrowth and irritable bowel syndrome: a bridge between functional organic dichotomy. Gut Liver. 2017;11(2):196–208. https://doi.org/10.5009/gnl16126.
105. Shepherd SJ, Parker FC, Muir JG, Gibson PR. Dietary triggers of abdominal symptoms in patients with irritable bowel syndrome: randomized placebo-controlled evidence. Clin Gastroenterol Hepatol. 2008;6(7):765–71. https://doi.org/10.1016/j.cgh.2008.02.058.
106. Skoog SM, Bharucha AE, Zinsmeister AR. Comparison of breath testing with fructose and high fructose corn syrups in health and IBS. Neurogastroenterol Motil. 2008;20(5):505–11. https://doi.org/10.1111/j.1365-2982.2007.01074.x.
107. Mazzawi T, Hausken T, Gundersen D, El-Salhy M. Effect of dietary management on the gastric endocrine cells in patients with irritable bowel syndrome. Eur J Clin Nutr. 2015;69(4):519–24. https://doi.org/10.1038/ejcn.2014.151.
108. Black CJ, Staudacher HM, Ford AC. Efficacy of a low FODMAP diet in irritable bowel syndrome: systematic review and network meta-analysis. Gut. 2022;71(6):1117–26. https://doi.org/10.1136/gutjnl-2021-325214.
109. Dionne J, Ford AC, Yuan Y, Chey WD, Lacy BE, Saito YA, Quigley EMM, Moayyedi P. A systematic review and meta-analysis evaluating the efficacy of a gluten-free diet and a low FODMAPs diet in treating symptoms of irritable bowel syndrome. Am J Gastroenterol. 2018;113(9):1290–300. https://doi.org/10.1038/s41395-018-0195-4.
110. Bellini M, Tonarelli S, Nagy AG, Pancetti A, Costa F, Ricchiuti A, de Bortoli N, Mosca M, Marchi S, Rossi A. Low FODMAP diet: evidence, doubts, and hopes. Nutrients. 2020;12(1):148. https://doi.org/10.3390/nu12010148.
111. Staudacher HM, Whelan K. The low FODMAP diet: recent advances in understanding its mechanisms and efficacy in IBS. Gut. 2017;66(8):1517–27. https://doi.org/10.1136/gutjnl-2017-313750. Epub 2017 Jun 7
112. Böhn L, Störsrud S, Liljebo T, Collin L, Lindfors P, Törnblom H, Simrén M. Diet low in FODMAPs reduces symptoms of irritable bowel syndrome as well as traditional dietary advice: a randomized controlled trial. Gastroenterology. 2015;149(6):1399–1407.e2. https://doi.org/10.1053/j.gastro.2015.07.054.
113. Talley NJ. Commentary: controversies in NICE guidance on irritable bowel syndrome. BMJ. 2008;336(7643):558–9. https://doi.org/10.1136/bmj.39504.409329.AD.
114. Staudacher HM, Rossi M, Kaminski T, et al. Long-term personalized low FODMAP diet improves symptoms and maintains luminal Bifidobacteria abundance in irritable bowel syndrome. Neurogastroenterol Motil. 2021;34(4):e14241. https://doi.org/10.1111/nmo.14241.
115. Lövdahl J, Störsrud S, Törnblom H. Editorial: gut-directed hypnotherapy or low FODMAP diet for

the treatment of irritable bowel syndrome? Aliment Pharmacol Ther. 2016;44(8):901–2. https://doi.org/10.1111/apt.13772.

116. Halmos EP, Christophersen CT, Bird AR, Shepherd SJ, Gibson PR, Muir JG. Diets that differ in their FODMAP content alter the colonic luminal microenvironment. Gut. 2015;64(1):93–100. https://doi.org/10.1136/gutjnl-2014-307264.
117. Reddel S, Putignani L, Del Chierico F. The impact of low-FODMAPs, gluten-free, and ketogenic diets on gut microbiota modulation in pathological conditions. Nutrients. 2019;11(2):373. https://doi.org/10.3390/nu11020373.
118. Staudacher HM. Nutritional, microbiological and psychosocial implications of the low FODMAP diet. J Gastroenterol Hepatol. 2017;32(Suppl 1):16–9. https://doi.org/10.1111/jgh.13688.
119. McKernan DP, Fitzgerald P, Dinan TG, Cryan JF. The probiotic Bifidobacterium infantis 35624 displays visceral antinociceptive effects in the rat. Neurogastroenterol Motil. 2010;22(9):1029–35., e268. https://doi.org/10.1111/j.1365-2982.2010.01520.x.
120. Agostini S, Goubern M, Tondereau V, Salvador-Cartier C, Bezirard V, Lévèque M, Keränen H, Theodorou V, Bourdu-Naturel S, Goupil-Feuillerat N, Legrain-Raspaud S, Eutamene H. A marketed fermented dairy product containing Bifidobacterium lactis CNCM I-2494 suppresses gut hypersensitivity and colonic barrier disruption induced by acute stress in rats. Neurogastroenterol Motil. 2012;24(4):376–e172. https://doi.org/10.1111/j.1365-2982.2011.01865.x.
121. Moloney RD, O'Leary OF, Felice D, Bettler B, Dinan TG, Cryan JF. Early-life stress induces visceral hypersensitivity in mice. Neurosci Lett. 2012;512(2):99–102. https://doi.org/10.1016/j.neulet.2012.01.066.
122. Distrutti E, Cipriani S, Mencarelli A, Renga B, Fiorucci S. Probiotics VSL#3 protect against development of visceral pain in murine model of irritable bowel syndrome. PLoS One. 2013;8(5):e63893. https://doi.org/10.1371/journal.pone.0063893.
123. López-Gómez L, Antón J, López-Tofiño Y, Pomana B, Uranga JA, Abalo R. Effects of commercial probiotics on colonic sensitivity after acute mucosal irritation. Int J Environ Res Public Health. 2022;19(11):6485. https://doi.org/10.3390/ijerph19116485.
124. Gou HZ, Zhang YL, Ren LF, Li ZJ, Zhang L. How do intestinal probiotics restore the intestinal barrier? Front Microbiol. 2022 Jul;14(13):929346. https://doi.org/10.3389/fmicb.2022.929346.
125. Liu Y, Tran DQ, Rhoads JM. Probiotics in disease prevention and treatment. J Clin Pharmacol. 2018;58 Suppl 10(Suppl 10):S164–79. https://doi.org/10.1002/jcph.1121.
126. Eutamene H, Lamine F, Chabo C, Theodorou V, Rochat F, Bergonzelli GE, Corthésy-Theulaz I, Fioramonti J, Bueno L. Synergy between lactobacillus paracasei and its bacterial products to counteract stress-induced gut permeability and sensitivity increase in rats. J Nutr. 2007;137(8):1901–7. https://doi.org/10.1093/jn/137.8.1901.
127. Moloney RD, Johnson AC, O'Mahony SM, Dinan TG, Greenwood-Van Meerveld B, Cryan JF. Stress and the microbiota-gut-brain axis in visceral pain: relevance to irritable bowel syndrome. CNS Neurosci Ther. 2016;22(2):102–17. https://doi.org/10.1111/cns.12490.
128. De Palma G, Collins SM, Bercik P, Verdu EF. The microbiota-gut-brain axis in gastrointestinal disorders: stressed bugs, stressed brain or both? J Physiol. 2014;592(14):2989–97. https://doi.org/10.1113/jphysiol.2014.273995.
129. García-Ródenas CL, Bergonzelli GE, Nutten S, Schumann A, Cherbut C, Turini M, Ornstein K, Rochat F, Corthésy-Theulaz I. Nutritional approach to restore impaired intestinal barrier function and growth after neonatal stress in rats. J Pediatr Gastroenterol Nutr. 2006;43(1):16–24. https://doi.org/10.1097/01.mpg.0000226376.95623.9f.
130. Urita Y, Goto M, Watanabe T, Matsuzaki M, Gomi A, Kano M, Miyazaki K, Kaneko H. Continuous consumption of fermented milk containing Bifidobacterium bifidum YIT 10347 improves gastrointestinal and psychological symptoms in patients with functional gastrointestinal disorders. Biosci Microbiota Food Health. 2015;34(2):37–44. https://doi.org/10.12938/bmfh.2014-017.
131. Zhang T, Zhang C, Zhang J, Sun F, Duan L. Efficacy of probiotics for irritable bowel syndrome: a systematic review and network meta-analysis. Front Cell Infect Microbiol. 2022;12:859967. https://doi.org/10.3389/fcimb.2022.859967.
132. Trivić I, Niseteo T, Jadrešin O, Hojsak I. Use of probiotics in the treatment of functional abdominal pain in children-systematic review and meta-analysis. Eur J Pediatr. 2021;180(2):339–51. https://doi.org/10.1007/s00431-020-03809-y.
133. Enck P, Zimmermann K, Menke G, Müller-Lissner S, Martens U, Klosterhalfen S. A mixture of Escherichia coli (DSM 17252) and Enterococcus faecalis (DSM 16440) for treatment of the irritable bowel syndrome--a randomized controlled trial with primary care physicians. Neurogastroenterol Motil. 2008;20(10):1103–9. https://doi.org/10.1111/j.1365-2982.2008.01156.x.
134. Chumpitazi BP, Cope JL, Hollister EB, Tsai CM, McMeans AR, Luna RA, Versalovic J, Shulman RJ. Randomised clinical trial: gut microbiome biomarkers are associated with clinical response to a low FODMAP diet in children with the irritable bowel syndrome. Aliment Pharmacol Ther. 2015;42(4):418–27. https://doi.org/10.1111/apt.13286.

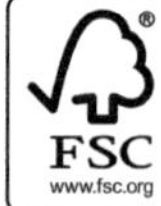

MIX
Papier aus verantwortungsvollen Quellen
Paper from responsible sources
FSC® C105338

If you have any concerns about our products,
you can contact us on
ProductSafety@springernature.com

In case Publisher is established outside the EU,
the EU authorized representative is:
Springer Nature Customer Service Center GmbH
Europaplatz 3, 69115 Heidelberg, Germany

Printed by Libri Plureos GmbH
in Hamburg, Germany